Neuroendocrinology of Reproduction
Physiology and Behavior

Neuroendocrinology of Reproduction
Physiology and Behavior

Edited by
NORMAN T. ADLER

University of Pennsylvania
Philadelphia, Pennsylvania

PLENUM PRESS · NEW YORK AND LONDON

Library of Congress Cataloging in Publication Data

Main entry under title:

Neuroendocrinology of reproduction.

Includes index.
1. Neuroendocrinology. 2. Reproduction. 3. Sexual behavior in animals. I.
Adler, Norman T. [DNLM: 1. Reproduction. 2. Endocrinology. 3. Hormones—
Physiology. 4. Neurophysiology. WQ 205 N495]
QP356.4.N4836   596′.016   80-28245
ISBN 0-306-40600-4   AACR2

© 1981 Plenum Press, New York
A Division of Plenum Publishing Corporation
233 Spring Street, New York, N.Y. 10013

Printed in the United States of America

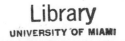

Contributors

Elizabeth Adkins-Regan, Department of Psychology and Section of Neurobiology and Behavior, Cornell University, Ithaca, New York 14853

Norman T. Adler, Department of Psychology, University of Pennsylvania, Philadelphia, Pennsylvania 19104

William R. Crowley, Department of Pharmacology, University of Tennessee Center for the Health Sciences, Memphis, Tennessee 38163

Jeffrey A. Elliott, Hopkins Marine Station, Department of Biological Sciences, Stanford University, Pacific Grove, California 93950

Harvey H. Feder, Institute of Animal Behavior, Rutgers University, Newark, New Jersey 07102

Bruce D. Goldman, Department of Bio-Behavioral Sciences, University of Connecticut, Storrs, Connecticut 06268

B. R. Komisaruk, Institute of Animal Behavior, Rutgers University, Newark, New Jersey 07102

Samuel McCann, Department of Physiology, University of Texas, Southwestern Medical School at Dallas, Dallas, Texas 75235

Bruce S. McEwen, Laboratory of Neuroendocrinology, The Rockefeller University, New York, New York 10021

Joan I. Morrell, Department of Psychology, The Rockefeller University, New York, New York 10021

Adrian Morrison, School of Veterinary Medicine, University of Pennsylvania, Philadelphia, Pennsylvania 19104

Donald W. Pfaff, Department of Psychology, The Rockefeller University, New York, New York 10021

Peter Reiner, School of Veterinary Medicine, University of Pennsylvania, Philadelphia, Pennsylvania 19104

J. F. Rodriguez-Sierra, Department of Anatomy, School of Medicine, University of Nebraska, Omaha, Nebraska 68105

E. Terasawa, Wisconsin Regional Primate Research Center, University of Wisconsin, Madison, Wisconsin 53706

John Woolsey, Leidy Laboratories, University of Pennsylvania, Philadelphia, Pennsylvania 19104

Frank P. Zemlan, Department of Pharmacology, University of Pennsylvania School of Medicine, Philadelphia, Pennsylvania 19104

Preface

The subject of this book is neuroendocrinology, that branch of biological science devoted to the interactions between the two major integrative organ systems of animals—the endocrine and nervous systems. Although this science today reflects a fusion of endocrinology and neurobiology, this synthetic approach is relatively recent. At the beginning of the 20th century, when the British physiologists, Bayliss and Starling, first proposed endocrinology to be an independent field of inquiry, they went to great lengths to establish the autonomy of chemical secretions in general and their independence from nervous control in particular (Bayliss, W. M., and Starling, E. H., 1902, The mechanism of pancreatic secretion, *J. Physiol.* **28**:325). They argued with Pavlov, who said that there was a strong influence of the nervous system on the gastrointestinal phenomena the endocrinologists were studying. For several decades, the English physiologists prevailed, at least in the West; and Pavlov's critique was not taken to heart by the practitioners of the newly emerging discipline of endocrinology.

Through the work of Harris, the Scharrers, Sawyer, Everett, and others, there has been something of a scientific detente in the latter half of this century; the hybrid field of neuroendocrinology is now regarded as one of the cornerstones of modern neural science and is of fundamental importance in basic and clinical endocrinology.

While these events in twentieth century *physiology* have been critical for the emergence of modern neuroendocrinology, the field has also developed because of discoveries in the behavioral sciences. From the classic work of Young, Beach, and Lehrman, it became clear that reproductive behavior is dependent on the animal's endocrine secretions and also that these endocrine secretions were influenced by behavior. It is now understood that neuroendocrine variables also intervene in aggression, feeding, drinking, learning, and cognitive-emotional states. With the nervous system as the final common path for behavior, students of psychology, animal behavior, and psychiatry discovered the same reciprocal influences between hormones and the nervous system that the physiologists recognized.

Neuroendocrinology is, therefore, basic to a modern understanding of how animals work. It is becoming increasingly apparent that neuroendocrine factors play a role in almost every realm of behavioral and physiological integration: reproduction, energy and water balance, biochemical homeostasis, biological rhythms, temperature regulation, and development. The chapters in this volume will deal primarily with the role of the neuroendocrine system in one of these realms: reproduction. We have restricted the subject to the reproduction of animals (and concentrated on vertebrates); however, we have tried to present as broad a biological treatment as possible. Basically, this book is meant to be something of a primer (defined by *Webster's New 20th Century Dictionary,* Second Edition, as "a textbook that gives the first principles of any subject"). The chapters are not intended to be advanced, specialized reviews for professionals working in the neuroendocrinology of reproduction; rather, they are directed to students, and workers in related disciplines, who want to become familiar with the problems, techniques, and contemporary state of knowledge of reproductive neuroendocrinology.

Because the neuroendocrinology of reproduction has developed so rapidly in recent years, each topic in this book has been discussed by an expert in his or her particular field. In order to make this a unified text suitable for students, however, each author has tried to deal with basic conceptual issues, has included something of the history of each subdiscipline, and has tried to integrate the presentation of results with notes on techniques and experimental method.

The book can be used as a text (or supplement) in courses in reproductive biology, neuroendocrinology, physiological psychology, hormones and behavior, and neurobiology. It presupposes that students have a basic background in chemistry and biology and is divided into four main sections and an appendix; this arrangement is intended to lead students from the chemical and biological foundations of neuroendocrinology, through the evolutionary and embryological development of reproductive systems in animals, to the physiological and biochemical control of reproductive neuroendocrinology in the adult organism.

Part I contains chapters on the chemical structure of pituitary and gonadal hormones. It also presents material on the histology of the pituitary and basic central nervous system neurochemistry.

Part II deals with the development of reproductive function. The embryological development of reproductive morphology, physiology, and behavior is discussed. In addition, there is a chapter on puberty as well as an overview of development from a comparative-evolutionary perspective.

Part III treats neuroendocrine control of reproduction in the adult. First, there is a chapter on the relationships between brain, pituitary, and ovary. The next two chapters discuss the ovarian cycle in mammals and the role of the central nervous system in mediating effects of the environment on the ovary. Finally, there is a chapter devoted to seasonal reproduction which explains the relationship between biological (especially circadian) rhythms and photoperiodism.

In Part IV, the authors discuss the cellular and chemical basis of reproductive neuroendocrinology. There are chapters on the central neurochemical control of pituitary function and mating behavior. Following these are chapters on the cellular biochemistry of hormone action in brain and pituitary, the autoradiography of hormone uptake in the brain, and electrophysiological effects of hormones on the brain.

While there are many diagrams, illustrations, and atlases of central nervous system structures involved in reproduction, there has not been a readily available dissection-oriented description of the peripheral nervous system associated with reproductive function in experimental animals. To amend this deficit, we have included a guide to the peripheral reproductive neuroanatomy of the rat as an appendix to this volume; we present this description (with the accompanying eight color figures) in the hope that students and research workers in reproductive neuroendocrinology will find it useful in their work.

Norman T. Adler

Philadelphia

Contents

3. Essentials of Steroid Structure, Nomenclature, Reactions, Biosynthesis, and Measurements
Harvey H. Feder

4. Neurotransmitter Systems: Anatomy and Pharmacology
William R. Crowley and Frank P. Zemlan

II. Development of Reproductive Function

5. Hormonal Actions on the Sexual Differentiation of the Genitalia and the Gonadotropin-Regulating Systems
Harvey H. Feder

6. Perinatal Hormones and Their Role in the Development of Sexually Dimorphic Behaviors
Harvey H. Feder

7. Early Organizational Effects of Hormones: An Evolutionary Perspective

Elizabeth Adkins-Regan

8. Puberty
Bruce D. Goldman

III. Control of Reproduction on the Organismic and Physiological Levels of Organization

9. Experimental Analysis of Hormone Actions on the Hypothalamus, Anterior Pituitary, and Ovary
Harvey H. Feder

10. Estrous Cyclicity in Mammals
Harvey H. Feder

11. How the Brain Mediates Ovarian Responses to Environmental Stimuli: Neuroanatomy and Neurophysiology
B. R. Komisaruk, E. Terasawa, and
J. F. Rodriguez-Sierra

12 Seasonal Reproduction: Photoperiodism and Biological Clocks
Jeffrey A. Elliott and Bruce D. Goldman

IV. Control of Reproduction on the Cellular and Chemical Level

13. CNS Control of the Pituitary: Neurochemistry of Hypothalamic Releasing and Inhibitory Hormones
Samuel McCann

14. The Neurochemical Control of Mating Behavior
William R. Crowley and Frank P. Zemlan

15. Cellular Biochemistry of Hormone Action in Brain and Pituitary
Bruce S. McEwen

16. Autoradiographic Technique for Steroid Hormone Localization: Application to the Vertebrate Brain

Joan I. Morrell and Donald W. Pfaff

I

Chemical Background of
Endocrine Function

Structure of Protein and Peptide Hormones

BRUCE D. GOLDMAN

I. INTRODUCTION

Protein and peptide hormones are produced by several glands in the verte-brates. These glands include the anterior pituitary, the pancreas, and, in some mammals, the placenta. There are also peptide hormones of neurosecretory origin that are secreted by the hypothalamus and the posterior pituitary gland (see Chapters 2, 4, and 13). Finally, some of the chemicals that transmit information between neurons—the neurotransmitters—are derivatives of simple amino acids, the fundamental components of proteins.

The basic amino acid structure is diagrammed in Fig. 1. A nitrogen-con-taining amino group and an organic acid are attached to the remainder of the organic molecule. These amino acids are linked into chains by peptide bonds that join the amino group of one amino acid to the carboxyl group of the next. As we shall see in this chapter, some proteins also contain carbohydrates (glycoproteins) or lipids (lipoproteins) (Ganong, 1978).

The linear order of the amino acids along the protein chain is termed the primary structure of a protein. These long chains are twisted or folded in complex ways; the term secondary structure refers to the resulting three-dimensional structure.

Most of the vertebrate peptide and protein hormones have undergone considerable evolution, so that both the structure and function of the mammal-

---

BRUCE D. GOLDMAN • Department of Bio-Behavioral Sciences, University of Connecticut, Storrs, Connecticut 06268.

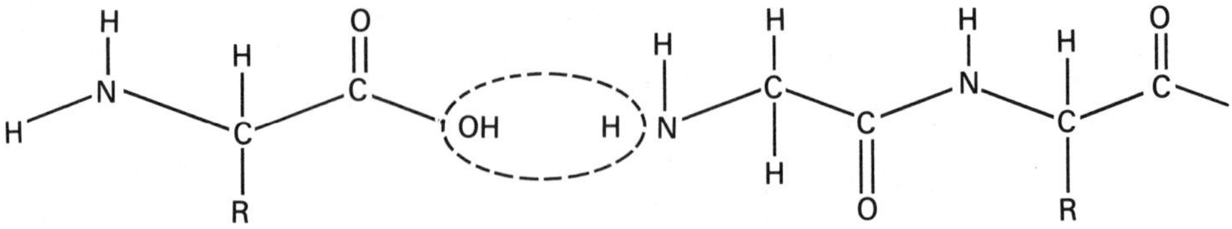

Figure 1. Amino acid structure and formation of peptide bonds. The dotted lines show how the peptide bonds are formed with the production of H_2O. R = remainder of amino acid. For example, in glycine, r = H; in glutamic acid, R = $-(CH_2)_2$ $-COOH$.

ian hormones are often somewhat different from those of the lower vertebrate classes.

II. PEPTIDE HORMONES

A. Posterior Pituitary

The peptide hormones that have been best studied with respect to evolution are the hormones of the posterior pituitary. These hormones are produced by cells of the supraoptic and paraventricular nuclei of the hypothalamus and are transported via axonal flow to sites of storage and release at the axon terminals in the pars nervosa.

Several posterior pituitary hormones are known, but any given species usually produces only two of them. All the hormones are octapeptides containing a five-membered ring (Fig. 2). A major breakthrough toward understanding the structural evolution of these compounds came when Vincent DuVigneaud and his associates determined the complete structure of the mammalian hormones oxytocin and vasopressin, and were able to synthesize them. Since that time, the structures of several lower vertebrate neurohypophyseal hormones have also been determined.

Vasotocin is found in the posterior pituitary in all vertebrate classes except mammals. Therefore, it may well represent a primitive hormone. Curiously, although vasotocin has not been found in the mammalian neurohypophysis, it has been extracted from the pineal glands of cows, cats, and rats. Vasopressin, also known as antidiuretic hormone (ADH), seems to have replaced vasotocin in the mammalian neurohypophysis. Most mammals produce arginine vasopressin, but some members of the pig family (*Suiformes*) produce lysine vasopressin, a compound that is very closely related both structurally and functionally. Vasopressin has not been found in any nonmammalian species, and arginine vasopressin differs structurally from vasotocin by a single amino acid replacement—vasopressin has phenylalanine instead of isoleucine at position 3. Therefore, it seems that the evolutionary shift from vasotocin to vasopressin resulted from a point mutation involving a single codon. Lysine vasopressin probably evolved from arginine vasopressin by another codon change, leading to the substitution of lysine for arginine at position 8 in the molecule. Thus, it may be that the vasotocin molecule was not altered through most of vertebrate evolution except in the line that gave rise to the mammals and in the *Suiformes* within the mammalian line of evolution.

The second hormonal component of the neurohypophyseal complex appears to have undergone a considerably greater degree of structural evolution. In mammals, birds, and some amphibians, this second hormone is oxytocin. However, several other hormones have been discovered, including isotocin (teleost fishes), mesotocin (amphibians, reptiles, lungfishes), and glumitocin (elasmobranchs). There may be some "missing links" in our current knowledge of the evolutionary chain that gave rise to oxytocin, and the probable sequence of mutations involved is not as clear as for the vasotocin–vasopressin sequence. The structures of some of the neurohypophyseal hormones are shown in Fig. 2.

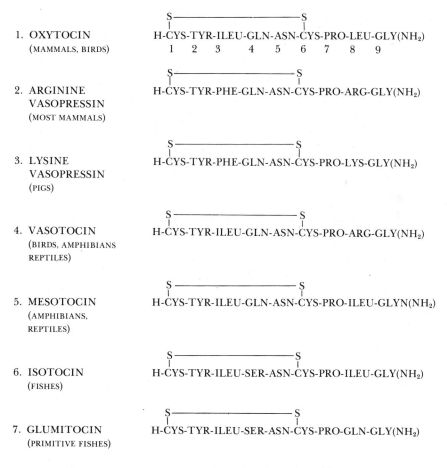

Figure 2. Structures of some of the neurohypophyseal hormones.

It is now known that the mammalian neurophypophyseal hormones, and probably those of other vertebrates as well, are always produced in association with much larger proteins called neurophysins. The hormonal peptide is chemically bound to the neurophysin during transport down the axon and is apparently cleaved free by protelolytic enzymatic action prior to release into the blood. Thus, it may be that neurophysins should be classified with the prohormones.

B. Hypothalamus

The hypothalamus produces several compounds that help to regulate the secretion of the various hormones produced by the anterior pituitary gland. These hypothalamic compounds have been referred to as releasing and inhibiting hormones (or releasing and inhibiting factors). They are probably produced by neurons and are released into the hypothalamic–pituitary portal system so that they reach the pituitary in high concentrations. It seems likely that all these hormones will prove to be peptides, although complete structural information is available for only three of them at present. These are as shown in Table 1.

Much of the difficulty in determining the structure of these hypothalamic hormones can be attributed to the uniqueness of their structures. Luteinizing hormone-releasing factor (LRF) and thyrotropin-releasing factor (TRF) have cyclized C-terminal glutamic acid residues, and the carboxyl group at the other end of the molecule is blocked by the formation of an amide. Somatostatin differs from the other known hypothalamic releasing hormones in that it contains a disulfide bond which forms the cyclic part of the molecule. The two termini are free. Since the hypothalamic releasing and inhibiting hormones and the neurohypophyseal hormones are all produced in the hypothalamus and are peptides, it has been suggested by Harris that they may be related with respect to evolution.

The elucidation of the structure of neurohypophyseal and hypothalamic peptide hormones has enabled scientists to synthesize these molecules and also

Table 1. Known Hypothalamic Peptide Hormones

Hormone	Function	Structure
Thyrotropin-releasing factor (TRF)	Stimulates the release of TSH	Tripeptide
Luteinizing hormone-releasing factor (LRF)	Stimulates the release of LH and possibly FSH	Decapeptide
Growth hormone inhibiting factor, somatostatin (GHIF, SHIF)	Inhibits release of GH; also inhibits insulin and glucagon secretion	14-Amino-acid peptide

has allowed for the controlled synthesis of hormone analogues that differ by only a single amino acid from the natural molecules. Comparisons among several such analogues for biological activity have shown that most amino acid substitutions result in a considerable loss of biological potency. These observations lead to the conclusion that there is no discrete active site per se on each molecule of peptide hormone but that the overall configuration of the molecule is important, probably for binding to the receptors in target tissues.

C. Anterior Pituitary

The anterior pituitary gland contains two polypeptide hormones. The best known of these is the adrenocorticotropic hormone, ACTH. This compound contains 39 amino acids, but by synthesizing and testing parts of the molecule, it has been shown that a fragment made up from the amino acid sequence 1–24 possesses potent biological activity. Any further reduction in the size of this fragment results in a considerable loss of activity. There is species variation in ACTH structure among the mammals, but the 1–24 amino acid sequence is identical in all species examined thus far. ACTH stimulates growth of the adrenal cortex and increases the rate of production of the adrenal steroid hormones (cortisol in the human, corticosterone in the rat). These adrenal hormones have an important role in the regulation of carbohydrate metabolism. It has also been suggested that ACTH or fragments of the molecule may exert some influence on the rate of extinction of certain learned behavioral responses (e.g., extinction of avoidance responses).

The intermediate lobe of the pituitary also produces a peptide hormone, the melanocyte-stimulating hormone (MSH). Actually, two forms of melanocyte-stimulating hormone are known; these are designated as α-MSH and β-MSH. The α-MSH contains 13 amino acids and is identical in structure to the amino acid sequence 1–13 of ACTH. Indeed, it appears that α-MSH is produced in the pars intermedia as a result of the action of specific proteolytic enzymes that cleave the ACTH molecule. In this case, ACTH may be thought of as a "prohormone." Humans do not have an intermediate lobe and are believed not to produce MSH. The β-MSH is an octapeptide. MSH stimulates the spreading out of pigment through the melanocyte cells in some of the lower vertebrates, and by this mechanism the hormone is able to induce a rapid darkening of the skin coloration.

D. Pancreas

The pancreatic hormones are also polypeptides. Insulin is composed of 51 amino acids, and the molecule is double-chained. The two chains are linked by two disulfide bridges. Insulin is first synthesized as a part of a larger prohormone, proinsulin. The active hormone is cleaved off from the proinsulin molecule by the action of peptidases in the pancreatic β cells. The structure of proinsulin has been established for several species, and the number of amino acids ranges from 81 to 86. Glucagon, the second pancreatic hormone, consists of 29 amino acid residues.

E. Blood

Angiotensin II is an octapeptide with potent vasopressor activity. It also has a role in stimulating the output of aldosterone from the adrenal cortex. More recently, it has been discovered that angiotensin II stimulates drinking in rats when injected peripherally or when placed in the subfornical region of the brain. All these actions seem to be related to maintenance of water and electrolyte balances. Angiotensin II is produced in the blood as a result of the cleavage of two terminal amino acids from a decapeptide precursor, angiotensin I. This cleavage is performed by the enzyme renin, which is secreted by the juxtaglomerular cells of the kidney. Renin is released when blood flow to the kidney is reduced, and this may result in hypertension.

III. PROTEIN HORMONES

A. Anterior Pituitary and Placenta

The anterior pituitary secretes five protein hormones. These can be placed into two classes based on structure and probably evolutionary origins. The first group is made up of growth hormone (GH) and prolactin. These hormones are proteins of molecular weight approximately 25,000. They share a number of common amino acid sequences, which suggests a close evolutionary relationship. In some instances, a certain amount of overlap has been detected in the biological activities of these respective hormones. Prolactin appears to have assumed more different functions during the course of vertebrate evolution than any other pituitary hormone. Mammalian prolactin has been shown to have some biological activity in every existing class of vertebrates except the cyclostomes. Therefore, it may be that prolactin function has evolved more extensively than has the structure of the molecule.

The second group of pituitary protein hormones includes the gonadotropins, LH and FSH, along with TSH. These hormones are all glycoproteins—i.e., the molecules include considerable carbohydrate components that are chemically bound to the protein backbone. The molecular weights of these hormones are about 22,000–25,000; carbohydrate accounts for approximately 10–20% of the total weight. An additional, and even more striking, similarity among LH, FSH, and TSH was revealed with the discovery that all three are double-chained molecules. Furthermore, in any given species it appears that the α chains are very similar or identical to each other. The β chains of these hormones are different and are mainly responsible for establishing the specificity of biological action. Even the β chains may show considerable similarity, however (as in the case of LH-β and TSH-β), and this is further evidence for evolutionary relationships (Papkoff, 1973). Neither the α nor β chains possess much biological activity when administered alone; they must be combined to show potent hormonal action.

Human chorionic gonadotropin is a glycoprotein hormone produced by the placenta. It is structurally and functionally similar to pituitary LH but contains a larger carbohydrate component comprising approximately 30% of the molecule. Pregnant mare serum gonadotropin (PMSG) is a glycoprotein produced by the endometrial cups of the mare during pregnancy. This molecule also has a high carbohydrate content and is unique in possessing both FSH-like and LH-like biological properties in easily detectable amounts.

The biological activities of most glycoprotein hormones are greatly reduced by exposing the molecule to the actions of either proteolytic or carbohydrate-attacking enzymes. Thus, it appears that both the protein and carbohydrate moieties are important for the biological function of the hormones. However, it should be noted that most of the tests for biological activity have been by *in vivo* bioassays. Neuraminidase-treated human chorionic gonadotropin retains biological activity in an *in vitro* test. Thus, it has been suggested that at least part of the function of the carbohydrate moiety may be to prevent the hormone from being broken down too rapidly *in vivo* (Winzler, 1973).

The complete amino acid sequences have been determined for a few of the protein and glycoprotein hormones. These discoveries are recent, but it is already apparent that some interspecies variation exists in the primary amino acid sequences for a given hormone—e.g., human and ovine LH are different. Earlier studies employing immunologic approaches also indicated species differences in protein hormone structure, even among closely related mammals. It has even been suggested that some heterogeneity, particularly for LH, may exist within a species (Papkoff, 1973). As a final variant on the theme of hormone heterogeneity, there is some evidence that castrated rats produce a somewhat different form of FSH than do intact rats and that androgen has an effect on the form in which FSH is produced.

Since species differences do exist with respect to protein hormone structures, it is of interest that the same hormones rarely show much evidence of species specificity among the mammals with respect to biological activity. Indeed, mammalian prolactin, LH, and TSH show considerable activity even in amphibians and fishes. These observations suggest that some amino acid substitutions can be made in these protein hormones without greatly affecting their biological potency. Also, it appears that evolutionary modifications may have occurred primarily in those segments of the molecules that are least crucial for biological activity.

IV. IODOPROTEINS

The thyroid gland produces a group of rather large protein molecules that are composed of several polypeptide chains that contain carbohydrate (8–10%) and iodine (0.2–1%). These proteins are referred to as thyroglobulins. When animals are subjected to conditions of iodine deficiency, the levels of iodine found in thyroglobulin may decrease markedly. In fact, noniodinated thyroglobulin has been isolated from hogs that were treated with methyl thiouracil, a compound which blocks the incorporation of iodide into thyroid hormones. Most of the iodine in thyroglobulin is found in four iodoamino acids. Two of these are derivatives of tyrosine and are designated as 3-monoiodotyrosine (MIT) and 3,5-diiodotryosine (DIT). The other two are derivatives of thyronine, 3,5,3'-triiodothyronine (T_3) and 3,5,3',5'-tetraiodothyronine or thyroxine (T_4). The structures of T_3 and T_4 are shown in Fig. 3. These hormones have potent hormonal activity, affecting brain development and metabolism in mammals and metamorphosis in amphibians.

The actual hormones are cleaved off from their precursor, thyroglobulin, by the action of a thyroid protease. After cleavage, the hormones are released into the blood. Normally, thyroglobulin itself does not enter the blood, and, in fact, thyroglobulins are highly antigenic. Hashimoto's disease is an apparent hypothyroid condition that results from autoimmunity to the thyroid. This is believed to develop as the result of a lesion or injury to the thyroid that allows thyroid proteins to enter the circulation and elicit an antigenic response.

Iodinated tyrosine has also been found in several invertebrates, including corals and sponges. Thyroxine and its precursors are also present in molluscs and insects. In *Amphioxus*, a prochordate considered to be related to the ancestral line leading to the vertebrates, iodoproteins are produced by a pharyngeal gland, the endostyle. This gland is also present in the *Ammocetes* larva of the

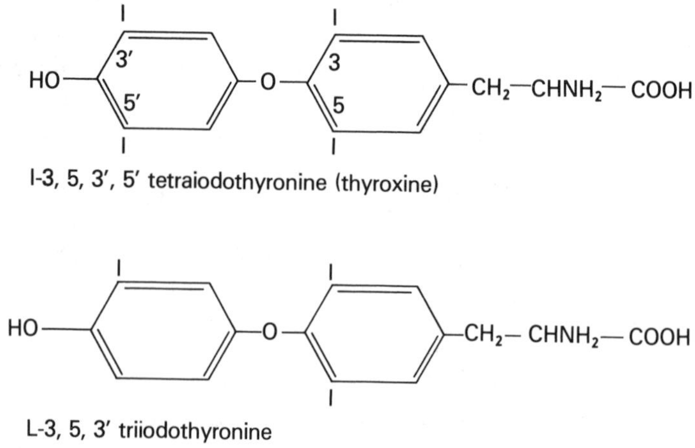

I-3, 5, 3', 5' tetraiodothyronine (thyroxine)

L-3, 5, 3' triiodothyronine

Figure 3. Structures of T_4 (thyroxine) and T_3 (triiodothyronine).

lamprey. The endostyle of *Ammocetes* drains its products into the pharynx via a duct. The endostylar duct closes at metamorphosis, and the endostyle differentiates into a thyroid in the adult lamprey (Gorbman, 1959).

V. CATECHOLAMINES AND INDOLEAMINES

Interestingly, there is strong evidence that dopamine and possibly norepinephrine may act directly on the mammotrophic cells of the pituitary to inhibit the secretion of prolactin. If so, this would indicate a hormonal role for molecules that serve as neurotransmitters as well. This would not be an unprecedented situation, since norepinephrine and epinephrine are secreted by nerve cells of the adrenal medulla into the peripheral circulation where they act as hormones in regulating glucose mobilization in the liver. Dopamine, norepinephrine, and epinephrine are all catecholamines with structures as shown in Fig. 4. The catecholamines are derivatives of the amino acid, tyrosine.

Melatonin, an indoleamine derived from serotonin, is produced by the pineal gland of various vertebrates and has often been suggested to have hormonal function. The physiological effects of melatonin are perhaps best known in amphibians where this compound apparently acts as a hormone to cause condensation of the melanin pigment in the melanocytes, resulting in lightening of the skin color. In mammals, melatonin has been suggested as a possible "antigonadal" hormone, but this has not yet been firmly established. In the sparrow, the pineal gland exerts a strong control on the circadian clock which controls the rhythm of activity. This is demonstrated by the observation that pinealectomized sparrows show random activity when placed in constant darkness, whereas intact birds show a free-running circadian rhythm when

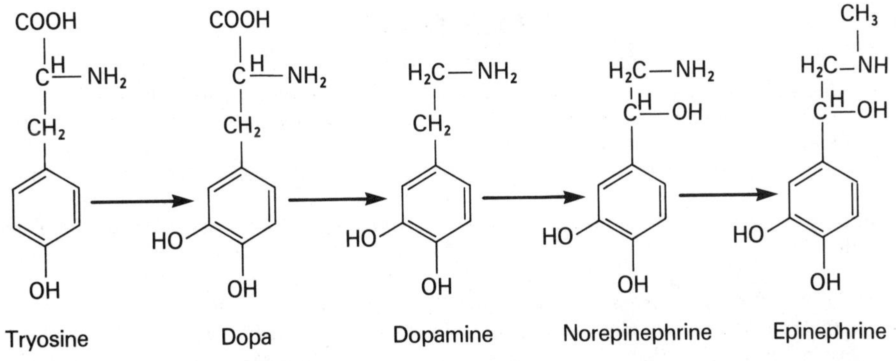

Figure 4. Biosynthesis of dopamine, norepinephrine and epinephrine. Tyrosine is first oxidized to form dopa. Dopa is subsequently decarboxylated and oxidized to yield dopamine and norepinephrine. Norepinephrine is methylated to form epinephrine. (Reproduced with permission from P. Karlson, 1963.)

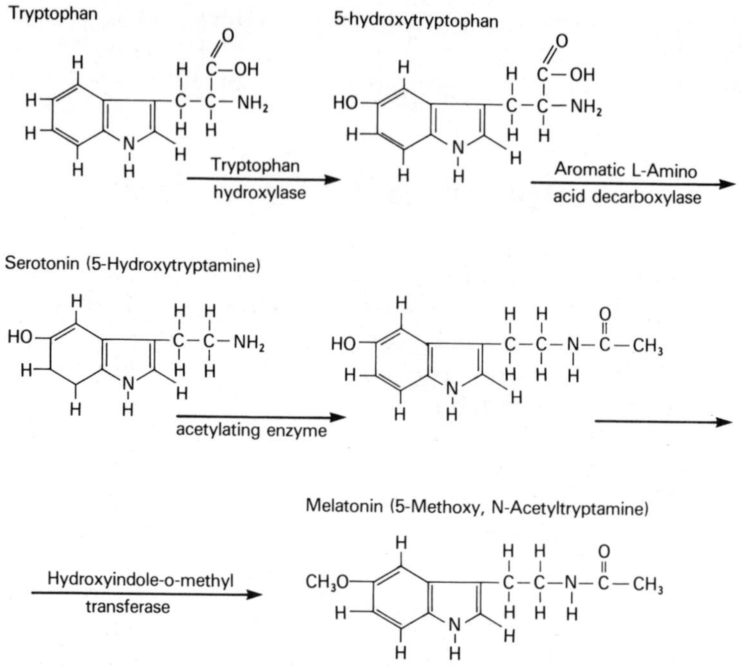

Figure 5. The structure of melatonin and its derivation from serotonin.

deprived of light cues (Zimmerman and Menaker, 1975). Exogenous melatonin has a marked effect on activity in the sparrow, so that it may well be that this compound is a pineal hormone with a role in the regulation of rhythmic behavior in birds. The structure of melatonin and its derivation from serotonin is shown in Fig. 5.

REFERENCES

DuVigneaud, V., Lawler, H. C., and Popenoe, E. A., 1953, Enzymic cleavage of glycinamide from vasopresson and a proposed sturcture for this pressor antidiuretic hormone of the posterior pituitary, *J. Am Chem. Soc.* **75**:4880–4881.

Ganong, W. F., 1978, *A Review of Medical Physiology,* Lange Medical Publications, Los Altos, California.

Gorbman, A., 1959, Problems in the comparative morphology and physiology of the vertebrate thyroid gland, in: *Comparative Endocrinology* (A. Gorbman, ed.), p. 266, John Wiley and Sons, New York.

Karlson, P., 1963, Introduction to Modern Biochemistry, Academic Press, New York.

Papkoff, H., 1973, The chemistry of the interstitial cell-stimulating hormone of ovine pituitary origin, in: *Hormonal Proteins and Peptides,* Vol. I (C. H. Li, ed.), pp. 59–100, Academic Press, New York.

Winzler, R. J., 1973, The chemistry of glycoproteins, in: *Hormonal Proteins and Peptides,* Vol. I (C. H. Li, ed.), pp. 1–15, Academic Press, New York.

Zimmerman, N.H., and Menaker, M., 1975, Neural connections of sparrow pineal: Role in circadian control of activity, *Science* **190**:477.

2

Histology of the Pituitary

BRUCE D. GOLDMAN

I. INTRODUCTION

In the previous chapter, we examined some characteristics of protein hormones, including those of the pituitary. In this chapter, we concentrate on the tissue structure of the pituitary and the relationship of this gland's morphology to its secretions.

II. POSTERIOR PITUITARY

The posterior pituitary gland, or neurohypophysis, originates from the infundibulum, which is an outpocketing from the hypothalamus. The neurohypophysis proper contains two cell types: axonal terminals and pituicytes. The pituicytes are fusiform cells and are regarded as homologues of neuroglial cells. Their function is not clear. However, it is believed that they may have some role in modulating the metabolism and/or hormone-secreting activities of the axons. The axon terminals of the posterior pituitary form a part of the magnocellular system of the hypothalamus. Their cell bodies lie in the supraoptic and paraventricular nuclei.

The hormones of the mammalian neurohypophysis are vasopressin, or antidiuretic hormone (ADH), and oxytocin. Both are octapeptides. ADH is found only in mammals. It appears that it evolved from another hormone, vasotocin, which has been found in the posterior pituitary in representatives of

BRUCE D. GOLDMAN • Department of Bio-Behavioral Sciences, University of Connecticut, Storrs, Connecticut 06268.

all classes of vertebrates except for the mammals. Vasotocin and ADH differ by only a single amino acid substitution. The hormones of the neurohypophysis appear to be synthesized in the cell bodies (in the paraventricular and supraoptic nuclei) and packaged in granules. The granules are transported down the axons to the posterior pituitary where they can be stored until they are released into the blood. If the posterior pituitary is removed, the hormones can be secreted from the severed axons. For this reason, removal of the neurohypophysis does not result in severe hormone deficiency. Indeed, the neurohypophysectomized animal may appear to be quite normal unless exposed to situations that require maximal secretion of the posterior pituitary hormones.

The neurohypophyseal hormones are bound to a large protein called neurophysin while they are being stored in secretion granules. They are apparently cleaved from the larger neurophysin molecule at the time of release into the blood. One of the problems that attracted the attention of several researchers was that of whether ADH and oxytocin are produced in the same cells or whether they are always synthesized in different cells. This problem has perhaps been solved through studies of a strain of rat called the Brattleboro strain. These animals appear to be unable to synthesize ADH, although oxytocin production remains normal. The trait is inherited as a single point mutation, perhaps of the gene that codes for the ADH molecule. When the magnocellular systems of Brattleboro rats were examined, it was found that about half of the posterior pituitary neurons appeared normal whereas the other half did not contain granules. Thus, it seems that each of the two hormones is synthesized in a separate cell type.

A second and related question is whether the two hormones of the neurohypophysis are synthesized in separate regions of the hypothalamus. It was shown that electrical stimulation of the supraoptic nuclei, but not of the paraventricular nuclei, led to an antidiuretic response (indicative of ADH release). In contrast, destruction of the paraventricular nuclei led to a marked reduction in the oxytocin content of the posterior pituitary with no significant decrement in ADH content. Destruction of the supraoptic nuclei led to polyuria (presumably reflecting decreased ADH secretion) but did not affect neurohypophyseal oxytocin content (Harris, 1947; Olivecrona, 1957). From these studies and further studies in the Brattleboro rat, it is now believed that the supraoptic nucleus is predominantly the site of ADH production and that the paraventricular nucleus is primarily responsible for the synthesis of oxytocin, but that the separation is not complete.

III. ANTERIOR PITUITARY

The anterior pituitary originates as an outpocketing of the pharyngeal epithelium. This embryonic outpocketing is called Rathke's pouch. It comes to lie in close association with the hypothalamus and with the neurohypophysis. In most mammals, the anterior pituitary is actually made up of two distinct lobes, the pars distalis and the pars intermedia, or intermediate lobe. The cells of the anterior pituitary have an abundant rough endoplasmic reticulum, a characteristic of protein-secreting cells. The cells also contain cytoplasmic granules, now known to contain hormones.

Since removal of the anterior pituitary, or hypophysectomy, results in a wide variety of physiological effects (e.g, thyroid, adrenal, and gonadal atrophy, growth retardation), it became evident to early workers that the gland must produce several hormones. Chemical isolation studies during the 1940s and 1950s revealed the presence of seven separate hormones.

At the same time that hormone isolation studies were proceeding, histologists were attempting to identify various cell types in the anterior pituitary. The one cell–one hormone theory postulated a separate cell type for each of the seven hormones of the gland. Most of the early histological studies consisted of attempts to distinguish among cell types based on differential staining with various dyes. It must be kept in mind that these dyes (e.g., acids, fuchsin, orange G, azocarmine) do not necessarily associate with the hormones themselves and can, therefore, only be considered as indirect methods for identifying cell types. Thus, the staining techniques had to be used in conjunction with other procedures to identify cells specifically. For example, it was known that gonadectomy led to increased secretion of gonadotropins (FSH and LH), whereas thyroidectomy led to increased secretion of TSH. It was observed that certain of the basophils (i.e., cells that tended to stain with basic, as opposed to acidic, dyes) became enlarged and showed other signs of hyperactivity following gonadectomy. Other basophils showed signs of hyperactivity after thyroidectomy. These observations led to the conclusion, since confirmed by other methods, that the gonadotropins and thyrotropin are produced by different types of basophilic cells. Other studies led to the conclusion that prolactin and growth hormone are produced by acidophils. For example, it was observed that acidophilic adenoma could be associated with human gigantism or acromegaly (GH hypersecretion) and that acidophils were absent from the pituitaries of genetically inbred dwarf mice (GH deficiency). By the use of many different staining procedures, several cell types were identified. However, some disagreement remained with respect to certain points; in particular, it was unclear whether the gonadotropins (LH and FSH) are produced in one cell or in different cells. The identity of the corticotropin-secreting cells was also disputed.

Electron microscopic studies revealed that different cells contained secretion granules of different sizes. It was possible to obtain a partial separation of different sized granules by the technique of density gradient ultracentrifugation. Bioassay of the hormonal activity in the various fractions showed that different hormones were associated with different sized granules in some cases (Costoff and McShan, 1969). Although this method did not lead to the identification of any new cell types or resolve the disputes referred to above, it did provide additional and more direct evidence confirming some of the histochemical findings.

A more recent method, and probably the most powerful tool for distinguishing cell types in the pituitary, is that of immunocytochemistry. Many variations of this method exist, but all depend on the complexing of hormone-specific antibodies to hormone within cells. The antibody is usually either tagged with a fluorescent compound or is complexed with an enzyme in such a way as to allow for later staining via enzymatic reaction. Thus, the immunochemical procedures provide for direct identification of specific cell types provided that certain criteria are met. These criteria include specificity of the antibodies and lack of hormone diffusion from one cell to another during the immunohistological procedure. In general, the results obtained with these methods have confirmed earlier conclusions. However, some new information seems to have been obtained in that the corticotrophs have been identified. Some doubt still remains regarding the identity of the gonadotrophs. It appears that there are some cells that produce only LH and others that synthesize only FSH; however, a few cells seem to contain both hormones.

When the pituitary is transplanted to a site distant from the hypothalamus, or when the pituitary stalk is sectioned so as to interrupt portal blood flow from the hypothalamus to the pars distalis, most of the pituitary cell types show signs of atrophy or at least decreased synthetic activity. This presumably occurs because of the reduced supply of hypothalamic releasing hormones such as LH-RH and TRH. However, the prolactin cells show indications of increased activity following pituitary transplantation. This correlates with the predominant role of a hypothalamic inhibitory factor (PIF) in the regulation of prolactin secretion.

Before the advent of sensitive radioimmunoassays for the pituitary hormones, scientists had to rely primarily on the less sensitive bioassays for quantitative measurement of the various hormones of the pituitary. In many cases, these bioassays were not sufficiently sensitive to detect the concentrations of hormones present in blood. Therefore, workers often had to rely on measurements of the amounts of hormones present in the pituitary gland itself. Attempts were made to draw conclusions about the effects of certain physiological manipulations on hormone secretion by measuring changes in glandular hormone content. However, it became apparent that this process could be fraught with error, since the relationship between changes in content and changes in secretion was not always predictable. For example, both pituitary and serum LH levels are elevated following castration in the male rat, but in the same animal serum FSH increases while pituitary FSH decreases. In the ovariectomized rat, both serum and pituitary FSH are increased as compared to the levels present in the intact female. More recent studies employing radioimmunoassay to measure growth hormone have showed that the administration of a dose of hypothalamic extract (GRF) sufficient to increase the rate of GH secretion severalfold results in release of only about 1% of the total pituitary GH content.

Most, but not all, mammals have a pars intermedia distinct from the pars distalis. The pars intermedia, or intermediate lobe, is the primary source of MSH synthesis. According to most workers, the pars intermedia is composed of light and dark cells. However, the clear differentiation of these two cell types may be dependent on the method of fixation of the tissue, and the functional significance of the cell types has not been established.

REFERENCES

Costoff, A., and McShan, W. H., 1969, Isolation and biological properties of secretory granules from rat anterior pituitary glands, *J. Cell Biol.* **43**:564.

Harris, G. W., 1947, The innervation and actions of the neurohypophysis; and investigation using the method of remote-control stimulation, *Phil. Trans. R. Soc. Lond.* [*Biol.*]. **232**:385.

Olivecrona, H., 1957, Paraventricular nucleus and pituitary gland, *Acta Physiol Scand.* [*Suppl.*] **136**:1.

Essentials of Steroid Structure, Nomenclature, Reactions, Biosynthesis, and Measurements

HARVEY H. FEDER

I. INTRODUCTION

The steroids are lipids with molecular weights of about 300. They are synthesized in the ovary, testis, adrenal cortex, and placenta. Since 1929, when the steroid estrone was first isolated, over 200 steroids have been isolated and identified in biological material. The purpose of this chapter is to provide a brief overview of the structure, nomenclature, reactions, biosynthesis, and measurement of some steroid hormones of interest to the neuro-endocrinologist. Because the remainder of this book concentrates on physiological and behavioral effects related to the hormones of reproduction, the overview will focus on the primary hormones of the gonads (progestins, androgens, and estrogens) and will omit detailed discussion of the adrenal corticoids. It should be recognized, however, that the gonads may produce corticoids and the adrenals secrete progestins, androgens, and estrogens.

II. BASIC STEROID STRUCTURE AND NOMENCLATURE

A. Cyclohexane and Stereochemistry

In order to understand the structural nature of steroid hormones, it is advisable to be acquainted with some of the properties of the atom that forms

HARVEY H. FEDER • Institute of Animal Behavior, Rutgers University, Newark, New Jersey 07102.

the backbone of steroids, carbon. Carbon occupies a position in the middle of the Periodic Table. Because carbon has four valence electrons, it has no more tendency to gain than to lose electrons and resists acquisition of either a positive or a negative charge. These properties account for the fact that when carbon is bound to other atoms, the type of binding is covalent rather than ionic. Covalent binding is that in which electrons are shared between atoms, whereas ionic binding is that in which electrons are completely transferred from one atom to another (Fig. 1).

The simplest conceivable hydrocarbon is methane, since it consists of one carbon (C) atom covalently bound to four hydrogen (H) atoms (Fig. 2). A series of methyl groups can be linked in a simple chain-like fashion or in branched chains (Fig. 3).

Note that although both of the butane compounds have the same molecular formula (C_4H_{10}), they have different physical and chemical properties attributable to their different structural formulae. This identity of molecular but not structural formulae is termed structural isomerism.

The chainlike hydrocarbons are known as aliphatic compounds. When each carbon atom in the chain has all of its four valences occupied by a linkage with a C or H, the compound is said to be saturated and is termed an alkane.

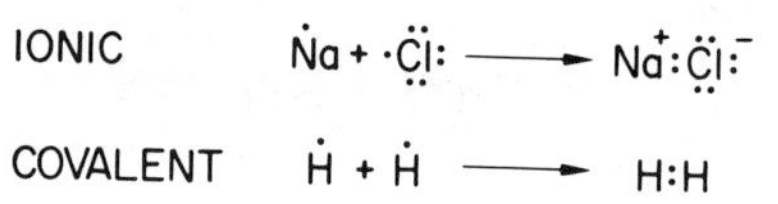

IONIC

COVALENT

Figure 1. Covalent and ionic binding.

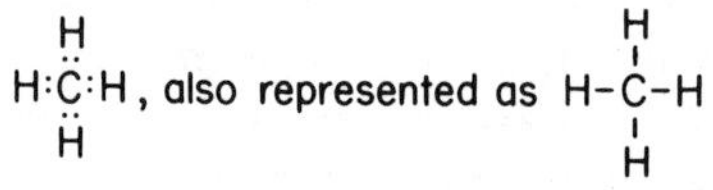

Figure 2. Methane.

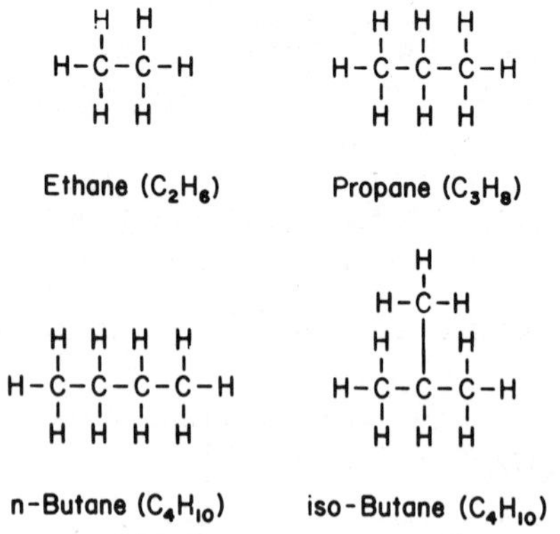

Ethane (C_2H_6)   Propane (C_3H_8)

n-Butane (C_4H_{10})   iso-Butane (C_4H_{10})

Figure 3. Linked series of methyl groups forming simple or branched chains.

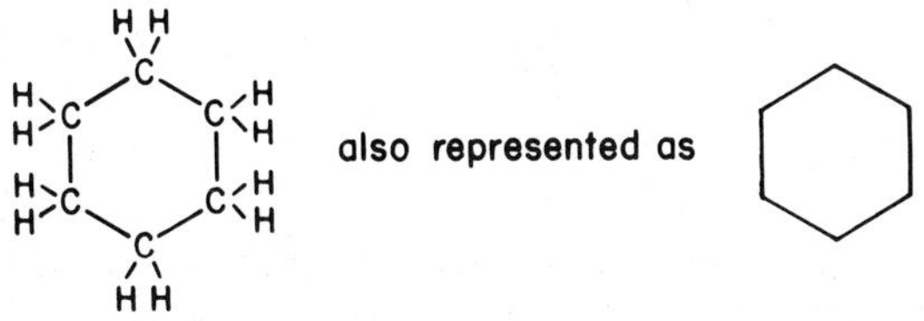

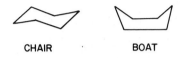

also represented as

Figure 4. Cyclohexane.

CHAIR   BOAT

Figure 5. "Chair" and "boat" forms of cyclohexane.

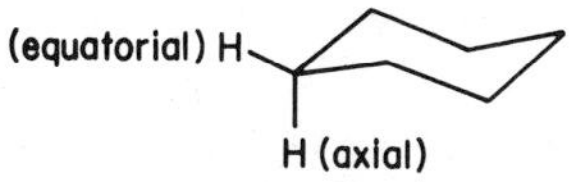

(equatorial) H

H (axial)

Figure 6. Equatorial and axial substituents.

If a ring, rather than a chain, structure is formed and is of the saturated type, it is termed a cycloalkane. One such cycloalkane is cyclohexane, a six-membered ring (Fig. 4).

The cyclohexane molecule is of particular importance because it has served as a model for the study of conformation. Conformation refers to the different possible arrangements of atoms in a single organic structure. Different arrangements are transformed into one another by rotating or twisting but not breaking of bonds. There are two possible extremes of conformation of cyclohexane, the "chair" and the "boat" forms (Fig. 5).

Stability of the molecule is greater when there is less repulsion between the nonbonded hydrogen substitutents. It happens that the boat form contains some H-to-H distances that are smaller than those in the chair form. The boat conformation is therefore less stable than the chain, and it is the chair form that cyclohexane predominantly assumes.

When cyclohexane is in the chair form, some of the H substituents are perpendicular to the plane of the ring, while others are more or less parallel to it. The substituents roughly perpendicular to the plane of the ring are termed axial, and those roughly parallel to the plane of the ring are called equatorial (Fig. 6). Generally, if a substituent is equatorial, it is more accessible for reaction than if it is axial.

Conformation is one aspect of stereochemistry. (Stereochemistry is the study of all aspects of chemistry dealing with spatial relations of atoms and molecules. Much of steroid chemistry depends on stereochemistry.) Another aspect is configuration. Each equatorial and axial substituent can project either towards the upper surface of the plane of the ring (β-configuration, denoted by solid line) or towards the under surface of the plane of the ring (α-configuration, denoted by dashed line).

If two cyclohexane rings are fused, they form a structure with a 10-carbon skeleton called a decalin. Decalins have two possible conformations, indicated by the terms *cis*- or *trans*-isomers. In the *cis* form, both substituents at the site of ring fusion are on the same side of the rings (Fig. 7). In the *trans* form, the substituents at the site of ring fusion are on opposite sides of the plane of the rings. The *trans* form of the decalin is the more stable.

B. The Steroid Nucleus

With these remarks to provide a general orientation, we can proceed to a discussion of steroids. The steroids are compounds that have a sterol-like skeleton. In turn, sterols are solid alcohols (stereos = solid) obtained from a portion of lipid extracts of tissue. A summary of the history of steroid structure determination may be found in Klyne (1957). According to Klyne, determination of the structure of steroids was made difficult because the steroid nucleus contains no atoms other than carbon and is therefore relatively invulnerable to chemical attack. However, by 1928, Wieland and Windaus had performed a series of stepwise degradations and determinations of ring sizes of sterols. They proposed that the basic sterol skeleton had two six-membered rings and two five-membered rings (Fig. 8). In 1932, Bernal noted that the Wieland–Windaus sterol structure could not account for X-ray crystallographic evidence that indicated the sterol skeleton was longer and flatter than the rather compact structure previously proposed. Also, in 1932, Diels found that dehydrogenation of the sterol cholesterol led to formation of the structure shown in Fig. 9.

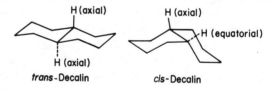

Figure 7. *Trans-* and *cis*-decalins.

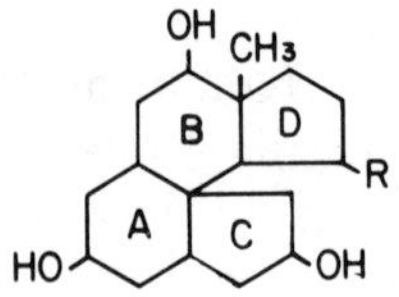

Figure 8. Wieland–Windaus model of a steroid molecule.

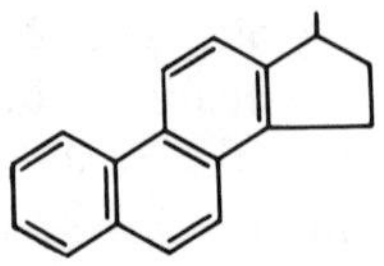

Figure 9. Diels's hydrocarbon.

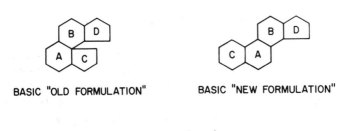

BASIC "OLD FORMULATION"   BASIC "NEW FORMULATION"

RELETTERED BASIC "NEW FORMULATION"

Figure 10. New model of steroid molecule proposed by Rosenheim and King.

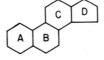

Figure 11. Benzene.

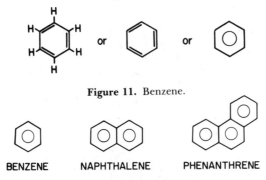

BENZENE   NAPHTHALENE   PHENANTHRENE

Figure 12. Series of fused benzene rings.

However, Diels interpreted this to mean that dehydrogenation led to a rearrangement of the Wieland–Windaus structure. In the same year, Rosenheim and King proposed that Diels's hydrocarbon was a normal degradation product that did not represent rearrangement of ring structure. To give their view of basic steroid structure, they merely transposed one ring of the Wieland–Windaus formula and made the transposed ring six-membered rather than five-membered (Fig. 10). The Rosenheim–King model became the accepted model for basic steroid structure.

This basic skeleton is said to be composed of the cyclopenteno-perhydrophenanthrene nucleus. To explain the derivation of this term, it is necessary to mention a second type of cyclic carbon ring that must be distinguished from the saturated cycloalkanes. This second type of cyclic structure is the aromatic ring, which is not saturated. The simplest aromatic ring is benzene (Fig. 11).

A series of benzene rings can be fused as illustrated in Fig. 12.

If a five-membered ring is then fused to phenanthrene, the compound is a cyclopenteno-phenanthrene. If all the double bonds are then saturated with hydrogen (perhydro-), the compound has the cyclopenteno-perhydro-phenanthrene structure, which is the nucleus of all sterols and steroids. The accepted numbering system for the carbons of the steroid molecule is shown in Fig. 13.

From this generalized picture of a steroid hormone, three hypothetical structures can be drawn that may be considered the "parent" compounds of the progestins (and corticoids), the androgens, and the estrogens. These parent compounds are pregnane, androstane, and estrane, respectively (Fig. 14). Pregnane has 21 carbons, androstane has 19 carbons, and estrane has 18 carbons.

The wavy line at the 5-position in Fig. 14 indicates that the configuration is unspecified. If we specify whether configuration at the 5-position is α or β, we generate two isomers from pregnane, two from androstane, and one structure from estrane (Fig. 15).

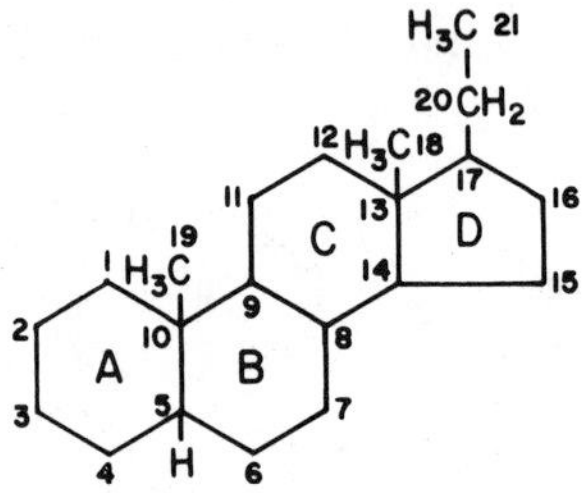

Figure 13. Numbering system for carbons of the steroid molecule.

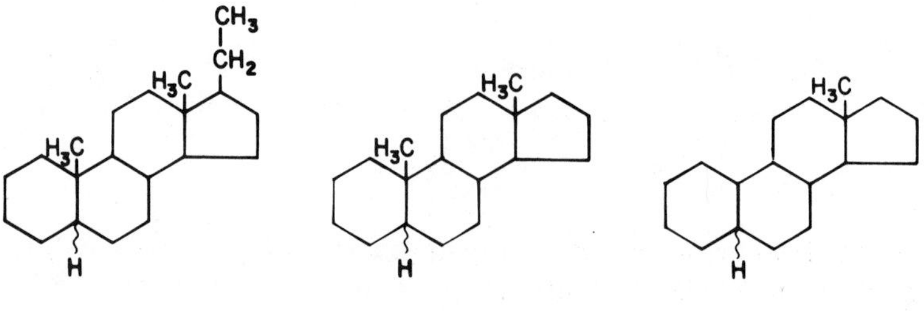

Pregnane   **Androstane**   **Estrane**

Figure 14. Hypothetical parent compounds of three categories of steroid hormones.

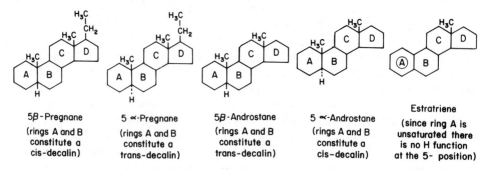

| 5β-Pregnane (rings A and B constitute a cis-decalin) | 5 α-Pregnane (rings A and B constitute a trans-decalin) | 5β-Androstane (rings A and B constitute a trans-decalin) | 5 α-Androstane (rings A and B constitute a cis-decalin) | Estratriene (since ring A is unsaturated there is no H function at the 5- position) |

Figure 15. 5α and 5β Configurations of pregnane and androstane and unsaturated ring A derivative of estrane.

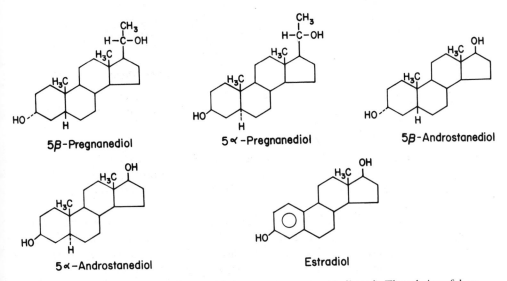

Figure 16. Examples of particular steroids (systematic names not indicated). The relation of these steroids to parent compounds can be appreciated by reference to Figs. 14 and 15.

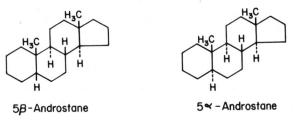

Figure 17. Basic relationships among substituents at ring junctions in typical steroids.

If various substitutions for the H atoms in the compounds of Fig. 15 are made, the structures of particular steroid hormones are generated. Examples of this are given in Fig. 16.

If we now review the disposition of atoms in a "parent" compound (androstane will be used, but the data apply to pregnane and estrane as well), we can summarize the basic structure, conformation, and configuration of all steroid hormones (Fig. 17).

First, note that all steroids are composed of three six-membered (all in the chair conformation) rings and one five-membered carbon ring. If the steroid is of the 5β-type, substituents at C-5 and C-10 are *cis* at the junction of rings A and B. If the steroid is of the 5α-type, substituents at C-5 and C-10 are *trans* at the A/B junction. At the B/C and C/D junctions, substituents are *trans* in all steroids. The links between rings A and C and between B and D are characterized by substituents that are *trans* to one another. Thus, the general picture that emerges is a series of *trans* relationships between substituents at adjacent ring functions along the "backbone" of the molecule (C-5-10-9-8-14-13); this yields a planar structure if the A/B junction is *trans*, but a somewhat more contorted structure if the A/B junction is *cis* (Fig. 18).

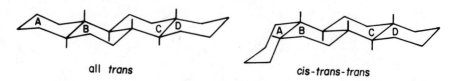

all *trans*   cis-*trans*-*trans*

Figure 18. Ring junctions and their influence on the shape of a steroid.

Another aspect of the stereochemistry of the steroid nucleus is that of the disposition of the substituents—are they α or β in configuration and are they axial or equatorial in conformation? These details of configuration and conformation are given in Table 1.

In naturally occurring steroids, there is sometimes a hydroxyl (-OH) substituent in place of hydrogen. The carbon positions at which -OH substituents most frequently occur are 3, 11, and 17. Table 2 shows the configuration and conformation of these hydroxyl groups when they occur in steriods.

Table 1. Configuration and Conformation of Nuclear Substituents of Steroids[a,b]

Position	5α Series (A/B *trans*)		5β Series (A/B *cis*)	
	α Configuration	β Configuration	α Configuration	β Configuration
1	a	e	e	a
2	e	a	a	e
3	a	e	e	a
4	e	a	a	e
5	a^{AB}	—	—	a^{A}e^B
10	—	a^{AB}	—	e^{A}a^B

	5α and 5β Series	
6	e	a
7	a	e
8	—	a
9	a	—
11	e	a
12	a	e
13	—	a
14	a	—
15	e$'^c$	a$'$
16	—^{d}	—^{d}
17	a$'$	e$'$

[a] Reproduced with permission from Klyne (1957).
[b] The letters a, e indicate axial and equatorial, respectively. a^{A}e^B indicates axial and equatorial with regard to rings A and B, respectively.
[c] a$'$, e$'$, quasi-axial and quasi-equatorial with respect to ring C.
[d] The terms axial and equatorial have no meaning for C-16.

Table 2. Configuration and Conformation of Commonly Occurring Hydroxyl
Groups on Steroids

Position of hydroxyl group	Configuration	Conformation
C-3	β in 5α series[a] α in 5β series[a] β in 4-ene series[a]	Equatorial
C-11	β	Axial
C-17	α	Axial

[a] These configurations are more usual than the alternatives, but the latter do occur.

C. Essentials of Steroid Nomenclature

The numbering of the steroid molecule is described in Fig. 13. The general form for systematic naming of particular steroids is the following.

1. When there are two or more substituents (other than H atoms) on the molecule, name the carbon(s) on which such substituents are found and give their configuration.

2. Indicate the substituent(s) by an appropriate prefix (e.g., hydroxy- for an alcohol, oxo- for a ketone).

3. If C-5 is saturated, state whether configuration of the H atom is α or β. This is because variation in stereochemistry at C-5 is more common than at other ring junctions.

4. Name the parent compound (e.g., pregnane, androstane, or estrane).

5. Denote the location of double bonds between carbons by changing the terminal "ane" of the parent compound to "-ene" (one double bond), "-adiene" (two double bonds), or "-yne" (triple bond). The terminal "e" of "-ane," "-ene," "-adiene," or "-yne" is deleted before a vowel (presence or absence of numerals has no effect on such deletions).

6. If only one substituent (other than H) is present on the steroid molecule, it is used as a suffix. If two or more substituents are present only one is used as a suffix. The choice of a suffix in decreasing order of preference is: 'onium salt, acid, lactone, ester, aldehyde, ketone, alcohol, amine, ether. The location of this substituent is indicated by the number of the carbon it is associated with, and the suffix is then added (e.g., suffix for ketone is "-one," for alcohol, "-ol").

Some examples will illustrate this method of naming steroids. Figure 19 illustrates an androstane-type steroid.

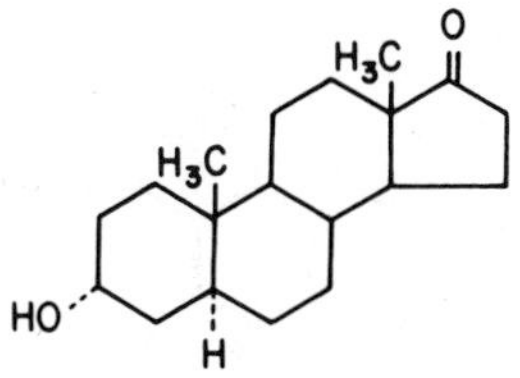

Figure 19. A steroid of the androstane family.

First, note that there are two substituents, a ketone at carbon-17 and an alcohol at carbon-3. Because ketones have preference over alcohols for the suffix position, the alcohol forms the prefix. The alcohol is 3α-, so it is called 3α-hydroxy-. The H atom at carbon-5 is α, and the compound is a C_{19} (androst-) saturated (-ane) compound. So far, our compound is called 3α-hydroxy- 5α-androstane. Next, the ketone (C=O) at C-17 is called -17-one (suffix). Because the suffix name begins with a vowel, the terminal "e" of "androstane" is dropped, and the complete name of the compound is therefore 3α-hydroxy-5α- androstan-17-one (commonly known as androsterone).

Figure 20 shows a steroid of the pregnane type with 21 carbons. In this case, there is only one type of substituent (ketone) represented at two carbons (C-3, C-20). Therefore, no prefix is called for. There is unsaturation at C-5, so no H atom is present. The location of the unsaturation is between C-4 and C-5, and this location is indicated by using only the lower number of the two sequential numbers. Because this steroid has 21 carbons, it is called a 4-pregnene. The two ketone groups are indicated in the suffix as 3,20-dione, giving a complete name for this steroid of 4-pregnene-3,20-dione (commonly known as progesterone).

Figure 21 shows a steroid of the estrane type, with 18 carbons. Again, only one type of substituent is present (alcohol groups at C-3 and C-17), so no prefix is called for. There is unsaturation at C-5. In fact, there are three double bonds in this 18-carbon molecule. The steroid is therefore a 1,3,5(10)-estratriene. Note that since the double bond at C-5 is associated with C-10, and 5 and 10 are not sequential numbers, the number 10 is indicated in parentheses after number 5. The two alcohol groups have β-configurations and form the suffix 3,17β-diol. The complete name of this compound is therefore 1,3,5(10)estratriene-3,17β-diol (commonly known as estradiol-17β).

Another complication in the naming of steroids is related to the stereochemistry of carbon 20 in pregnane compounds (Fig. 22). Figure 22 illustrates

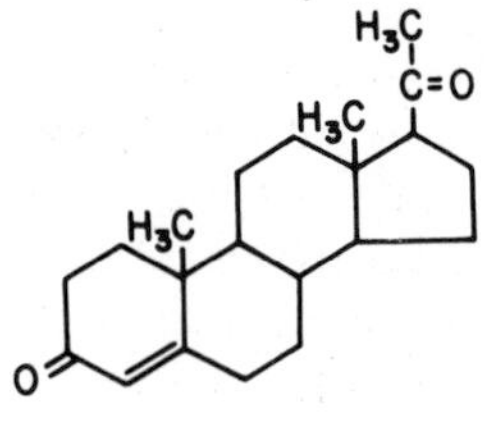

Figure 20. A steroid of the pregnane family.

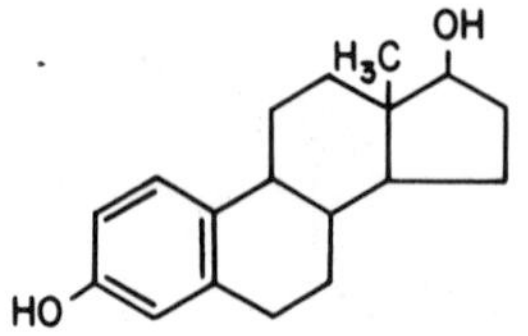

Figure 21. A steroid of the estrane family.

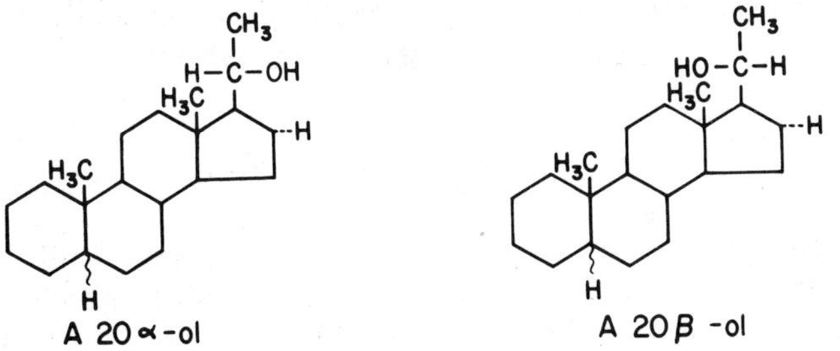

Figure 22. Nomenclature of C-20 substituents. Substituents shown to the right of C-20 are termed α, while those to the left are termed β.

that substituents shown to the right of C-20 are termed α-, and those to the left are termed β (these particular α-and β- notations therefore do not refer to whether a substituent is below or above the plane of the steroid).*

In addition to these rules for systematic naming of steroids, there are several "trivial" terms that are commonly used to describe steroids. Among these are several prefixes:

1. *allo*—Formerly used to denote 5α- configuration (no longer acceptable).
2. *epi*—Denotes inversion of a substituent other than at the C-5 position.
3. *dehydro*—Loss of 2H from adjacent carbon atoms with formation of a double bond, or loss of 2H from a CHOH group with formation of carbonyl or keto group.
4. Δ—Denotes a double bond within a steroid ring (no longer acceptable).
5. *deoxo* (or *desoxo*)—Loss of a C=O group by saturation with H (C=O→CH$_2$).
6. *deoxy* (or *desoxy*)—Loss of an oxygen (COH→CH).
7. *dihydro*—Addition of 2H to a double bond.
8. *nor*—Elimination of a methylene group from a steroid side chain. *Nor* is preceded by the number of the carbon atom that is eliminated.

These prefixes are used in conjunction with "trivial" names of steroids, such as testosterone, estradiol, progesterone, etc., yielding terms such as 19-nor-testosterone or 5α-dihydroprogesterone.

---

*The Sequence Rule should actually be used for nomenclature of substituents in the C-17 side chain. According to this rule, a 20α-hydroxy group is called 20S- (S for sinister or left) and a 20β-hydroxy group is called 20R- (R for rectus or right). As an aid to understanding the various aspects of conformation and configuration discussed in this chapter, I suggest inspecting models constructed from sets that are commercially available.

III. FUNCTIONAL GROUPS IN STEROIDS AND THEIR CHEMICAL REACTIONS

A. Simple Functional Groups

In discussing the nomenclature of steroids, we noted that the steroid molecule consists of a backbone of C–C linkages with possibilities for other types of linkages projecting above or below this backbone. It is the reactions of these individual linkages that give to a steroid its chemical properties. This is a major point that is clearly summarized in two quotations from Klyne (1957):

> It is entirely misleading to think or speak of the reactions of individual compounds—e.g., "the reactions of testosterone." One should think in terms of the reactions of a ketone group (at position 3) and more specifically in terms of a Δ^4-3 ketone group, which differ in detail but not in principle from those of similar ketone groups in other positions on steroid molecules or other molecules. One should also think of the reactions of a 17β-hydroxyl group, which differ in detail but not in principle from hydroxyl groups in other positions and in other configurations. . . .

> The chemical properties of a steroid like those of any other organic compound should be considered as being essentially reactions of the functional groups contained in it. As in all other fields of organic chemistry, it is true, as a first approximation, that each functional group undergoes its own reactions with little or no interference by other groups present. The fascination of complex natural products, such as the steroids, depends on the exceptions and refinements to this general statement.

The most important simple functional groups on steroids are hydroxyls, phenols, carbonyls, and double bonds within the rings of the steroid. Using the approach of Klyne (1957), we shall briefly review the reactions of these simple functional groups that are of most concern to reproductive endocrinologists.

1. Hydroxyl Groups

Nearly all steroids have an oxygen function at C-3, so reactions at this position have a special importance.

a. Esterification

The general form of this reaction is shown in Fig. 23. Particular types of esterifications of interest to reproductive endocrinologists include those shown in Fig. 24. These steroid esters are important because they retain biological activity longer than native forms of steroids. (Generally, the longer the group added to the steroid, the longer the steroid takes to be metabolized.)

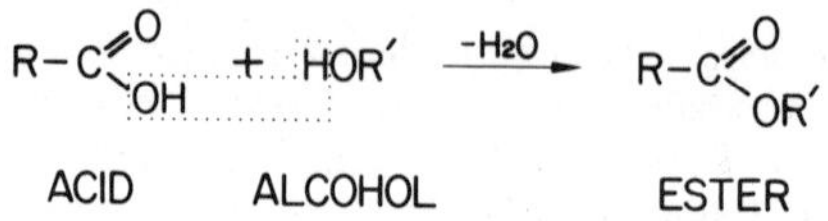

Figure 23. General form of an esterification reaction.

b. Replacement

This is a reaction in which the hydroxyl is replaced by a halogen with either retention or inversion of configuration (or a mixture of both). Certain synthetic compounds in current use are halogenated derivatives. The general form of the reaction is shown in Fig. 25.

c. Epimerization

This is a reaction in which axial hydroxyl groups are epimerized (epimers are a pair of isomers that correspond in configuration at all but one carbon) (Fig. 26).

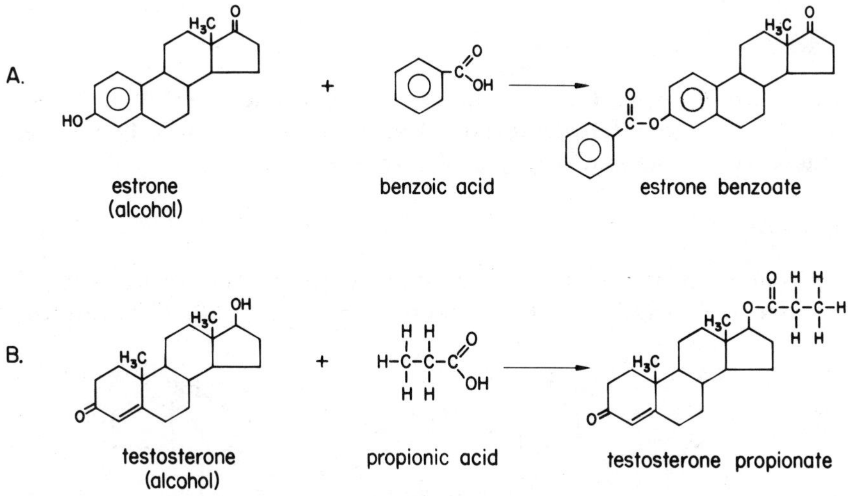

A.

estrone
(alcohol)

benzoic acid

estrone benzoate

B.

testosterone
(alcohol)

propionic acid

testosterone propionate

Figure 24. Typical esterifications of estrone and testosterone.

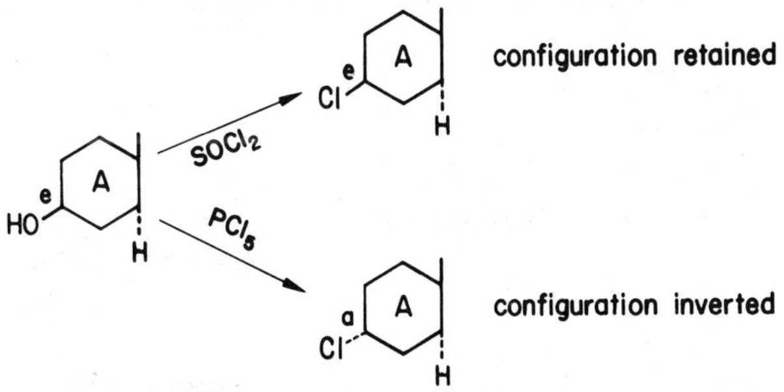

configuration retained

configuration inverted

Figure 25. Typical halogenation reactions.

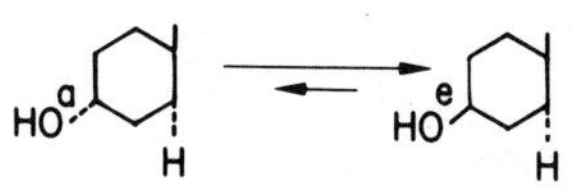

Figure 26. Epimerization.

2. Phenolic Groups

Phenols are a special group of hydroxylated compounds with the hydroxyl group on an aromatic (benzene type) ring. Estrogens are phenolic compounds. Reactions of phenolic groups include formation of sodium salts—estrogens dissolve in dilute sodium hydroxide with formation of sodium salts (Fig. 27)— and formation of methyl ethers—this reaction is important in the case of steroids with multiple hydroxyl groups, only one of which the investigator wishes to esterify. The formation of a methyl ether prior to esterification "protects" that site from esterification. A specific example, using estradiol-17β, is given in Fig. 28. After the 17β-hydroxyl of the 3-methyl ether derivative has been formed, the compound can be demethylated, yielding a steroid that is selectively esterified at the C-17 position.

3. Carbonyl Groups

Carbonyl groups are of two types, ketones and aldehydes. With the exception of aldosterone, aldehydes do not normally occur in steroids. Therefore, we shall limit remarks about reactions of carbonyls to ketones.

a. Reductions

A commonly used reduction reaction takes the general form shown in Fig. 29. A specific illustration of this reaction is given in Fig. 30. The reduction of

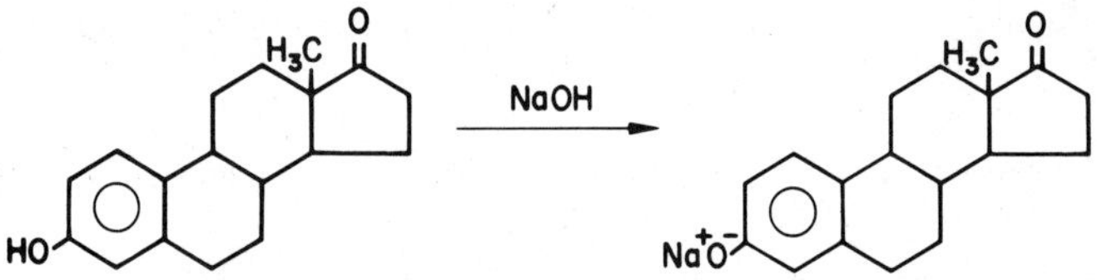

Figure 27. Formation of sodium salt of estrone.

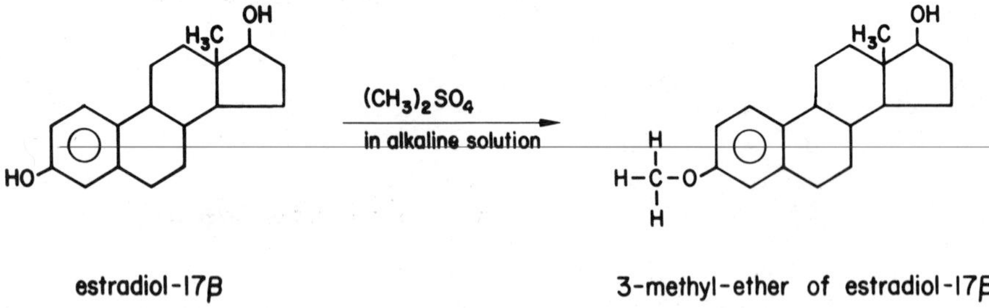

estradiol-17β   3-methyl-ether of estradiol-17β

Figure 28. Formation of 3-methyl ether of estradiol-17β.

KETONE

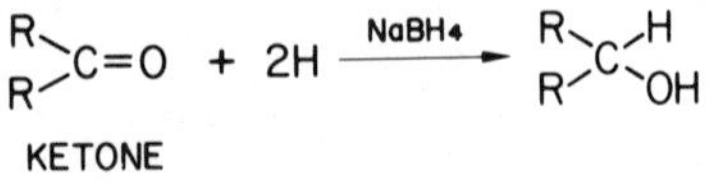

Figure 29. General form of one type of reduction reaction.

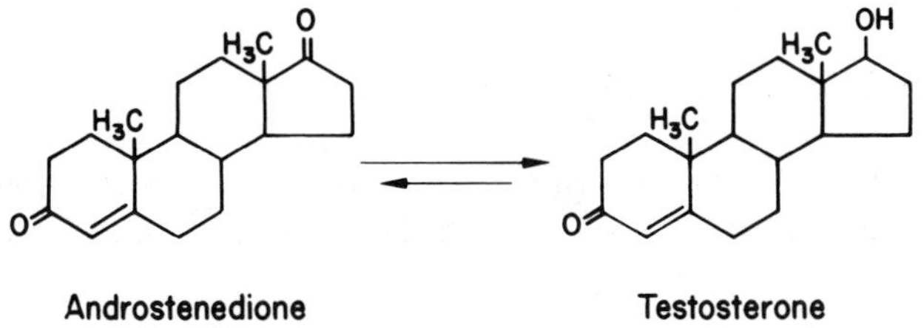

Androstenedione   **Testosterone**

Figure 30. Reduction of androstenedione to testosterone.

the carbonyl group of androstenedione (or other steroids) by sodium borohydride has been used in order to form a hydroxylated steroid that can then be esterified. Certain types of esters (e.g., monochloroacetates) have properties that make them amenable to measurement by gas–liquid chromatography with electron capture detection (see Section VI).

b. Formation of Nitrogenous Derivatives

Two such derivatives are semicarbazones and oximes, which have been used in steroid measurement by double-isotope derivative techniques and radioimmunoassay techniques (see Section VI). General and particular forms of the reactions that yield these derivatives are given in Figs. 31 and 32.

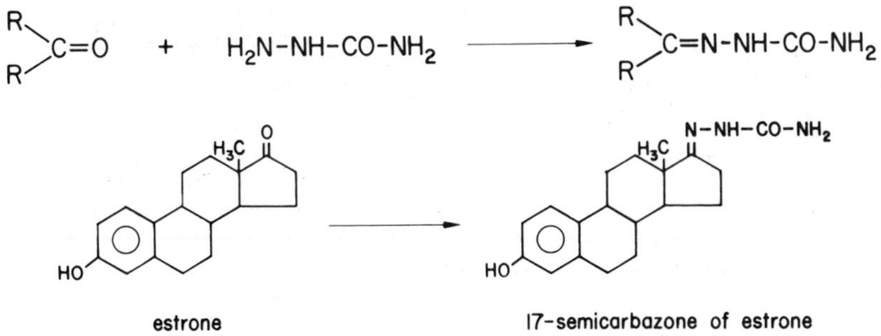

estrone   17-semicarbazone of estrone

Figure 31. Formation of semicarbazone of estrone.

testosterone

testosterone o-carboxy methyl oxime

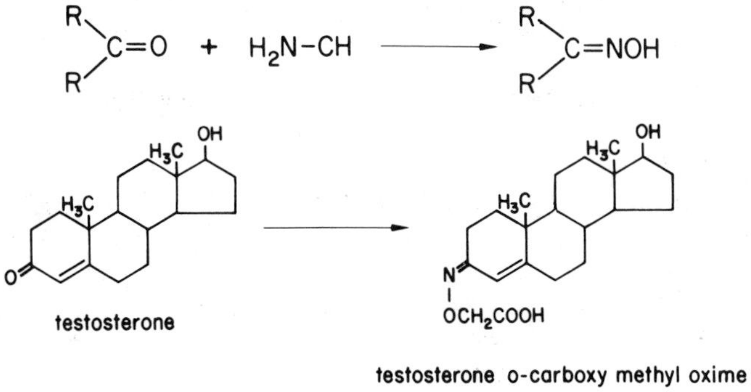

Figure 32. Formation of oxime derivative of testosterone.

c. Reaction with Girard Reagent

This is illustrated in Fig. 33. The reaction is useful for separating ketones from nonketones. Ketones will form a water-soluble derivative, whereas other unconjugated steroids that are nonketones will not react and will not be water soluble. This reaction has been particularly useful with ketones at the 3- or 17-position.

d. Enolization

Keto groups exist in reversible equilibrium in two forms (Fig. 34). This is important because the enol form (see Fig. 34) can be esterified.

e. Oxidation

This has had importance in the past because oxidation of a ketone of a ring structure involves fission of the ring.

f. Condensation of Methylene Group Adjacent to Ketone

This reaction actually involves a group adjacent to a ketone rather than alteration of the ketone itself. The particular condensation reaction shown in Fig. 35 is known as the Zimmermann reaction. It has been widely used in

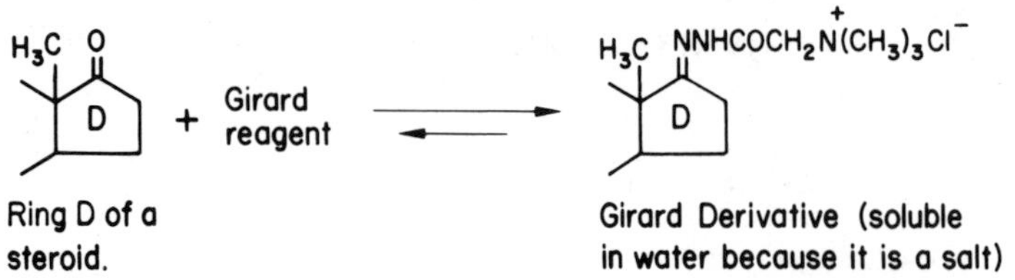

Figure 33. Girard reaction with ketone at C-17 of a steroid.

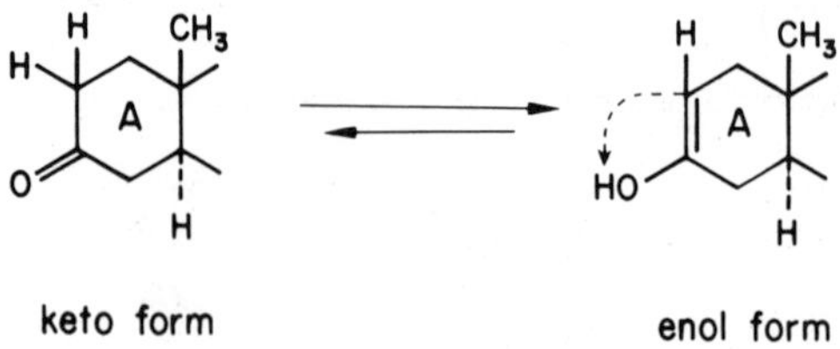

keto form   enol form

Figure 34. Enolization.

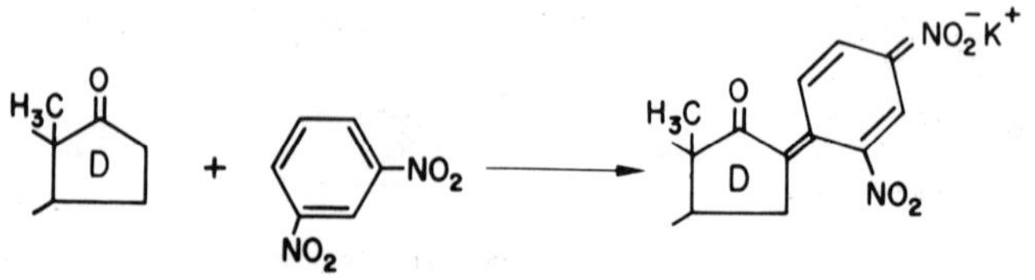

Figure 35. Zimmermann reaction.

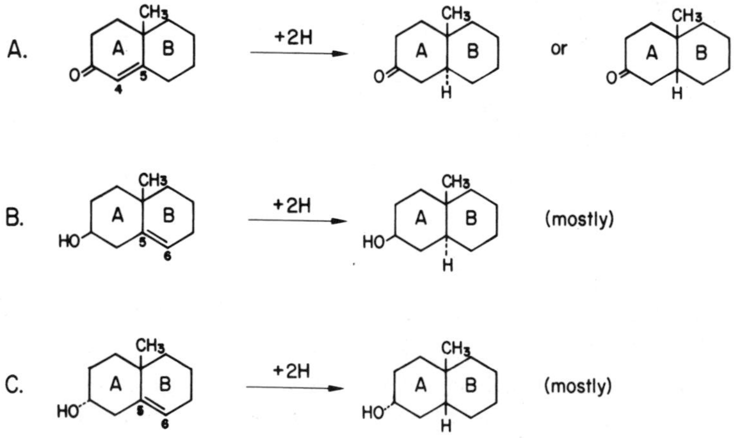

A.   +2H   or

B.   +2H   (mostly)

C.   +2H   (mostly)

Figure 36. Examples of hydrogenation of double bonds at the 4–5 and at the 5–6 positions.

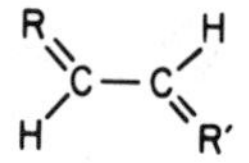

Figure 37. Conjugated double bonds.

spectrophotometric determinations of urinary androgens with a keto group at position C-17 (urinary ketosteroids). However, the Zimmermann reaction is not entirely specific.

4. Double Bonds within the Steroid Rings

Among the reactions of the double bond, the most important for discussion here is hydrogenation. The most relevant of these reactions involve reduction of the double bond between C-4 and C-5, and between C-5 and C-6 (Fig. 36a–c).

B. Complex Functional Groups

One very important refinement of the rule that simple functional groups behave similarly in all molecules comes about when two simple functions are so close together in a molecule that they greatly influence one another's properties. In this case, it is best to consider the two simple groups together as a single complex function. The most important complex function that occurs in gonadal steroids is the conjugated ketone.

1. Conjugated Ketones

A conjugated double bond is one in which a single C-to-C bond is surrounded on both sides by double bonds (Fig. 37).

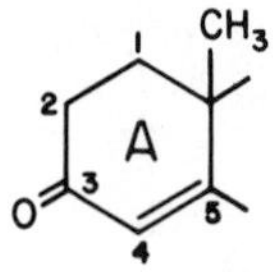

Figure 38. Conjugated double bonds on ring A of a steroid.

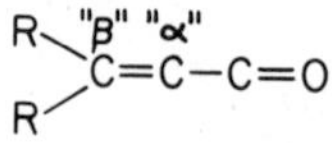

Figure 39. "α" and "β" Carbons of conjugated double bonds.

Many physiologically active steroids contain a conjugated double bond on ring A. This conjugated double bond is of the type shown in Fig. 38. Since a ketone group accounts for one of the two double bonds, these are called conjugated ketones. Another term, somewhat less satisfactory but widely used, is "α, β unsaturated ketones." In this case α and β do not refer to configuration but denote the atoms next to ("α") and next but one ("β") to carbon of the ketone group (Fig. 39).

A variety of chemical techniques not necessary to be discussed here can be used to saturate either of the double bonds selectively or to saturate both double bonds. However, there are two properties of conjugated 4-en-3-ones that are of considerable interest. The 4-en-3-one is more stable than the corresponding 4–5 saturated compound with a keto group in the 3 position. This is because of the greater electronic stability of conjugated systems over systems containing only one double bond or systems with unconjugated multiple double bonds. The 4-en-3-one compounds absorb ultraviolet light, at about 240 nm. This physical property is of enormous value in visualizing the position of 4-en-3-ones on paper or on thin-layer chromatographic strips by merely looking at the strips under UV light. A minimum of about 5 μg of steroid is necessary for such direct visualization.

C. Steroid Sulfates and Glucuronides

Until now, we have spoken only of pregnanes and androstanes (sometimes referred to as "neutral" steroids) and estranes (sometimes referred to as "phenolic" steroids) in their "free" forms.* Such free steroids readily dissolve in organic solvents such as benzene, ether, or ethyl acetate but do not dissolve in water (except estriol). In contrast to the "free" forms of these steroids are certain water-soluble derivatives. These derivatives are of two types, the sulfates and the glucuronides. They are urinary excretion products and are referred to as "conjugated" steroids (the term conjugation has a different

---

*Actually, almost all "free" steroid in the blood is not free at all but is loosely bound to serum proteins. This topic is covered in Pincus *et al.* (1966) and in Westphal (1970).

meaning here than that discussed previously in the context of conjugated ketones). The most significant properties of conjugated steroids are summarized below.

1. Sulfates

These conjugated steroids (Fig. 40) are (a) easily separable from free steroids because of their solubility in water and (b) easily hydrolyzed by dilute aqueous acids, giving the free steroid plus sulfate ion (SO_4^{2-}).

2. Glucuronides

Glucuronides, or glucosiduronic acids, are also acidic (Fig. 41) and soluble in water or alcohols such as butanol and thus are similar to sulfates. Like the sulfates, the glucuronides are hydrolyzed by acid, but not as readily. Sulfates and glucuronides are separable from each other by at least two methods: glucuronides can be acetylated to form a triacetyl derivative that is soluble in benzene whereas sulfates remain unaffected and insoluble in benzene; and specific enzymes called β-glucuronidases (sources are spleen, bacteria, and snails) hydrolyze the glucuronides without affecting the sulfates (except that the snail glucuronidase also has some sulfatase activity).

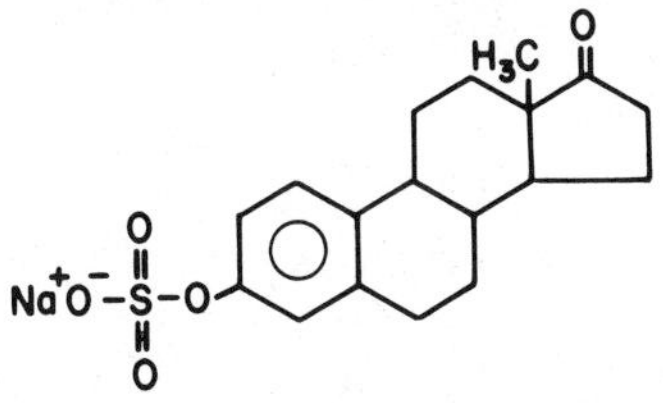

Figure 40. Estrone sulfate.

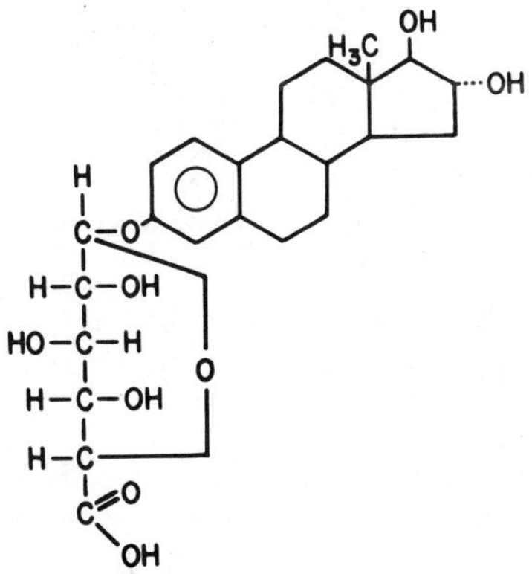

Figure 41. Estriol glucuronide.

It should be understood that all classes of gonadal hormones—the preg-nanes, androstanes, and the estranes—form metabolites that are sub-sequently conjugated with either sulfate or glucuronic acid. In contrasting the so-called "free" steroids with the conjugated steroids, one should also bear in mind that "free" steroids are usually bound to proteins in the blood. The term "free" is meant only to indicate absence of conjugation to sulfate or glucuronide.

IV. ENZYMES AND STEROID TRANSFORMATIONS

We have now discussed some of the chemical reactions that simple and complex functional groups on the steroid molecule can undergo. These chemi-cal reactions were seen to be of value in determining steroid structure and in providing quantitative data on steroid concentrations.

Under physiological conditions, the functional groups also react, and these reactions are catalyzed by enzymes. These enzymes are therefore responsible for the biosynthesis and the breakdown of steroid hormones.

The enzymes may be classified into the following types: oxidoreductases such as hydroxylases, dehydrogenases and reductases,* lyases (formerly termed desmolases), conjugation and deconjugation enzymes, and miscellane-ous enzymes (e.g., isomerases). We shall briefly review some of the properties of these enzymes.

A. Hydroxylases

The hydroxylases introduce an -OH group onto a steroid (Fig. 42), usually irreversibly (hydroxylation at C-21 is reversible). Hydroxylation could theoret-ically occur at any position on the steroid molecule. In fact, in addition to the commonly occurring hydroxyl groups at positions C-3α, 3β, and 17β, hydroxy-lation in mammalian systems has been demonstrated at positions C-2 and C-4 (in phenolic steroids, with formation of catechol estrogens), 2α, 6α, 6β, 7α, 11β, 15α, 16α (16α is involved in formation of estriol), 17α, 18, 19 (19 is involved in aromatization of androgen to estrogen), and 21 (21 is involved in formation of corticosterone). Cholesterol can be hydroxylated at the 20α- and the 22R-† positions.

All hydroxylases that have been studied catalyze reactions with retention of configuration at the sites of reaction (e.g., Bergstrom *et al.*, 1958). Another

---

*Oxidoreductases have been categorized and systematized according to IUPAC rules. However, for convenience, only the trivial names of oxidoreductases such as hydroxylases, dehydrogenases, and reductases will be used in this chapter.
†See footnote p. 29.

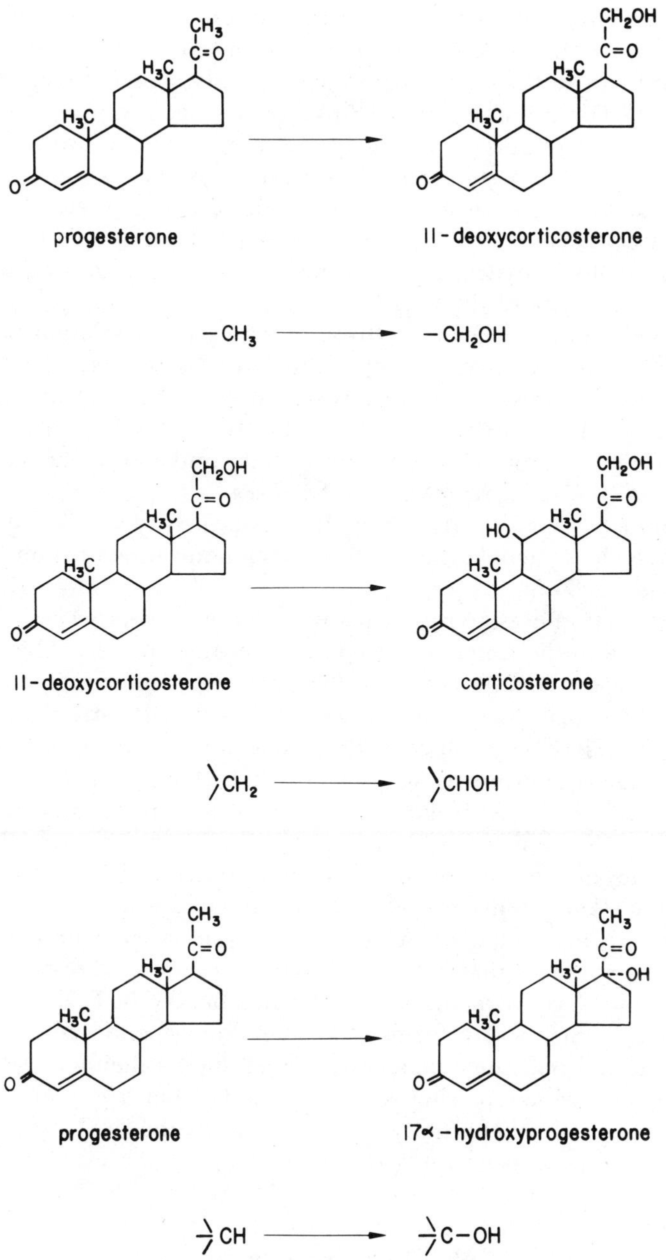

progesterone   II-deoxycorticosterone

$-CH_3 \longrightarrow -CH_2OH$

II-deoxycorticosterone   corticosterone

$>CH_2 \longrightarrow >CHOH$

progesterone   17∝-hydroxyprogesterone

$\overset{}{\underset{}{\rangle}}CH \longrightarrow \overset{}{\underset{}{\rangle}}C-OH$

Figure 42. Hydroxylations.

property of hydroxylases is their specificity. This specificity is probably imposed by a lock-and-key type of relationship between enzyme and steroid. In a general way, this would account for the inability of, for example, 7α-hydroxylating enzyme to affect other positions on a steroid. However, this is speculative, since the three-dimensional relationships of the enzyme–steroid coupling are still unknown. Hydroxylases are also specific with respect to conformation. For example, the 11β-hydroxylase does not hydroxylate the 11α- position to any degree. Specificity with respect to conformation may be related to whether the position to be hydroxylated is axial or equatorial. In the case of an impending axial hydroxylation (e.g., 11β-), the site of maximum electron density is either above or below the plane of the ring. In the case of an impending equatorial hydroxylation (e.g., 11α-), the site of maximum electron density is in the plane of the ring.

The biochemical mechanism through which hydroxylation takes place consists of a complex series of steps elucidated by the use of adrenal cell fractions. The mechanism is known as reversed electron transport and involves NADPH, a flavoprotein dehydrogenase specific to NADPH, a protein that contains nonheme iron, a cytochrome system, and molecular oxygen (see Schulster *et al.*, 1976 for review and references).

It should be mentioned that hydroxylase activity can be affected by anesthetics, such as phenobarbital, that are commonly used in animal research (Conney *et al.,* 1965).

Of particular interest to reproductive endocrinologists is a set of hydroxylations involved in the conversion of androgens to estrogens. This process is known as aromatization. Aromatase activity has been demonstrated not only in tissues such as placenta, ovary, testis, and adrenal cortex, but also in hypothalamic cells of certain species. Because an unsaturated ring A is required for aromatization, androgens such as adrostenedione and testosterone are aromatizable, whereas androgens such as 5α-dihydrotestosterone are not aromatizable. The steps involved in the aromatization process are schematized in Fig. 43. They include hydroxylation of one of the three hydrogens at C-19 of an androgen. The 19-hydroxy-4-en-3-one formed is an obligatory intermediate for aromatization. A second hydroxylation then occurs, giving a 19,19-dihydroxysteroid that presumably is then reversibly dehydrated to form a 19-oxosteroid. A conformational change then breaks the C-10 to C-19 bond with release of formic acid or formaldehyde. A double bond is formed between C-1 and C-2, and rearrangement of the resulting 1,4-dienone yields a compound with a benzene-type ring A. Loss of the C-19 methyl group combined with appearance of a benzene-type ring A means that a C_{18} steroid of the estrogen category has been formed.

B. Dehydrogenases

The dehydrogenases may be divided into two types, the hydroxysteroid dehydrogenases and the reductases.

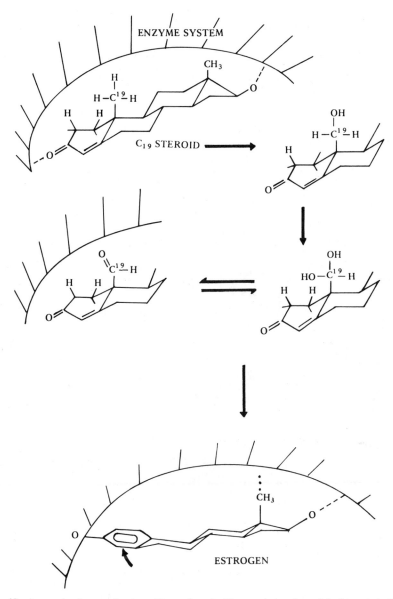

Figure 43. Aromatization mechanism. (Reproduced with permission from Schulster *et al.*, 1976.)

The relevant hydroxysteroid dehydrogenases are those that catalyze reactions of 5-en-3β-ols, 3β-ols, 4-en-3α- or β-ols, 17α- and 17β-ols, and 20α- and 20β-ols. The reactions catalyzed are shown in Fig. 44.

These reactions are crucially involved in steroid biosynthesis. For example, the type of reaction illustrated in Fig. 44A is important in the biosynthesis of progesterone from pregnenolone. Note that there are two steps involved and that the second is irreversible. Figure 44D shows the type of reaction involved

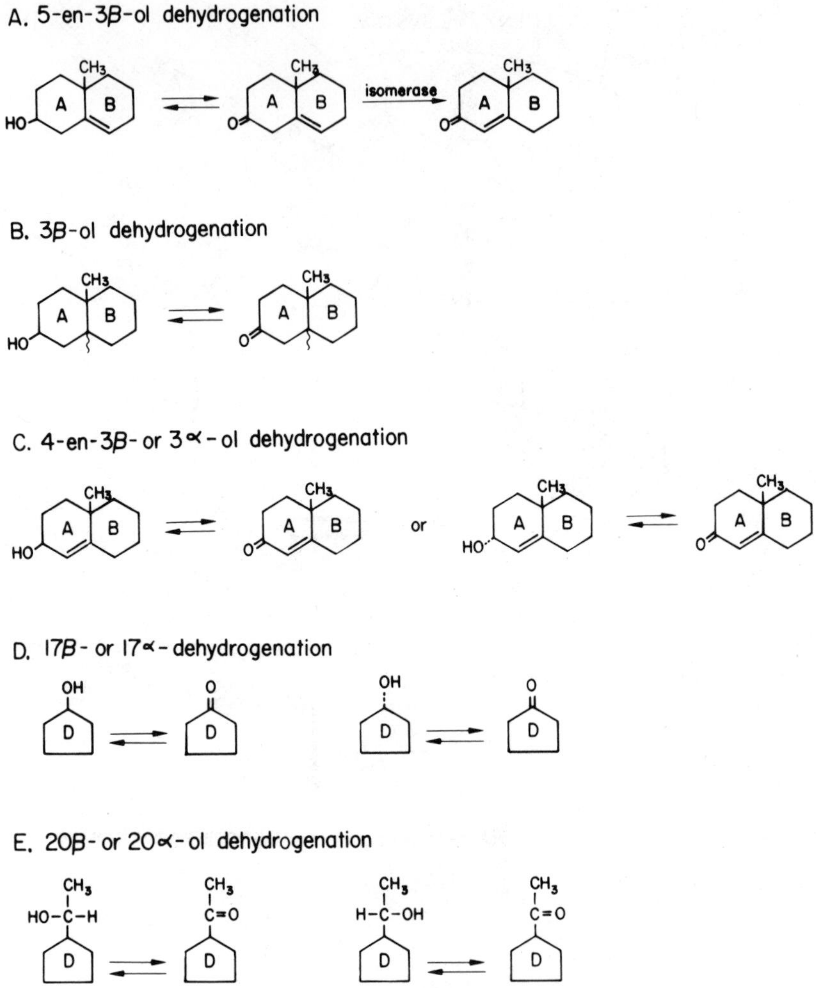

A. 5-en-3β-ol dehydrogenation

B. 3β-ol dehydrogenation

C. 4-en-3β- or 3∝-ol dehydrogenation

D. 17β- or 17∝-dehydrogenation

E. 20β- or 20∝-ol dehydrogenation

Figure 44. Dehydrogenation reactions.

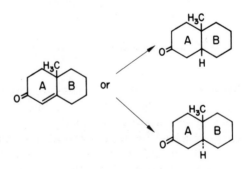

Figure 45. Reduction of the 4–5 double bond.

in the interconversion between testosterone (a 17β-ol) and androstenedione, and between estradiol-17β and estrone. The enzymes involved are not necessarily the same for the androgens and for the estrogens. In Fig. 44E are seen the types of reactions involved in interconversion between 20β-dihydroprogesterone and progesterone or between 20α-dihydroprogesterone and progesterone.

The relevant reductases are those that catalyze the reduction of the 4–5 double bond to either 5β- or 5α-ring A saturated steroids (Fig. 45). This type of reaction occurs when testosterone is reduced to 5α- or 5β-dihydrotestosterone. Corresponding reactions occur with progesterone, and these are also of biological significance.

C. Lyases

These are enzymes that cause splitting of a side chain or loss of methyl groups. The most significant steroid lyases are:

1. *10,19 lyase*—Splits off C-19 as part of aromatization process (conversion of androgens to estrogens).
2. *17α,20 C-21 lyase*—Splits off C-20 and C-21 from 17α-hydroxyprogesterone as part of pathway from progestins to androgens (Fig. 46).
3. *20α,22 C-27 lyase*—Splits off the side chain of cholesterol as part of the pathway to pregnenolone (Fig. 47).

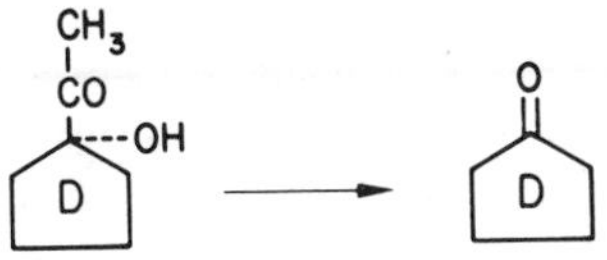

Figure 46. Reaction catalyzed by the 17α,20-C$_{21}$ lyase system.

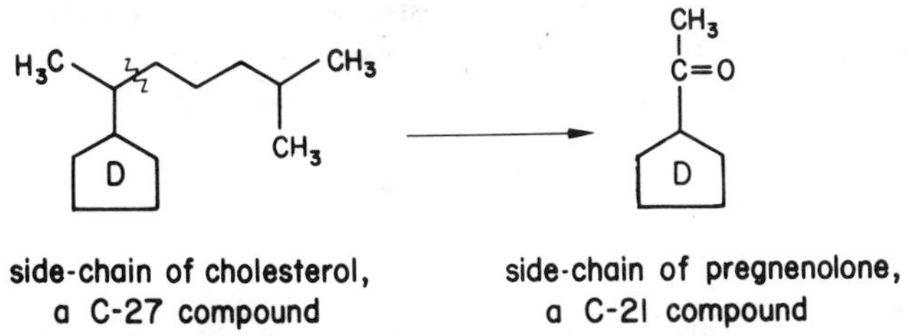

side-chain of cholesterol,
a C-27 compound

side-chain of pregnenolone,
a C-21 compound

Figure 47. Reaction catalyzed by the 20α,22-C$_{27}$ lyase system. Squiggly line on side chain of cholesterol indicates site of splitting of side chain.

D. Conjugation and Deconjugation Enzymes

There appear to be at least two distinct sulfation systems (sulfotransferases). One is active for estrogens and the other for 3β-hydroxy neutral steroids. Current methods do not permit a conclusion as to whether individual steroids have individual sulfotransferases.

There are also enzymes that are responsible for glucuronide formation. Most steroid conjugates are excreted as glucuronides because glucuronides are cleared rapidly through the kidneys.

The deconjugation enzymes are the sulfatases and glucuronidases.

E. Miscellaneous Enzymes

Among other enzymes of interest to reproductive endocrinologists are isomerases and esterases. The action of an isomerase is illustrated in Fig. 44A.

Esterases are enzymes that hydrolyze esterified steroids such as testosterone propionate or estradiol-17β-3-benzoate to the native forms. The esterase may be present in mammalian tissue and/or in microorganisms present in mammals. The significance of the esterases in neuroendocrine research is well-illustrated in an article by Goodman (1978).

V. BIOSYNTHESIS OF STEROIDS

In the previous section we reviewed various enzymatic reactions that occur with respect to functional groups in steroids. In this section we shall discuss how these enzymatic reactions are utilized in the biosynthetic pathways to the steroid hormones. We shall begin the discussion of biosynthetic pathways by describing the pathway to the production of pregnenolone, the steroid that is the precursor of all other steroids.

A. Biosynthesis of Pregnenolone

The biosynthesis of pregnenolone proceeds by a similar route in a variety of endocrine tissues. This route can be considered in two sections, the conversion of acetate to cholesterol and the conversion of cholesterol to pregnenolone.

1. Conversion of Acetate to Cholesterol

Acetate is a ubiquitous small molecule (2 carbons) derived from the breakdown of lipids and carbohydrates. Cholesterol is a 27-carbon compound that is also distributed throughout all tissues of the body. The story of the process whereby cholesterol is synthesized from acetate was unravelled by three groups of workers: Bloch and his colleagues (U.S.), Lynen (Germany), and Popják and Cornforth (U.K.) (see Popják and Cornforth, 1960). Their work was characterized by brilliant intuitive insights and elegant experimental verifications of these insights.

Perhaps the best place to begin is in 1937 with an experiment by Rittenberg and Schoenheimer. These workers fed deuterium-labeled water to mice over a prolonged period and subsequently extracted cholesterol from the carcasses. They found that the extracted cholesterol had a high deuterium content. This would not have been expected if cholesterol were biosynthesized by (a) conversion of ingested sterols or steroids directly into cholesterol, or (b) conversion of already-existing long-chain fatty acids (e.g., oleic acid) directly into cholesterol. (This was supported by the finding that feeding animals a high-fat diet did not stimulate cholesterol synthesis to a significant degree.) Rittenberg and Schoenheimer therefore concluded that cholesterol was biosynthesized by the coupling of a large number of small molecules. This would require many reactions with the consequence that there would be frequent opportunities for deuterium to be incorporated into cholesterol.*

Which small molecules could serve as the precursor for cholesterol? In the 1940s Bloch discovered that injection of radioactive acetate in an *in vivo* or *in vitro* system led to the production of cholesterol labeled at all carbons. Furthermore, labeled cholesterol arose only from those injected substances that were known to be metabolized via acetate. Now, several questions regarding the role of acetate in cholesterol synthesis could be posed. (a) Are both the side chain and the nucleus of cholesterol formed from acetate? (b) Acetate consists of two carbon atoms—do both of them contribute to sterol synthesis? (c) If both carbons of acetate are involved in sterol synthesis, is it possible to assign to particular carbons in cholesterol an origin from either the carboxyl or the methyl carbon of acetate (Fig. 48)?

---

*Recent work indicates that two-thirds of the cholesterol in human plasma is contained within low-density lipoprotein (LDL). Cell-membrane-receptor-mediated endocytosis permits hydrolysis of the protein of LDL to amino acids and hydrolysis of cholesteryl esters contained in LDL to free cholesterol. The unesterified cholesterol is then available for steroid synthesis (Brown, M. S., and Goldstein, J. L., 1979, *Proc. Nat. Acad. Sci. USA* **76**:3330). Thus, LDL-derived cholesterol and acetate are both important substrates for steroid synthesis.

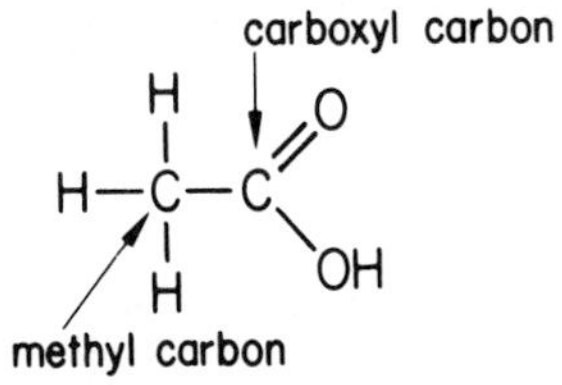

Figure 48. Acetate.

Administration of labeled acetate and subsequent degradation of the resulting radioactive cholesterol into small fragments led to the finding that both the nucleus and side-chain carbons of cholesterol were derived from acetate. Block (1957) then did the ingenious experiment of feeding double-labeled acetate ($^{14}CH_3{}^{13}CO_2Na$) to rats. He found that the ratio of $^{14}C/^{13}C$ in the resulting cholesterol was 5 : 4. If all 27 carbons of cholesterol are derived from acetate, this means that 15 of them originate from the methyl group and 12 originate from the carboxyl group. Exactly which carbons of cholesterol are derived from the methyl or carboxyl carbons of acetate was determined by degrading the synthesized cholesterol atom by atom. This impressive work was carried out by Popják and Cornforth (1960) (Fig. 49).

When this structural basis of cholesterol was appreciated, Bloch noticed that there were three places on cholesterol where a type of structure similar to isoprene (Fig. 50) could be formed. These isoprenelike units (or isoprenoid units) are indicated in Fig. 49. On the basis of finding these isoprenoid units in cholesterol, Bloch (1957) suggested that cholesterol arose from an intermediate consisting entirely of isoprenoid units, only some of which survived in the final cholesterol molecule. Such a compound exists and is called squalene (Fig. 51).

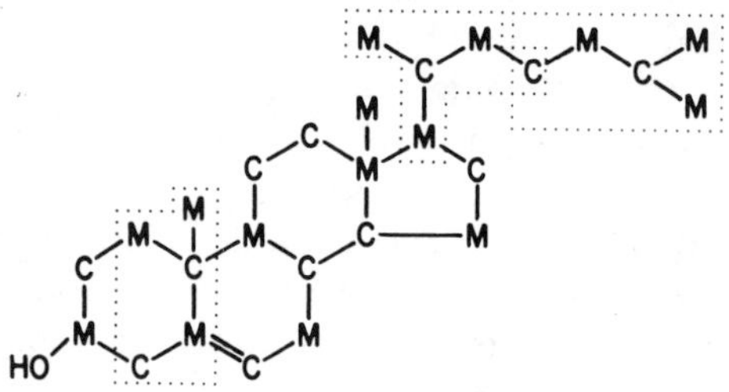

Figure 49. Origins of carbon atoms on cholesterol from the carbons of acetate (M = methyl carbon; C = carboxyl carbon of acetate). Stippled areas are isoprenoid units.

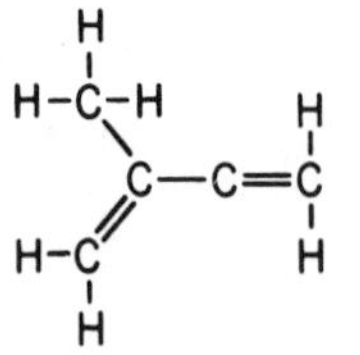

Figure 50. Isoprene.

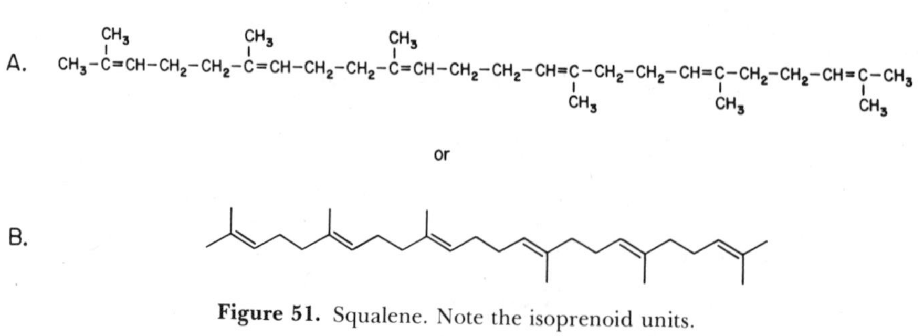

Figure 51. Squalene. Note the isoprenoid units.

Bloch was able to marshall evidence for his hypothesis that acetate molecules build up the squalene molecule and that squalene, in turn, is a precursor of cholesterol. Older evidence had shown an increased cholesterol content in the livers of rabbits fed squalene. Bloch (1957) also found that squalene was synthesized entirely from acetate in rat liver. Finally, he showed that labeled squalene, when administered to rats, served as a precursor for labeled cholesterol. Even though the conversion of squalene to cholesterol gave a yield of only about 10%, this was a higher yield than for any other precursor that had been previously tried. So far, then, the sequence of cholesterol synthesis was: acetate → squalene → cholesterol. But it was obvious that there must be many intermediate steps. For example, squalene is a long-chain, 30-carbon substance, whereas cholesterol is 4-ring system having only 27 carbons. What intermediates were there between squalene and cholesterol?

It was hypothesized that an enzyme catalyzed the cyclization of squalene to a 30-carbon, 4-ring compound. At about the same time, the compound lanosterol was isolated from wool fat. Lanosterol has the structure shown in Fig. 52. It differs from cholesterol only in that it contains (a) methyl groups at C-4 and C-14, (b) a double bond at C-8 to C-9 rather than at C-5 to C-6, and (c) a double bond in the side chain. Lanosterol was immediately suggested as an intermediate, and Bloch (1957) supported this idea by showing that labeled lanosterol served as an efficient precursor for labeled cholesterol. The methyl groups at 4 and 14 could then be removed to form zymosterol [8,24-(5α)-cholestadien-3β-ol]. The primary pathway from zymosterol to cholesterol is still not entirely worked out, but it probably includes desmosterol (5,24-cholestadien-3β-ol). Desmosterol is identical to cholesterol except that it contains a double bond (at C-24) in the side chain.

The events occurring between acetate and squalene had not been clarified at that point. What was the source of isoprenoid (C_5) units needed for the building up of the squalene molecule? No real progress occurred on this point until the accidental discovery of a compound called mevalonic acid (Fig. 53) by a group of workers studying an entirely different problem in bacterial metabolism (see reviews by Bloch, 1957; Popják and Cornforth, 1960).

The evidence that mevalonic acid was a precursor of cholesterol included the facts that (a) 2-^{14}C-labeled mevalonic acid gave labeled squalene and cholesterol in high yield; (b) degradation of labeled squalene revealed the pattern of labeling shown in Fig. 54. This coincided with the pattern to be expected from a

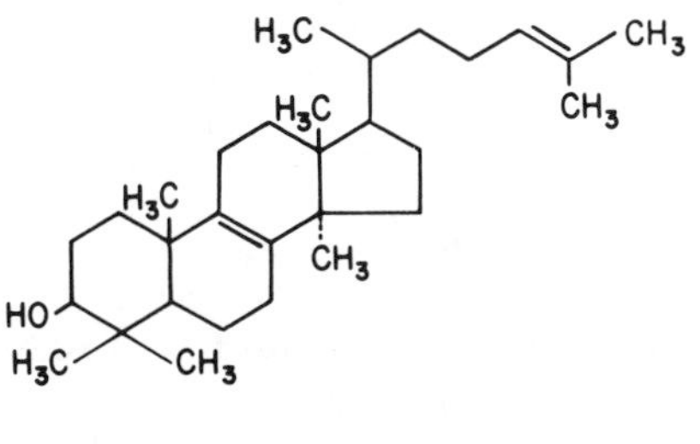

Figure 52. Lanosterol.

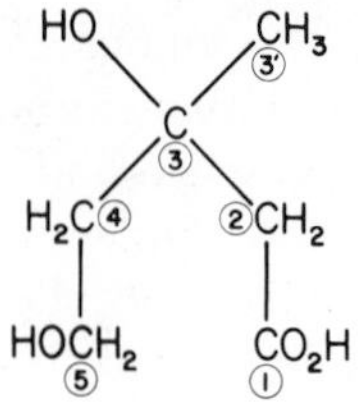

Figure 53. Mevalonic acid.

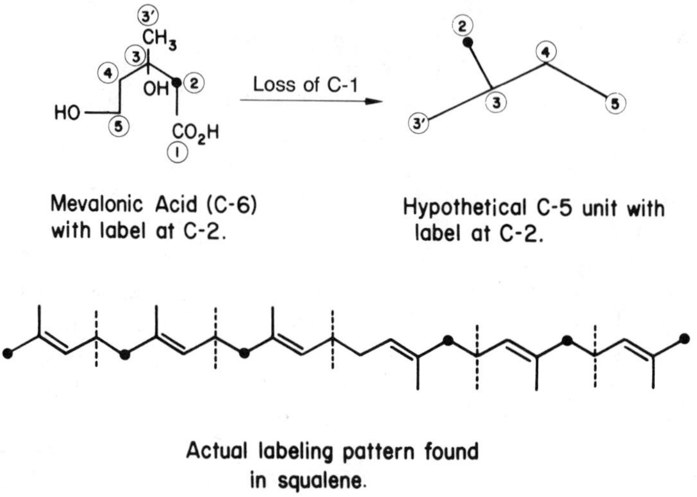

Mevalonic Acid (C-6)
with label at C-2.

Hypothetical C-5 unit with
label at C-2.

Actual labeling pattern found
in squalene.

Figure 54. Synthesis of squalene from mevalonic acid.

hypothetical C_5 unit labeled at the 2-position and derived from mevalonic acid, and it provided the key to understanding the early stages of cholesterol biogenesis. The sequence could now be represented in detail as shown in Fig. 55.

Note that phosphorylated mevalonic acid gives rise to isopentenyl pyrophosphate, which is a source of isoprenoid units. Geranyl pyrophosphate is a condensation product of two isoprenoid units (for a total of 10 carbons), and farnesyl pyrophosphate is a condensation product of three isoprenoid units (for a total of 15 carbons). Squalene, a 30-carbon compound, represents a condensation product of two molecules of farnesyl pyrophosphate.

This completes the consideration of the biosynthesis of cholesterol from acetate. Although many details are still uncertain, the basic pattern has been worked out.

2. Conversion of Cholesterol to Pregnenolone

Starting from cholesterol, a C_{27} compound, we wished to arrive at progesterone, a C_{21} compound. The steps involved in this conversion began to be

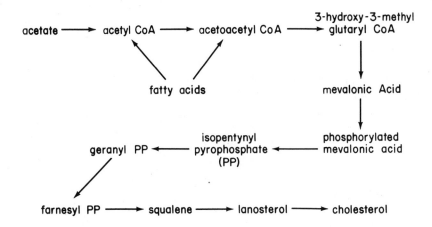

Figure 55. Basic synthetic pathway from acetate to cholesterol.

understood about 25 years ago. Radioactive cholesterol labeled in the 26-position with ^{14}C was incubated with enzyme preparations from adrenals, ovaries, and testes. After incubation, a radioactive compound containing six carbons was isolated. At first, this six-carbon compound was thought to be isocaproic acid [$(CH_3)_2CH(CH_2)_2COOH$], but it has more recently been found that isocaproaldehyde is initially formed, and this is subsequently oxidized to the acid (Schulster *et al.*, 1976).

Later work showed that when cholesterol was labeled in the 4-position instead of the 26-position, the radioactive product was pregnenolone (3β-hydroxy-5-pregnen-20-one). From these data, it was evident that enzymes within endocrine glands could cleave six carbons from the side chain of cholesterol (Fig. 56). The side chain cleavage enzyme (a lyase) has the following

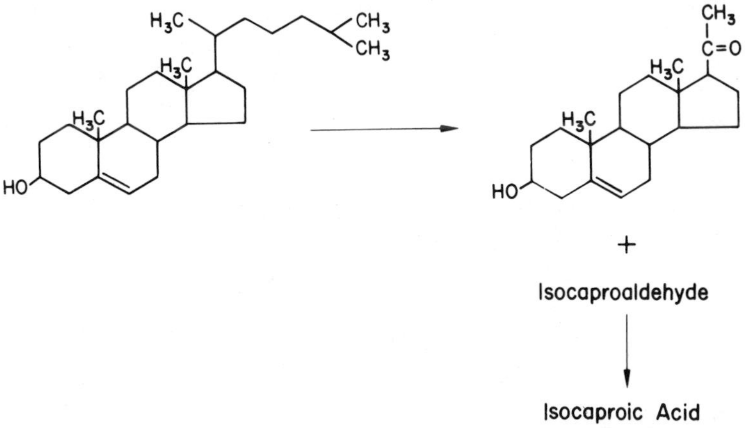

$$\text{(cholesterol structure)} \longrightarrow \text{(pregnenolone structure)}$$

+

Isocaproaldehyde

↓

Isocaproic Acid

Figure 56. Lyase cleavage of cholesterol side chain to produce pregnenolone plus isocaproaldehyde.

properties: (a) it is found in mitochrondria of ovary, testis, placenta, and adrenal cortex; (b) it requires NADPH and O₂. Since the conversion of cholesterol to pregnenolone would appear to require several intermediate steps, the requirement for NADPH and O₂ is an important clue. These substances are required for hydroxylation reactions, so there are probably hydroxylated intermediates between cholesterol and pregnenolone.

Work in the 1950s (Sulimovici and Boyd, 1969) suggested two possible intermediates according to two lines of evidence: (a) incubation of cholesterol-4-^{14}C with enzyme preparations led to isolation of 20α-hydroxycholesterol and 20α,22R-dihydroxycholesterol (b) labeled 20α-hydroxycholesterol and 20α,22R-dihydroxycholesterol incubated with appropriate enzyme preparations led to production of pregnenolone and isocaproic acid. On the basis of these data the sequence shown in Fig. 57 was proposed (See Schulster *et al.*, 1976 for reviews). This was a widely accepted theory of pregnenolone formation, but more recently Burstein and Gut (1971) suggested that an alternative pathway occurs at a higher rate (Fig. 58). Burstein and colleagues favor 22R-hydroxycholesterol, rather than 20α-hydroxycholesterol, as an important intermediate in pregnenolone synthesis for several reasons including (a) that 20α-hydroxycholesterol can act as an inhibitor of pregnenolone synthesis, and (b) that 22R-hydroxycholesterol is a better substrate for production of pregnenolone than 20α-hydroxycholesterol. However, this research area is still somewhat controversial, and some authors favor the view that the true intermediates are not hydroxylated derivatives of choles-

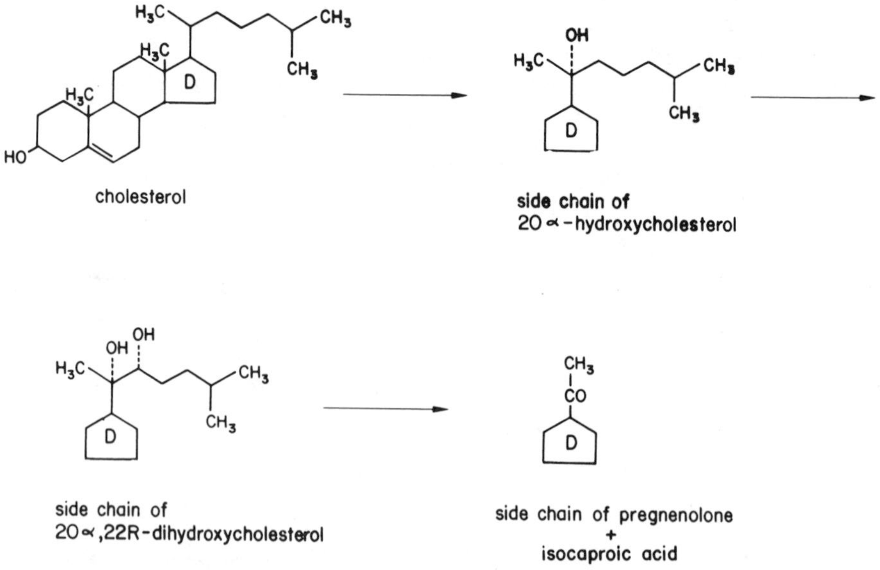

Figure 57. One theory of route of synthesis of pregnenolone from cholesterol.

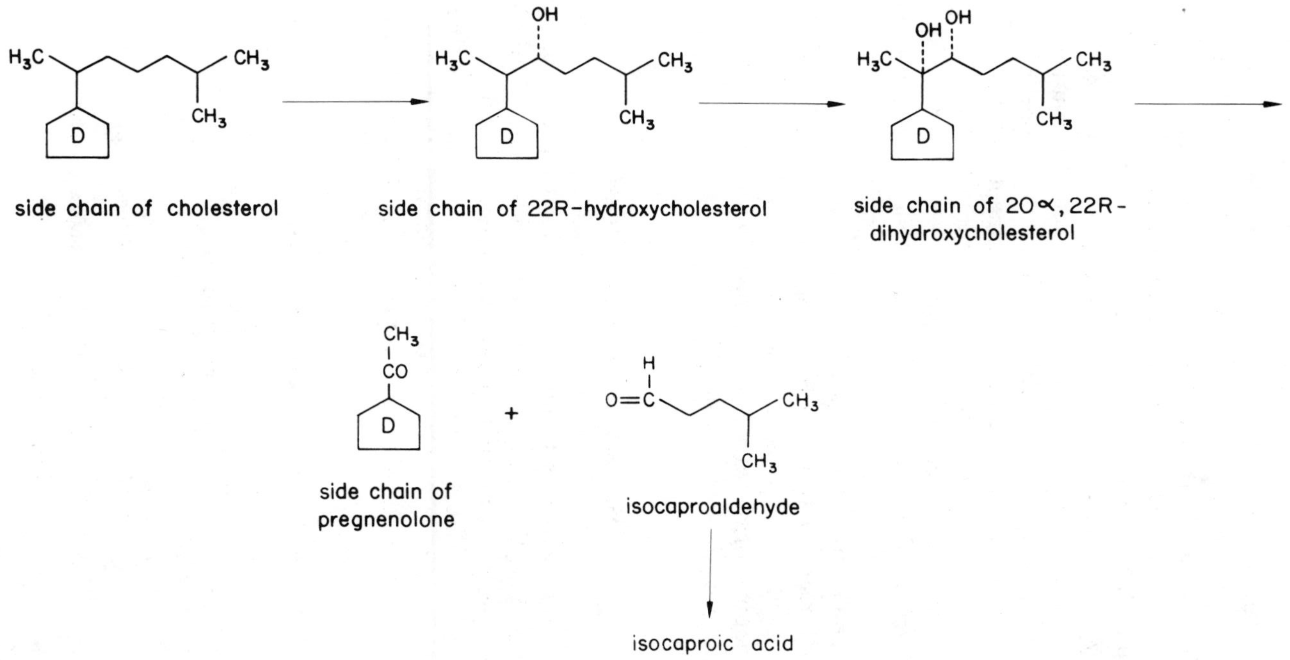

Figure 58. A more recent proposal for the route of synthesis of pregnenolone from cholesterol.

terol but are transient, nonisolatable compounds that produce pregnenolone from cholesterol by a rapid, concerted process (Schulster *et al.*, 1976).

The series of reactions that produces pregnenolone from cholesterol is of great biological importance because it constitutes the rate-limiting step in the production of steroids and is the primary site of action of LH, ACTH, and possibly FSH. Some interesting speculations have been made regarding the mechanism of trophic hormone stimulation of the conversion of cholesterol to pregnenolone. It has been proposed (Schulster *et al.*, 1976) that the side-chain-splitting enzyme system actually consists of a series of linked reactions similar to that of the hydroxylase systems. The enzyme complex consists of one flavo-protein, one nonheme iron-containing compound, and one heme compound. These three proteins are separable by experimental means, and enzymatic activity can be restored by recombining all three proteins. It appears that trophic hormones exert their primary effect on steroid synthesis by stimulating adenylate cyclase. This causes increased production of cyclic AMP, which subsequently causes an increase in the synthesis of the lyase that splits the side chain from cholesterol. Another action of the trophic hormones that may be of significance for steroid synthesis is stimulation of production of "free" choles-terol from intracellular pools of cholesterol esters. It should also be borne in mind that trophic hormones may have some effects on steroid synthesis beyond the point of pregnenolone synthesis.

B. Biosynthesis of Progestins

Once pregnenolone is formed, it serves as the precursor for all other steroids (Fig. 59). The first category of steroids whose synthesis we shall examine has pregnane as the hypothetical parent compound. Pregnenolone itself belongs to this category. Pregnenolone is converted to another important steroid in this category, progesterone, by a relatively simple and irreversible process. The enzymes involved in this process are a 5-ene-3β-hydroxysteroid

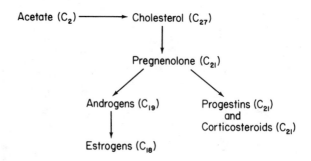

Figure 59. The key role of pregnenolone as a precursor in steroid biosynthesis. (Modified with permission from Schulster *et al.*, 1976.)

dehydrogenase and a C-5 to C-4-en isomerase. Progesterone then serves as a major precursor for a variety of steroids of the C_{21} type. These include (a) the adrenal corticoids, corticosterone and aldosterone, (b) 5α-, 5β-, 20α-, and 20β-reduced derivatives of progesterone, and (c) 17α-hydroxyprogesterone (itself an important precursor of cortisol and of androgens and estrogens). These relationships are diagrammed in Fig. 60.

C. Biosynthesis of Androgens

A major pathway to the androgens (C_{19} compounds) is via 17α-hydroxyprogesterone, with another important pathway via the 17α-hydroxylated derivative of pregnenolone. Among the biologically significant androgens formed are androstenedione, testosterone, and dehydroepiandrosterone. Testosterone may be reduced at the C-5 position to yield nonaromatizable 5α- or 5β-dihydrotestosterone. These relationships are shown in Fig. 61. The 5α-derivative has important effects on a variety of steroid target tissues.

It may be mentioned that androgens can also be generated from corticosteroids such as cortisol. Androgens of this type possess an oxygen function (hydroxyl or ketone) at the C-11 position.

D. Biosynthesis of Estrogens

Testosterone and androstenedione serve as major precursors of the estrogens estradiol-17β and estrone, respectively. Estradiol-17β and estrone are interconvertible. Estriol is formed from estrone by a nonreversible process, with aromatization of dehydroepiandrosterone constituting another possible pathway to estriol. Of interest to neuroendocrinologists is the formation of catecholestrogens by hydroxylation of estradiol-17β and estrone at the C-2 position (Fig. 62).

A detailed analysis of the catabolism and excretion of steroids is beyond the scope of this chapter, and books such as that by Dorfman and Ungar (1965) should be consulted. It may be mentioned that the general route of steroid catabolism utilizes reduction of double bonds and hydroxylation. The steroids are usually excreted as glucuronides and sulfates.

VI. SELECTED METHODS OF STEROID MEASUREMENT

If one wishes to measure a steroid in a biological fluid or tissue, the first step is to extract the steroid from the fluid or tissue. This is accomplished by shaking the biological material (tissues must first be homogenized in an aqueous medium) with an organic solvent such as diethyl ether, dichloromethane,

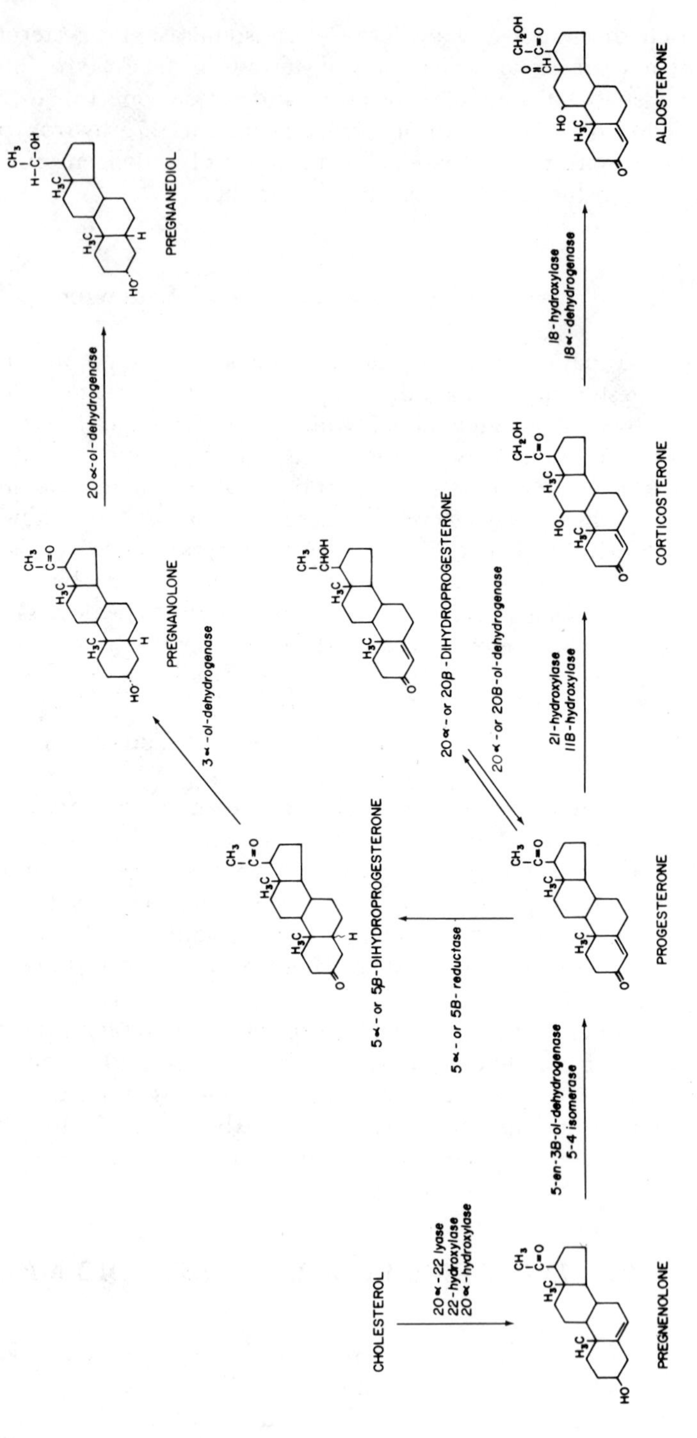
CHOLESTEROL
20α-22 lyase
22-hydroxylase
20α-hydroxylase
PREGNENOLONE
5-en-3B-ol-dehydrogenase
5-4 isomerase
PROGESTERONE
5α- or 5B- reductase
5α- or 5β-DIHYDROPROGESTERONE
3α-ol-dehydrogenase
PREGNANOLONE
20α-ol-dehydrogenase
PREGNANEDIOL
20α- or 20B-ol-dehydrogenase
20α- or 20β-DIHYDROPROGESTERONE
21-hydroxylase
11B-hydroxylase
CORTICOSTERONE
18-hydroxylase
18α-dehydrogenase
ALDOSTERONE

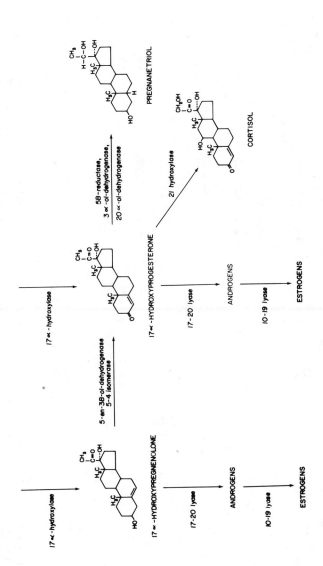

Figure 60. Basic routes of biosynthesis and catabolism of C₂₁ steroids (progestins and corticoids). Note that only trivial names of steroids are given. By use of the rules of nomenclature, the reader should be able to give the systematic names of all compounds in Figs. 60–62.

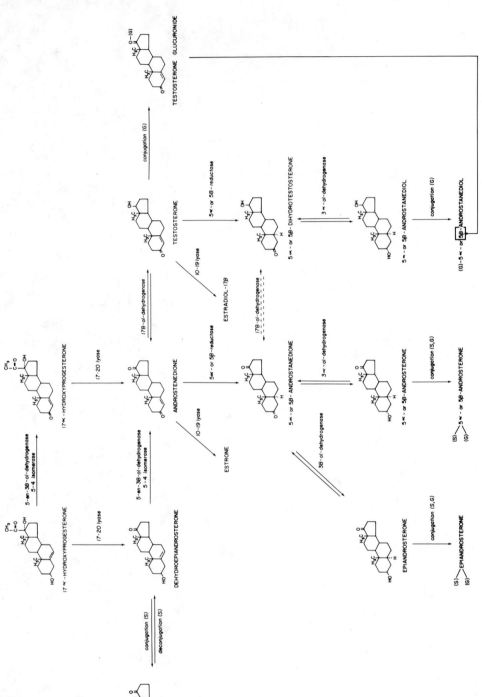

Figure 61. Basic routes of biosynthesis and catabolism of C_{19} steroids (androgens). Note that catabolic processes include reductions and hydroxylations (see also Figs. 60, 62).

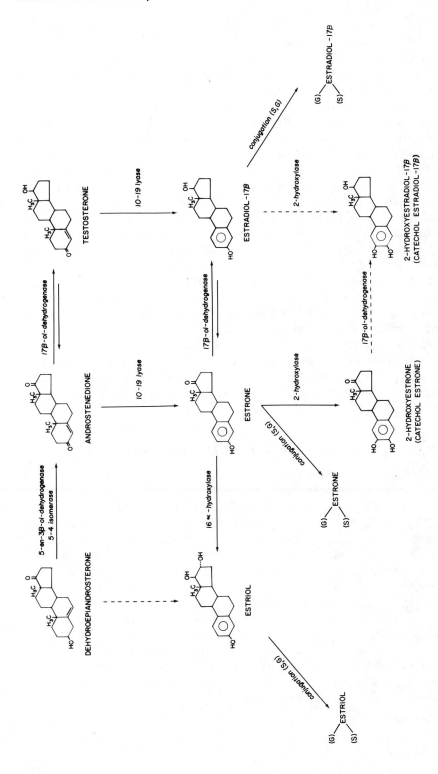

Figure 62. Basic routes of biosynthesis and catabolism of C_{18} steroids with aromatic ring A (estrogens). In addition to the catechol estrogens shown in the figure, 4-hydroxyestrone and 4-hydroxyestradiol have been identified.

or benzene. This procedure will extract the "free"* steroids but will not be successful for conjugated steroids which are more water soluble. If one wishes to measure conjugated steroids, the conjugates can be hydrolyzed (by acid or specific enzymes) to the "free" forms. Subsequently, organic solvents of the type mentioned can be used to extract the steroids.

Once the steroids are extracted, a particular steroid can be separated from other steroids by a variety of techniques that include chromatography on columns (of materials such as silica, alumina, polyacrylamide, or dextran gels), thin layers (of silica or alumina applied to a glass or plastic plate), or specifically treated paper strips. Such separation techniques can be used in conjunction with transformation of the steroid into a known derivative. For example, progesterone can be converted to a 20β-dihydroprogesterone derivative. This derivative can then be rechromatographed (it will have chromatographic properties different from the original progesterone), thereby giving the investigator increased confidence in the purity of the progesterone extract to be measured.

The actual quantification of an extracted steroid is possible by a number of means. Older methods relied on bioassay or colorimetric reactions. Although some bioassay systems can be very sensitive, they are often deficient in specificity and precision. The colorimetric techniques are usually rather insensitive and require relatively large amounts of steroid for accurate measurements to be made. In recent years, three sensitive, specific, and precise methods have been developed for the measurement of steroids in biological materials. These are double isotope derivative assays, gas–liquid chromatography, and saturation analysis.

A. Double Isotope Derivatives

In this procedure, to a sample of steroid from an organism is added a small known amount of the same steroid containing a radioactive label. For all practical purposes, the unlabeled and labeled material will be identical in properties relating to extraction, separation, and quantification. The mixture of labeled and unlabeled steroid is then converted to a derivative by use of a reagent labeled with a different isotope. The two isotopes (tritium and ^{35}S are often used) have different properties and can be measured independently of one another. Because the steroid and reagent combine in a precisely known proportion, it is possible to quantify the amount of the steroid in the biological sample. It is usually not necessary to subtract the contribution of the labeled steroid that was added to the sample, because the mass of labeled steroid added is negligible compared to the mass of the steroid in the sample.

Although this method is sensitive in the nanogram (ng = 10^{-9} g) range and is highly reliable in terms of specificity, precision, and accuracy, it is quite expensive and time-consuming (Baird et al., 1968).

*See footnote p. 36.

B. Gas–Liquid Chromatography

Typically, in this method, a sample of steroid from an organism is mixed with a small amount of labeled (usually tritium) steroid of the type to be quantified. The mixture is then extracted and separated by column, thin-layer, or paper chromatography. Often, a derivative will also be formed. At the end of this process, the amount of radioactivity left in an aliquot of the sample is measured. This gives an accurate estimate of procedural losses, and an appropriate correction can be made for these losses in the calculation of the amount of unlabeled steroid. For example, if 33.3% of the labeled material were lost, it would be necessary to multiply the amount of unlabeled steroid measured by 3/2.

The steroid can then be injected into a gas–liquid chromatograph (GLC). The GLC system consists essentially of a glass or metal column filled with an inert solid material coated with a nonvolatile liquid. The column is enclosed in a heated (200 to 250°C) oven. The steroid injected into the GLC is volatized and is carried through the column by a stream of inert gas (e.g., nitrogen or helium). The physiochemical properties of the steroid will determine the rate at which the steroid moves through the column to a detector at the end of the column. The type of detector can vary, but the two most commonly used are the flame-ionization and electron-capture detectors. In the flame-ionization system, the outflow from the column is mixed with hydrogen and burned between two electrodes. The current thus generated is measured and recorded. The electroncapture detector is more sensitive but more limited in applicability to steroid measurement because not all steroids can be put into the form of derivatives with properties that allow them to be measured by electron capture. The electron-capture detector system consists of two parallel plates of stainless steel (electrodes) separated by an insulator. The sample (carried by gas flow) enters the detector chamber through a tube leading to the anode and departs through a hole in the cathode. The source of ionizing radiation consists of a disk coated with titanium tritide. When carrier gas (e.g., nitrogen, N_2) without sample flows through the detector chamber, electrons (e^-) emitted by the radiation source react with the carrier gas molecules to produce positive ions and electrons (e.g., $N_2 + e^- \rightarrow N_2^+ + e^- + e^-$). If a sample (S) now flows into the detector and captures electrons (not all types of sample have this capability), relatively slow-moving negative molecular ions are formed in place of the more mobile electrons (e.g., $S + e^- \rightarrow S^-$). The lower mobility of the negative molecular ion increases the possibility that charges will be neutralized (e.g., $N_2^+ + S^- \rightarrow N_2 + S$). This decreases the current flowing in the detector, and this decrease is quantitatively recorded. The result is translatable into a measurement of concentration of steroid in a sample by means of comparison of the drop of current caused by the sample to decreases in current caused by known amounts of steroid from a standard curve.

Derivatives that capture electrons include chloroacetates (Fig. 63) and heptafluorobutyrates. For example, progesterone can be measured by electron

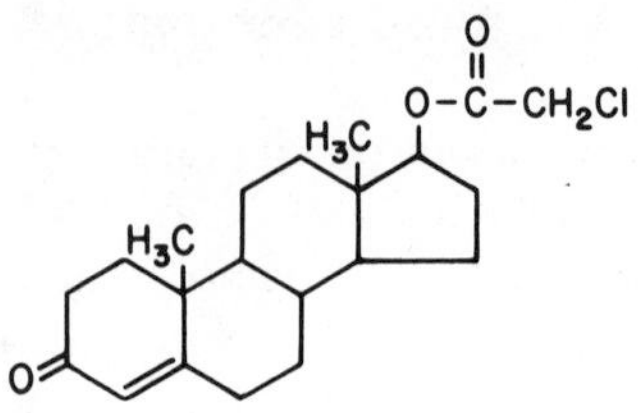

Figure 63. Electron-capturing chloroacetate derivative of testosterone.

capture if it is first reduced to 20β-dihydroprogesterone and then esterified to form a monochloroacetate at the 20β-hydroxy position. Similarly, testosterone can be measured by making a monocloroacetate at the 17-hydroxy position. Androstenedione can be measured by first reducing it to testosterone through a borohydride reaction. Heptafluorobutyrates may also be used as derivatives, and these have been particularly useful in the measurement of estrogens.

There are procedural losses between the time the steroid is injected into the GLC and the time the steroid reaches the detector. These losses cannot be gauged by use of a radioactive tracer because GLC does not measure radioactivity. The only way to gauge these procedural losses is to mix another steroid (with similar, but not identical properties to the steroid of interest) and inject the mixture into the GLC. Appropriate corrections can then be made for these losses.

Gas–liquid chromatography is highly reliable in terms of specificity, precision, and accuracy when properly utilized. Sensitivity is in the nanogram range, and GLC is especially useful in this range when electron-capture detection is employed. However, GLC is very time-consuming and is not readily applicable to all steroids (see Wotiz and Clark, 1966; Eik-Nes and Horning, 1968).

C. Saturation Analysis

Currently, the most convenient way to measure small quantities of steroid is by some form of saturation analysis. The techniques are relatively simple and can be performed in a short time span. Moreover, specificity, accuracy, and precision are (or can be) quite adequate, and sensitivity is in the picogram range (pg = 10^{-12} g).

The most extensively used form of saturation analysis for steroids is radioimmunoassay (RIA). A typical procedure would include addition of a very small, known quantity of tritium-labeled steroid [e.g., about 5 pg, containing about 2000 disintegrations per minute (dpm)] to the biological sample, extraction of the sample, separation of steroid to be measured by column chromatography, and assessment of procedural losses by measurement of the radioactive tracer. The sample is then ready for quantification. To the sample are added (unlabeled) antibody to the steroid and a small, known quantity of radioactive steroid (e.g., about 50 pg, containing about 30,000 dpm). This time, radioactive steroid is not used as an indicator of procedural losses. The role of the radioactive steroid added at this time will become apparent in the next paragraph. A standard curve is constructed by adding various concentrations of steroid to a separate set of test tubes. To these tubes are also added antibody and the same quantity of radioactive steroid that was added to the biological samples. All tubes are shaken and "incubated" for several hours. Then an adsorbent such as dextran-coated charcoal is added to the tubes, and the tubes are shaken, "incubated" briefly, and centrifuged. An aliquot of supernatant above the charcoal layer is then counted in a liquid scintillation counter.

The steroid in the biological sample and the radioactive steroid compete for a limited number of binding sites on the antibody. The more unlabeled steroid there is in the biological sample, the more labeled steroid will be displaced from the antibody by competition. The amount of radioactively tagged steroid bound to and/or not bound to the antibody can then be assessed. This is accomplished by separating bound and unbound steroid. The bound steroid will be in the supernatant fraction (because steroid bound to antibody forms a relatively large complex that is not adsorbed onto the charcoal), whereas the unbound steroid is adsorbed because it is a small molecule. Other methods of separation of bound and unbound steroid (e.g., precipitation of the bound steroid by ammonium sulfate) are also sometimes employed. The amount of steroid in the biological sample can then be calculated by reference to the standard curve.

Because steroids by themselves will not provoke production of antibodies, the manufacture of antibody to a steroid hormone involves: (a) making a derivative of the steroid, such as an oxime or a hemisuccinate (Fig. 64), and (b) covalent coupling of the derivative to a large protein such as bovine serum albumin. This steroid–protein conjugate can then be used to provoke antibody production in an animal such as a rabbit, ewe, or guinea pig. After purification, the antibody produced can be used in the RIA of steroid hormones. Although it is usually necessary to perform some separation technique to purify the biological sample to be assessed for steroid content, in some instances the separation procedures can be dispensed with (e.g., when steroids other than the one the investigator wishes to measure are present in negligible quantities in the sample or do not cross-react with the antibody to a significant degree).

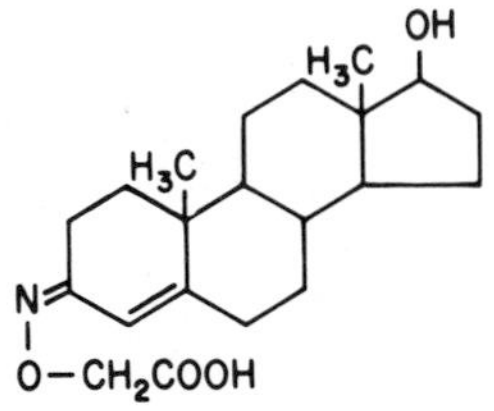

Figure 64. An oxime derivative of testosterone used in RIA of testosterone.

Other methods of saturation analysis include competitive protein binding (CPB) and radioligand receptor assays, but these have not been used as extensively as RIA for steroid measurements. Competitive protein binding assays use certain naturally occurring proteins of blood plasma (e.g., corticosteriod-binding globulin) as the protein for which labeled and unlabeled steroid compete. In general, CPB is a less specific and less sensitive technique of steroid measurement than RIA. Radioligand receptor assays use naturally occurring protein receptors for steroid hormones as the competition site. Such receptors are found in steroid target tissues (e.g., estrogen receptor in uterus). The receptor method for steroid measurement is still being developed (See Péron and Caldwell, 1970; Odell and Daughaday, 1971; Chard, 1978 for discussion of saturation analysis techniques.)

VII. SUMMARY

The study of the structure of steroids is akin to the study of the structure of tissues or organs. The data from such studies do not tell us how the steroids exert their effects or how tissues function. But an understanding of structure is a crucial antecedent to the understanding of function. It is unlikely that neuroendocrinologists will derive a sense of excitement from a chapter that describes the structure, reactions, synthesis, and measurement of steroids. However, it is my hope that this chapter will provide a basis for deeper appreciation of the exciting work now being carried out on the mechanisms through which steroids influence reproductive physiology and behavior.

ACKNOWLEDGMENTS. I am very grateful to Christian Reboulleau for his critical comments on the manuscript. Nancy Jachim, Winona Cunningham, and Cindy Banas provided invaluable help with preparation of the manuscript. The author is supported by NIH Research Grant HD-04467 and NIMH Research Scientist Development Award MH-29006. Contribution No. 318 of the Institute of Animal Behavior.

REFERENCES

Baird, D. T., 1968, A method for the measurement of estrone and estradiol-17β in peripheral human blood and other biological fluids using ^{35}S pipsyl chloride, *J. Clin. Endocrinol. Metab.* **28**:244.

Bergstrom, S., Lindstredt, S., Samuelsson, B., Corey, E. J., and Gregoriou, G. A., 1958, Stereochemistry of 7α-hydroxylation in the biosynthesis of cholic acid from cholesterol, *J. Am. Chem. Soc.* **80**:2337.

Bloch, K., 1957, The biological synthesis of cholesterol, *Vitam. Horm.* **15**:119.

Burstein, S., and Gut, M., 1971, Kinetic studies on the transformation of cholesterol to pregnenolone in adrenal tissue, in: *Hormonal Steroids, Proceedings of the Third International Congress* (V. H. T. James, ed.), pp. 15–16 Excerpta Medica, Princeton.

Chard, T., 1978, *An Introduction to Radioimmunoassay and Related Techniques*, North-Holland, New York.

Dorfman, R. I., and Ungar, F., 1965, *Metabolism of Steroid Hormones*, Academic Press, New York.

Eik-Nes, K. B., and Horning, E. C., 1968, *Gas Phase Chromatography of Steroids*, Springer-Verlag, New York.

Goodman, R. L., 1978, The site of the positive feedback action of estradiol in the rat, *Endocrinology* **102**:151.

Klyne, W., 1957, *The Chemistry of the Steroids*, Methuen, London.

Odell, W. D., and Daughaday, W. H. (eds.), 1971, *Principles of Competitive Protein-Binding Assays*, J. B. Lippincott, Philadelphia.

Péron, F. G., and Caldwell B. V. (eds.), 1970, *Immunologic Methods in Steroid Determination*, Appleton-Century-Crofts, New York.

Pincus, G., Nakao, T., and Tait, J., 1966, *Steroid Dynamics*, Academic Press, New York.

Popják, G., and Cornforth, J. W., 1960, The biosynthesis of cholesterol, *Adv. Enzymol.* **22**:281.

Rittenberg, D., and Schoenheimer, R., 1937, Deuterium as an indicator in the study of intermediary metabolism, *J. Biol. Chem.* **121**:235.

Schulster, D., Burstein, S., and Cooke, B. A., 1976, *Molecular Endocrinology of the Steroid Hormones*, John Wiley and Sons, New York.

Sulimovici, S. I., and Boyd, G. S., 1969, The cholesterol side-chain cleavage enzymes in steroid hormone-producing tissues, *Vitam. Horm.* **27**:199.

Westphal, U., 1970, Binding of hormones to serum proteins, in: *Biochemical Actions of Hormones* (G. Litwack, ed.), pp. 209–265, Academic Press, New York.

Wotiz, H. H., and Clark, S. J., 1966, *Gas Chromatography in the Analysis of Steroid Hormones*, Plenum Press, New York.

BIBLIOGRAPHY

Breuer, H., 1962, Metabolism of the natural estrogens, *Vitam. Horm.* **20**:285.

Bush, I. E., 1961, *The Chromatography of Steroids*, Pergamon Press, New York.

Conney, A. H., Schneidman, K., Jacobson, M., and Kuntzman, R., 1965, Drug-induced changes in steroid metabolism, *Ann. N.Y. Acad. Sci.* **123**:98.

Determann, H., 1969, *Gel Chromatography*, Springer-Verlag, New York.

Djerassi, C., 1963, *Steroid Reactions*, Holden-Day, San Francisco.

Eik-Nes, K. B. (ed.), 1970, *The Androgens of the Testis*, Marcel Dekker, New York.

Fieser, L., and Fieser, M., 1959, *Steroids*, Rheinhold, New York.

Heftmann, E., and Mosettig, E., 1960, *Biochemistry of Steroids*, Rheinhold, New York.

IUPAC-IUB Rules, 1969, *Steroids* **13**:117.

Loraine, J. A., and Bell, E. T., 1971, *Hormone Assays and their Clinical Application*, Williams and Wilkins, Baltimore.

Samuels, L. T., 1960, Metabolism of steroid hormones, in: *Metabolic Pathways*, Vol. 1 (D. M. Greenberg, ed.), pp. 431–480, Academic Press, New York.

Shoppee, C. W., 1964, *Chemistry of the Steroids*, Butterworths,·Washington.

Stahl, E. (ed.), 1969, *Thin-Layer Chromatography*, Springer-Verlag, New York.

Talalay, P., 1963, Hydroxysteroid dehydrogenases, in *The Enzymes*, Vol. 7 (P. D. Boyer, H. Lardy, and K. Myrback, eds.), pp. 177–202, Academic Press, New York.

Neurotransmitter Systems

Anatomy and Pharmacology

WILLIAM R. CROWLEY and FRANK P. ZEMLAN

I. INTRODUCTION

In recent years, our understanding of chemical synaptic transmission has advanced considerably. Underlying these advances have been research on the biochemistry of neurotransmitters, the development of drugs that affect these substances in relatively specific ways, and the use of various histological procedures that reveal in detail the anatomical projections of neurons containing specific neurotransmitters. These achievements enable physiological psychologists who are concerned with brain–behavior relations in general to approach the study of behavior from a neurochemical and neuropharmacological perspective.

Many recent studies of sexual, ingestive, aggressive, operant, and other motivated behaviors have addressed themselves to the question of which neurotransmitter systems mediate a particular set of related behaviors. Most psychopharmacological studies have employed drugs that affect four neurotransmitters, acetylcholine (ACh), norepinephrine (NE), dopamine (DA), and 5-hydroxytryptamine (5-HT; serotonin). Norepinephine and dopamine are catecholamines whose molecular structure consists of a catechol ring (benzene ring with two hydroxyl groups) and a side chain with an amine group (NH_2) (see Figs. 1 and 2). Serotonin is an indoleamine, containing an indole ring

WILLIAM R. CROWLEY • Department of Pharmacology, University of Tennessee Center for the Health Sciences, Memphis, Tennessee 38163.   FRANK P. ZEMLAN • Department of Pharmacology, University of Pennsylvania School of Medicine, Philadelphia, Pennsylvania 19104.

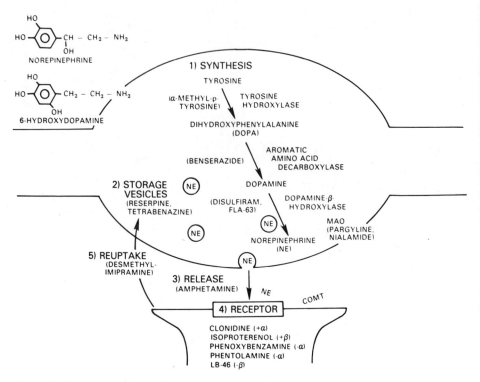

Figure 1. Schematic diagram of a noradrenergic synapse. Drugs are shown by the numbered process they affect. Abbreviations: MAO, monoamine oxidase; COMT, catechol-O-methyltransferase.

structure with a hydroxyl group and an amine group on the side chain (see Fig. 3). Norepinephrine, DA, and 5-HT also are known collectively as monoamines, i.e., compounds containing one amine group. As seen in Figs. 1–3, the monoamines are synthesized from precursor amino acids. Other amino acids, including glycine, aspartate, glutamate, and the glutamate derivative γ-amino butyric acid (GABA) have also been proposed as central neurotransmitters. However, because fewer drugs are available to affect these systems, there have not been as many studies of their role in behavior.

As a prelude to discussions of the involvement of neurotransmitters in the mediation of male and female mating behavior patterns (Chapter 14), the present chapter will describe (a) how drugs increase or decrease functional activity in cholinergic and monoaminergic neurons and (b) the anatomical organization of monoaminergic and cholinergic pathways. One of the most active areas in neurobiology today is the study of a possible transmitter function for small peptides. The anatomy section will review briefly the neural distribution of several peptides that appear to have a role in neuroendocrine processes and behavior. The present review is selective in that emphasis is placed on those drugs shown to affect sexual behavior. For a more complete background on the physiology and biochemistry of synaptic transmission and the biochemical

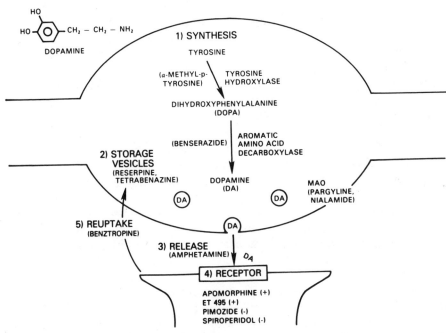

Figure 2. Schematic diagram of a dopaminergic synapse with drugs that affect DA neurotransmission.

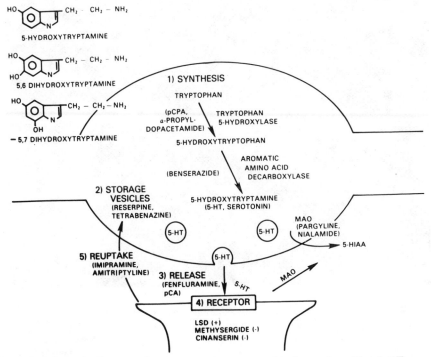

Figure 3. Schematic diagram of a serotonergic synapse with drugs that affect 5-HT neurotransmission. 5-HIAA, 5-hydroxyindoleacetic acid.

mechanisms of psychoactive drug action, useful references are the books by McLennan (1970), Cooper *et al.* (1978), and Lipton *et al.* (1978), and review articles by Krnjevic (1974), Haefely *et al.* (1976), and Carlsson (1975 a–c).

Monoaminergic and cholinergic neurons are multipolar; that is, numerous processes emerge from their cell bodies. These processes contain swellings or varicosities (see Fig. 4) that are thought to be the active nerve terminals from which the transmitter is released.

Figures 1–3 and 5 are schematic representations of monoaminergic and cholinergic synapses and depict the processes susceptible to pharmacological intervention. Synthesis of the neurotransmitter takes place primarily in the presynaptic nerve terminal varicosity and proceeds as depicted in the figures. The transmitter is stored within synaptic vesicles and released by nerve action potentials into the synaptic cleft. The released transmitter then occupies receptor sites on the postsynaptic membrane. There is growing evidence that the subsequent postsynaptic events, at least in some transmitter systems, involve changes in the structure of the postsynaptic membrane resulting in the flow of ions through the membrane so that it becomes depolarized or hyperpolarized (Nathanson, 1977). The postsynaptic action of the transmitter may be terminated by enzymatic degradation, recapture by the presynaptic nerve terminal (reuptake), or by diffusion away from the synapse and subsequent degrada-

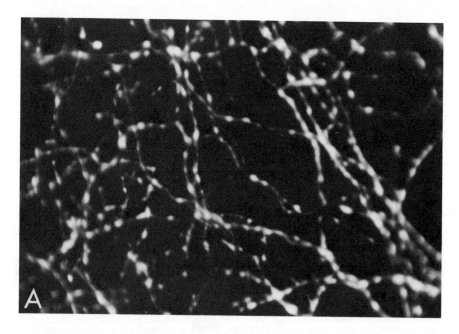

Figure 4. A: Sympathetic noradrenergic innervation of the rat iris. Note varicose swellings on the axons. B: Dense noradrenergic innervation of the hypothalamic paraventricular nucleus. Arrows show varicosities on axons. V, 3rd ventricle. C: The tuberoinfundibular DA system. Arrows show fluorescing arcuate DA cell bodies (A 12) and terminals along capillary plexus in median eminence. Fluorescence photomicrographs courtesy Dr. D. M. Jacobowitz, National Institute of Mental Health.

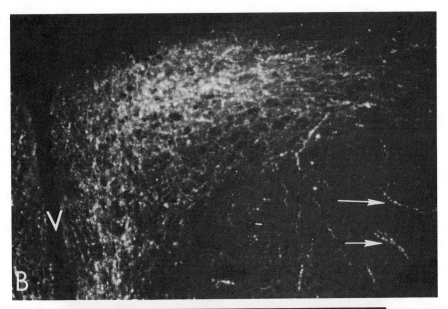

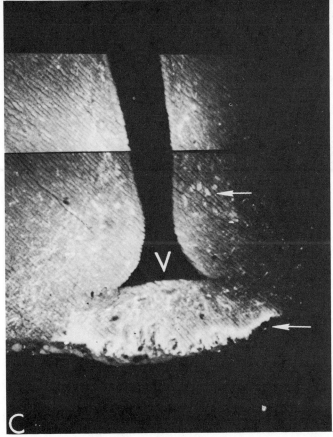

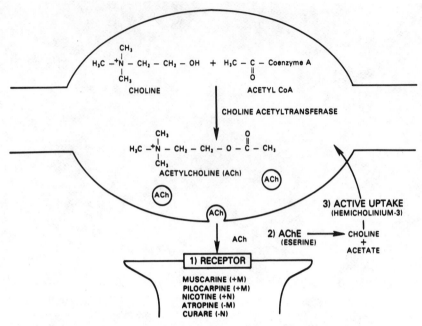

Figure 5. Schematic diagram of a cholinergic synapse with drugs that affect ACh neurotransmission.

tion. As seen in Figs. 1–3 and 5, a number of drugs are available to influence these various processes.

Turnover refers to the overall utilization, i.e., synthesis, release, degradation, resynthesis, etc., of the transmitter. Turnover studies provide an estimate of the functional state of the system; a fast turnover rate generally indicates an active, and a slow turnover rate indicates an inactive system. Anton-Tay and Wurtman (1971) and Weiner (1974) have critically reviewed the various techniques used to study turnover, and in Chapter 14, we shall discuss the effects of gonadal hormones on monoamine turnover.

Neurons require a readily available supply of neurotransmitter for release. To insure this supply, a variety of mechanisms serve to regulate the amount of neurotransmitter present within the nerve terminal (see Axelrod, 1974, 1977). For example, increased neuronal activity can lead to an increase in the activity and/or synthesis of enzymes responsible for the synthesis of the neurotransmitter (Roth *et al.*, 1978; Reis *et al.*, 1974). Postsynaptic receptors that have not been stimulated for some time develop a "supersensitivity," so that the neuron can be affected by less than normal amounts of the transmitter or a drug. This may actually occur through an increase in receptor sites (Creese *et al.*, 1977).

There are also mechanisms to prevent overactivation of the system. Catecholamines inhibit several of the enzymes responsible for their own synthesis (end product inhibition). Excess intraneuronal monoamines can be metabolized by enzymes such as monoamine oxidase (MAO, see Figs. 1–3).

In addition, there appear to be several types of transsynaptic regulations for local control. Cells innervated by a specific neurotransmitter system may modulate that input by sending their own axons to innervate the presynaptic neurons. There may also be presynaptic receptors on the neuron, known as autoreceptors, that are sensitive to the cell's own neurotransmitter. Such auto-receptors have been described for brain monoaminergic systems (Bunney and Aghajanian, 1975; Aghajanian and Wang, 1978). When the neuron fires, its recurrent collaterals (axons that have branched from the main route to return to their own or adjacent cell bodies) may inhibit further firing by stimulating autoreceptors on the cell body or dendrites. There may be autoreceptors on the nerve terminals as well. As the transmitter is released, it occupies both pre- and postsynaptic receptors, and stimulation of presynaptic autoreceptors inhibits the further release of the transmitter (Starke, 1977). Finally, the postsynaptic cell may release substances that feed back and affect release of the neuro-transmitter. For example, there is evidence that prostaglandins can be released postsynaptically after stimulation to inhibit further presynaptic release of norepinephrine (see Hedqvist, 1977). Other suggested presynaptic modulators include ACh, angiotensin II, and the enkephalins (Starke, 1977; Westfall, 1977).

The next section reviews how drugs may change activity in monoaminergic and cholinergic systems (see also Table 1). We have emphasized the best-known or documented action of each drug, but the reader should bear in mind the fact that no drug is completely specific or selective in its effects and that many drug effects depend on such variables as dosage, route of administration, or species tested.

II. METHODOLOGY OF PSYCHOPHARMACOLOGY

A. Mode of Action of Neuropharmacological Agents

1. Neurotransmitter Agonists

a. Increased Supply and Release of Transmitter

When administered systematically, neither ACh, NE, nor DA penetrate to the brain in appreciable amounts. Central monoamine levels may be elevated by systemic administration of precursors, such as dihydroxyphenylalanine (DOPA), a precursor of NE and DA (Figs. 1, 2), or tryptophan or 5-hydroxy-tryptophan (5-HTP), the precursors to 5-HT (Fig. 3). The behavioral effects of these exogenously supplied precursors may be potentiated by protecting them from metabolism before they reach their site of conversion to the transmitter in the nerve terminal. This may be accomplished by pretreatment with inhibitors of MAO which converts monoamines to inactive metabolites.

Table 1. Summary of Actions of Neuropharmacological Agents

Transmitter	Agonists	Antagonists
Norepinephrine	Receptor stimulants Clonidine (α) Isoproterenol (β)	Receptor blockers Phentolamine (α) Phenoxybenzamine (α) LB-46 (β) Yohimbine (α_2)
	Releasers Amphetamine	Storage blockers Reserpine Tetrabenazine
	Reuptake inhibitors Amphetamine Desmethylimipramine	Synthesis inhibitors α-Methyl-p-tyrosine Disulfiram FLA-63
	MAO inhibitors Pargyline Nialamide	Toxin 6-OHDA
Dopamine	Receptor stimulants ET-495 Apomorphine	Receptor blockers Pimozide Spiroperidol Haloperidol
	Releasers Amphetamine	Storage blockers Reserpine Tetrabenazine
	Reuptake inhibitors Amphetamine Benztropine	Synthesis inhibitors α-Methyl-p-tyrosine
	MAO inhibitors Pargyline Nialamide	Toxin 6-OHDA
5-Hydroxytryptamine (Serotonin)	Receptor stimulants LSD Quipazine	Receptor blockers Methysergide Cinanserin
	Releasers p-Chloroamphetamine Fenfluramine	Storage blockers Reserpine Tetrabenazine
	Reuptake inhibitors Imipramine	Synthesis inhibitors pCPA
	MAO inhibitors Paragyline Nialamide	Toxins 5,6-DHT 5,7-DHT p-Chloroamphetamine Fenfluramine
Acetylcholine	Receptor stimulants Muscarine (M) Pilocarpine (M) Nicotine (N) AChE inhibitors Eserine (Physostigmine) Neostigmine	Receptor blockers Atropine (M) Scopolamine (M) Curare (N)

The enzymes for the synthesis of catecholamines are also present within the sympathetic nervous system and may act to convert exogenously administered DOPA to NE or DA before it can reach the brain. Thus, to facilitate the entry of DOPA into central nerve terminals, animals may be pretreated with inhibitors of aromatic amino acid decarboxylase (Figs. 1–3) in dosages that will affect only peripheral enzymes.

It is also possible to enhance the release of endogenous transmitter. Amphetamine promotes the release of NE and DA, and fenfluramine and p-chloroamphetamine (PCA) can release 5-HT stores.

b. Prolongation of Neurotransmitter Action

Several techniques are available to prolong the action of the neurotransmitter at the receptor site. ACh is hydrolyzed by the postsynaptic enzyme acetylcholinesterase (AChE) (see Fig. 5). If this enzyme is inhibited by eserine, the action of ACh at the receptor is potentiated.

In monoaminergic neurons, a "membrane pump" actively removes the neurotransmitter from the synapse and causes it to reenter the presynaptic nerve terminal. This membrane pump reuptake process can be blocked by various drugs, including the stimulants cocaine and amphetamine. Imipramine, chlorimipramine, and fluoxetine are effective blockers of reuptake of 5-HT, and the related drugs desmethylimipramine and protriptyline are inhibitors of NE reuptake.

c. Receptor Stimulants

Selective increases in the activity of a neurotransmitter system may be achieved by administration of drugs that directly stimulate postsynaptic receptors. These agents mimic the effect of the endogenous transmitter at the receptor. Generally, they are more resistant to enzymatic degradation or reuptake than the naturally occurring transmitter and therefore produce a prolonged increase in functional activity. There are two types of cholinergic receptors, muscarinic and nicotinic. In the peripheral nervous system, muscarinic receptors are found on organs innervated by postganglionic parasympathetic nerves, whereas nicotinic receptors are found on the ganglionic cell bodies of sympathetic and parasympathetic neurons and also at the neuromuscular junction. Both types probably are present within the brain. Figure 5 indicates that muscarinic receptors are stimulated by muscarine or pilocarpine ($+M$), whereas the action of ACh at nicotinic receptors is mimicked by nicotine ($+N$).

Distinct alpha (α) and beta (β) noradrenergic receptor types have been described in the peripheral and central nervous system. Clonidine is a potent stimulant of α receptors ($+\alpha$), and isoproterenol excites β receptors ($+\beta$) (Fig. 1). ET-495 and apomorphine are relatively specific DA receptor stimulants (Fig. 2). Drugs that enhance 5-HT receptor activity include hallucinogens such as LSD, *N, N'*-dimethyltryptamine (DMT), and the hallucinogenic amphetamines, and nonhallucinogens such as quipazine.

In doses usually lower than those required to stimulate postsynaptic receptors, some monoamine receptor agonists such as clonidine, apomorphine, and LSD also stimulate presynaptic autoreceptors (Bunney and Aghajanian, 1975; Aghajanian and Wang, 1978). As discussed in Section I, this leads to an inhibition of transmitter release and an overall inhibition, rather than excitation, of the system. Strömböm (1975) has summarized behavorial and biochemical experiments demonstrating these dual effects, and in Chapter 14, we shall review some apparently paradoxical drug effects on sexual behavior that may be explained by this mechanism.

2. Neurotransmitter Antagonists

a. Synthesis Inhibition

The supply of releasable neurotransmitter can be depleted in several ways. Inhibition of neurotransmitter synthesis can produce a major decrease in monoaminergic neural activity. Catecholamine synthesis is blocked at the rate-limiting step (tyrosine → DOPA) by α-methyl-p-tyrosine, a competitive inhibitor of tyrosine hydroxylase (Fig. 1). Norepinephrine synthesis may be selectively reduced by blocking the conversion of DA to NE with disulfiram or FLA-63, drugs that inhibit dopamine-β-hydroxylase. p-Chlorophenylalanine (pCPA) blocks the formation of 5-HTP from tryptophan (Fig. 3), producing a long-lasting depletion in brain 5-HT. Acetylcholine synthesis can be inhibited by blocking the uptake of precursor choline with hemicholinium-3 (Fig. 5).

b. Blockade of Vesicular Storage

A second technique used to decrease neurotransmitter levels involves interference with their binding to storage granules. Reserpine and tetrabenazine deplete brain monoamines by displacing them from synaptic vesicles, allowing the intraneuronally released amines to be rapidly degraded by MAO.

c. Blockade of Postsynaptic Receptors

Drugs may prevent the neurotransmitter from occupying its receptor and thereby reduce the functional activity of that system. Selective α and β noradrenergic receptor blockers (Fig. 1) ($-\alpha$; $-\beta$) are in use, as are nicotinic ($-N$) and muscarinic ($-M$) antagonists (Fig. 5). Dopamine receptors are blocked by "neuroleptics," such as haloperidol, pimozide, and spiroperidol (Fig. 2), which are used clinically as antipsychotic agents. A number of agents, including methysergide, cinanserin, and methiothepin, are employed as 5-HT receptor blockers, but their efficacy and specificity in brain remain to be established.

Receptor antagonists may also block presynaptic autoreceptors, and, therefore, they may increase release of transmitter (Starke, 1977). Some catecholamine receptor blockers appear to have differential affinity for pre- and postsynaptic receptors, and, for this reason, α and β receptors may be further subdivided. For example, phenoxybenzamine is a potent nor-adrenergic antagonist at postsynaptic (α_1) receptor sites, whereas yohimbine appears to be more selective towards presynaptic (α_2) sites (Strömböm, 1975).

d. Neurotoxins

Recently, much interest has focused on the use of neurotoxins to create neurotransmitter-specific lesions within the CNS. The best known such drug is 6-hydroxydopamine (6-OHDA) which, because of its molecular similarity to NE and DA (see Fig. 1), accumulates in catecholamine neurons. Its destructive action probably results from formation of toxic products. When administered systemically, this agent damages the sympathetic noradrenergic system but does not penetrate to the brain to any great extent. To deplete central cate-cholamines, 6-OHDA has been injected into the cerebroventricular system or directly into areas containing catecholamine cell bodies, tracts, or nerve termi-nals. Although there is some disagreement as to the nature and extent of nonspecific damage to noncatecholamine neurons after central administration (Hökfelt and Ungerstedt, 1973; Bloom, 1975; Butcher, 1975; Javoy *et al.*, 1976), the consensus appears to be that with proper usage, this drug may produce specific lesions of central catecholamine systems and thus may be a valuable tool in investigating the role of catecholamines in behavior. Authorita-tive reviews on the methodology, mechanisms of action, and on the behavioral and biochemical effects of 6-OHDA are available (Kostrezewa and Jacobowitz, 1974; Sachs and Jonsson, 1975; Ungerstedt, 1971a).

Serotonergic systems may be lesioned in a similar manner by 5,6- or 5,7-dihydroxytryptamine (Fig. 3). These drugs appear to be more toxic and less specific than 6-OHDA (see Baumgarten and Björklund, 1976, for review). Recently, it has been suggested that *p*-chloroamphetamine (Fig. 3) and fenfluramine are also 5-HT neurotoxins (Harvey and McMaster, 1975; Sanders-Bush and Massari, 1977). These drugs have the advantage of reaching the brain after systemic administration. Their acute effects include release of 5-HT, most likely from damaged nerve endings, followed by a long-lasting depletion of 5-HT.

B. Psychopharmacological Techniques

1. Systemic and Central Administration of Drugs

Systemic administration of drugs is a useful first step in analyzing the role of neurotransmitters in behavior. However, it is possible to deliver drugs directly to brain tissue. This has several advantages over systemic injection.

First, one may study the effects of substances, such as the transmitters themselves, that do not readily cross the blood–brain barrier. Secondly, intracranial administration can localize the effect of a drug to discrete areas, perhaps facilitating development of a "neurochemical anatomy" of behavior. With regard to the study of reproductive behaviors, intracranial drug administration has been limited mainly to the placement of crystalline steroid hormones into a few diencephalic and mesencephalic sites. Only a handful of studies on sexual behavior have employed central administration of neuropharmacological agents of the type described in this chapter. This remains a relatively unexplored and potentially rewarding area of research. A large number of such studies have, however, been done on ingestive behaviors, with the result that several controversies have arisen. Most of the disputes in the literature center around methodological considerations such as the use of aqueous solutions versus crystalline forms of drug and problems in controlling volume, dosage, and pH.

Whether studies use systemic or central routes of injection, the battery of pharmacological agents described above may be used to affect neurotransmission in a variety of ways. A pharmacologically consistent picture should emerge from the use of receptor stimulants, blockers, transmitter releasers, etc. All of these topics have been treated in detail elsewhere, and the reader is referred to Dews (1972) for a discussion of behavioral pharmacology, to Pelligrino and Cushman (1971) for details on the general methods of stereotaxic neurosurgery, and to Myers (1971, 1974) and Routtenberg (1972) for specific reviews on the techniques and controversies concerning chemical stimulation of the brain.

III. NEUROANATOMY OF CHOLINERGIC AND MONOAMINERGIC PATHWAYS

It is a great advantage for those working on neuropharmacology and behavior that a detailed mapping of monoaminergic neurons is available, at least for the rat. This information is important in guiding experimentation. One may inject drugs into areas known to contain the transmitter, or one may lesion or stimulate these systems specifically. This section will review briefly the major known neurotransmitter pathways. The reader should consult the following papers for greater detail: Dahlström and Fuxe (1964); Fuxe (1965); Fuxe and Jonsson (1974); Hökfelt et al. (1974; 1976b; 1977b); Jacobowitz (1978); Jacobowitz and Palkovits (1974); Palkovits and Jacobowitz (1974); Lindvall and Björklund (1974); Shute and Lewis (1966); Moore and Bloom (1978, 1979); Ungerstedt (1971b). Several of these references, [Ungerstedt (1971b), the review by Jacobowitz (1978), and the two papers by Jacobowitz and Palkovits (1974)], have presented monoaminergic and cholinergic neuroanatomy in the form of stereotaxic atlases. This facilitates the types of surgical interventions mentioned above.

NE, DA, and 5-HT have been visualized directly by fluorescence histochemistry. In this technique, brain tissue is exposed to paraformaldehyde vapor or glyoxylic acid. The fluorescent compounds that form from monoamines may then be viewed under a fluorescence microscope (Fig. 4). More recently, immunologic techniques have been developed for the histochemical detection of neurons that contain peptide transmitters or the enzymes in the biosynthetic pathways of monoamines. Cholinergic neurons have been observed after staining for AChE (Fig. 5). A valuable adjunct to these histological procedures is the technique of biochemical mapping (Kobayashi *et al.*, 1974; O'Donohue *et al.*, 1979), wherein specific lesions of transmitter systems are made, and discrete brain regions are removed and assayed for the transmitter or for enzyme activity. This procedure identifies structures receiving specific monoamine input and is quantitatively more sensitive than fluorescence histochemistry.

A. The Norepinephrine Systems

Groups of cell bodies in the medullary and pontine reticular formation give rise to descending and ascending axonal systems (Fig. 6). These axons have numerous collateral branches and a large network of terminals. In the caudal midbrain, two ascending noradrenergic systems have been described. The dorsal NE bundle arises from cell bodies of the locus coeruleus in the dorsal pontine tegmentum (A6). This bundle innervates the thalamus, and its fibers turn ventrally and continue on to terminate in parts of the hypothalamus, basal telencephalon, limbic structures such as amygdala and hippocampus, and the

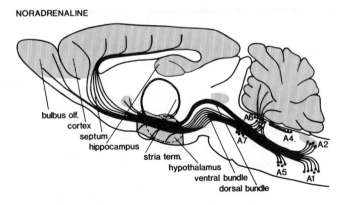

Figure 6. Saggital diagram of noradrenergic projections in the rat brain. Striped areas show NE nerve terminals. (Reprinted from Ungerstedt, 1971b, with permission of the author and *Acta Physiologica Scandinavica.*)

neocortex. The cerebellar cortex, lower brainstem, and spinal cord also receive input from the NE neurons of the locus coeruleus. The second system, the ventral NE bundle or central tegmental tract, courses ventrally in its ascent. Its axons are formed from cell bodies in the other brainstem clusters (A1,A2,A5,A7) and provide dense input to the hypothalamus and basal telencephalon.

B. The Epinephrine System

Immunohistochemical techniques have revealed the existence of central neurons that contain phenylethanolamine-N-methyltransferase, an enzyme that converts NE to epinephrine. This suggests that these neurons use epinephrine or a similar substance as a transmitter. The cell bodies are concentrated in the A1 and A2 cell groups in the medulla. Nerve terminals can be detected in the spinal cord, cranial nerve nuclei, locus coeruleus, periventricular gray of the midbrain and thalamus, and perifornical, paraventricular, and arcuate nuclei of the hypothalamus. Biochemical assays for epinephrine confirm its existence in these areas of the CNS (Van der Gugten *et al.,* 1976).

C. The Dopamine Systems

The major dopaminergic system in rat brain is in the nigrostriatal pathway (Fig. 7). Dopamine cell bodies in the compact part of the midbrain substantia nigra (A9) and adjacent tegmentum (A8) send axons through the far lateral hypothalamus to provide massive innervation of the caudate–putamen complex or neostriatum. The mesolimbic DA system (Fig. 7) originates from perikarya (A10) that surround the interpeduncular nucleus of the midbrain. Its axons project through the lateral hypothalamus and terminate in the olfac-

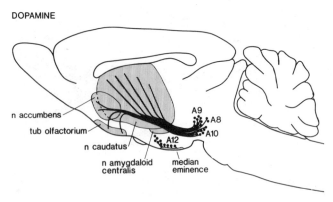

Figure 7. Saggital diagram of dopaminergic projections in the rat brain. (Reprinted from Ungerstedt, 1971b, with permission of the author and *Acta Physiologica Scandinavica.*)

tory tubercle, interstitial nucleus of the stria terminalis, areas within the septum and diagonal band, nucleus accumbens, and frontal cortex. There are also DA cell groups in the diencephalon. Of particular interest to the field of neuroendocrinology are the tuberohypophyseal systems. One of these, the tuberoinfundibular tract, arises from cells in the arcuate and ventral periventricular nuclei (A12); its axons terminate along the capillary plexus of the median eminence (Fig. 4).

D. The Serotonin Systems

Most 5-HT-containing neurons are found within and around the raphe nuclei of the brainstem (B1–8, Fig. 8). The most rostral of these in the pons and mesencephalon are the origin for ascending 5-HT projections. The route of these ascending axons has been described by Moore *et al.* (1978). Fluorescence studies suggest a medial pathway that innervates the hypothalamus and a lateral pathway that supplies terminals to the neostriatum, hippocampus, and neocortex (Fuxe and Jonsson, 1974).

E. The Acetylcholine Systems

Nerve terminals that show a dense stain for acetylcholinesterase generally are assumed to be cholinergic. Especially dense concentrations of AChE-containing nerve terminals appear in the neostriatum and nucleus accumbens. Clusters of cell bodies staining for AChE appear throughout the brain. It is not known whether these are truly cholinergic, i.e., use ACh as a transmitter, or cholinoceptive, i.e., receive presynaptic cholinergic innervation, or both. Some AChE-containing cells appear in the substantia nigra and locus coeruleus in the same locations as catecholamine cell bodies. Because AChE-containing termi-

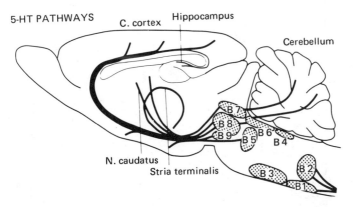

Figure 8. Saggital diagram of serotonergic pathways in the rat brain. (Reprinted from Fuxe and Jonsson, 1974, with permission of the authors and Raven Press.)

Table 2. Structure, Neural Localization, and Behavioral Effects of Some Brain Peptides

Peptide	Localization[a]	Behavioral effects	Representative references
LH-releasing hormone (LRH) (Pyro) Glu-His-Trp-Ser-Tyr-Gly-Leu-Arg-Pro-Gly-NH₂	Cell bodies: Preoptic area, arcuate N. Terminals: Lateral median eminence, vascular organ of lamina terminalis	Facilitation of Lordosis	King & Gerall, 1976; Setalo et al., 1976; McCann and Moss, 1975; Sternberger and Hoffman, 1978
Thyrotropin-releasing hormone (TRH) (Pyro) Glu-His-Pro-NH₂	Cell bodies: Hypothalamus Nerve terminals: Median eminence, nuclei of cranial nerves III, V, VII, X, XII, spinal cord ventral horn, sympathetic lateral column	Inhibition of Lordosis; arousal	Krulich et al., 1977; Havlicek et al., 1976; Hökfelt et al., 1975, 1978a
Somatotropin-inhibiting hormone (Somatostatin) H-Ala-Gly-Cys-Lys-Asn-Phe-Phe-Trp-Lys-Thr-Phe-Thr-Ser-Cys-OH	Cell bodies: Periventricular N., amygdala, zona incerta, spinal dorsal root ganglia Terminals: Median eminence, vascular organ of lamina terminalis, preoptic, ventromedial, arcuate N., spinal cord laminae I and II	Motor disorders	Havlicek et al., 1976; Parsons et al., 1976; Hökfelt et al., 1976a, 1978a
Substance P H-Arg-Pro-Lys-Pro-Gln-Gln-Phe-Phe-Gly-Leu-Met-NH₂	Cell bodies: Spinal dorsal root ganglia, globus pallidus, hypothalamus, central gray, raphe magnus Terminals: Substantia nigra reticulata, spinal cord dorsal horn, central gray, hypothalamus	Pain transmission	Leeman and Mroz, 1974; Mroz et al., 1977; Brownstein, 1977b; Hökfelt et al., 1976a, 1977a, 1978a

ACTH$_{4-10}$ Met-Glu-His-Phe-Arg-Trp-Gly		Acquisition and retention of avoidance responses, sexual arousal, stretching and yawning, grooming	DeWied, 1977
Endorphins Met^5-enkephalin Tyr-Gly-Gly-Phe-Met-OH Leu^5-Enkephalin Tyr-Gly-Gly-Phe-Leu-OH	Cell bodies: Central gray, raphe magnus, laminae I–V of spinal cord, caudate N., lateral septum, bed nucleus of stria terminalis, medial preoptic N., paraventricular N., arcuate N., ventromedial N., N. reticularis gigantocellularis, N. solitary tract Nerve terminals: Spinal laminae I and II, cranial nuclei of V, X, XII, locus coeruleus, central gray, medial thalamus, periventricular N., central amygdala, globus pallidus, caudate N., N. accumbens, bed nucleus of stria terminalis, lateral septum, hypothalamus, median eminence	Analgesia	Frederickson, 1977; Hökfelt *et al.*, 1977a,c; Johansson *et al.*, 1978
β-Endorphin β-Lipotropin (61–91)	Anterior and intermediate lobes of pituitary Cell bodies: arcuate nucleus Terminals: Hypothalamus, central gray, locus coeruleus	Analgesia, akinesia	Bloom *et al.*, 1977, 1978

[a] Mainly obtained in rats.

nals also appear in these regions, these cells are most likely cholinoceptive. Shute and Lewis (1966) have suggested three major cholinergic systems. (a) The dorsal tegmental pathway arises from the nucleus cuneiformis of the midbrain and supplies terminals to the tectum and thalamus. (b) The ventral tegmental pathway originates in the midbrain tegmentum and courses through the lateral hypothalamus to innervate various telencephalic areas. Along their route, some of these neurons synapse with hypothalamic and telencephalic AChE-containing cells. These cells, in turn, send their axons into neocortical areas. (c) Cholinergic neurons also appear to form key links in some classically recognized limbic system interconnections, such as from medial septum to hippocampus.

F. The Peptidergic Systems

It has been known for some time that administration of various peptides results in behavioral effects (see DeWied, 1977, for review). It now appears that some peptides of neural origin may serve as neurotransmitters or neuromodulators. Table 2 summarizes the localization and behavorial effects of some important neuropeptides. Table 2 also shows that the distribution of three hypothalamic hormones, LRH, TRH, and somatostatin, strongly suggests that they have functions other than control of pituitary secretions. Much interest has focused recently on the endorphins, now thought to be the endogenous ligands for the opiate receptors that mediate the effects of opiate drugs on behavior. Similarly, ACTH may serve as a prohormone for the behaviorally active fragment $ACTH_{4-10}$. In addition to the references in the table, the reader should consult Brownstein (1977a) and Hökfelt et al. (1978b).

REFERENCES

Aghajanian, G. W., and Wang, R. Y., 1978, Physiology and pharmacology of central serotonergic neurons, in: *Psychopharmacology: A Generation of Progress* (M. A. Lipton, A. DiMascio, and K. F. Killam, eds.), pp. 171–184, Raven Press, New York.

Anton-Tay, F., and Wurtman, R. J., 1971, Brain monoamines and endocrine function, in: *Frontiers in Neuroendocrinology* (L. Martini and W. F. Ganong, eds.), pp. 45–66, Oxford University Press, New York.

Axelrod, J., 1974, Regulation of the neurotransmitter norepinephrine, in: *The Neurosciences Third Study Program* (F. O. Schmitt, and F. G. Worden, eds.), pp. 863–876, MIT Press, Cambridge, Massachusetts.

Axelrod, J., 1977, Regulation of the synthesis, release and actions of catecholamine neurotransmitter, in: *First European Symposium on Hormones and Cell Regulation* (T. Dumont and A. Nunez, eds.), pp. 137–155, Elsevier, Amsterdam.

Baumgarten, H. G. and Björklund, A., 1976, Neurotoxic indoleamines and monoamine neurons, *Annu. Rev. Pharmacol. Toxicol.* **16**:101.

Bloom, F. E., 1975, Monoaminergic neurotoxins: Are they selective? *J. Neural. Trans.* **37**:183.

Bloom, F. E., Battenberg, E., Rossier, J., Ling, N., Leppaluoto, J., Vargo, T. M., and Guillemin, R., 1977, Endorphins are located in the intermediate and anterior lobes of the pituitary gland, not in the neurohypophysis, *Life Sci.* **20**:43.

Bloom, F. E., Rossier, J., Battenberg, E. L. F., Bayon, A., French, E., Henriksen, S. J., Siggins, G., Segal, D., Browne, R., Ling, M., and Guillemin, R., 1978, β-Endorphin: Cellular localization, electrophysiological and behavioral effects, *Adv. Biochem. Psychopharmacol.* **18**:89.

Brownstein, M. J., 1977a, Biologically active peptides in the mammalian central nervous system, in: *Peptides in Neurobiology* (H. Gainer, ed.), pp. 145–170, Plenum Press, New York.

Brownstein, M. J., 1977b, Neurotransmitters and hypothalamic hormones in the central nervous system, *Fed. Proc.* **36**:1960.

Bunney, B. S., and Aghajanian, G. K., 1975, Evidence for drug actions on both pre- and post-synaptic catecholamine receptors in the CNS, in: *Pre- and Postsynaptic Receptors* (E. Usdin and W. E. Bunney, eds.), pp. 89–122, Marcel Dekker, New York.

Butcher, L. L., 1975, Degenerative processes after punctate intracerebral administration of 6-hydroxydopamine, *J. Neural. Trans.* **37**:189.

Carlsson, A., 1975a, Monoamine precursors and analogues, *Pharmacol. Ther.* [B] **1**:381.

Carlsson, A., 1975b, Monoamine-depleting drugs, *Pharmacol. Ther.* [B] **1**:393.

Carlsson, A., 1975c, Drugs acting through dopamine release, *Pharmacol. Ther.* [B] **1**:401.

Cooper, J. R., Bloom, F. E., and Roth, R. H., 1978, *The Biochemical Basis of Neuropharmacology*, Third Edition, Oxford University Press, New York.

Creese, I., Burt, D. R., and Snyder, S. H., 1977, Dopamine receptor binding enhancement accompanies lesion-induced behavioral supersensitivity, *Science* **197**:596.

Dahlström, A., and Fuxe, K., 1964, Evidence for the existence of monoamine-containing neurons in the central nervous system. I. Demonstration of monoamines in the cell bodies of brain stem neurons, *Acta Physiol. Scand.* [Suppl.] **232**:1.

DeWied, D., 1977, Peptides and behavior, *Life Sci.* **20**:195.

Dews, P. B., 1972, Assessing the effects of drugs, in: *Methods in Psychobiology*, Vol. 2 (R. D. Meyers, ed.), pp. 4–124, Academic Press, New York.

Frederickson, R. C. A., 1977, Enkephalin pentapeptides—A review of current evidence for a physiological role in vertebrate neurotransmission, *Life Sci.* **21**:23.

Fuxe, K., 1965, Evidence for the existence of monoamine-containing neurons in the CNS. IV. The distribution of monoamine nerve terminals in the CNS, *Acta Physiol. Scand.* [Suppl.] **247**:36.

Fuxe, K., and Jonsson, G., 1974, Further mapping of central 5-hydroxytryptamine neurons: Studies with the neurotoxic dihydroxytryptamines, *Adv. Biochem. Psychopharmacol.* **10**:1.

Haefely, W., Bartholini, G., and Pletscher, A., 1976, Monoaminergic drugs: General pharmacology, *Pharmacol. Ther.* [B] **2**:185.

Harvey, J. A., and McMaster, S. E., 1975, Fenfluramine: Evidence for a neurotoxic action on midbrain and a long term depletion of serotonin, *Psychopharmacol. Commun.* **1**:217.

Havlicek, U., Rezek, M., and Freisen, H., 1976, Somatostatin and thyrotropin releasing hormone: Central effect on sleep and motor system, *Pharmacol. Biochem. Behav.* **4**:455.

Hedqvist, P., 1977, Basic mechanisms of prostaglandin action on autonomic neurotransmission, *Annu. Rev. Pharmacol. Toxicol.* **17**:259.

Hökfelt, T., and Ungerstedt, U., 1973, Specificity of 6-hydroxydopamine induced degeneration of central monoamine neurones: An electron and fluorescence microscopic study with special reference to intracerebral injection on the nigro-striatal dopamine system, *Brain Res.* **60**:269.

Hökfelt, T., Fuxe, K., Goldstein, M., and Johansson, O., 1974, Immunohistochemical evidence for the existence of adrenaline neurons in the rat brain, *Brain Res.* **66**:235.

Hökfelt, T., Fuxe, K., Johansson, O., Jeffcoate, S., and White, N., 1975, Thyrotropin releasing hormone (TRH)-containing nerve terminals in certain brain stem nuclei and in the spinal cord, *Neurosci. Lett.* **1**:133.

Hökfelt, T., Elde, R., Johansson, O., Luft, R., Nilsson, G., and Arimura, A., 1976a, Immunohisto-chemical evidence for separate populations of somatostatin-containing and substance P-containing primary afferent neurons in the rat, *Neuroscience* **1**:131.

Hökfelt, T., Johansson, O., Fuxe, K., Goldstein, M., and Park, D., 1976b, Immunohistochemical studies on the localization and distribution of monoamine neuron systems in the rat brain. I. Tyrosine hydroxylase in the mes- and diencephalon, *Med. Biol.*, **54**:427.

Hökfelt, T., Elde, R., Johansson, O., Terenius, L., and Stein, L., 1977a, The distribution of enkephalin-immunoreactive cell bodies in the rat central nervous system, *Neurosci. Lett.* **5**:25.

Hökfelt, T., Johansson, O., Fuxe, K., Goldstein, M., and Park, D., 1977b, Immunohistochemical studies on the localization and distribution of monoamine neuron systems in the rat brain. II. Tyrosine hydroxylase in the telencephalon, *Med. Biol.* **55**:21.

Hökfelt, T., Ljungdahl, Å., Terenius, L., Elde, R., and Nilsson, G., 1977c, Immunohistochemical analysis of peptide pathways possibly related to pain and analgesia: Enkephalin and substance P, *Proc. Natl. Acad. Sci. USA* **74**:3081.

Hökfelt, T., Elde, R., Fuxe, K., Johansson, O., Ljungdahl, A., Goldstein, A., Luft, R., Efendic, S., Nilsson, G., Terenius, L., Ganten, D., Jeffcoate, S. L., Rehfeld, J., Said, S., Perez de la Mora, M., Passani, L., Tapia., R., Teran, L., and Palacios, R., 1978a, Aminergic and peptidergic pathways in the nervous system with special reference to the hypothalamus, in: *The Hypothalamus* (S. Reichlin, R. J. Baldessarini, and J. B. Martin, eds.), pp. 69–135, Raven Press, New York.

Hökfelt, T., Elde, R., Johansson, O., Ljungdahl, A., Schultzberg, M., Fuxe, K., Goldstein, M., Nilsson, G., Pernow, B., Terenius, L., Ganten, D., Jeffcoate, S. L., Rehfeld, J., and Said, S., 1978b, Distribution of peptide containing neurons, in: *Psychopharmacology: A Generation of Progress* (M. A. Lipton, A. DiMascio, and K. F. Killam, eds.), pp. 39–66, Raven Press, New York.

Jacobowitz, D. M., 1978, Monoaminergic pathways in the central nervous system, in: *Psychopharmacology: A Generation of Progress* (M. A. Lipton, A. DiMascio, and K. F. Killam, eds.), pp. 119–129, Raven Press, New York.

Jacobowitz, D. M. and Palkovits, M., 1974, Topographic atlas of catecholamine and acetylcholinesterase-containing neurons in the rat brain. I. Forebrain (telencephalon, diencephalon), *J. Comp. Neurol.* **157**:13.

Javoy, F., Sotelo, C., Herbet, A., and Agid, Y., 1976, Specificity of dopaminergic neuronal degeneration induced by intracerebral injection of 6-hydroxydopamine in the nigrostriatal dopamine system, *Brain Res.* **102**:201.

Johansson, O., Hökfelt, T., Elde, R. P., Schultzberg, M., and Terenius, L., 1978, Immunohistochemical distribution of enkephalin neurons, *Adv. Biochem. Psychopharmacol.* **18**:51.

King, J. C., and Gerall, A. A., 1976, Localization of luteinizing hormone-releasing hormone, *J. Histochem. Cytochem.* **24**:829.

Kobayashi, R. M., Palkovits, M., Kopin, I. J., and Jacobowitz, D. M., 1974, Biochemical mapping of noradrenergic nerves arising from the rat locus coeruleus, *Brain Res.* **77**:269.

Kostrezewa, R., and Jacobowitz, D. M., 1974, Pharmacological actions of 6-hydroxydopamine, *Pharmacol. Rev.* **26**:199.

Krnjevic, K., 1974, Chemical nature of synaptic transmission in vertebrates, *Physiol. Rev.* **54**:418.

Krulich, L., Quijada, M., Wheaton, J. E., Illner, P., and McCann, S. M. 1977, Localization of hypophysiotropic neurohormones by assay of sections from various brain areas, *Fed. Proc.* **36**:1953.

Leeman, S. E., and Mroz, E. A., 1974, Substance P, *Life Sci.* **15**:2033.

Lindvall, O., and Björklund, A., 1974, The organization of the ascending catecholamine neuron systems in the rat brain as revealed by the glyoxylic acid fluorescence method, *Acta Physiol. Scand. [Suppl.]* **412**:1.

Lipton, M. A., DiMascio, A., and Killam, K. H., 1978, *Psychopharmacology: A Generation of Progress*, Raven Press, New York.

McCann, S. M., and Moss, R. L., 1975, Putative neurotransmitters involved in discharging gonadotropin releasing neurohormones and the action of LH releasing hormone on the CNS, *Life Sci.* **16**:833.

McLennan, H., 1970, *Synaptic Transmission*, W. B. Saunders, Philadelphia.

Meyers, R. D., 1971, Methods for chemical stimulation of the brain, in: *Methods in Psychobiology*, Vol. 1 (R. D. Meyers, ed.), pp. 247–279, Academic Press, New York.

Meyers, R. D., 1974, *Handbook of Drug and Chemical Stimulation of the Brain*, Van Nostrand–Reinhold, New York.

Moore, R. Y., and Bloom, F. E., 1978, Central catecholamine neuron systems: Anatomy and physiology of the dopamine systems, *Annu. Rev. Neurosci.* **1**:129.

Moore, R. Y., and Bloom, F. E., 1979, Central catecholamine neuron systems: Anatomy and physiology of the norepinephrine and epinephrine systems, *Annu. Rev. Neurosci.* **2**:113.

Moore, R. Y., Halaris, A. E., and Jones, B. E., 1978, Serotonin neurons of the midbrain raphe: Ascending projections, *J. Comp. Neurol.* **180**:417.

Mroz, E. A., Brownstein, M. J., and Leeman, S. E., 1977, Evidence for substance P in the striato–nigral tract, *Brain Res.* **125**:305.

Nathanson, J. A., 1977, Cyclic nucleotides and nervous system function, *Physiol. Rev.* **57**:157.

O'Donohue, T. L., Crowley, W. R., and Jacobowitz, D. M., 1979, Biochemical mapping of the noradrenergic ventral bundle projection sites: Evidence for a noradrenergic–dopaminergic interaction, *Brain Res.* **172**:87.

Palkovits, M., and Jacobowitz, D. M., 1974, Topographic atlas of catecholamine and acetyl-cholinesterase-containing neurons in the rat brain II. Hindbrain (mesencephalon, rhomb-encephalon), *J. Comp. Neurol.* **157**:29.

Parsons, J. A., Erlandsen, S. L., Hegre, O. D., McEvoy, R. C., Elde, R. P., 1976, Central and peripheral localization of somatostatin; immunoenzyme immunocytochemical studies, *J. Histochem. Cytochem.* **24**:872.

Pelligrino, L. J., and Cushman, A. J., 1971, Use of the stereotaxic technique, in: *Methods in Psychobiology*, Vol. 1 (R. D. Meyers, ed.), pp. 67–90, Academic Press, New York.

Reis, D. J., Joh, T. H., Ross, R. A. and Pickel, V. M., 1974, Reserpine selectively increases tyrosine hydroxylase and dopamine-β-hydroxylase enzyme protein in central noradrenergic neurons, *Brain Res.*, **81**:380.

Roth, R. H., Salzman, P. M., and Nowycky, M. C., 1978, Impulse flow and short term regulation of transmitter biosynthesis in central catecholaminergic neurons, in: *Psychopharmacology: A Generation of Progress* (M. A. Lipton, A. DiMascio, and K. F. Killam, eds.), pp. 185–198, Raven Press, New York.

Routtenberg, A., 1972, Intracranial chemical injection and behavior: A critical review, *Behav. Biol.* **7**:601.

Sachs, C., and Jonsson, G., 1975, Mechanisms of action of 6-hydroxydopamine, *Biochem. Pharmacol.* **24**:1.

Sanders-Bush, E., and Massari, V. J., 1977, Actions of drugs that deplete serotonin, *Fed. Proc.* **36**:2149.

Setalo, G., Vigh, S., Schally, A. V., Arimura, A., and Flerko, B., 1976, Immunohistological study of the origin of LH-RH-containing fibers of the rat hypothalamus, *Brain Res.* **103**:597.

Shute, C. C. D., and Lewis, P. R., 1966, Cholinergic and monoaminergic pathways in the hypothalamus, *Br. Med. Bull* **22**:221.

Starke, K., 1977, Regulation of noradrenaline release by presynaptic receptor systems, *Rev. Physiol. Biochem. Pharmacol.* **77**:1.

Sternberger, L. A., and Hoffman, G. E., 1978, Immunocytology of luteinizing hormone-releasing hormone, *Neuroendocrinology* **25**:111.

Strömböm, U., 1975, On the functional role of pre- and postsynaptic catecholamine receptors in brain, *Acta Physiol. Scand.* [*Suppl.*] **431**:1.

Ungerstedt, U., 1971a, Histochemical studies on the effect of intracerebral and intraventricular injections of 6-hydroxydopamine on monoamine neurons in the rat brain, in: *6-Hydroxydopamine and Catecholamine Neurons* (T. Malmfors and H. Thoenen, eds.), pp. 101–134, American Elsevier, New York.

Ungerstedt, U., 1971b, Stereotaxic mapping of the monoamine pathways in the rat brain, *Acta Physiol. Scand.* [*Suppl.*] **367**:1.

Van Der Gugten, J., Palkovits, M., Wijnen, H. L. J. M., and Versteeg, D. H. G., 1976, Regional distribution of adrenaline in rat brain, *Brain Res.* **107**:171.

Weiner, N. I., 1974, A critical assessment of methods for the determination of monoamine synthesis turnover rates *in vivo*, *Adv. Biochem. Psychopharmacol.* **12**:143.

Westfall, T. C., 1977, Local control of adrenergic neurotransmission, *Physiol Rev.* **57**:659.

II

Development of Reproductive Function

Hormonal Actions on the Sexual Differentiation of the Genitalia and the Gonadotropin-Regulating Systems

HARVEY H. FEDER

I. BRIEF HISTORY OF THE PROBLEM

In 1903, Bouin and Ancel proposed that substances produced by the testes controlled differentiation of the embryonic genital structures. Their observation that there was a very well-developed secretory interstitium in the testes of pig embryos at the time of genital tract differentiation indirectly supported this notion. The idea of hormonal regulation of the process of sexual differentiation was given further impetus by studies of a phenomenon known as freemartinism. Freemartinism occurs in cows, sheep, goats, and pigs (Short, 1972). Descriptions of the syndrome in cattle include the following: (a) the freemartin calf is a sexually abnormal chromosomal female born as a twin to an apparently normal male; (b) about 90% of female cattle born as twins to males are sterile; (c) external genitalia of the freemartin are of the female type, and there is mammary gland development; (d) there is variable development of the internal genital tracts; and (e) the gonads are atrophic but resemble testes more than they resemble ovaries (Burns, 1961). To account for the occurrence of freemartinism, a "hormone theory" was devised by Keller and Tandler (1916) and

HARVEY H. FEDER • Institute of Animal Behavior, Rutgers University, Newark, New Jersey 07102.

by Lillie (1917). According to this theory, androgenic hormones produced by the male fetus are able to reach the female twin because of fusion of some of the placental blood vessels that supply the twins. The evidence in support of this view included the findings that such vascular anastomoses occurred in cattle (Fig. 1) and that in the 10% or so of cases in which a female twin of a male was fertile in adulthood, the placental anastomoses had been obliterated. That the blood-borne factor responsible for freemartinism was produced by the male was adduced from the facts that the male twin seemed normal and that the prenatal testis was apparently (by histological examination) active before the ovary.

These observations stimulated research, but today the position that freemartinism is explicable in terms of the "hormone theory" seems untenable. Experimental freemartins have never been produced after administration of androgens to pregnant cows (Jost *et al.*, 1963). In fact, after exposure to androgens prenatally, female fetuses were found to have ovaries, internal genitalia of a predominantly female type, and masculinized external genitalia. Table 1 summarizes the substantial differences between freemartins and female mammalian fetuses exposed to exogenous androgens. More recent theories of the origin of freemartinism implicate an exchange of cells between twins in early pregnancy (Herschler and Fechheimer, 1967) or passage from the male to the female fetus of a nonsteroidal factor that favors testicular development (Short, 1970), but details of these ideas need not concern us here.

Because criticisms of the "hormone theory" did not arise immediately after its formulation, early interpretations of the etiology of freemartinism, though probably misguided, had ample time to focus attention on the gonadal steroids as agents of genital sexual differentiation. During the 1920s gonadal grafting and parabiosis techniques were used to alter the course of sexual differentiation, with avian and amphibian preparations preferred (Minoura, 1921; Humphrey, 1928). In the 1930s, crystalline steroid hormones became available and were widely used as agents for altering differentiation in placental mammals

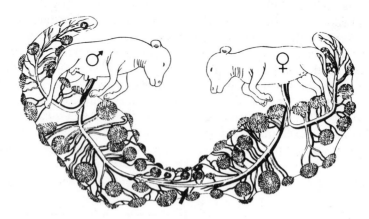

Figure 1. Vascular connections in twin fetal calves removed from the uterus. The freemartin is on the right. (Reproduced with permission from R. V. Short, 1972, after F. R. Lillie, 1917.)

Table 1. Differences between Freemartins and Female Mammalian Fetuses Exposed to Exogenous Androgens

	Type of gonad	Type of internal genitalia	Type of external genitalia
Freemartin	Atrophic (but may resemble testis more than ovary)	Male	Female
Androgenized female	Female	Female	Male (if dosage of androgen is sufficiently high)

and marsupials (Burns, 1939; Moore, 1941; Green, 1942). Still later, in the 1940s and 1950s, surgical (Jost, 1947; Wells, 1950; Raynaud, 1950; Wells *et al.*, 1954), chemical (Greene, 1942), and irradiation (Raynaud and Frilley, 1947) techniques were developed for use in fetal animals to erase or diminish their gonadal secretions. In these ways, the role of the gonads in directing sexual differentiation could be more easily assessed, and the objection could not be made that administration of exogenous hormones altered sexual development merely by nonspecific or pharmacological means. (For a more complete review of the history of the study of sex differentiation, see Burns, 1961.) The results of all of these manipulations led to several clear conclusions. To understand these conclusions, we must first be familiar with the normal embryology of the genital system. This digression into normal embryology will include some discussion of the experimental manipulations to which I have alluded. Thus, "as we are digressing we will also hopefully be progressing" (Sterne, 1759) toward a complete picture of the prenatal forces that mold the genitalia.

II. NORMAL EMBRYOGENESIS OF THE GENITAL SYSTEM

A. Sex Determination and Differentiation of the Gonads

The primary step in the process of sex differentiation occurs at fertilization. An ovum can be fertilized either by a Y chromosome- or an X chromosome-bearing sperm. This process, termed sex determination, has consequences for the differentiation of the embryonic gonads. Each individual, whether XX or XY, contains a thickened ridge of tissue on the ventromesial surface of the mesonephros* known as the genital ridge (Fig. 2). The genital ridge is the primordium of the gonad, and early in development it appears to have the potential to develop into either an ovary or a testis (Burns, 1961).

*In higher vertebrates, the mesonephros serves the embryo as a temporary excretory organ. The mesonephros consists of a series of tubules. When the tubules enlarge, they bulge into the coelom and produce a urogenital ridge. The urogenital ridge then divides into a medial genital ridge and a more lateral mesonephric ridge.

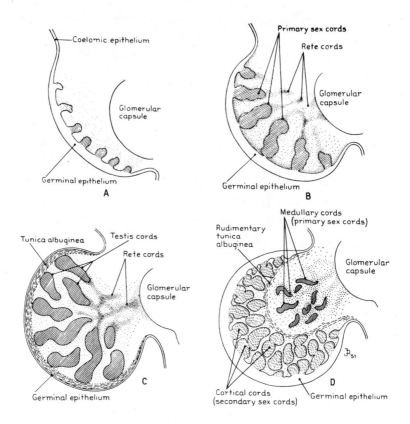

Figure 2. Differentiation of the genital ridge into a gonad. A: Origin of the primary sex cords (medullary cords) from the germinal epithelium. B: Gonad at the indifferent stage of sexual differentiation; the well-developed primary sex cords represent the male or medullary component, whereas the germinal epithelium represents, potentially, the cortical component. C: Differentiation of a testis consists in the further development of the primary sex cords and the reduction of the germinal epithelium to a thin, serous membrane, accompanied by development of the tunica albuginea. D: Differentiation of an ovary consists in reduction of the primary sex cords to medullary cords of the ovary, whereas the cortex is formed by continued development of cortical cords from the germinal epithelium. (Reproduced with permission from R. K. Burns, 1955b.)

Thus, each individual embryo is theoretically sexually bipotential with regard to the type of gonad that will develop. The direction of gonadal differentiation is guided by the presence or absence of male-determining genes. Male-determining genes may be located on the Y chromosome (Welshons and Russel, 1959), or they may be located on the X chromosome but be capable of activation only if a Y chromosome is present (Hamerton, 1968). The active male-determining genes cause the selective persistence of the central portion, or medulla, of each genital ridge. The mechanism by which the Y chromosome causes testicular differentiation is not known, but Mittwoch (1970) has proposed that the Y chromosome causes increases in the number of cell divisions in the gonad. This notion is consistent with the somewhat controversial claim that testicular growth occurs sooner than ovarian growth during differentiation (Mittwoch, 1967). As the medulla of the genital ridge develops, it is said to produce a nonsteroidal inductor substance, "medullarin," that inhibits the growth of the outer portion, or cortex, of each genital ridge (Witschi, 1957). The medulla of the genital ridge is the precursor of the fetal testis. When male-determining genes are absent or in a latent state because of the absence of a Y chromosome, the genital ridge cortex develops and is said to produce "corticin," a nonsteroidal inductor substance that is an antagonist of medullary development (Witschi, 1957). The cortex of the genital ridge is the forerunner of the fetal ovary.

The medullarin–corticin hypothesis has been questioned by Jost (1972). Recent attention to the problem of how the medulla differentiates into a testis and the cortex into an ovary has centered on the possibility that H-Y antigen (a cell surface component present in all mammalian males) is the inducer substance responsible for differentiation of the indifferent gonad into a testis (Wachtel, 1977; Wilson, 1978).

The genital ridges consist not only of somatic mesodermal and epithelial tissue, but also of germ cells that have migrated from the yolk sac to reside in the ridges. The germ cells accomplish this migration by the use of pseudopodia, perhaps by the release of lytic enzymes that break down obstructive membranes, and perhaps by passive transport in the vascular system. An unidentified chemotactic substance ("telopheron") is thought to emanate from the genital ridge and attract the germ cells. The germ cells colonize the ridges, and their number increases. In general, they pass into the medulla if the genital ridge is to differentiate into a testis and into the cortex if the ridge is to differentiate into an ovary (Baker, 1972). The numbers of germ cells that colonize the medulla do not influence the endocrine activity of the testis, but the female germ cells induce development of follicle cells that ultimately are involved in estrogen secretion (Short, 1972). The events summarized thus far are depicted in Fig. 2. In their specifics, the descriptions of these events apply only to mammals. Some interesting differences exist between mammalian and nonmammalian forms with regard to sex determination and gonadal differentiation.

First, in mammals the male is the heterogametic sex. In reptiles and birds, it is the female that is heterogametic. In fish and amphibia, there are some species in which the male is heterogametic and some in which the female is heterogametic. A general principle that emerges for vertebrates is that the sex that is heterogametic determines the direction of gonadal differentiation (Beatty, 1970). Thus, in mammals, the Y chromosome of the heterogametic (XY) male causes differentiation of the testis, whereas in birds, the W chromosome of the heterogametic (ZW) female induces differentiation of the ovary. In invertebrates (e.g., *Drosophila*), the situation is again different. The balance between autosomes (male-determining) and X chromosomes (female-determining) decides whether the gonads are to be of the male or female type (Bridges, 1939).

A second important difference between mammalian and nonmammalian forms is the lability of the gonadal primordia or of the differentiated gonads. In a number of species of fish and amphibia, complete sex reversal of the gonadal primordia can be brought about by the addition of minute amounts of water-soluble estrogen or androgen preparations to aquaria (Yamamoto, 1962, 1975) or by gonadal grafts (Gallien, 1965). Other agents, such as temperature change, also may bring about complete sex reversal in these nonmammalian forms during differentiation (reviewed in Burns, 1961). This lability of gonadal structure can continue well after the larval period, as strikingly illustrated by the change in gonadal sex seen in members of a species of "cleaner fish" (*Labroides dimidiatus*) when a change in social hierarchy occurs (Robertson, 1972), or by the existence of "hermaphrodites in time" among fish (Chan, 1970; Reinboth, 1975). Sex reversal of the gonads can also occur in birds. This occurrence is no doubt favored by the normal persistence of testicular elements in the right gonad of females of some species of birds (Burns, 1961).

These findings may be contrasted with those for mammals. When hermaphroditism occurs in mammals, it is always referable to some distortion of the normal process of embryogenesis, and it does not arise as the result of postparturitional forces. Despite repeated attempts to cause sex reversal of gonads in mammals by means of steroid treatments during sexual differentiation, there is no convincing evidence for an effect of such treatment. Only Burns (1955a) has reported substantial reversal of gonadal sex after use of massive doses of estrogen in differentiating marsupials. The biochemical and anatomical bases of the high degree of resistance to sex reversal exhibited by the mammalian gonad remain to be discovered. Short (1972) has proposed the teleological argument that viviparity in mammals, with its accompanying exposure of prenatal animals to maternal steroids, requires a mechanism of gonadal differentiation resistant to the actions of steroids.

To summarize, the sexually bipotential genital ridge is induced to form a testis when the mammalian embryo is XY and to develop into an ovary in the absence of a contribution from the Y chromosome. A number of chemically undefined, nonsteroidal substances (medullarin, corticin, telopheron) have been posited to play a role in gonadal differentiation, but steroids do not affect the course of gonadal differentiation in mammals. Therefore, chromosomal constitution has crucial consequences for the course of gonadal differentiation. We see in the next section that the direction of gonadal differentiation dictates the development or demise of the genital ducts.

B. Differentiation of the Genital Ducts

Each embryo, regardless of genetic sex, contains two bilaterally represented sets of genital ducts. Therefore, at some stage of development, each individual is sexually bipotential with regard to the genital duct systems. For most of its length, the more lateral duct is the Müllerian duct. Medial to this is the Wolffian or mesonephric duct. The Müllerian ducts are anlagen of the oviduct, uterus, and a portion of the vagina, whereas the Wolffian ducts are the primordia of the epididymis, vas deferens, and seminal vesicles (Fig. 3). The now classic experiments of Jost (1947, 1953) and of others (Brewer, 1962; Picon, 1969; Price, 1970) have unequivocally demonstrated that in the presence of functional testes the Wolffian ducts develop and differentiate but the Müllerian ducts regress. Testicular grafts *in vivo* or *in vitro* during the period of genital duct differentiation cause Wolffian duct development and Müllerian duct regression regardless of the chromosomal sex of the target tissue ducts. Castration of genetic males prior to the growth or regression of these duct systems results in subsequent regression of the Wolffian ducts and retention and differentiation of the Müllerian ducts. The presence or absence of ovaries plays no role in the fate of the ducts. Thus, regardless of chromosomal sex, the

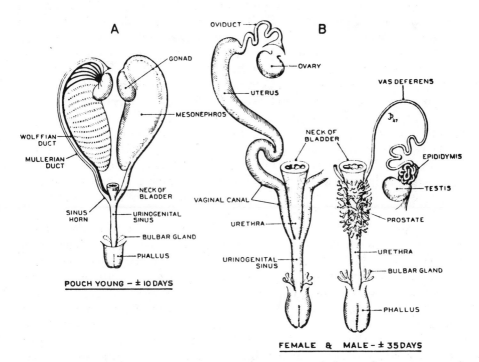

Figure 3. Early development and sexual differentiation in the genital tracts of young opossums. A: The bisexual stage of development in a female embryo ±10 days of age showing the paired gonaducts of both sexes, the sexually indifferent stage of the urinogenital sinus, and the undifferentiated genital tubercle or phallus. B: Male and female at about 35 days, when sexual differentiation is far advanced, showing the structures that develop from the primitive sex ducts and dimorphic development of the sinus region. The phallus shows chiefly a difference in size without marked morphologic divergence. (Reproduced with permission from R. K. Burns, 1955a.)

testis determines, by virtue of its presence or absence, whether a male or a female type of duct system will be fashioned. Further investigation has questioned whether the testicular factor that favors Wolffian duct development is identical to the testicular factor that inhibits Müllerian duct development.

Basically, findings have indicated that testosterone and some related androgens stimulate development of the Wolffian ducts (Wilson, 1975) and that synthetic antiandrogens suppress Wolffian duct differentiation in at least some mammalian species (Elger, 1966; Jost, 1966). However, it has rarely been claimed (Greene and Ivy, 1937) that androgens significantly inhibit the growth of mammalian Müllerian ducts. Rather, it is hypothesized that a separate, nonsteroidal substance figures in the inhibition of the Müllerian ducts. The chemical identity of the Müllerian duct-inhibiting factor is not yet established, but recent work by Josso (1973) and colleagues (1975) suggests that it is a nondialyzable compound produced by the seminiferous tubules during the fetal–neonatal period.

If a nonsteroidal substance of testicular origin inhibits the Müllerian ducts, and an androgen of testicular origin promotes growth of the Wolffian ducts, another question arises. Which specific androgen is responsible for Wolffian duct differentiation? This problem has been approached in a number of ways. A variety of exogenous androgens has been administered to mammals during the period of genital duct differentiation. Two androgens shown to be active in favoring Wolffian duct development in rat fetuses are testosterone and 5α-dihydrotestosterone (Schultz and Wilson, 1974). A more refined technique than administration of exogenous hormones involves the measurement of endogenous androgens during fetal life. In studies of humans (Reyes *et al.*, 1974), rhesus macaques (Resko *et al.*, 1973), pigs (Meusy-Dessolle, 1974), calves (Challis *et al.*, 1974), and rabbits (Veyssiere *et al.*, 1975), testosterone appears to be a major androgen in the circulation of developing male fetuses, thereby suggesting a role for this hormone in genital duct differentiation. However, a conclusion based on these data would be premature, because a plethora of evidence shows that testosterone is converted extensively to its 5α-reduced derivative, 5α-dihydrotestosterone, in several target tissues of the adult (Wilson and Gloyna, 1970). A stronger argument for the direct participation of testosterone (rather than one of its metabolic products) is that in the rabbit fetus, enzyme activity that catalyzes the 5α reduction of testosterone does not appear in the Wolffian ducts until after the onset of gonadal androgen production and after differentiation of the Wolffian tissue is quite advanced (Wilson, 1973).

To summarize, anlagen of masculine and feminine genital tract structures are present in prenatal mammals of both sexes. The male genital tract primordium, or Wolffian duct, develops under the influence of testicular androgen, probably testosterone. The female genital tract primordium, or Müllerian duct, is inhibited by a testicular product of a nonsteroid nature and develops in the absence of this testicular product. The rules of differentiation of the anlagen of the prostate, vagina, phallus, scrotum, clitoris, and labia bear some resemblance to those for differentiation of the genital ducts, but are not identical, as we see in the next section.

C. Differentiation of the Urogenital Sinus and Genital Tubercle

The urogenital sinus is, in its undifferentiated state, a short canal extending from the neck of the bladder to its exterior opening at the base of the genital elevation (Burns, 1961). The genital elevation is an external eminence in the midline of the embryo. It develops with a centrally prominent elevation, the genital tubercle. The tubercle is immediately flanked by paired folds (genital folds) and, farther laterally, flanked by rounded swellings (genital swellings) (Patten, 1958). In the male, the urogenital sinus is the primordium of the prostate gland and prostatic urethra (Fig. 4). The genital tubercle is the anlage of the penis, and the genital folds and genital swellings are anlagen of the prepuce and the scrotal pouches, respectively (Fig. 4). In the female, the entire urethra and a portion of the vagina develop from the urogenital sinus, the clitoris forms from the genital tubercle, and the labia minora and labia majora differentiate from the genital folds and genital swellings, respectively (Fig. 4).

The rules of differentiation of these structures differ in four important respects from those governing differentiation of the genital ducts. First, to paraphrase Beach, the development of normal male or female structures derived from the urogenital sinus represents mutually exclusive alternatives. The same imperative applies to the development of normal male or female structures derived from the genital elevation. For example, because the labia majora and scrotal sacs develop from identical anlagen (the genital swellings), only one or the other can be produced (Beach, 1971). In contrast, it is theoretically possible for a single individual to possess differentiated Wolffian and Müllerian ducts (i.e., if androgen is present but Müllerian duct inhibitor is absent), to be lacking differentiated Wolffian and Müllerian ducts (i.e., if no androgenic stimulation is present but Müllerian duct inhibitor is present), or to possess differentiated representatives of one or the other duct system (as is normally the case).

Second, the differentiation of the urogenital sinus and genital elevation is regulated by a single factor, the presence or absence of testicular androgen. This is in contrast to the situation for the genital ducts, whose differentiation requires two factors.

Third, the differentiation of the urogenital sinus and genital elevation requires that circulating androgens act at a distance from their site of secretion from the testes. On the contrary, the effects of testicular secretions on the differentiation of Wolffian and Müllerian ducts are local, not systemic. This is shown by the occurrence of "lateral gynandromorphs" in certain strains of mice, hamsters, and pigs (Hollander *et al.*, 1956; Kirkman, 1958; Short, 1972). These animals have a small testis on one side and a small ovary on the other side of the body. The Wolffian duct develops, and the Müllerian duct regresses on the side on which the testis is located. On the side containing the ovary, the Wolffian duct regresses and the Müllerian duct differentiates. It is also shown by unilateral testis transplant studies with rabbits, in which the Wolffian duct differentiates only on the side on which the testis transplant is located (Short, 1972).

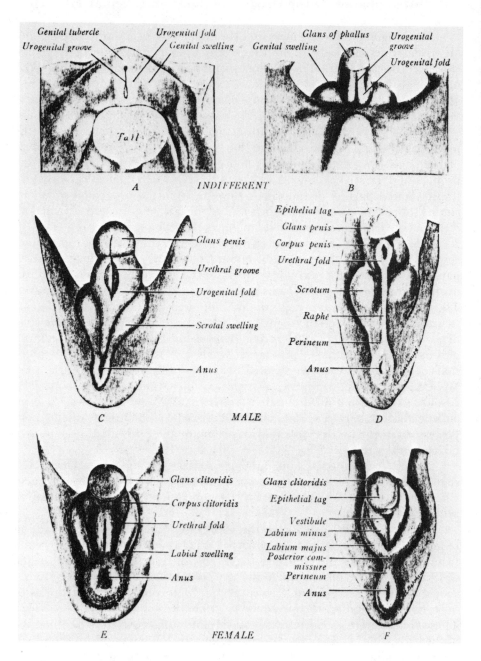

Figure 4. Differentiation of the human external genitalia (after Spaulding). A, B: at nearly 7 and nearly 8 weeks (×15). C, D: the male at 10 and 12 weeks (×8). E, F: the female at 10 and 12 weeks (×8). (Reproduced with permission from L. B. Arey, 1954.)

Finally, enzyme activity responsible for conversion of testosterone to 5α-dihydrotestosterone is present in the urogenital sinus and genital elevation prior to differentiation of these primordia. Dihydrotestosterone derived from testosterone probably mediates masculinization of the urogenital sinus and genital elevation (Siiteri and Wilson, 1974), whereas unconverted testosterone mediates masculinization of the Wolffian ducts (Wilson, 1973).

Despite these differences, there are some significant respects in which the differentiation of the urogenital sinus and genital elevation is similar to the differentiation of the genital duct system. Each individual embryo is, at first, bipotential with respect to the direction of development of the urogenital sinus and genital elevation, just as each individual is sexually bipotential with respect to the direction of genital duct development. All three sets of anlagen (ducts, urogenital sinus, genital elevation) develop in a masculine direction in the presence of appropriate testicular secretions, and all three develop in a feminine direction in the absence of such secretions. Each of them is sensitive to the effects of testicular products during periods of prenatal (and, for differentiation of external genitalia in short-gestation rodents, neonatal) development. None of them are dependent on the fetal ovaries for their differentiation. In all of these respects, another tissue, mammary tissue, follows the same course of development.

D. Differentiation of the Mammary Glands

The anlagen of the mammary glands are budlike growths of epidermal epithelium that extend down to the mesoderm. In normal females, or (as shown in experiments with rodents) in males deprived of androgen stimulation before mammary gland differentiation, the buds retain their connection with the epidermis, and nipple development ensues (Raynaud, 1950; Goldman and Neumann, 1969; Neumann et al., 1970; Goldman et al., 1973). In normal male rodents, or in female rodents treated during fetal development with androgen, the buds break their connection with the epidermis and become isolated nodules in the mesoderm, and nipple formation is inhibited (Greene et al., 1941). Thus, in rodents, the absence or presence of testicular androgen determines whether mammary gland primordia will develop or not. Recent results demonstrate that testosterone is more potent than its 5α-reduced metabolites in masculinization of the mammary glands of rats (Goldman et al., 1976a). It should be borne in mind that there is not the same clear-cut histological difference between the breasts of embryonic human males and females as there is between rodent males and females. In fact, there does not appear to be a difference in histological structure of the breasts in humans until puberty (Pfaltz, 1949). This accounts for the ability of human males to undergo breast development in response to hormones in adulthood.

With these observations, we close our discussion of the normal differentiation and development of the genitalia and mammary glands. In the course of this digression, we have mentioned experimental work in which androgens have been administered to chromosomal females (see reviews by Burns, 1961; Jost, 1970) and in which androgens have been withdrawn from chromosomal males during differentiation. The androgen withdrawal experiments have utilized methodologies as diverse as castration (Wells *et al.*, 1954), irradiation of the testes (Raynaud and Frilley, 1947) and administration of synthetic anti-androgens (Neumann *et al.*, 1970) or antibodies to testosterone (Goldman *et al.*, 1972). Decapitation (Jost, 1950) and administration of antibodies to gonado-tropins (Goldman and Mahesh, 1970) have also been used in mammalian fetuses as techniques to diminish pituitary stimulation of the testes. Further-more, descriptive studies have been carried out on the testicular content of androgens in perinatal animals (Resko *et al.*, 1968; Attal, 1969; Stewart and Raeside, 1976), on the androgen-synthesizing capability of the fetal testes *in vitro* (Price and Ortiz, 1965; Bloch *et al.*, 1974; Picon, 1976), and on the concentration of androgen in the fetal blood plasma (Mizuno *et al.*, 1968; Brown-Grant, 1974; Resko, 1974) or in the amniotic fluid (Giles *et al.*, 1974). These experimental and descriptive studies have clearly and consistently impli-cated fetal testicular androgens as crucial factors in the virilization of the internal genitalia (except for the gonads and Müllerian duct derivatives) and the external genitalia. However, this insight into normal development has been blurred by some puzzling data on the effects of exogenous estrogens on the course of mammalian sexual differentiation. If the ovaries normally have no role in differentiation of the sexual accessory structure of mammals, would we not predict that estrogens would fail to influence development of these struc-tures?

III. THE EFFECTS OF EXOGENOUS ESTROGENS ON EMBRYOGENESIS OF THE GENITAL SYSTEM

When estrogen preparations were administered during fetal life to geneti-cally male mammals, the Müllerian ducts developed in some species (oppos-sum, rabbit, rat, mouse) but not in others (field mouse, hamster, man). Some-times there was regression and sometimes slight stimulation of the Wolffian ducts, depending on estrogen dosage. Prostatic development was suppressed, and the penes of estrogen-treated male fetuses were small and often incom-pletely formed, resulting in a condition called hypospadias (a defect in the development of the urethra such that the canal is open on the undersurface of the penis) (these data are reviewed by Burns, 1961). If we consider these consequences of estrogen treatment one at a time, we arrive at the realization that estrogen did not bring them about through one mechanism only. First, the fact that the Müllerian duct develops in some species suggests that, at the doses used in these species, Müllerian duct-inhibiting substance is not active to its normal extent. Alternatively, exogenous estrogen may compensate for any loss of Müllerian inhibitor that it caused. In species in which fetal estrogen treatment failed to prevent Müllerian duct regression, it may be presumed that the estrogen treatment failed to prevent the secretion or action of Müllerian inhibitor. The finding that there was sometimes stimulation of the Wolffian ducts may be termed a "paradoxical effect" of estrogen. Paradoxical effects of hormones occur when excessively high doses are used. In this instance, estrogen may have been given in a large enough quantity to mimic some action of testicular androgen. It has long been known that in castrated adult mammals exogenous estrogen stimulates at least some morphological responses in the male genital tract (Burrows, 1949). Furthermore, structures such as the seminal vesicle take up and retain significant quantities of radioactive estradiol (Marrone and Feder, 1977). It is unlikely, however, that testicular androgens must be converted (aromatized) to estrogens in order to stimulate Wolffian duct differentiation. (In Chapter 6, we shall see that aromatization of androgens may play an obligatory role in brain differentiation.)

That Wolffian duct, prostatic, and penile development should have been inhibited by fetal estrogen treatment seems contradictory to the finding that estrogen sometimes stimulates the Wolffian ducts. The explanation of this inhibition lies either in an indirect action of estrogen mediated by the testis, or in a direct effect of estrogen on the Wolffian duct, urogenital sinus, and genital tubercle. That is, estrogen treatment of the fetus may have caused a "functional castration" or "chemical castration" by interference with the secretion of testicular androgens. If this were so, the sexual accessory anlagen would have suffered a deficit of androgen stimulation. Consistent with this idea, it has been demonstrated that treatment of perinatal rats with estrogen results in severely decreased testicular size (Kincl et al., 1963; Feder, 1967) and decreased testicular secretion of androgen in adulthood (Jean et al., 1975). An alternative, but not mutually exclusive notion is that estrogen acts as an antiandrogen within the Wolffian ducts, urogenital sinus, and genital elevation by diminishing their ability to take up androgens. In the urogenital elevation, estrogen might also interfere with conversion of testosterone to 5α-dihydrotestosterone (Yanaihara and Troen, 1972; Denef et al., 1973). Such direct interference, if it exists (Wilson, 1975), would not be compensated for by the presence of even large quantities of exogenous estrogen, because these anlagen depend on non-aromatizable 5α-dihydrotestosterone for their differentiation.

Estrogens were also administered to female rodent fetuses, with the results that the Müllerian duct derivatives showed hypertrophy, there was some stimulation (depending on dosage) of the Wolffian ducts, and the urogenital sinus and genital elevation differentiated into a vagina, clitoris, and labia majora and minora (reviewed by Burns, 1961). Consideration of these effects of estrogen in females buttresses the conclusions about estrogen action derived from work on males. The fact that the Müllerian ducts differentiate in females given estrogen is not surprising, because the testicular Müllerian duct-inhibiting substance is not present. The hypertrophy of Müllerian duct derivatives in estrogenized females indicates that estrogen receptors are present in uterine tissue rather early in development. (Clark and Gorski, 1970, demonstrated uterine estrogen receptors in neonatal rats.) Stimulation of Wolffian duct growth in females is truly a paradoxical effect forced by nonphysiological dose ranges of estrogen, because such growth does not normally occur in females. As expected, differentiation of the vagina, clitoris, and labia is not prevented by administration of estrogen to fetal females. Such differentiation occurs if androgens are absent, and the presence or absence of estrogen is irrelevant to this process.

Despite the temporary confusion arising from results with fetal estrogen treatments, the work of experimental embryologists since the time of Bouin and Ancel (1903) has rather consistently pointed to the following principles of sex differentiation in mammals.

1. Each individual, regardless of genotype, is sexually bipotential early in prenatal life.
2. Each sexual accessory structure passes through an early stage of development during which it is not yet competent to respond to steroid stimulation.
3. Later in prenatal development, the sexual accessory structures pass through a period during which they are able to respond to steroids. This period coincides with the time that the fetal testis is an active secretory gland.
4. The steroids released by the testis cause masculinization of sexual accessory tissues, whereas the absence of testicular secretions results in morphological feminization.
5. Afterward, the newly differentiated tissues are stabilized, and their course of development can no longer be reversed.

Each step of the normal sexual differentiation process that we have discussed can, and sometimes does, go wrong. Because the process consists of a linked chain of events (Fig. 5), distortion of one of the events early in the process may cause distortions of all subsequent aspects of sexual differentiation. We have already mentioned freemartinism, and this is one example of normal differentiation gone astray. In the following sections, a few representative abnormalities of sex determination, gonadal development, and sexual accessory tissue development will be selected and analyzed.

IV. DISTURBANCES IN EMBRYOGENESIS OF THE GENITAL SYSTEM

A. Disturbances of the Sex Determination Process

A widely known disturbance in the mammalian sex determination process is attributable to a sex chromosome abnormality that results in an XXY constitution (Klinefelter's syndrome). Because the presence of the Y chromosome

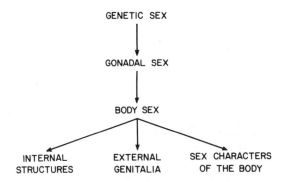

Figure 5. Linkage of events in sexual differentiation. (Reproduced with permission from Jost, 1970.) The figure is somewhat misleading in that genetic factors may be significant not only at the first stage but as an interactive element thoughout the entire period of development.

is somehow crucial (with the exceptions described in Section IV. B) for testicular differentiation, we anticipate the XXY individuals will have testes and will be phenotypic males. In fact, XXY human males present the following symptoms in adulthood: small testes, variable penile development, masculine genital duct derivatives that are smaller than normal, a small prostate, and, frequently, gynecomastia. These individuals are sterile (Overzier, 1963). Thus, the presence of the Y chromosome is compatible with differentiation of a testis and consequent masculinization of the internal and external genitalia. However, the presence of the extra X chromosome somehow prevents total functional normality of the testes, and the sexual accessory tissues are thereby reduced in size.

Another syndrome that has been brought to light relatively recently involves humans with XYY constitutions. These individuals apparently possess normal male genitalia, are taller than normal, and score lower on certain IQ tests than normal subjects. However, such men are no more likely than XXY males to be abnormally aggressive (Witkin *et al.*, 1976). Both the XXY and XYY syndromes conform to the rule that presence of the Y chromosome confers a masculine pattern of gonadal differentiation upon mammals.

B. Disturbances of Gonadal Differentiation

The view that the Y chromosome is solely responsible for gonadal masculinization in mammals will almost certainly have to be modified in the light of recent evidence to the contrary. Humans with 46,XX karyotypes but having both testicular and ovarian tissue (true hermaphroditism) accompanied by a basically male phenotype with regard to internal and external genitalia have been found (Rosenberg *et al.*, 1963). Similarly, instances of goats (Hamerton *et al*., 1969) and mice (Cattanach *et al*., 1971) lacking a Y chromosome but having testicular rather than ovarian tissue have been described. It is thought that an autosomal gene is responsible for these examples of testicular differentiation in the absence of the Y chromosome. We have already mentioned that in *Drosophila*, the autosomes play a role in sex determination.

There are also examples of failure of gonads to develop beyond rudimentary "streaks" (gonadal dysgenesis) in humans with 46,XY constitution (Federman, 1973). These individuals appear as phenotypic females because of their failure to produce adequate quantities of androgen and Müllerian duct inhibitor from the rudimentary gonads. It is thought that a gene on the X chromosome is defective in these individuals, and that normal testis differentiation requires the participation of this X chromosome factor (Goldstein and Wilson, 1973). These data fit well with Hamerton's (1968) idea, discussed earlier, that male-determining genes are actually located on the X chromosome but are normally activated by the presence of the Y chromosome. The existence of these gonadally dysgenic 46,XY individuals proves that the presence of a Y chromosome is not sufficient to insure full testicular development, just as the absence of the Y chromosome does not automatically rule out differentiation of testicular tissue in 46,XX individuals.

Gonadal dysgenesis may also occur in individuals with other genotypes, such as 46,XX. The existence of this anomaly in humans has been interpreted as implying the participation of an autosomal factor in normal ovarian differentiation (Goldstein and Wilson, 1973). A widely recognized form of gonadal dysgenesis in humans occurs in the context of an XO constitution (commonly referred to as Turner's syndrome). Individuals with an XO chromosomal pattern have rudimentary gonads that are basically of ovarian structure, but they lack germ cells and follicles. The internal and external genitalia are of the female type, but they are hypoplastic and infantile because of lack of estrogenic stimulation (Hauser, 1963). In mice, XO individuals have ovaries with germ cells and are fertile (Short, 1972).

C. Disturbances of Androgen Action

Androgen activity during sexual differentiation can be unusually low or unusually high. There are several ways in which each of these abnormalities may come about.

1. Unusually Low Androgen Activity

We have seen that testosterone and its metabolite, 5α-dihydrotestosterone, both have roles in genital differentiation. One obvious way in which low androgen activity can occur is through defective synthesis of these androgens during sexual differentiation. Experiments with fetal rats have used synthetic steroid analogues to inhibit enzymatic processes that lead to the synthesis of testosterone. The production of male pseudohermaphrodites that are phenocopies* of human syndromes arising from genetically caused defects in these enzymatic processes is reported (Goldman *et al.*, 1976b). Goldstein and Wilson (1973) review a number of papers that indicate that insufficient testosterone synthesis occurs as a result of deficient enzyme action at any one of five points in the metabolic pathway from cholesterol to testosterone. These enzyme deficiencies are transmitted via autosomal recessive genes in humans. In XY individuals, such defects in androgen synthesis lead to pseudohermaphroditism, whereas in XX individuals, there is no pseudohermaphroditism. These findings are concordant with the hypothesis, derived from work with nonprimate mammals, that adequate androgen stimulation is required for masculinization of the genitalia, and absence of androgen permits differentiation of the genitalia in a feminine direction.

If testosterone synthesis is abnormally low, one would expect 5α-dihydrotestosterone synthesis, for which testosterone is a substrate, to be subnormal. However, there are also instances in which testosterone formation is normal, but the enzyme responsible for conversion of testosterone to 5α-dihydrotestosterone is somehow deficient. A fascinating account of such an enzyme deficiency in humans has appeared (Imperato-McGinley *et al.*, 1974). In the Dominican Republic, 24 male pseudohermaphrodites (46,XY) were studied. These individuals were raised as girls. At birth, each had a labial-like scrotum, a blind vaginal pouch, a clitoral-like phallus, bilateral testes, and no Müllerian structures. At puberty, the voice deepened, muscle mass increased, the phallus enlarged to become a penis, breast development was absent, spermatogenesis was present, and postpubertal psychosexual orientation was masculine. However, the prostate remained small, and beard growth was scanty. The authors of this account demonstrated that 5α-dihydrotestosterone conversion was subnormal and concluded that the female-like appearance of external genitalia at birth and the lack of prostatic and beard growth at puberty were attributable to this defect.

Hormone action depends not only on the nature and quantity of hormone, but on the nature and state of the tissues with which the hormone reacts. Thus, deficiency of androgen action may result not only from inadequate androgen synthesis but also from a lack of responsivity of the target tissues for androgen. The most outstanding and instructive example of tissue unresponsiveness to androgen is found in the syndrome known as "testicular feminization." This syndrome occurs in humans and has close analogues in certain strains of androgen-insensitive mice (Lyon and Hawkes, 1970) and rats (Stanley *et al.*, 1973). In the human, the complete form of testicular feminization is inherited as an X-linked recessive or X-limited dominant trait (Federman, 1967). The individual is a phenotypic female with female external genitalia, female body build, and breast development (Fig. 6). There is an absence of internal female

---

*A phenocopy is an environmentally induced change in an organism that is similar to a mutation but is nonhereditary.

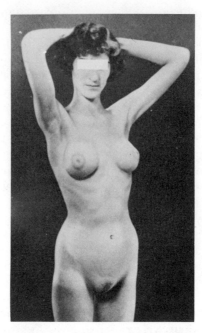

Figure 6. A 21-year-old with testicular feminization syndrome. Note well-developed breasts, no axillary hair, scanty pubic hair. (Reproduced with permission from Hauser, 1963.)

genitalia. The individual is genetically male (46,XY) and has bilateral testes that often remain within the abdomen. There is a lack of facial, axillary, and pubic hair. The behavior and gender identity of these individuals are unambiguously female (Hauser, 1963).

An understanding of the physiological basis of this disorder came gradually. At first, it was thought that the synthesis of androgen might be subnormal. Measurements of testosterone in adults with testicular feminization showed that plasma values were within the normal range for males (Southern *et al.*, 1965). Next, it was thought that conversion of testosterone to estrogen might be abnormally high in affected individuals. This too was found not to be the case (French *et al.*, 1966). Nor did lack of conversion of testosterone to 5α-dihydrotestosterone seem to be involved (Strickland and French, 1969). Investigators then turned from examination of the hormones to study of the target tissues to understand this remarkable syndrome. Studies with animal preparations were performed. Because androgen-insensitive male mice and rats lack seminal vesicles and prostates, other potential target tissues for androgens such as the preputial gland, kidney, and submandibular gland were used as test substrates (reviewed by Chan and O'Malley, 1976). From these studies, it was concluded that the primary defect in rodent target tissue androgen responsiveness resided in the inability of cells of these tissues to transfer 5α-dihydrotestosterone from the cytoplasm to the nucleus. In humans, fewer data are available, but they indicate that "testicular feminization results from a mutation of an X-linked gene specifying a dihydrotestosterone receptor" (reviewed by

Chan and O'Malley, 1976). All of these data fit well with the deduction made by Wilkins (1950) that testicular feminization is basically a disorder of end organ responsiveness to androgens rather than a disturbance of androgen secretion.

2. Unusually High Androgen Activity

If subnormal androgen activity caused by hormonal or tissue factors results in genital feminization of differentiating genetic males, one might expect that hypernormal androgen activity would result in genital masculinization of differentiating genetic females. Findings that support this contention have been reported.

In humans, overproduction of adrenal androgens sometimes occurs during gestation. Figure 7 outlines the sequence of events leading to this disruption

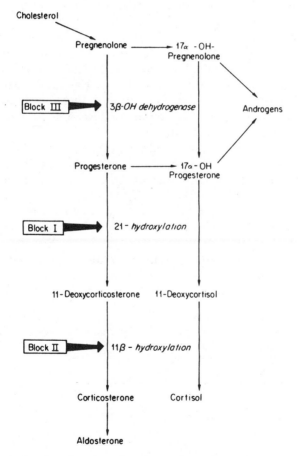

Figure 7. Deficiencies in adrenal enzymes found in various adrenogenital syndromes. (Reproduced with permission from Schulster *et al.*, 1976.) Note that Blocks I and III result in increased androgen production. The increased androgen production by the adrenal does not result in inhibition of ACTH secretion, so adrenal androgen continues to be produced at high levels.

of normal development. If the fetus is female, the external genitalia will be masculinized to a variable degree, depending on the severity of adrenal androgen overproduction. In such cases of "adrenogenital syndrome," genetic females retain a uterus and Fallopian tubes (no testes are present, so there is no Müllerian duct inhibitor produced) and do not possess highly masculinized internal genitalia (the adrenal androgens begin to be produced too late to effectively masculinize the internal genitalia). Furthermore, adrenal androgens such as androstenedione are less potent virilizers than testicular androgens such as testosterone (Goldstein and Wilson, 1973; Schultz and Wilson, 1974). Unfortunately, some human female fetuses have been exposed to exogenous synthetic compounds (progestins) with androgenic properties. The rationale for such treatment was prevention of abortion, but the consequence was dose-dependent masculinization of the developing external genitalia, as in the adrenogenital syndrome (Money and Ehrhardt, 1972).

Clemens (1974) has reported another way in which excessive androgens may reach the developing female fetus and cause genital masculinization. He demonstrated, in rats, that female fetuses adjacent to male fetuses had longer anogenital distances and larger phalluses (characteristics of males) than female fetuses adjacent to other females (Table 2). Presumably, androgens produced by the male fetuses affected the female siblings. However, the manner in which the androgens were transferred between fetuses was not established, and the relationship of this phenomenon to human development under conditions of multiple birth remains uncertain.

In this discussion of abnormally high androgen activity in developing females, examples of overabundance of androgen have been given. At this time, no examples of human syndromes that reflect a supersensitivity of differentiating genital tissues in the female to the actions of normal quantities of androgen have been described. However, animal models in which there are strain differences in responsiveness to androgen are available (Price and Williams-Ashman, 1961). From the preceding discussion, one might suppose that wide variations in tissue sensitivity to androgen among differentiating human females may eventually be found to exist.

Table 2. Relation of Anogenital Distance (AgD) in Female Rats to the Location of a Male Fetus *in Utero*[a]

Uterine position	N	$\bar{x}$AgD ± S.D. (cm)
F	5	2.9 ± 0.1
FFFM	6	2.6 ± 0.2
FFM	14	3.0 ± 0.1
FM	36	3.1 ± 0.1
MFM	14	3.3 ± 0.1

[a] Means refer to females designated *F* in the first column. F, female fetus; M, male fetus. Data taken from Clemens (1974).

D. Disturbances of Müllerian Duct Inhibitor Action

The existence of another type of disturbance might also be inferred from the foregoing material on normal differentiation. That is, a genetic male with androgen-secreting testes may have a defect in production of Müllerian duct inhibitor substance or a defect in the ability of Müllerian duct derivatives to respond to the inhibitor substance. Indeed, a syndrome has been described in humans wherein genetic males with testes, differentiated Wolffian ducts, and normal external genitalia also possess a uterus and Fallopian tubes (Nilson, 1939; Potashnik et al., 1977).

It is conceivable that absence of a uterus and Fallopian tubes in otherwise normal human females (Hauser and Schreiner, 1961) may result from production of a Müllerian duct inhibitor substance by nontesticular tissue. Alternatively, the existence of an abnormal gene that prevents Müllerian duct differentiation might be posited (Goldstein and Wilson, 1973).

With this brief review of abnormalities of the differentiation process, consideration of the rules of development for the genital tissues is completed. However, some major principles of genital differentiation that have been discussed may also apply to the development of another sexually dimorphic character, namely, the pattern of gonadotropin release.

V. DIFFERENTIATION OF GONADOTROPIN RELEASE SYSTEMS

In 1936, Carroll Pfeiffer wrote a classic paper in endocrinology that clearly showed that differentiation of gonadotropin release patterns in the adult was dependent on gonadal influences exerted early in life. His studies, using rats as experimental subjects, are summarized in Table 3. Examination of the data indicates that they are similar, in certain respects, to those obtained in experiments dealing with differentiation of genitalia. That is, at some early stage of development the presence of testes insures a masculine, tonic pattern of gonadotropin release, one that is incapable of mediating ovulation in rats given ovarian transplants in adulthood. The absence of testicular secretions during early development leads to a feminine, cyclic pattern of gonadotropin release, one that can mediate ovulation in genetic females as well as in genetic, perinatally castrated males given ovarian transplants in adulthood. The presence or absence of the ovary during early development is inconsequential in that a feminine pattern of gonadotropin release develops as long as the adult is given an ovarian transplant.* Although these major conclusions were clear, details

*Döhler (1978) proposes that ovarian hormones are involved in the differentiation of female characteristics. According to his model, low levels of estrogens may "imprint" a female differentiation of neural tissues subserving reproduction, and higher levels of estrogen (derived from aromatization of testicular androgens) may "imprint" a male differentiation of these tissues.

Table 3. Summary of Results Obtained by Pfeiffer (1936) after Experimental Manipulation of Perinatal Rats

Sex	Treatment at birth	Treatment in adulthood	Evidence of ovulation
♂	Gonadectomy	Receives ovarian transplant	Yes
♀	Gonadectomy	Receives ovarian transplant	Yes
♂	Receives testis transplant	Receives ovarian transplant	No
♀	Receives testis transplant	None	No
♂[a]	None	Gonadectomized and receives ovarian transplant	No

[a] This group was tested by Goodman (1934).

were lacking. For example, at what age did the testis exert its masculinizing action on tissues that regulate ovulation? Could androgens or other steroids substitute for the testis in the masculinization of gonadotropin secretion patterns? Where did the testicular product act in order to produce an anovulatory state? Did the developing female mammal possess mechanisms that "protected" it from masculinization of the gonadotropin release system?

A. Age Factors in Differentiation of Gonadotropin Release Patterns

In the 1940s, several workers administered testosterone to female rats prenatally and during the first month of postnatal life. Rats injected prenatally usually ovulated in adulthood, but females that received their first androgen injection within the first two weeks of postnatal life usually did not ovulate in adulthood (Bradbury, 1941; Huffman, 1941; Wilson *et al.*, 1941). The analysis of the limits of the period of susceptibility to androgen was greatly aided by Barraclough's technique of administration of a single injection of testosterone propionate to female rats of various ages (Barraclough, 1961). Results indicated that testosterone propionate (dosage = 1 .25 mg/rat) given on postnatal day 2 or 5 caused anovulatory sterility in adult female rats. When injection was delayed until day 10, some but not all, females were rendered anovulatory. Injection on day 20 did not cause anovulatory sterility. These data suggested that a "critical period" or "period of maximal susceptibility" for masculinization of gonadotropin release patterns occurred within the first 5 days of postnatal life in rats.

Still further refinement of the analysis of temporal factors was provided by the elegant work of Yazaki (1960) and of Harris (1970). Yazaki found that castration of male rats on postnatal days 1–3 resulted in a female pattern of cyclic release of hormones. This was assessed by grafts of vaginal and ovarian tissue into the castrated males in adulthood and observations of the occurrence of cycles of vaginal cornification. Apparently, males castrated within the first 3 days of postnatal life released gonadotropins in a cyclic manner. This induced cycles of ovarian function that were reflected in cycles of vaginal cornification.

Castration of males at 5 days of age did not lead to cyclic activity of ovarian and vaginal grafts in adulthood.

Thus, maximal sensitivity to masculinizing effects of testicular secretions on gonadotropin release appeared to occur within the first 3 days of postnatal life in rats. Harris' data suggested that the very first day of postnatal life in rats was most critical. He castrated male rats at 1 day of age and, in adulthood, performed intraocular transplants of ovarian tissue. The transplants showed evidence of cyclic ovulation in 58/61 cases. When castration was performed on day 2, the ratio was 7/33, and when castration was carried out on day 3 or later, the ratio was 0/33. These combined data suggest that the secretions of the testis are more effective in masculinization of the pattern of gonadotropin release within 24 hr after birth in rats, but that exogenous androgen, if given in large enough quantities over the first 5 days of life, can cause such masculinization in almost all individuals.

Obviously, there is a dosage–time interaction that determines the limits of the period during which masculinization of gonadotropin release patterns can occur (Gorski, 1966; Tarttelin *et al.*, 1975). In related studies, it has been found that administration of low doses of testosterone propionate (e.g., 10–30 μg) given during the first few days of postnatal life to female rats gives rise to a syndrome in which there are some ovulatory cycles followed by a state of permanent anovulatory sterility. This is known as the delayed anovulation syndrome (Swanson and van der Werff ten Bosch, 1964; Gorski, 1968).

In short-gestation species such as mice (Barraclough and Leathem, 1954), masculinization of gonadotropin release patterns is also accomplished most readily by hormone manipulations within the first few days after birth. However, in long-gestation rodents such as guinea pigs, anovulatory sterility is induced by prenatal androgen treatment. In guinea pigs, such treatment is most effective when initiated on day 33 of pregnancy (Brown-Grant and Sherwood, 1971).

The situation appears to be even more radically different in primates. Prenatal androgenization of female rhesus macaque monkeys delays menarche but does not ultimately prevent the occurrence of ovulation (Wells and van Wagenen, 1954; Goy, 1970). In humans, females affected by the adrenogenital syndrome or inadvertent prenatal androgenization are still capable of ovulation in adulthood (Money and Ehrhardt, 1972). Thus, there are considerable species differences of a quantitative and qualitative nature in the ability of androgens to induce a tonic pattern of gonadotropin release. Some of these species differences will be discussed in more detail in Sections V. B–D.

B. Steroidal Factors in Differentiation of Gonadotropin Release Patterns

We have just discussed some experiments in which exogenous testosterone preparations were effective in masculinization of gonadotropin release patterns in female rodents. Thus, it is apparent that certain testosterone preparations can mimic the effects of testicular secretions on differentiation of the gonadotropin system (Harris, 1964). The finding that injection of estradiol preparations, even in rather low doses, to neonatal female rats also causes anovulatory sterility (Gorski, 1963; Zucker and Feder, 1966; Dörner et al., 1971) eventually led to the hypothesis that androgen secreted by the neonatal rat testis is converted within the brain to estrogen (Reddy et al., 1974; Weisz and Gibbs, 1974) and that this estrogen is directly responsible for masculinization of the gonadotropin regulatory system.

The hypothesis receives solid support from the finding that synthetic antiestrogens block the masculinizing action of androgens on the patterning of gonadotropin release in rats (McDonald and Doughty, 1972). In addition, androgens that are convertible to estrogens (aromatizable androgens) are more effective than nonaromatizable androgens in virilization of the gonadotropin regulatory system (McDonald and Doughty, 1974). Nonetheless, some caution should be exercised before the hypothesis is accepted. Unconverted androgen may still be capable of reaching and being bound by neural and pituitary tissues involved in gonadotropin regulation (Sheridan et al., 1974). Androgens that are not converted to estrogens (e.g., 5α-dihydrotestosterone) may permanently affect gonadotropin release systems in rats under special circumstances (Gerall et al., 1976). Species other than rats may rely on testosterone or other androgens, rather than on estrogen, for masculinization of the gonadotropin release system. This is to be expected particularly among species that do not possess adequate enzymes for conversion of androgen to estrogen in the brain. Compounds that cannot be converted to either androgen or estrogen (e.g., adrenal corticoids) have, on occasion, been shown to masculinize gonadotropin control systems in rats (Takewaki, 1962).

One reason for this apparent nonspecificity (androgens, estrogens, and corticoids have been shown to virilize gonadotropin patterns) may reside in the nature of the response being studied. The response that is being observed is a failure to ovulate in adulthood. That is, some mechanism responsible for mediation of ovulation is being experimentally manipulated and disrupted. It is easy to see that disruption of a biological process such as ovulation might occur in many ways, some of them not directly related to one another or to normal physiological processes. In this sense, the study of differentiation of gonadotropin release patterns is more likely to be clouded by artifact than either the study of genital differentiation or the investigation of sex behavior differentiation. For the genital system, there are independent measures of masculinization (e.g., development of the Wolffian ducts) and feminization (e.g., development of Müllerian ducts). Even when a single anlage differentiates in a masculine or femine direction, the response to hormone manipulation is graded rather than all-or-none (e.g., differentiation of genital tubercle).

For sex behavior, differentiations of male and female capacities are independent processes (see Chapter 6), and these capacities, in at least some respects, are related to perinatal androgen dosage in a graded fashion. However, for the differentiation of gonadotropin control systems, the same perinatal treatment that "masculinizes" also "defeminizes" these systems. There are not two independent processes of masculinization and feminization for the gonadotropin release pattern. Furthermore, the usually observed response of the gonadotropin release system to perinatal hormone manipulation is an all-or-none rather than a graded one. With the exception of the delayed anovulation syndrome, ovulation either occurs in adulthood in an individual or it does not.

C. Site of Action of Hormones Involved in Differentiation of Gonadotropin Release Patterns

When Pfeiffer interpreted his data on the differentiation of gonadotropin release patterns, he was influenced by a prevailing opinion that steroids produced by the gonads acted on the anterior pituitary, and this gland regulated gonadal activity by a negative feedback or "push–pull" mechanism (Moore and Price, 1932). Not surprisingly, Pfeiffer opined that the site of action of testicular steroids in the masculinization of gonadotropin release pattern was the anterior pituitary gland. This hypothesis was shown to be erroneous. For example, Harris and Jacobsohn (1952) and Martinez and Bittner (1956) demonstrated that the rodent anterior pituitary gland is not sexually differentiated. They took normal adult male pituitaries and transplanted them under the median eminence of hypophysectomized adult females. Estrous cycles resumed in these females, indicating there was no intrinsic lack of ability of pituitaries exposed to perinatal androgens (as is the case for pituitaries from normal males) to mediate cyclic patterns of gonadotropin release adequate for ovulation. Subsequent work has demonstrated that pituitaries of perinatally androgenized female rats are as sensitive as pituitaries of nonandrogenized rats to the actions of GnRH (Mennin et al., 1974).

In 1961, Barraclough and Gorski, and in 1963, Gorski and Barraclough demonstrated that the masculinizing actions of perinatal androgen on gonadotropin release patterns in rats were exerted on the brain rather than directly on the pituitary gland. Female rats were given either 1250 or 10 μg of testosterone propionate on day 5 of postnatal life. In adulthood, these animals failed to ovulate. However, electrical stimulation of the arcuate–ventromedial nucleus area (Arc–Vmn) of the hypothalamus stimulated ovulation in some animals of the 10-μg dosage group. When progesterone treatment was given to the adult females prior to electrical stimulation, the 1250-μg dosage group ovulated when the electrodes were in the Arc-Vmn, and the 10-μg dosage group ovulated when the electrodes were in either the Arc-Vmn or suprachiasmatic nucleus–preoptic area (Scn–POA).

The authors concluded that the low (10 μg) dose of testosterone propionate primarily affected the Scn–POA, whereas the high (1250 μg) dose affected both the Scn–POA and Arc–Vmn areas in such a way as to inhibit the abilities of these areas to mediate ovulation. Further work by these authors suggested the notion that in normal females the Scn–POA area is responsible for cyclic discharges that affect the tonic activity of the Arc–Vmn region. The Arc–Vmn region is thereby driven to act cyclically by the Scn–POA and to synthesize and release GnRH in a cyclic manner. The cyclic release of GnRH causes cyclic release of ovulatory hormone from the pituitary. According to this scheme, secretions of the testes during the perinatal period (or exogenous steroids) permanently dampen the ability of the Scn–POA to induce cyclic activity of the Arc–Vmn and thereby produce an exclusively tonic, or masculinized pattern of gonadotropin release that is generally incapable of mediating ovulation (Fig. 8).

This idea has had a significant impact on sex differentiation research, and it is concordant with a mass of data that implicates the Scn in rhythmic neural function (Zucker *et al.*, 1976). It also fits well with data that show that lesions of the Scn–POA inhibit ovulation in rats and that knife cuts that disrupt pathways between the Scn–POA and Arc–Vmn inhibit ovulation in rats (Halász and Gorski, 1967; Blake *et al.*, 1972; Neill, 1972; Norman *et al.*, 1972). However, it must be borne in mind that other experiments suggest that the inability of perinatally androgenized female rats to ovulate in response to electrochemical stimulation may have been attributable to decreased sensitivity of the ovaries to LH (Mennin *et al.*, 1974) or to diminished sensitivity of the neuroendocrine system to exogenous progesterone (Clemens *et al.*, 1969, 1970) rather than to

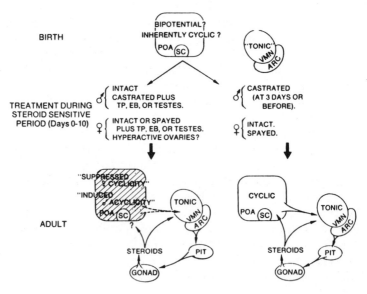

Figure 8. A model proposed to account for the influence of perinatal hormones on sexual differentiation of the hypothalamic regulation of LH secretion. ARC, arcuate nucleus; EB, estradiol benzoate; PIT, pituitary; POA, preoptic area; SC, suprachiasmatic nucleus; TP, testosterone propionate; VMN, ventromedial nucleus. (Reproduced with permission from Gorski and Wagner, 1965.)

differences in sensitivity to electrochemical stimulation between normal and perinatally androgenized rats (Kubo *et al.*, 1975).

Intracranial implantation of testosterone or estradiol pellets into neonatal female rats has also been performed, and this technique has implicated both the POA and Arc–Vmn regions in the differentiation of gonadotropin control. Thus, inhibition of ovulatory capacity was observed when such implants were located either in the POA or Arc–Vmn region (Wagner *et al.*, 1966; Nadler, 1973; Hayashi and Gorski, 1974; Döcke and Dörner, 1975). These implants may cause decreases in the ability of hypothalamic tissues to respond to estrogen stimulation in adulthood. Failure of perinatally androgenized hypothalamic tissues to respond to estrogen is indicated by the finding that such tissues do not mediate a surge of prolactin release as is normally the case in female rats after exposure to estrogen in adulthood (Neill, 1972). Several studies also suggest a reduction of the ability of adult hypothalamic tissue to concentrate estrogen as a consequence of perinatal exposure of the nervous system to testicular steroids (Whalen and Massicci, 1975; Marrone and Feder, 1977) or to exogenous androgen or estrogen (Flerkó *et al.*, 1969; McGuire and Lisk, 1969; Anderson and Greenwald, 1969).

In addition to the hypothalamus and preoptic area, other brain regions such as the amygdala and hippocampus have been implicated in gonadotropin regulation. For example, after perinatal androgenization, the gonadotropin-stimulating activity of the amygdala has been observed to be diminished (Kawakami and Terasawa, 1972).

We have previously noted (see Section V.A) that prenatal androgenization of rhesus monkeys or humans does not preclude the occurrence of ovulation in adulthood. It has been shown that massive surges of LH release can be induced in adult, castrated male rhesus macaques after administration of estradiol (Karsch *et al.*, 1973). Furthermore, disruption of pathways from POA–anterior hypothalamus to the Arc–Vmn region in adult rhesus monkeys does not prevent release of substantial quantities of LH in response to estradiol (Krey *et al.*, 1975a,b) as it does in adult rats.

These and related data have led some workers to propose that brain mechanisms that regulate gonadotropin release in rhesus monkeys and humans are not masculinized by the actions of prenatal steroids (Knobil, 1974). Failure of normal male rhesus monkeys or men to release massive surges of LH once every 28 days or so may be, according to this argument, attributable to the lack of corresponding periodic increases in estrogen secretion from the male gonad (testis). Such periodic increases of estrogen secretion are, of course, provided by the female gonad (ovary). Because formation of mammalian gonadal tissue is generally resistant to disturbance by steroids (Burns, 1961), prenatal androgenization of female primates does not lead to anovulatory sterility. Thus, to speak of "masculinization" of brain mechanisms that regulate gonadotropin release in rhesus monkeys and in humans as a result of prenatal androgenization of females may be inappropriate. Perhaps there are no naturally occurring sex differences in such mechanisms in primates. On the other hand, Norman *et al.* (1976) showed that bilateral destruction of the ventral POA–anterior hypothalamus compromises the ability of the hypothalamus to mediate release of LH in response to estrogen in female rhesus macaques. Steiner *et al.* (1976) also presented evidence that although male and prenatally androgenized female rhesus monkeys show a positive feedback of LH in response to estrogen in adulthood, these animals may be less sensitive than normal females to the negative feedback actions of estrogen on LH secretion. Possibly, this represents a partial "masculinization" of the rhesus brain by prenatal androgen, but other interpretations are also tenable.

D. Mechanisms for the Protection of Female Fetuses from Masculinizing Agents

We have seen that prenatal androgens and estrogens can masculinize brain tissues that mediate gonadotropin release in at least some species. Viviparity in mammals carries with it the potential danger that androgens and estrogens produced by the pregnant female might cross the placenta, reach brain receptors that can distinguish between androgen and estrogen (Fox, 1974; Attardi *et al.*, 1976), and masculinize the brains of female fetuses. A variety of protective mechanisms has evolved to diminish this danger.

In rats (Aussel *et al.*, 1973; Uriel *et al.*, 1975) and perhaps in humans (Arnon *et al.*, 1973; Nunez *et al.*, 1974; Savu *et al.*, 1974; Swartz and Soloff, 1974), a blood-borne protein, α-fetoprotein, binds estrogen and inactivates it. α-Fetoprotein is not only present during gestation, but its concentration is high during the first few critical days of postnatal life in rats. It declines to negligible levels by day 20. This has led to the supposition that α-fetoprotein protects developing rats (Plapinger and McEwen, 1975) not only from maternal estrogens but from estrogens that may be secreted by the neonate (Weisz and Gunsalus, 1973).

In guinea pigs, α-fetoprotein does not appear to exist (Savu *et al.*, 1974; Plapinger *et al.*, 1977). Instead, guinea pigs may rely on antiestrogenic and antiandrogenic properties of progesterone secreted by the corpora lutea of the pregnant female (Diamond and Young, 1963). It is conceivable that progesterone also serves this role in rats (Kincl and Maqueo, 1965; Dorfman, 1967). Some species, e.g., the guinea pig, convert large proportions of the highly potent estrogen, estradiol-17β, to other forms of estrogen such as estrone or estrogen sulfates and glucuronides (Freeman and Hobkirk, 1976; Goutte-Couissieu *et al.*, 1976) or, in the case of the human produce greatly increased quantities of weakly estrogenic estriol during pregnancy (Hopper *et al.*, 1968). Possibly, estrone and estriol compete for neural sites with estradiol and thereby dampen the effects of estradiol.

In primates, a genetic factor that insures resistance of neural circuits that mediate positive feedback effects of estrogen on LH release and resistance of neural circuits that mediate expression of behaviors with copulatory and social functions (e.g., the presenting posture in rhesus macaques) to the actions of prenatal hormones may be involved (R. W. Goy, personal communication).

None of these protective mechanisms, (a) inactivation of circulating steroids by protein binding in blood plasma, (b) antagonism of estrogen and androgen by progesterone, (c) metabolism of potent estrogens or androgens to less powerful forms, and (d) genetically dictated high resistance of neural tissues to hormone action during development, are mutually exclusive. It would not be surprising to find more than one type of protective mechanism at work in the same animal. Indeed, it would be reasonable to expect that the extremely important job of prevention of anovulatory sterility in females would not be entrusted to a single mechanism.

Some investigators have attempted to understand the mechanism of action of perinatal hormones on neural tissues destined to mediate gonadotropin release by means of administration of compounds that counteract the perinatal hormones. A wide range of compounds given concurrently with androgen or estrogen in the perinatal period has been found to prevent or ameliorate steroid-induced anovulatory sterility in rats. Such "protective" compounds include tranquilizers (reserpine, chlorpromazine), barbiturates (pentobarbital, phenobarbital), antiandrogens (cyproterone acetate, progesterone), anesthetics (progesterone), and some blockers of RNA synthesis (Gorski, 1971). From this work, Gorski (1971) has estimated that a period of more than 48 hr of exposure of the nervous system of the perinatal rat to exogenous androgen is required for masculinization of the gonadotropin release system.

VI. SUMMARY

In this chapter, the rules for differentiation of the genital system and the neural tissues that mediate gonadotropin release were discussed. Androgen from the interstitial cell compartment of the testis masculinizes the Wolffian ducts, urogenital sinus, and external genital anlagen. Absence of testicular androgen during crucial periods of development results in rudimentary Wolffian ducts and feminization of the urogenital sinus and external genitalia. The testis also secretes a nonsteroidal compound from the seminiferous tubule compartment that inhibits development of the Müllerian ducts. The ovary normally plays no significant role in differentiation of the genital system. Thus, although each individual embryo is bipotential with regard to genital tract development, the presence or absence of the testis dictates whether the genital tract will be masculinized or feminized.

The presence or absence of the testis during neural differentiation also determines whether a masculine (tonic) or feminine (cyclic) pattern of gonadotropin release will be apparent in adulthood, in at least some species. In contrast to their role in genital tract and neural differentiation, steroids play little or no role in the differentiation of gonadal sex. This is genetically regulated.

ACKNOWLEDGMENTS. I am indebted to Dr. Jean Wilson for his critical reading of the manuscript, his many helpful comments, and his encouragement. I also thank Drs. I. T. Landau, Auri Naggar, and Christina Williams for their valuable suggestions. Thanks are also due to Ms. W. Cunningham, Ms. N. Jachim, and Ms. C. Banas for preparation of the manuscript.

The author was supported by NIH Research Grant HD-04467 and by Research Scientist Development Award NIMH-K2-29006. Contribution Number 299 of the Institute of Animal Behavior.

REFERENCES

Anderson, C. H., and Greenwald, G. S., 1969, Autoradiographic analysis of estradiol uptake in the brain and pituitary of the female rat, *Endocrinology* **85**:1160.

Arey, L. B., 1954, *Developmental Anatomy*, Sixth Edition, W. B. Saunders, Philadelphia.

Arnon, R., Teicher, E., Bustin, M., and Sela, M., 1973, Preparation of antisera to α-fetoprotein making use of estradiol affinity column, *FEBS Lett.* **32**:335.

Attal, J., 1969, Levels of testosterone, androstenedione, estrone and estradiol-17β in the testes of fetal sheep, *Endocrinology* **85**:280.

Attardi, B., Geller, L. M., and Susumu, O., 1976, Androgen and estrogen receptors in brain cytosol from male, female and testicular feminized (tfm/y ♂) mice, *Endocrinology* **98**:864.

Aussel, C., Uriel, J., and Mercier-Bodard, C., 1973, Rat alpha-fetoprotein: Isolation, characterization and estrogen-binding properties, *Biochimie* **55**:1431.

Baker, T. G., 1972, Primordial germ cells, in: *Reproduction in Mammals, Book I, Germ Cells and Fertilization* (C. R. Austin, and R. V. Short, eds.), pp. 1–13, Cambridge University Press, New York.

Barraclough, C. A., 1961, Production of anovulatory, sterile rats by single injections of testosterone propionate, *Endocrinology* **34**:62.

Barraclough, C. A., and Gorski, R. A., 1961, Evidence that the hypothalamus is responsible for androgen-induced sterility in the female rat, *Endocrinology* **68**:68.

Barraclough, C. A., and Leathem, J. H., 1954, Infertility induced in mice by a single injection of testosterone propionate, *Proc. Soc. Exp. Biol. Med.* **85**:673.

Beach, F. A., 1971, Hormonal factors controlling the differentiation, development, and display of copulatory behavior in the ramstergig and related species, in: *The Biopsychology of Development* (E. Tobach, L. R. Aronson, and E. Shaw, eds.), pp. 249–296, Academic Press, New York.

Beatty, R. A., 1970, Genetic basis for the determination of sex, *Phil. Trans. R. Soc. Lond.* [*Biol.*] **259**:3.

Blake, C. A., Weiner, R. I., Gorski, R. A., and Sawyer, C. H., 1972, Secretion of pituitary luteinizing hormone and follicle stimulating hormone in female rats made persistently estrous or diestrous by hypothalamic deafferentation, *Endocrinology* **90**:855.

Bloch, E., Gupta, C., Feldman, S., and Van Damme, O., 1974, Testosterone production by testes of fetal rats and mice, in: *Endocrinologie Sexuelle de la Période Périnatale*, Vol. 32 (M. G. Forest and J. Bertrand, eds.), pp. 177–189, INSERM, Paris.

Bouin, P., and Ancel, P., 1903, Sur la signification de la glande interstitielle du testicule embryonnaire, *C. R. Soc. Biol. (Paris)* **55**:1682.

Bradbury, J. T., 1941, Permanent after-effects following masculinization of the infantile female rat, *Endocrinology* **28**:101.

Brewer, N. L., 1962, Sex differentiation of the fetal mouse *in vitro*, Ph.D. thesis, University of Chicago, Chicago.

Bridges, C. B., 1939, Cytological and genetic basis of sex, in: *Sex and Internal Secretions* (E. Allen, ed.), pp. 15–63, Baillière, Tindall and Cox, London.

Brown-Grant, K., 1974, On "critical periods" during the post-natal development of the rat, in: *Endocrinologie Sexuelle de la Période Périnatale,* Vol. 32 (M. Forest and J. Bertrand, eds.), pp. 357–375, INSERM, Paris.

Brown-Grant, K., and Sherwood, M. R., 1971, The "early androgen syndrome" in the guinea-pig, *J. Endocrinol.* **49**:277.

Burns, R. K., 1939, Sex differentiation during the early pouch stages of the opossum (*Didelphys virginiana*) and a comparison of the anatomical changes induced by male and female sex hormones, *J. Morphol.* **65**:497.

Burns, R. K., 1955a, Experimental reversal of sex in the gonads of the opossum, *Didelphys virginiana, Proc. Natl. Acad. Sci. USA* **41**:669.

Burns, R. K., 1955b, Urogenital system, in: *Analysis of Development* (B. H. Willier, P. A. Weiss, and V. Hamburger, eds.), W. B. Saunders, Philadelphia.

Burns, R. K., 1961, Role of hormones in the differentiation of sex, in: *Sex and Internal Secretions,* Third Edition (W. C. Young, ed.), pp. 76–158, Williams & Wilkins, Baltimore.

Burrows, H., 1949, *Biological Actions of Sex Hormones*, Cambridge University Press, New York.

Cattanach, B. M., Pollard, C. E., and Hawkes, S. G., 1971, Sex reversed mice: XX and XO males, *Cytogenetics* **10**:318.

Challis, J. R. G., Kim, C. K., Naftolin, F., Judd, H. L., Yen, S. S. C., and Benirschke, K., 1974, The concentrations of androgens, oestrogens, progesterone and luteinizing hormone in the serum of foetal calves throughout the course of gestation, *J. Endocrinol.* **60**:107.

Chan, L., and O'Malley, B. W., 1976, Mechanism of action of the sex steroid hormones, *N. Eng. J. Med.* **294**:1322,1372,1430.

Chan, S. T. H., 1970, Natural sex reversal in vertebrates, *Phil. Trans. R. Soc. Lond.* [*Biol.*] **259**:59.

Clark, J. H., and Gorski, J., 1970, Ontogeny of the estrogen receptor during early uterine development, *Science* **169**:76.

Clemens, L. G., 1974, Neurohormonal control of male sexual behavior, in: *Reproductive Behavior* (W. Montagna and W. A. Sadler, eds.), pp. 23–53, Plenum Press, New York.

Clemens, L. G., Hiroi, M., and Gorski, R. A., 1969, Induction and facilitation of female mating behavior in rats treated neonatally with low doses of testosterone propionate, *Endocrinology* **84**:1430.

Clemens, L. G., Shryne, J., and Gorski, R. A., 1970, Androgen and development of progesterone responsiveness in male and female rats, *Physiol Behav.* **5**:673.

Denef, C., Magnus, C., and McEwen, B. S., 1973, Sex differences and hormonal control of testosterone metabolism in rat pituitary and brain, *J. Endocrinol.* **59**:605.

Diamond, M., and Young, W. C., 1963, Differential responsiveness of pregnant and non-pregnant guinea pigs to the masculinizing action of testosterone propionate, *Endrocrinology* **72**:429.

Döcke, F., and Dörner, G., 1975, Anovulation in adult female rats after neonatal intracerebral implantation of oestrogen, *Endokrinologie* **65**:375.

Döhler, K. D., 1978, Is female sexual differentiation hormone-mediated?, *Trends Neurosci.* **1**:138.

Dorfman, R. I., 1967, The antiestrogenic and antiandrogenic activities of progesterone in the defense of a normal fetus, *Anat. Rec.* **157**:547.

Dörner, G., Döcke, F., and Hinz, G., 1971, Paradoxical effects of estrogen on brain differentiation, *Neuroendocrinology* **7**:146.

Elger, W., 1966, Die Rolle der fetalen Androgene in der Sexualdifferenzierung des Kaninchens und ihre Abgrenzung gegen andere hormonale und somatische Faktoren durch Anwendung eines starken Antiandrogens, *Arch. Anat. Microsc. Morphol. Exp.* **55**:657.

Feder, H. H., 1967, Specificity of testosterone and estradiol in the differentiating neonatal rat, *Anat. Rec.* **157**:79.

Federman, D. D., 1967, *Abnormal Sexual Development*, W. B. Saunders, Philadelphia.

Federman, D. D., 1973, Genetic control of sexual difference, in: *Progress in Medical Genetics*, Vol. IX (A. G. Steinberg and A. G. Bearn, eds.), pp. 215–235, Grune and Stratton, New York.

Flerkó, B., Mess, B., and Illei-Donhoffer, A., 1969, On the mechanism of androgen sterilization, *Neuroendocrinology* 4:164.

Fox, T. O., 1975, Androgen- and estrogen-binding macromolecules in developing mouse brain: Biochemical and genetic evidence, *Proc. Natl. Acad. Sci. USA* 72:4303.

Freeman, D. J., and Hobkirk, R., 1976, Metabolites of estradiol-17β in guinea pig uterus late in pregnancy, *Steroids* 28:613.

French, F. S., Van Wyk, J. J., Baggett, B., Easterling, W. E., Talbert, L. M., Johnston, F. R., Forchielli, E., and Dey, A. C., 1966, Further evidence of a target organ defect in the syndrome of testicular feminization, *J. Clin. Endocrinol. Metab.* 26:493.

Gallien, L. G., 1965, Genetic control of sexual differentiation in vertebrates, in: *Organogenesis* (R. L. de Haan and H. Ursprung, eds.), pp. 583–610, Holt, Rinehart and Winston, New York.

Gerall, A. A., Dunlap, J. L., and Wagner, R. A., 1976, Effects of dihydrotestosterone and gonadotropins on the development of female behavior, *Physiol. Behav.* 17:121.

Giles, H. R., Lox, C. D., Heine, W., and Christian, C. D., 1974, Intrauterine fetal sex determination by radioimmunoassay of amniotic fluid testosterone, *Gynecol. Invest.* 5:317.

Goldman, A. S., and Neumann, F., 1969, Differentiation of the mammary gland in experimental congenital adrenal hyperplasia due to inhibition of Δ^5, 3β;hydroxysteroid dehydrogenase in rats, *Proc. Soc. Exp. Biol. Med.* 132:237.

Goldman, A. S., Baker, M. K., Chen, J. C., and Wieland, R. G., 1972, Blockade of masculine differentiation in male rat fetuses by maternal injection of antibodies to testosterone-3-bovine serum albumin, *Endocrinology* 90:716.

Goldman, A. S., Shapiro, B. S., and Root, A. W., 1973, Inhibition of fetal masculine differentiation in the rat by maternal administration of antibodies to bovine LH, cyanoketone, or antibodies to testosterone-3-bovine serum albumin, *Proc. Soc. Exp. Biol. Med.* 143:422.

Goldman, A. S., Shapiro, B. H., and Neumann, F., 1976a, Role of testosterone and its metabolites in the differentiation of the mammary gland in rats, *Endocrinology* 99:1490.

Goldman, A. S., Eavey, R. D., and Baker, M. K., 1976b, Production of male pseudohermaphroditism in rats by two new inhibitors of steroid 17α-hydroxylase and C17-20 lyase, *J. Endocrinol.* 71:289.

Goldman, B. D., and Mahesh, V. B., 1970, Induction of infertility in male rats by treatment with gonadotropin antiserum during neonatal life, *Biol. Reprod.* 2:44.

Goldstein, J. L., and Wilson, J. D., 1973, Hereditary disorders of sexual development in man, in: *International Congress Series No. 310, Birth Defects, Proceedings Fourth International Conference, Vienna, Austria, September 1973* (A. G. Motulsky and W. Lentz, eds.), pp. 165–173, Excerpta Medica, Amsterdam.

Goodman, L., 1934, Observations on transplanted immature ovaries in the eyes of adult male and female rats, *Anat. Rec.* 59:223.

Gorski, R. A., 1963, Modification of ovulatory mechanisms by postnatal administration of estrogen to the rat, *Am. J. Physiol.* 205:842.

Gorski, R. A., 1966, Localization and sexual differentiation of the nervous structures which regulate ovulation, *J. Reprod. Fertil.* [*Suppl.*]1:67.

Gorski, R. A., 1968, Influence of age on the response to perinatal administration of a low dose of androgen, *Endocrinology* 82:1001.

Gorski, R. A., 1971, Gonadal hormones and the perinatal development of neuroendocrine function, in: *Frontiers in Neuroendocrinology* (L. Martini and W. F. Ganong, eds.), pp. 237–290, Oxford University Press, New York.

Gorski, R. A., and Barraclough, C. A., 1963, Effect of low doses of androgen on the differentiation of hypothalamic regulatory control of ovulation in the rat, *Endocrinology* 73:210.

Gorski, R. A., and Wagner, J. W., 1965, Gonadal activity and sexual differentiation of the hypothalamus, *Endocrinology* 76:226.

Goutte-Coussieu, C., Adessi, G., and Jayle, M.-F., 1976, Etude *in vitro* du métabolisme du (6,7−^{3}H) oestradiol-17β par le placenta de cobaye, *C. R. Acad. Sci. [D] (Paris)* **283**:1437.

Goy, R. W., 1970, Experimental control of psychosexuality, *Phil. Trans. R. Soc. Lond. [Biol.]* **259**:149.

Greene, R. R., 1942, Hormonal factors in sex inversion: The effects of sex hormones on embryonic sexual structures of the rat, *Biol. Symp.* **9**:105.

Greene, R. R., and Ivy, A. C., 1937, The experimental production of intersexuality in the female rat with testosterone. *Science* **86**:200.

Greene, R. R., Burrill, M. W., and Ivy, A. C., 1941, Experimental intersexuality: The effects of combined estrogens and androgens on the embryonic sexual development of the rat, *J. Exp. Zool.* **87**:211.

Halász, B., and Gorski, R. A., 1967, Gonadotrophic hormone secretion in female rats after partial or total interruption of neural afferents to the medial basal hypothalamus, *Endocrinology* **80**:608.

Hamerton, J. L., 1968, Significance of sex chromosome derived heterochromatin in mammals, *Nature* **219**:910.

Hamerton, J. L., Dickson, J. M., Pollard, C. E., Grieves, S. A., and Short, R. V., 1969, Genetic intersexuality in goats, *J. Reprod. Fertil. [Suppl.]* **7**:25.

Harris, G. W., 1964, Sex hormones, brain development and brain function, *Endocrinology* **75**:627.

Harris, G. W., 1970, Hormonal differentiation of the developing central nervous system with respect to patterns of endocrine function, *Phil. Trans. R. Soc. Lond. [Biol.]* **259**:165.

Harris, G. W., and Jacobsohn, D., 1952, Functional grafts of the anterior pituitary gland, *Proc. R. Soc. Lond. [Biol.]* **139**:263.

Hauser, G. A., 1963, Testicular feminization, in: *Intersexuality* (C. Overzier, ed.), pp. 255–276, Academic Press, New York.

Hauser, G. A., and Schreiner, W. E., 1961, Das Mayer-Rokitansky-Küster-Syndrom: Uterus bipartitus solidus rudimentarius cum vagina solida, *Schweiz, Med. Wochenschr.* **91**:381.

Hayashi, S., and Gorski, R. A., 1974, Critical exposure time for androgenization by intracranial crystals of testosterone propionate in neonatal female rats, *Endocrinology* **94**:1161.

Herschler, M. S., and Fechheimer, N. S., 1967, The role of sex chromosome chimerism in altering sexual development of mammals, *Cytogenetics* **6**:204.

Hollander, W. F., Gowen, J. W., and Stadler, J., 1956, A study of 25 gynandromorphic mice of the Bagg albino strain, *Anat. Rec.* **124**:233.

Hopper, B. R., Tullner, W. W., and Gray, C. W., 1968, Urinary estrogen excretion during pregnancy in a gorilla (*Gorilla gorilla*), *Proc. Soc. Exp. Biol. Med.* **129**:213.

Huffman, J. W., 1941, Effect of testosterone propionate in reproduction in the female, *Endocrinology* **29**:77.

Humphrey, R. R., 1928, The developmental potencies of the intermediate mesoderm of amblystoma when transplanted into ventrolateral sites in other embryos: The primordial germ cells of such grafts and their role in the development of a gonad, *Anat. Rec.* **40**:67.

Imperato-McGinley, J., Guerrero, T., Gautier, T., and Peterson, R. E., 1974, Steroid 5α-reductase deficiency in man: An inherited form of male pseudohermaphroditism, *Science* **186**:1213.

Jean, C., André, M., Jean, C., Berger, M., DeTurckheim, M., and Véyssiere, G., 1975, Estimation of testosterone and androstenedione in the plasma and testes of cryptorchid offspring of mice treated with oestradiol during pregnancy, *J. Reprod. Fertil.* **44**:235.

Josso, N., 1973, *In vitro* synthesis of Müllerian-inhibiting hormone by seminiferous tubules isolated from the calf fetal testis, *Endocrinology* **93**:829.

Josso, N., Forest, M. G., and Picard, J., 1975, Müllerian-inhibiting activity of calf fetal testes: Relationship to testosterone and protein synthesis, *Biol. Reprod.* **13**:163.

Jost, A., 1947, Recherches sur la différenciation de l'embryon de lapin. III. Rôle des gonades foetales dans la différenciation sexuelle somatique, *Arch. Anat. Microsc. Morphol. Exp.* **36**:271.

Jost, A., 1950, Sur le contrôle hormonal de différenciation sexuelle du lâpin, *Arch. Anat. Microsc. Morphol. Exp.* **39**:577.

Jost, A., 1953, Problems of fetal endocrinology: The gonadal and hypophyseal hormones, *Recent Prog. Horm. Res.* **8**:379.

Jost, A., 1966, Steroids and sex differentiation of the mammalian fetus, in: *Excerpta Medica International Congress Series, No. 132, Proceedings Iind International Congress in Hormonal Steroids, Milano* (L. Martini, F. Fraschini, and M. Motta, eds.), pp. 74–81, Excerpta Medica, Amsterdam.

Jost, A., 1970, Hormonal factors in the sex differentiation of the mammalian foetus, *Phil. Trans. R. Soc. Lond. [Biol.]* **259**:119.

Jost, A., 1972, A new look at the mechanisms controlling sex differentiation in mammals, *Johns Hopkins Med. J.* **130**:38.

Jost, A., Chodkiewicz, M., and Mauleon, P., 1963, Intersexualité du foetus de veau produite par des androgénes comparaison entre l'hormone foetale responsable du freemartinisme et l'hormone testiculaire adulte, *C. R. Acad. Sci. [D] (Paris)* **256**:274.

Karsch, F. J., Dierschke, D. J., and Knobil, E., 1973, Sexual differentiation of pituitary function: Apparent differences between primates and rodents, *Science* **179**:484.

Kawakami, M., and Terasawa, E., 1972, A possible role of the hippocampus and the amygdala in the androgenized rat: Effect of electrical or electro-chemical stimulation of the brain on gonadotropin secretion, *Endocrinol. Jpn.* **19**:349.

Keller, K., and Tandler, J., 1916, Über des Verhalten der Eihäute bei der Zwillingssträchtigkeit des Rindes. Untersuchungen über die Enstenhungsursache der geschlechtlichen Unterentwicklung von weiblichen Zwillingskälbern, welche neben einem männlichen Kalbe zur Entwicklung gelangen, *Wien Tierartz. Wochenschr.* **3**:513.

Kincl, F. A., and Maqueo, M., 1965, Prevention by progesterone of steroid-induced sterility in neonatal male and female rats, *Endocrinology* **77**:859.

Kincl, F. A., Folch-Pi, A. and Herrera Lasso, L., 1963, Effect of estradiol benzoate treatment in the newborn male rat, *Endocrinology* **72**:966.

Kirkman, H., 1958, A hypophysectomized gynandromorphic Syrian hamster, *Anat. Rec.* **131**:213.

Knobil, E., 1974, Maturation of the neuro-endocrine control of gonadotropin secretion in the Rhesus monkey in: *Endocrinologie Sexuelle de la Période Périnatale*, Vol. 32 (M. Forest and J. Bertrand, eds.), pp. 205–218, INSERM, Paris.

Krey, L. C., Butler, W. R., and Knobil, E., 1975a, Surgical disconnection of the medial basal hypothalamus and pituitary function in the rhesus monkey. I. Gonadotropin secretion, *Endocrinology* **96**:1073.

Krey, L. C., Lu, K. H., Butler, W. R., Hotchkiss, J., Piva, F., and Knobil, E., 1975b, Surgical disconnection of the medial basal hypothalamus and pituitary function in the rhesus monkey. II. GH and cortisol secretion, *Endocrinology* **96**:1088.

Kubo, K., Mennin, S. P., and Gorski, R. A., 1975, Similarity of plasma LH release in androgenized and normal rats following electrochemical stimulation of the basal forebrain, *Endocrinology* **96**:492.

Lillie, F. R., 1917, The freemartin: A study of the action of sex hormones in the fetal life of cattle, *J. Exp. Zool.* **23**:371.

Lyon, M. F., and Hawkes, S. G., 1970, X-linked gene for testicular feminization in the mouse, *Nature* **227**:1217.

Marrone, B. L., and Feder, H. H., 1977, Characteristics of (^{3}H)-estrogen and (^{3}H)-progestin uptake and effects of progesterone on (^{3}H)-estrogen uptake in brain, anterior pituitary and peripheral tissues of male and female guinea pigs, *Biol. Reprod.* **17**:42.

Martinez, C., and Bittner, J. J., 1956, A non-hypophysial sex difference in estrous behaviour of mice bearing pituitary grafts, *Proc. Soc. Exp. Biol. Med.* **91**:506.

McDonald, P. G., and Doughty, C., 1972, Inhibition of androgen-sterilization in the female rat by administration of an anti-oestrogen, *J. Endocrinol* **55**:455.

McDonald, P. G., and Doughty, C., 1974, Effect of neonatal administration of different androgens in the female rat: Correlation between aromatization and the induction of sterilization, *J. Endocrinol.* **61**:95.

McGuire, J. L., and Lisk, R. D., 1969, Oestrogen receptors in androgen or oestrogen sterilized female rats, *Nature* **221**:1068.

Mennin, S. P., Kubo, K., and Gorski, R. A., 1974, Pituitary responsiveness to luteinizing hormone releasing factor in normal and androgenized female rats, *Endocrinology* **95**:412.

Meusy-Dessolle, N., 1974, Evolution du taux de testostérone plasmatique au cours de la vie foetale chez le porc domestique (*Sus scrofa L.*), *C. R. Acad. Sci.* [*D*] (Paris) **278**:1257.

Minoura, T., 1921, A study of testis and ovary grafts on the hen's egg and their effects on the embryos, *J. Exp. Zool.* **33**:1.

Mittwoch, U., 1967, *Sex Chromosomes*, Academic Press, New York.

Mittwoch, U., 1970, How does the Y chromosome affect gonadal differentiation, *Phil. Trans. R. Soc. Lond* [*Biol.*] **259**:113.

Mizuno, M., Lobotsky, J., Lloyd, C. W., Kobayashi, T., and Murasawa, A., 1968, Plasma androstenedione and testosterone during pregnancy and in the newborn, *J. Clin. Endocrinol. Metab.* **28**:1133.

Money, J., and Ehrhardt, A. A., 1972, *Man and Woman Boy and Girl,* Johns Hopkins University Press, Baltimore.

Moore, C. R., 1941, On the role of sex hormones in sex differentiation in the opossum (*Didelphys virginiana*), *Physiol Zool.* **14**:1.

Moore, C. R., and Price, D., 1932, Gonad hormone functions, and the reciprocal influence between gonads and hypophysis with its bearing on the problem of sex-hormone antagonism, *Am. J. Anat.* **50**:13.

Nadler, R. D., 1973, Further evidence on the intrahypothalamic locus for androgenization of female rats, *Neuroendocrinology* **12**:110.

Neill, J. D., 1972, Sexual differences in the hypothalamic regulation of prolactin secretion, *Endocrinology* **90**:1154.

Neumann, F., von Berswordt-Wallrabe, R., Elger, W., Steinbeck, H., Hahn, J. D., and Kramer, M., 1970, Aspects of androgen-dependent events as studied by antiandrogens, *Recent Prog. Horm. Res.* **26**:337.

Nilson, O., 1939, Hernia uteri inguinalis beim Manne, *Acta Chir. Scand.* **82**:231.

Norman, R. L., Blake, C. A., and Sawyer, C. H., 1972, Effects of hypothalamic deafferentation on LH secretion and the estrous cycle in the hamster, *Endocrinology* **91**:95.

Norman, R. L., Resko, J. A., and Spies, H. G., 1976, The anterior hypothalamus: How it affects gonadotropin secretion in the rhesus monkey, *Endocrinology* **99**:59.

Nunez, E., Vallette, G., Banassayag, C., and Jayle, M. F., 1974, Comparative study on the binding of estrogen by human and rat serum proteins in development, *Biochem. Biophys. Res. Commun.* **57**:126.

Overzier, C., 1963, The so-called true Klinefelter's syndrome, in: *Intersexuality* (C. Overzier, ed.), pp. 277–297, Academic Press, New York.

Patten, B. M., 1958, *Foundations of Embryology*, McGraw-Hill, New York.

Pfaltz, C. R., 1949, Das embryonale und postnatale Verhalten der männlichen Brustdrüse beim Menschen. II. Das Mammarorgan im Kindes-, Junglings-, Mannes und Greisenalter, *Acta Anat.* **8**:293.

Pfeiffer, C. A., 1936, Sexual differences of the hypophyses and their determination by the gonads, *Am. J. Anat.* **58**:195.

Picon, R., 1969, Action du testicule foetal sur le développement *in vitro* des canaux de Müller chez le rat, *Arch. Anat. Microsc. Morphol. Exp.* **58**:1.

Picon, R., 1976, Testosterone secretion by foetal rat testes *in vitro, J. Endocrinol.* **71**:231.

Plapinger, L., and McEwen, B. S., 1975, Immunochemical comparison of estradiol-binding molecules in perinatal rat brain cytosol and serum, *Steroids* **26**:255.

Plapinger, L., McEwen, B., Landau, I. T., and Feder, H. H., 1977, Characteristics of estradiol-binding macromolecules in fetal and adult guinea pig brain cytosols, *Biol. Reprod.* **16**:586.

Potashnik, G., Sober, I., Inbar, I., and Ben-Aderet, N., 1977, Male Müllerian hermaphroditism: A case report of a rare cause of infertility, *Fertil. Steril.* **28**:273.

Price, D., 1970, *In vitro* studies on differentiation of the reproductive tract, *Phil. Trans. R. Soc. Lond.* [*Biol.*] **259**:133.

Price, D., and Ortiz, E., 1965, The role of fetal androgen in sex differentiation in mammals, in: *Organogenesis* (R. L. deHaan and H. Ursprung, eds.), pp. 629–652, Holt, Rinehart and Winston, New York.

Price, D., and Williams-Ashman, H. G., 1961, The accessory reproductive glands of mammals, in:

Sex and Internal Secretions, Vol. I, Third Edition, (W. C. Young, ed.), pp. 366–448, Williams & Wilkins, Baltimore.

Raynaud, A., 1950, Recherches expérimentales sur le développement de l'appareil génital et le fonctionnement des glandes endocrines des foetus de souris et de mulot, *Arch. Anat. Microsc. Morphol. Exp.* **39**:518.

Raynaud, A., and Frilley, M., 1947, Destruction des glandes génitales de l'embyron de souris par une irradiation au moyen des rayons x, à l'âge de 13 jours, *Ann. Endocrinol.* **8**:400.

Reddy, V. V., Naftolin, F., and Ryan, K. J., 1974, Conversion of androstenedione to estrone by neural tissues from fetal and neonatal rats, *Endocrinology* **94**:117.

Reinboth, R. (ed.), 1975, *Intersexuality in the Animal Kingdom, Papers from a Symposium, Mainz, Germany, July, 1974,* Springer Verlag, New York.

Resko, J. A., 1974, Sex steroids in the circulation of the fetal and neonatal rhesus monkey: A comparison between male and female fetuses, in: *Endocrinologie Sexuelle de la Période Périnatale,* Vol. 32 (M. Forest and J. Bertrand, eds.), pp. 195–204, INSERM, Paris.

Resko, J. A., Feder, H. H., and Goy, R. W., 1968, Androgen concentrations in plasma and testis of developing rats, *J. Endocrinol.* **40**:485.

Resko, J. A., Malley, A., Begley, D., and Hess, D. L., 1973, Radioimmunoassay of testosterone during fetal development of the rhesus monkey, *Endrocrinology* **93**:156.

Reyes, F. I., Boroditsky, R. S., Winter, J. S. D., and Faiman, C., 1974, Studies on human sexual development. II. Fetal and maternal serum gonadotrophins and sex steroid concentrations, *J. Clin. Endocrinol. Metab.* **38**:612.

Robertson, D. R., 1972, Social control of sex reversal in a coral-reef fish, *Science* **177**:1007.

Rosenberg, H. S., Clayton, G. W., and Hsu, T. C., 1963, Familial true hermaphrodism, *J. Clin. Endocrinol. Metab.* **23**:203.

Savu, L., Vallette, G., Nunez, E., Azria, M., and Jayle, M. F., 1974, Etude comparative de la liason entre proteines seriques et les oestrogenes libres au cours du développement de diverses espèces animales, in: *L'Alphafoetoproteine* (R. Masseyeff, ed.), pp. 75–83, INSERM, Paris.

Schulster, D., Burstein, S., and Cooke, B. A., 1976, *Molecular Endocrinology of the Steroid Hormones,* John Wiley and Sons, New York.

Schultz, F. M., and Wilson, J. D., 1974, Virilization of the Wolffian duct in the rat fetus by various androgens, *Endocrinology* **94**:979.

Sheridan, P. J., Sar, M., and Stumpf, W. E., 1974, Interaction of exogenous steroids in the developing rat brain, *Endocrinology* **95**:1749.

Short, R. V., 1970, The bovine freemartin: A new look at an old problem, *Phil. Trans. R. Soc. Lond* [*Biol.*] **259**:141.

Short, R. V., 1972, Sex determination and differentiation, in: *Reproduction in Mammals,* Vol. 2, *Embryonic and Fetal Development* (C. R. Austin and R. V. Short, eds.), pp. 43–71, Cambridge University Press, New York.

Siiteri, P. K., and Wilson, J. D., 1974, Testosterone formation and metabolism during male sexual differentiation in the human embryo, *J. Clin. Endocrinol. Metab.* **38**:113.

Southren, A. L., Ross, H., Sharma, D. C., Gordon, G., Weingold, A. B., and Dorfman, R. I., 1965, Plasma concentration and biosynthesis of testosterone in the syndrome of feminizing testes, *J. Clin. Metab.* **25**:518.

Stanley, A. J., Gumbreck, L. G., Allison, J. E., 1973, Male pseudohermaphroditism in the laboratory Norway rat, *Recent Prog. Horm. Res.* **29**:43.

Steiner, R. A., Clinton, D. K., Spies, H. G., and Resko, J. A., 1976, Sexual differentiation and feedback control of luteinizing hormone secretion in the rhesus monkey, *Biol. Reprod.* **15**:206.

Sterne, L., 1759, *The Life and Opinions of Tristram Shandy, Gentleman* (reissued), Penguin Books, Baltimore.

Stewart, D. W., and Raeside, J. I., 1976, Testosterone secretion by the early fetal pig testes in organ culture, *Biol. Reprod.* **15**:25.

Strickland, A. L., and French, F. S., 1969, Absence of response to dihydrotestosterone in the syndrome of testicular feminization, *J. Clin. Endocrinol. Metab.* **29**:1284.

Swanson, H. E., and van der Werff ten Bosch, J. J., 1964, The "early-androgen" syndrome, its development and the response to hemispaying, *Acta Endocrinol.* **45**:1.

Swartz, S. K., and Soloff, M. S., 1974, The lack of estrogen binding by human α-fetoprotein,*J. Clin. Endocrinol. Metab.* **39**:589.

Takewaki, K., 1962, Some aspects of hormonal mechanism involved in persistent estrus in the rat, *Experientia* **18**:1.

Tarttelin, M. F., Shryne, J. E., and Gorski, R. A., 1975, Pattern of body weight change in rats following neonatal hormone manipulation: A "critical period" for androgen-induced growth increases, *Acta Endocrinol.* **79**:177.

Uriel, J., Bouillon, D., and Dupiers, M., 1975, Affinity chromatography of human, rat and mouse α-fetoprotein on estradiol–Sepharose adsorbents, *FEBS Lett.* **53**:305.

Veyssiere, G., Berger, M., Jean-Faucher, C., DeTurckheim, M., and Jean, C., 1975, Dosage radioimmunologique de la testostérone dans le plasma, les gonades et les surrénales de foetus en fin de gestation et de nouveau-nés chez le lapin, *Arch. Int. Physiol. Biochim.* **83**:667.

Wachtel, S. S., 1977, H-Y Antigen and the genetics of sex determination, *Science* **198**:797.

Wagner, J. W., Erwin, W., and Critchlow, V., 1966, Androgen sterilization produced by intracerebral implants of testosterone in neonatal female rats, *Endocrinology* **79**:1135.

Weisz, J., and Gibbs, C., 1974, Conversion of testosterone and androstenedione to estrogens *in vitro* by the brain of female rats, *Endocrinology* **94**:616.

Weisz, J., and Gunsalus, P., 1973, Estrogen levels in immature female rats: True or spurious— Ovarian or adrenal?, *Endocrinology* **93**:1057.

Wells, L. J., 1950, Hormones and sexual differentiation in placental mammals,*Arch. Anat. Microsc. Morphol. Exp.* **39**:499.

Wells, L. J., and van Wagenen, G., 1954, Androgen-induced female pseudohermaphroditism in the monkey (*Macaca mulatta*): Anatomy of the reproductive organs, *Contrib. Embryol.* **35**: 93.

Wells, L. J., Cavanaugh, M. W., and Maxwell, E. L., 1954, Genital abnormalities in castrated fetal rats and their prevention by means of testosterone propionate, *Anat. Rec.* **118**:109.

Welshons, W. J., and Russell, L. B., 1959, The Y chromosome as the bearer of male determining factors in the mouse, *Proc. Natl. Acad. Sci. USA* **45**:560.

Whalen, R. E., and Massicci, J., 1975, Subcellular analysis of the accumulation of estrogen by the brain of male and female rats, *Brain Res.* **89**:255.

Wilkins, L., 1950, *The Diagnosis and Treatment of Endocrine Disorders in Childhood and Adolescence,* Charles C. Thomas, Springfield, Illinois.

Wilson, J. D., 1973, Testosterone uptake by the urogenital tract of the rabbit embryo,*Endocrinology* **92**:1192.

Wilson, J. D., 1975, Metabolism of testicular androgens, in: *Handbook of Physiology,* Sect. 7, Vol. 5 (D. W. Hamilton and R. O. Greep, eds.), pp. 491–508, American Physiological Society, Washington.

Wilson, J. D., 1978, Sexual diffe.entiation, *Annu. Rev. Physiol.* **40**:249.

Wilson, J. D., and Gloyna, R. E., 1970, The intranuclear metabolism of testosterone in the accessory organs of reproduction, *Recent Prog. Horm. Res.* **26**:309.

Wilson, J. G., Hamilton, J. B., and Young, W. C., 1941, Influence of age and presence of the ovaries on reproductive function in rats injected with androgens, *Endocrinology* **29**:784.

Witkin, H. A., Mednick, S. A., Schulsinger, F., Bakketstrom, E., Christiansen, K. O., Goodenough, D. R., Hirschhorn, J., Lundsteen, C., Owen, D. R., Philip, J., Rubin, D. B., and Stocking, M., 1976, Criminality in XYY and XXY men, *Science* **193**:547.

Witschi, E., 1957, The inductor theory of sex differentiation,*J. Fac. Sci. Hokkaido Univ., Ser. VI, Zool.* **13**:428.

Yamamoto, T.-O., 1962, Hormonic factors affecting gonadal sex differentiation in fish,*Gen. Comp. Endocrinol. [Supp.]* **1**:341.

Yamamoto, T.-O., 1975, A YY male goldfish from mating estrone-induced XY female and normal male, *J. Hered.* **66**:2.

Yanaihara, T., and Troen, P., 1972, Studies of the human testis. II. Effect of estrogen on testosterone formation in human testis *in vitro, J. Clin. Endocrinol.* **34**:968.

Yazaki, I., 1960, Further studies on endocrine activity of subcutaneous ovarian grafts in male rats by daily examination of smears from vaginal graft, *Annot. Zool. Jpn.* **33**:217.

Zucker, I., and Feder, H. H., 1966, The effect of neonatal resperine treatment on female sex behaviour of rats, *J. Endocrinol.* **35**:423.

Zucker, I., Rusak, B., and King, R. G., Jr., 1976, Neural basis for circadian rhythms in rodent behavior, in: *Advances in Psychobiology*, (A. H. Riesen and R. F. Thompson, eds.), pp. 35–74, Wiley, New York.

Perinatal Hormones and Their Role in the Development of Sexually Dimorphic Behaviors

HARVEY H. FEDER

I. BRIEF HISTORY OF THE PROBLEM

In the previous chapter, we saw that steroid hormones have long been known to play an important role in the morphological differentiation of genital tissues. It is only more recently that the idea of an influence of steroids on the differentiation of neural substrates for sexual behavior has been brought forward and systematically examined. The purpose of this chapter is to survey the evidence on which the notion of behavioral differentiation is based. But first, let us ask why the idea that perinatal steroids affect the differentiation of neural tissues regulating adult behavior has been so slow to take root. Three major conceptual confusions can be cited as obstacles.

First, in the early years of endocrine research, the type of sexual behavior displayed was thought to depend primarily, if not exclusively, on the nature of the hormone administered. The character of the substrate on which the hormone acted was all but ignored. For example, it was believed that testicular hormone stimulated the expression of masculine behavior equally well in males and females, and that ovarian hormone stimulated the expression of feminine behavior equally well in females and in males (Steinach, 1940). This belief that the nature of the steroid was of primary importance in determining the nature

HARVEY H. FEDER • Institute of Animal Behavior, Rutgers University, Newark, New Jersey 07102.

of the behavior displayed was taken to its ultimate length with the claim that adult gonadectomized animals given simultaneous grafts of a testis and an ovary displayed alternating bouts of masculine and feminine behavior (Sand, 1919). Of the pioneer workers, Goodale (1918) was among the few to emphasize that the sex of the animal was at least as significant as the type of hormone administered in determining the nature and intensity of a behavioral response. Later, other workers, notably Ball (1937), Beach (1948), and Young (1961), extended Goodale's insight from work with avian species to mammals. A generalization from this work is that it is easier to produce complete and intense masculine responses to male hormones in males than in females and that it is easier to produce complete and intense feminine responses to female hormones in females than in males. Thus, the character of the substrate or soma on which a hormone acts is an important determining factor in the behavioral outcome of a hormonal treatment. On the basis of published research, one can now readily accept that genome (Luttge and Hall, 1973; McGill and Haynes, 1973), age (Jakubczak, 1964; Goy et al., 1967), conditions of rearing (Valenstein et al., 1955), experience (Rosenblatt and Aronson, 1958), nutritional state (Leathem, 1961), and testing situation (Edwards, 1969) are factors that influence the character or state of the soma and thereby help to determine the quality of the behavioral response an adult animal will display after steroid hormone treatment. It was not until about 20 years ago that it was realized that the steroid environment in which the fetal or perinatal animal develops is also a factor in determining somatic character.

Second, an early prevailing view based on work with adult animals was that after steroid hormones had acted over a period of hours or days, some increase in sexual behavior could be detected, and that this sexual activity declined fairly rapidly when the hormones were withdrawn. That is, the influence of the steroids was transitory, and there was a more or less concurrent relation between the presence of a hormone and a change in frequency of sexual activity (see reviews by Beach, 1948, 1971; Young, 1961). This principle of concurrency might be assumed to operate at all stages of development. However, when injections of testosterone or estradiol preparations were given to neonatal rats, it was noted that the neonates did not show concurrent increases in sexual behavior (they did not possess the requisite neuromuscular coordination to do so*) or precocity of sexual behavior (Wilson et al., 1941; Wilson, 1943; Wilson and Wilson, 1943), and it was concluded that neonates were insensitive to the conventional behavior-influencing actions of steroid hormones. Moreover, sex steroid injections into neonatal female rats had an effect that could not be understood readily in the context of concurrency in which most experimenters' thoughts were grounded. Specifically, estrogen or androgen given to neonatal female rats apparently permanently diminished the tendency to display feminine behavior in adulthood (Wilson et al., 1941; Wilson, 1943). Here then was a nontransitory, nonconcurrent effect of hormones on be-

---

*Dr. Christina Williams (personal communication) has recently demonstrated that neonatal (6-day-old) rats are capable of displaying lordosis in response to estradiol as long as behavioral testing is conducted at 34° ± 1°C.

havior. Its discovery outpaced an appreciation of its significance by more than 20 years.

A third reason that the influence of steroid hormones on the shaping of the soma during prenatal or perinatal periods was not recognized resides in findings from studies on neonatal animals lacking gonadal tissue. For example, Beach (1945) found in his laboratory colony a rat with congenital absence of gonadal tissue. This animal was able to exhibit feminine behavior when given appropriate hormone treatment in adulthood. Beach and Holz (1946) reported that neonatally castrated male rats showed no deficits in mounting behavior when given androgen replacement therapy in adulthood. Although such animals revealed decrements in the frequency of intromission and ejaculation behavior, the decrements were ascribed to the deficient penile development of the neonatally castrated males. These findings suggested that perinatal gonadectomy had no effects on central neural tissues that would be reflected in adult patterns of homotypical sexual behavior. It was therefore concluded that endogenous testicular steroids had no permanent central nervous system actions related to the display of sex behavior. This conclusion was premature, for the early investigators did not test endogenous or exogenous perinatal hormones for their ability to influence the expression of heterotypical sexual behavior patterns in adults (e.g., lordosis behavior in males).

II. PRENATAL HORMONES AND THEIR EFFECTS ON THE SEX BEHAVIOR OF ADULT GUINEA PIGS

One of the first clues that prenatal hormone* administration might permanently alter heterotypical patterns of sexual behavior came from the work of Vera Dantchakoff (1938a,b). She observed that female guinea pigs given androgen during prenatal life showed increased masculine behavior in adulthood. However, because Dantchakoff was primarily interested in the effects of prenatal androgens on the morphology of the genitals, her behavioral descriptions were casual and unquantified.

W. C. Young and his colleagues decided to reexamine this problem by using more controlled methods of behavioral observation, and in 1959, Phoenix et al. published their classic study. The experiments consisted of administering large doses of testosterone propionate to pregnant guinea pigs throughout almost the entire 68-day period of gestation. At birth, some of the female offspring from these pregnancies had external genitalia that were indistinguishable from males. These females were designated hermaphrodites (actually they are pseudohermaphrodites). Another group of females which had received smaller doses of the androgen prenatally, had no visible abnor-

---

*At various points in the text, I have used the terms "prenatal hormones" or "prenatal androgens" as a shorthand for "hormones present during the prenatal period." I do not mean to imply by this shorthand notation that the hormones of the prenatal or perinatal period are necessarily qualitatively different from the hormones secreted during adulthood.

malities of the external genitalia, and these females were referred to as unmodified females. In adulthood, both groups of females as well as the control males and females that did not receive androgen prenatally were gonadectomized and given estrogen and progesterone therapy in order to stimulate the display of female sexual reponses. The results are summarized in Table 1. Afterward, some of the same animals were given injections of testosterone propionate in order to stimulate the expression of malelike sexual behavior (mounting). The data from this experiment are summarized in Table 2.

The conclusions that could be drawn from these and related data in the same paper were that exogenous androgen administered during prenatal life (a) decreased the ability of female guinea pigs to display lordosis behavior in response to estrogen–progesterone therapy in adulthood, (b) enhanced the ability of female guinea pigs to display mounting behavior in response to testosterone therapy in adulthood, and (c) had no deleterious effect on mounting and other masculine behavior patterns in males. A fourth finding was that exogenous androgen given early in postnatal life to guinea pigs did not decrease the ability of females to display lordosis in adulthood.

This experiment with guinea pigs stimulated research on the influence of hormones on the differentiation of neural tissues destined to mediate mating behaviors. Not only were the data of considerable interest, but the conceptual framework in which the authors chose to cast them was wide and rich.

The authors made the following speculations. (a) A clear distinction could be drawn between the prenatal action of hormones in causing differentiation or "organization" of neural substrates for behavior and the action of hormones of adulthood in causing "activation" of these substrates. (b) There might be a critical period of perinatal development during which an animal is maximally susceptible to the organizing actions of steroids on neural tissues. (c) The organization of neural tissues mediating mating behavior was in some ways analogous to the differentiation of the genital tracts. That is, prenatal androgens induced differentiation of the Wolffian ducts and the neural substrates for masculine behavior. The absence of prenatal androgens was consistent with the differentiation of female genital anlagen and neural substrates for feminine behavior. (d) The nature of the organizing effect of steroid hormones on prenatal neural tissues might be subtle and be reflected in an alteration in "function rather than in visible structure." (e) The prenatal hormones might have a general or localized organizing effect on neural tissues. (f) Testosterone or a metabolite of testosterone might be the prenatal factor responsible for permanently altering neural function or structure. (g) Prenatal androgens might influence the "masculinity or femininity of an animal's behavior beyond that which was purely sexual." (h) The idea of an organizing action of prenatal hormones on the neural substrates for behavior in rodents has possible implications for the study of the behavior of primates, including humans. Each of these eight speculations will now be examined in turn in the light of subsequent research.

Table 1. Duration of Heat and Lordosis in Gonadectomized Guinea Pigs Given Different Amounts of Estradiol and 0.2 mg of Progesterone[a]

Subjects	Tests[b] N	Tests positive for estrus (%)	Mean latency (hr)	Mean duration of heat (hr)	Median duration of maximum lordosis (sec)
1.66 μg estradiol					
Control females	19	89	5.7	5.7	11.5
Unmodified females	20	65	6.5	2.8	8.5
Hermaphrodites	9	22	8.5	2.5	2.0
Castrated males	8	38	6.0	1.2	2.0
3.32 μg estradiol					
Control females	33	94	4.4	7.3	12.3
Unmodified females	38	68	5.6	2.8	5.1
Hermaphrodites	18	22	8.0	2.0	3.0
Castrated males	16	31	4.5	3.2	2.7
6.62 μg estradiol					
Control females	28	96	3.7	7.2	9.3
Unmodified females	22	77	5.8	3.3	6.0
Hermaphrodites	18	22	9.2	2.0	2.0
Castrated males	16	0	—	—	—

[a] From Phoenix et al. (1959).
[b] All animals were given one or more tests at each level of hormone.

Table 2. Masculine Behavior in Gonadectomized Adult Guinea Pigs
Injected with Testosterone Propionate[a]

Animals	Mean mounts per test	Median number of tests to the first display of mounting	Median dose of testosterone propionate prior to the display of mounting (mg)
Spayed untreated females	5.8	7.0	30.0
Spayed pseudohermaphrodites	15.4	3.0	10.0
Males castrated prepuberally	20.5	1.5	3.8

[a]From Phoenix *et al.* (1959) with minor modifications.

III. EIGHT QUESTIONS REGARDING "ORGANIZING" EFFECTS OF HORMONES

A. Are There "Organizing" and "Activating" Effects of Hormones? A Matter of Terminology

In order to distinguish the effects of prenatal hormone treatment on the behavior of adult guinea pigs from the effects of hormonal treatment given during adulthood, a terminology had to be devised. Phoenix *et al.* (1959) chose the terms "organizational" and "activational" to describe, respectively, these two different actions of hormones. The word organizational was borrowed from embryologists who used the term "organizer" to refer to substances that acted over extremely short distances to induce an altered course of structural differentiation in embryonic cells (Spemann, 1938). Choice of the word organizational was not meant to imply that steroid hormone action on neural tissues during prenatal life was identical to the action of organizer substances (e.g., hormones, unlike organizer substances, could act on distant tissues), but rather was meant to call attention to a previously unrecognized analogy. The analogy was extended to include not only the action of steroid hormones on neural tissues mediating behavior but also the action of steroids on the differentiation or organization of the genital tracts. Thus, some parallels between the development of the nervous system and the development of the genitalia could begin to be discerned (see Section III.C).

Another advantage to the adoption of the word organizational was that the term did not prejudge issues such as whether the effects of prenatal steroids on the nervous system were structural or functional, general or localized, or were limited to a sensitization or desensitization of neural elements to the actions of the hormones of adulthood. However, in a recent review, Beach (1971) argued vehemently against the use of the term organization* and recommended

---

*Beach's objections to the term "organization" are varied, with one of the objections being that the meaning of the term seems continually to be shifting. I think that these shifts do not reflect so

abandoning this hypothetical construct for "quantitative statements . . . based upon directly observable S–R relationships." Laudable as this resolution may be, it should be apparent that hypothetical constructs have provided valuable conceptual frameworks within which experiments have been designed to test the strengths of the constructs. In the words of Max Black: "Perhaps every science must start with metaphor and end with algebra; and perhaps without the metaphor there would never have been any algebra" (1962). In this particular case, for instance, the setting up of a hypothetical neurological mechanism that is organized by prenatal hormones encouraged neuroanatomists to seek evidence for structural changes in brain tissue exposed to steroid hormones perinatally (Raisman and Field, 1973).

In summary, the word organizational will be taken to refer to the action of steroid hormones during fetal and/or neonatal life on neural tissues destined to mediate sexual behavior. The word activational will refer to the more or less concurrent facilitation of sexual activity by hormones in adulthood. W. C. Young likened the activational role of hormones to that of a photographic developer. By this analogy, an animal may be considered to be like an exposed but undeveloped photographic film. The developer merely serves to bring out or activate the pattern already existing on the film. The perinatal hormones, on the other hand, are among the factors that form or organize the pattern.

B. Are There Critical Periods or Periods of Maximal Susceptibility to Perinatal Hormones?

The experiment of Phoenix *et al.* (1959) utilized a design in which androgen was injected into pregnant guinea pigs from the tenth through the 68th day of gestation (gestation period is 68 days). Further work had to be done to determine whether such a long injection schedule was necessary to cause behavioral consequences in adulthood. Goy *et al.* (1964) showed that maximal susceptibility to prenatal androgen occurred when injections were initiated 30 days after fertilization and terminated between days 45 and 55 of gestation. Female fetuses given such treatment displayed diminished lordosis responses when gonadectomized and given estrogen–progesterone therapy in adulthood. They also exhibited increased mounting behavior even in the absence of steroid hormones in adulthood. Furthermore, injections of testosterone pro-

---

much an inadequacy of the term as an unavoidable difficulty in "pinning down" a concept that has not yet completely emerged. R. G. Collingwood beautifully depicts this problem:

> The proper meaning of a word (I speak not of technical terms, which kindly godparents furnish soon after birth with neat and tidy definitions, but of words in a living language) is never something upon which the word sits perched like a gull on a stone; it is something over which the word hovers like a gull over a ship's stern. Trying to fix the proper meaning in our minds is like coaxing the gull to settle in the rigging, with the rule that the gull must be alive when it settles: one must not shoot it and tie it there. The way to discover the proper meaning is to ask not, "What do we mean?" but, "What are we trying to mean?" And this involves the question "What is preventing us from meaning what we are trying to mean?" (Collingwood, 1958).

pionate to female guinea pigs for the first 80 days of postnatal life did not permanently suppress lordosis later in adulthood (Phoenix *et al.*, 1959). The data therefore suggest that in guinea pigs the period of maximal susceptibility to organizing actions of androgen extends from about prenatal day 30 to day 45 and does not extend into postnatal life.

Experiments with other rodents yielded results which, at first glance, seemed quite different. For instance, some work indicated that perinatal androgen most effectively suppressed the adult rat's lordosis response when it was administered as repeated injections over the first 2 to 4 weeks of postnatal life; prenatal injections were relatively ineffective in this respect (Wilson *et al.*, 1941; Revesz *et al.*, 1963). However, this does not mean that prenatally administered androgen was completely ineffective (Ward and Renz, 1972). The work with rats and with other short-gestation species was greatly aided by the discovery that a single injection of androgen at an appropriately early postnatal stage could permanently diminish the probability of occurrence of lordosis in rats (Barraclough and Gorski, 1962). By use of this single-injection technique, it was found that in short-gestation rodents such as rats (21- to 22-day gestation), hamsters (16- to 17-day gestation), and mice (18- to 20-day gestation), maximal susceptibility to organizing actions of androgens on sexual behavior occurred during about the first 5 days of postnatal life (Feder, 1967; Edwards and Burge, 1971; Carter *et al.*, 1972).

The apparent discrepancy between these data and the guinea pig data is resolved when it is realized that the crucial factor in susceptibility to organizing actions of hormones is the status of neural development at the time of exposure to hormone and not whether an animal happens to be prenatal or postnatal at the time of hormone administration. Thus, a fairly close correspondence in the periods of maximal susceptibility among guinea pigs, rats, mice, and hamsters is arrived at when number of days after fertilization is used as an index, because this takes developmental stage into account in the comparison between short- and long-gestation species. An even closer correspondence is obtained when the number of days since the onset of testicular differentiation is used as an index (Table 3).

Nonrodent mammals may follow somewhat different rules in the timing of the maximally susceptible period. For example, beagle dogs, with a gestation period of 58–63 days, are sensitive to organizing actions of androgen through an extended period spanning prenatal and early postnatal life (Beach and Kuehn, 1970). On the other hand, short-gestation rabbits (30 to 32-day gestation) did not show a decreased tendency to display lordosis in adulthood when they were given androgen early in postnatal life (Campbell, 1965). Sheep (145-day gestation) given androgen between days 20 and 60 of pregnancy did not display female behavior in adulthood and exhibited increased masculine behavior. Initiation of prenatal androgen treatment on day 80 of pregnancy did not have these behavioral consequences (Short, 1974).

In this discussion, I have preferred the term "period of maximal susceptibility" (Goy *et al.*, 1964) over the term "critical period" in describing the timing

Table 3. Time Periods When Androgen Treatment Will Suppress Female Mating Behavior (Lordosis) or Facilitate Male Mating Behavior in Four Rodent Species[a]

Species	Length of gestation (days)	Androgen suppresses lordosis (postcoital age, days)	Postcoital age for TD[b] (days)	Androgen suppresses lordosis (days from TD)	Androgen facilitates mounting (days from TD)
Hamster	16	16–21	11.5	4.5–7.5	4.5–7.5
Laboratory mouse	19–20	20(?)	12.5	7.5(?)	—
Rat	21–22	18–28	13.0	5.0–14.0	—
Guinea pig	68	30–35	25.0	5.0–11.0	5.0–11.0

[a]This Table, with minor modifications, is taken from Clemens (1973).
[b]TD, testicular differentiation.

of perinatal hormone effects. The justifiability of this preference may be recognized by the fact that by increasing the dosage of perinatal hormone, it is possible to lengthen the interval over which perinatal hormones exert organizing effects on behavior (Edwards, 1970). A second semantic point is that each tissue or regulatory system has its own period of maximal susceptibility to organizing actions of hormones. Thus, differentiation of the internal genitalia, the external genitalia, and differentiation of neural tissues regulating gonadotropin release, lordosis behavior, other female behaviors, mounting behavior, intromission and ejaculation behavior, and nonreproductive behavior may be separable processes that in some cases happen to run on the same developmental schedule.

C. Are There Parallels between Genital Differentiation and Neural Organization?

Regardless of genetic sex, every mammalian fetus possesses an undifferentiated genital tubercle during fetal life. If the genital tubercle develops in the presence of adequate androgenic substances, it will differentiate into a penis. If androgenic stimulation is absent or minimal, the tubercle will develop into a clitoris (see Chapter 5). Thus far, in the discussion of behavioral systems, the effects of giving androgens to female fetuses or neonates have been emphasized. Such androgen administration is said to suppress the tendency to display feminine behavior and, in some experiments with rats, to enhance the tendency to display masculine behaviors (Barraclough and Gorski, 1961; Harris and Levine, 1965; Gerall and Ward, 1966; Whalen and Edwards, 1967).

This appears to be analogous to the situation for differentiation of the genital tubercle but not for the genital duct systems. If there is some further parallel between the rules for differentiation of the genital tubercle and organization of the nervous system, one would predict that withdrawal of male hormones from males during the organizational period of maximal susceptibility would result in an enhanced tendency to display feminine behaviors and a diminished tendency to exhibit masculine behaviors in adulthood.

This prediction was first tested by using a short-gestation species (the rat) whose neural organization was incomplete at birth. Withdrawal of gonadal androgens during the period of maximal susceptibility was accomplished by castration of neonatal male rats. The results of this landmark experiment by Grady et al. (1965) were as follows. When compared with males castrated at later ages, male rats castrated within the first 5 days of neonatal life exhibited (a) increased tendency to display lordosis after being given estrogen–progesterone therapy in adulthood (Table 4), and (b) decreased tendency to display intromission and ejaculation response (but no decrease in tendency to mount) after being given testosterone treatment in adulthood (Table 5).

At first glance, these results appear to confirm the idea that the rules of steroid-induced organization of the neural substrates for sexual behavior

Table 4. Relationship of Lordosis Quotients to Quantities of Estradiol Benzoate in Neonatally Castrated Rats[a]

Group	3.3 μg Estradiol benzoate[b]			6.6 μg Estradiol benzoate			165 μg Estradiol benzoate		
	N	% Tests Ss were mounted	LQ[c]	N	% Tests Ss were mounted	LQ	N	% Tests Ss were mounted	LQ
Spayed females	9	97	0.452	7	100	0.787	4	88	0.696
Day-1 males	8	88	0.301	7	100	0.572	6	100	0.604
Day-5 males	8	78	0.253	6	96	0.183	6	83	0.501
Day-10 males	5	75	0.000	6	88	0.028	5	90	0.206
Day-20 males	7	79	0.003	7	89	0.056	—	—	—
Day-30 males	7	71	0.000	7	89	0.085	—	—	—
Day-50 males	8	84	0.000	7	96	0.053	5	90	0.081
Day-90 males	7	78	0.000	7	100	0.038	—	—	—

[a] From Grady et al. (1965) with minor modifications.
[b] All animals were given 0.5 mg progesterone 40 hr after estradiol benzoate injection and tested for lordosis beginning 1 hr after progesterone.
[c] LQ, mean lordosis-to-mount ratio.

Table 5. Mean Rates of Mounting and Intromission in 30-min Tests by Castrated Rats Given 200 μg TP/100 g Body Weight per Day in Adulthood[a]

Day of castration	N	Mean mounts/min	Mean intromission/min	% Ejaculating
Day 1	6	2.44	0.01	0
Day 5	8	1.85	0.18	25
Day 10	9	1.59	0.59	88
Day 30	8	1.46	0.53	88
Day 90	7	1.98	0.76	86

[a]Table taken from Grady *et al.* (1965)

parallel the rules of steroid-induced differentiation of the genital tubercle. But there are two major objections to jumping to this simple conclusion. First, it must be recognized that neonatal castration of male rats results in deficient penile development (Beach and Holz, 1946). Perhaps the reduced tendency of such castrates to display intromission and ejaculation patterns in adulthood is the result of inadequate penile development rather than (or in addition to) inadequate organization of central neural substrates mediating intromission and ejaculation responses. Second, it is unclear from the foregoing experiment whether the increase in feminine behavior seen in neonatally castrated rats occurs at the expense of intromission and ejaculation responses. Indeed, if the analogy to the differentiation of the genital tubercle is to be accepted, a single neural substrate mediating both male and female sexual behavior would be assumed. Logically, any increase in capacity to display one type of sexual behavior would then have to occur at the expense of the other type. Both of these questions have been put to experimental test, and the following subsections will deal with the results of these experiments in some detail.

1. Does Perinatal Androgen Enhance the Tendency to Display Intromission and Ejaculation in Adulthood by Acting on the CNS, the Penis, or Both?

A number of experiments demonstrate incontestably that castration of neonatal rats results in decreased penile size (Beach and Holtz, 1946; Beach *et al.*, 1969) and that perinatal administration of androgens to female rodents results in increased clitoral size (Goy *et al.*, 1964; Ward, 1969; Table 6). Although such experiments also generally yield a good positive correlation between phallic size and tendency to display masculine behaviors, this cannot be taken as proof that androgens exert no organizing actions on central neural tissues mediating masculine behaviors.

In fact, several studies using a variety of techniques indicate such actions at the central level. First, some workers have noted that correlations between tendency to display the behaviors of mounting or intromission and phallic size of perinatally treated rats are not always perfect. For example, Ward and Renz

Table 6. Morphologic Measures for Guinea Pigs Given Prenatal
Treatment with Testosterone Propionate (TP)[a]

TP treatment given during prenatal days	N	% with male urethra	Mean length of phallus (mm)
Untreated females	11	0	11.7
15–30	9	0	10.9
15–40	8	0	12.2
15–45	11	18.2	13.8
15–60+	10	10.0	13.6
20–65	10	10.0	14.1
25–40	13	84.6	17.2
30–45	6	66.7	15.8
30–55	6	66.7	18.3
30–65	11	81.8	20.0
35–65	9	22.2	14.3
40–65	9	0	13.6
50–65	3	0	12.7
Untreated males	7	100.0	23.7

[a] Taken from Goy *et al.* (1964) with modifications.

(1972) showed that female rats given the antiandrogen cyproterone acetate prenatally and postnatally had normal clitoral size yet exhibited decrements in mounting behavior in adulthood. And Ward (1969) showed that ability to perform ejaculatory responses was not directly related to increases in clitoral length in female rats given testosterone prenatally. Second, some workers have injected androgenic or estrogenic substances into neonatally castrated male rats or hamsters and have demonstrated a lack of correlation between phallic size and male behaviors. Some of these substances (e.g., fluoxymesterone, dihydrotestosterone) had the property of enhancing phallic size without enhancing the tendency to perform intromission or ejaculation patterns in adulthood (Whalen and Luttge, 1971; Hart, 1972). Conversely, other substances (e.g., estradiol-17β, diethylstilbestrol) had the property of facilitating the tendency to perform mounting, intromission, or ejaculatory responses without stimulating full penile development (Levine and Mullins, 1964; Paup *et al.*, 1972; Table 7). Third, preoptic area implants of testosterone into neonatal female rats stimulated the tendency to display mounting behavior in adulthood, even though this method of delivery of the androgen did not result in leakage into the general circulation with consequent stimulation of phallic development (Christensen and Gorski, 1975). All of these approaches therefore suggest that perinatal androgens may not act to enhance the tendency to display intromission or ejaculation patterns merely by insuring adequate phallic development. Rather, a central neural component also seems to be involved.

Table 7. Mounting Behavior in Female Hamsters Treated Days 2–4 after Birth with Androgens or Diethylstilbestrol[a]

Neonatal treatment	N	Dose (μg/day)	Mean mount frequency[b]	N	Mean os + cartilage length (mm)
Sesame oil	10	—	0.7	7	2.6
Testosterone	10	25	6.1	9	3.2
Androsterone[c]	19	25	0.2	18	3.0
Androsterone	5	100	0.2	5	3.4
Diethylstilbestrol	8	25	13.8	8	2.7

[a] Data taken from Table 1 and Fig. 2 of Paup *et al.* (1972).
[b] Sum of rear, head, and side mounts after 28 days of testosterone propionate (300 μg/day) injections in adulthood.
[c] A nonaromatizable androgen.

2. Are the Central Neural Substrates Mediating Male and Female Behavior Identical? Does One Behavior Develop at the Expense of the Other?

As Beach (1971) stated: ". . . the development of normal male or female external genitals in mammals represents mutually exclusive alternatives." If the analogy between behavioral differentiation and genital tubercle differentiation is accurate, then the development of the tendencies to display normal male behavior and normal female behavior should also represent mutually exclusive alternatives. However, this is clearly not the case. Numerous experiments with rodents show that males exposed to normal endogenous secretions of androgen during perinatal life are still capable of displaying lordosis responses in adulthood under appropriate testing conditions (Pfaff, 1970; Södersten and Larsson, 1974). The extent to which this occurs is species-dependent, with adult male hamsters particularly capable of exhibiting lordosis, and male rats and guinea pigs less so (Tiefer, 1970; Eaton, 1970; Swanson, 1971). Furthermore, female rodents that have undergone a normal differentiation can be induced to display mounting, intromission, and even ejaculation patterns by appropriate hormonal treatment during adulthood (Beach and Rasquin, 1942; Emery and Sachs, 1975). Additionally, intracerebral lesions that disrupt masculine behavior do not necessarily have adverse effects on lordosis behavior in adult rats (Singer, 1968; Hitt *et al.*, 1970).

The most direct test of whether masculine behavioral capacity develops at the expense of feminine behavioral capacity was carried out by Goldfoot *et al.* (1969) and independently by Stern (1969). In both experiments, neonatally castrated male rats were given injections of androstenedione neonatally, and in both experiments this resulted in the ability to display high frequencies of lordosis as well as mounting, intromission, and ejaculation behavior after appropriate hormone treatment in adulthood (Table 8). That is, the an-

Table 8. Lordosis Responses and Intromissions Displayed by Adult Male Rats Castrated on Day 1, Day 20, or Castrated on Day 1 and Given Androstenedione (Δ^4) on Days 1 through 20[a]

	Tests following exogenous estradiol and progesterone		Tests following exogenous testosterone propionate in adulthood—mean frequency of intromissions
	N	Mean lordosis quotient[b]	
Day 1	6	90	0.75
Day 20	5	12	6.00
Day 1 + Δ^4	7	78	8.15

[a] From Goldfoot *et al.* (1969) with minor modifications.
[b] The quotient is obtained by the ratio of the number of lordoses to the number of times mounted multiplied by 100.

drogenic actions of androstenedione on female and male behavioral capacities are actions on two independent processes that do not occur at each other's expense.

It is abundantly clear that differentiation of the genital tubercle does not provide a good analogy for organization of the nervous system. Originally, Phoenix *et al.* (1959) proposed that a suitable analogy for neural organization is the differentiation of the genital tracts rather than the genital tubercle. In a sense, this is the more suitable analogy because there are two sets of primordia for the genital tracts, and one set does not develop at the expense of the other (see Chapter 5). However, such analogizing, although appropriate earlier in the history of the subject, is no longer helpful in framing questions regarding neural organization and may even be counterproductive.

D. Organizational Effects—Structural or Functional?

In his influential review, Beach (1971) ridicules the notion that perinatal steroids cause alterations in the organization of the nervous system in the sense of causing structural changes. However, recent experiments have demonstrated such steroid-induced structural changes. For example, Pfaff (1966) found that nerve cell nuclear area and nucleolar area were similar in neonatally castrated male rats and in female rats, and these two categories of animals corresponded more closely to each other than to normal males. Dörner and Staudt (1969) also found effects of neonatal castration or neonatal androgenization on nuclear sizes in the hypothalamic ventromedial nucleus of the rat. In a recent abstract it was shown that testosterone or estradiol can enhance neuronal maturation and myelinogenesis in hypothalamus and preoptic area *in vitro* (Toran-Allerand, 1975). Perhaps the most striking evidence for steroid-induced structural changes in the CNS comes from the work of Raisman and

Field (1973).* These workers demonstrated that the distribution of synapses in the preoptic area is sexually dimorphic in rats (there is a higher proportion of synapses on dendritic shafts than on dendritic spines in males) and that neonatal castration of males results in a female-type pattern of distribution in the preoptic area (Table 9).

Even if such structural changes in anatomy had not been found, the idea that perinatal steroids organize neural tissues could still be considered plausible. The organizing action might occur at a biochemical rather than at an anatomical level. Indeed, despite a rather confusing literature on the subject, there seems to be some evidence for a decreased uptake of radioactive estradiol into hypothalamic cell nuclei (Vertes and King, 1971; Whalen and Massicci, 1975) in male as compared to female rats. However, this sex difference is usually not seen in hypothalamic whole homogenates (Green *et al.*, 1969). Administration of androgen to neonatal female rats is said to cause decreases in ability to take up estradiol even in whole homogenates of the hypothalamus (Flerkó *et al.*, 1969; McGuire and Lisk, 1969; McEwen and Pfaff, 1970; Maurer and Woolley, 1971). Other biochemical effects of perinatal hormones may include alterations of testosterone metabolism (Kraulis and Clayton, 1968), reductions in brain uridine uptake (Clayton *et al.*, 1970), long-term changes in RNA synthesis (Shimada and Gorbman, 1970), stimulation of methionine incorporation into protein in lateral amygdaloid nucleus (MacKinnon, 1970), inhibition of amino acid incorporation into brain protein (Litteria, 1973; Litteria and Thorner, 1974), and changes in brain indoleamines (Ladosky and Gaziri, 1970).

Other experiments indicate that male rats are less sensitive to the lordosis-promoting actions of estradiol and progesterone than are female rats (Davidson, 1969; Davidson and Levine, 1969; Arén-Engelbrektsson *et al.*, 1970). Treatment of neonatal female rats with testosterone results in decrements of behavioral sensitivity to both estrogen and progesterone (Gerall and Kenny, 1970; Clemens *et al.*, 1970). The bases of these functional differences in adult responsiveness to hormones are unknown. The functional differences may be related to the sex differences in neuroanatomical structure or in the neural uptake of estrogens that have already been mentioned. There may be other bases for these differences in responsiveness that result from as yet undiscovered sex differences in neural tissue or to sex differences in the handling of steroids by nonneural tissues (e.g., liver: Denef and De Moor, 1972). For example, how is one to account for the diminished responsiveness of males to progesterone when there appears to be no evidence for a diminution

---

*The major objective of this chapter is to provide a historical framework in which to place research on behavior sex differentiation. Bibliographic work for this chapter was completed in 1975, and a few more recent references were added after completion of the manuscript. For additional evidence of structural changes in the CNS induced by perinatal administration of steroids see *Brain Res.* 126:63, 1977, and *Brain Res.* 148:333, 1978. An excellent recent monograph, *Sexual Differentiation of the Brain* (R. W. Goy and B. S. McEwen, eds., MIT Press, Cambridge, 1980) should also be consulted.

Table 9. The Incidences per Grid Square (Mean ± Standard Error) of the Four Types of Synapse in the Preoptic Area (POA) and Ventromedial Nucleus (VMH) in the Six Groups of Animals[a]

| | Endocrine status[b] | | | | | |
| | Cyclic | | | Noncyclic | | |
	F(16)	F16 (7)	M0 (9)	M (11)	M7 (7)	F4 (14)
POA						
Nonstrial shaft	50.0 ± 2.0	53.1 ± 3.0	54.3 ± 3.0	55.2 ± 1.4	52.6 ± 1.3	48.4 ± 2.4
spine	5.3 ± 0.3	5.4 ± 0.5	5.0 ± 0.3	3.3 ± 0.2	3.9 ± 0.4	3.5 ± 0.2
Strial shaft	1.2 ± 0.1	1.0 ± 0.1	1.2 ± 0.1	1.2 ± 0.1	0.7 ± 0.1	0.9 ± 0.1
spine	1.6 ± 0.2	1.4 ± 0.3	1.8 ± 0.2	1.7 ± 0.1	1.3 ± 0.1	1.6 ± 0.2
VMH						
Nonstrial shaft	46.3 ± 1.8	44.4 ± 1.6	43.6 ± 1.6	42.4 ± 1.5	42.3 ± 1.4	42.8 ± 1.8
spine	12.9 ± 0.7	12.6 ± 0.8	13.2 ± 0.9	12.0 ± 0.7	13.9 ± 0.9	13.1 ± 0.9
Strial shaft	2.3 ± 0.2	1.6 ± 0.2	1.9 ± 0.3	1.9 ± 0.3	1.8 ± 0.2	1.9 ± 0.2
spine	6.2 ± 0.5	6.2 ± 0.6	6.6 ± 0.5	7.0 ± 0.6	6.7 ± 0.4	6.5 ± 0.5

[a] From Raisman and Field (1973).
[b] The cyclic group consists of F (normal females), F16 (females treated with androgen on day 16), and M0 (males castrated within 12 hr of birth); the noncyclic group consists of M (normal males), M7 (males castrated on day 7), and F4 (females androgenized on day 4). Number of rats given in parentheses.

of neural uptake of this steroid in males as compared to females (Wade and Feder, 1972)?*

In summary, there is evidence for induction of functional as well as structural changes by perinatal steroid hormones. The relationships between the structural and biochemical effects of the perinatal steroids on neural tissues and the eventual behavioral effects of the perinatal steroids are still unclear. A final point may be made. The perinatal steroids appear to act by changing thresholds for behavioral responses rather than by grossly changing the course of neural pathways. Thus, perinatally androgenized female rats can be shown to suffer decrements in lordosis behavior under certain test conditions (Barraclough and Gorski, 1962), but these decrements can be overcome by prolonged testing (Brown-Grant, 1975). Similarly, although it is usually difficult to elicit lordosis in male rats or ejaculation movements in female rats, the potential for these behaviors exists, and the behaviors can be brought out under appropriate hormonal and environmental testing circumstances (Beach, 1948). That is, the essential "wiring" for these behaviors persists. Similar considerations hold for the induction of massive surges of LH secretion in males and in neonatally androgenized females (Gorski and Barraclough, 1963; Naftolin et al., 1975). In this sense, Beach (1971) was correct in questioning the idea that perinatal steroids change the essential structure of the nervous system. However, even the earliest paper of the proponents of the "organizational theory" anticipated

*We have recently demonstrated that male guinea pigs are less sensitive than females to the induction of hypothalamic cytoplasmic progestin receptors by estradiol (J. Blaustein, H. Ryer, and H. Feder, Neuroendocrinology, 1980, in press).

that the effects of the perinatal hormones on the nervous system would be subtle rather than gross (Phoenix *et al.*, 1959).

E. Perinatal Hormones—Are Their Effects on the Nervous System General or Localized?

The finding that perinatal hormones affect behavior led Nadler (1968) to attempt to localize the anatomical site of action of these hormones. In this pioneering experiment, Nadler gave intracranial implants of testosterone preparations to newborn female rats. He learned that hypothalamic implants caused an increase in male behavior and an acyclic pattern of female behavior. Cerebral cortical or amygdaloid implants did not have as marked effects as the hypothalamic implants. The interpretation of these data was made difficult by the possibility of leakage of the implanted androgen into the systemic circulation. More recently, Christensen and Gorski (1975) found that neonatal intracranial implants of testosterone or estradiol into rat preoptic area caused an increase in mounting behavior in adulthood in the absence of any detectable leakage of the steroid into the systemic circulation.

The results, of course, should not be taken to mean that the hypothalamus and preoptic area are the only neural sites on which the perinatal steroids act. Hart (1968) has presented evidence that testicular androgen in the neonate exerts effects at the spinal level. Thus, male rats castrated at 4 days of age and given androgen therapy in adulthood did not show ejaculatory movements to manual stimulation of the penis when spinal transection was carried out. In contrast, males castrated after the period of maximal susceptibility and given comparable treatment did show ejaculatory movements. Workers studying ovulation have also implicated the amygdala as a possible site of perinatal hormone action (Velasco and Taleisnik, 1969), and this site may be relevant for sexual behavior as well.

In summary, it would be premature to ascribe the major effects of perinatal hormones exclusively to their actions on hypothalamic cells.

F. What Is the Effective Perinatal Hormone—Is It Testosterone or a Metabolite of Testosterone?

Indirect evidence suggests that the concentration of testicular hormone during prenatal stages, even in short-gestation species, is related to the potential for display of masculine behaviors in adulthood. For example, Clemens and Coniglio (1971) and Gandelman *et al.* (1977) found a direct relationship between the number and position of fetal male siblings and the ability of fetal female siblings to display male behaviors in adulthood. That is, in rats and in mice, a female fetus that is immediately adjacent to two male fetuses is more likely to display male behaviors in adulthood than a female fetus that is immediately adjacent to other female fetuses. Ward (1972) showed that prenatal stress causes decreases in mounting behavior of genetic male rats in adulthood. This effect may be a result of stress-induced alteration in fetal androgen secretion (Ward and Weisz, 1980).

More direct chemical evidence supports the notion that fetal rat testes are capable of producing androgens (Noumura *et al.*, 1966). Prenatal male sheep (Attal, 1969) and rhesus monkeys (Resko, 1970) have been shown to secrete testosterone in higher quantities than their female counterparts. The period of maximal susceptibility to organizing actions of steroid hormones extends into the postnatal period in short-gestation species, and heightened testosterone secretion in male rats during the early postnatal period has been demonstrated (Resko *et al.*, 1968; Brown-Grant, 1974). In a recent publication, Döhler and Wuttke (1975) reported evidence for increased secretion of androgens other than testosterone during the postnatal period in male rats. The nature of these other substances is unknown, but it is unlikely that either androstenedione or 5α-dihydrotestosterone are potent factors. Androstenedione levels are low in rats in early neonatal life (Resko *et al.*, 1968), and this substance, given neonatally, is rather ineffective in decreasing lordosis in adult rats (Goldfoot *et al.*, 1969; Stern, 1969). 5α-Dihydrotestosterone also does not appear to be present in large quantities in the circulation during early postnatal life (Döhler and Wuttke, 1975), and this substance also seems ineffective, when given neonatally, in suppressing lordosis in adulthood (Whalen and Rezek, 1974). However, more recent data suggest that the lack of a behavioral effect of 5α-dihydrotestosterone may be because of reduced bioavailability (e.g., it may be rapidly metabolized) of the injected material rather than because of an intrinsic inability of this substance to affect neural tissues involved in sex behavior (Gerall *et al.*, 1976).

The possibility that perinatal 5α-dihydrotestosterone has consequences for behavior is important. ' 5α-Dihydrotestosterone is a nonaromatizable metabolite of testosterone. One of the most intriguing suggestions in the recent literature is that androgen must be aromatized to estrogen in order to exert its perinatal effects (Reddy *et al.*, 1974).

Several independent lines of evidence suggest that aromatization may indeed be a significant factor in perinatal neural differentiation. First, estradiol given perinatally to rodents tends to suppress lordosis and enhance mounting in adulthood (Whalen and Nadler, 1963; Levine and Mullins, 1964; Feder and Whalen, 1965). That is, estradiol mimics the effects of testosterone and the effects of the perinatal testis. Defeminizing effects of estradiol on behavior and on gonadotropins can be seen even after low doses of the compound (Zucker and Feder, 1966). Second, aromatization of androgen has been shown to occur in limbic structures of perinatal as well as adult rats (Weisz and Gibbs, 1974; Reddy *et al.*, 1974; Lieberburg and McEwen, 1975). Third, neonatally administered aromatizable androgens have, in general, been shown to be more effective than nonaromatizable androgens in inducing later behavioral effects (Paup *et al.*, 1972; Coniglio *et al.*, 1973). Fourth, the neonatal rat and mouse brain can concentrate radioactive estrogen in the hypothalamus (Sheridan *et al.*, 1974a; Fox, 1975). Fifth, antiestrogens can block the defeminizing effects of perinatal androgens on gonadotropin release patterns and adult sexual behavior (McDonald and Doughty, 1972; review by Plapinger and McEwen, 1978).

According to proponents of the aromatization hypothesis, testosterone secreted by the testis acts as a prohormone. It enters the systemic circulation without being inactivated by α-fetoprotein that interacts with and inactivates circulating estrogens in young rats (Raynaud *et al.*, 1971; Nunez *et al.*, 1971; Plapinger *et al.*, 1973). Indeed, several workers have demonstrated that considerable quantities of estrogen are present in neonatal rats (Weisz and Gunsalus, 1973; Meijs-Roelofs *et al.*, 1973; Döhler and Wuttke, 1975). Testosterone then enters hypothalamic cells and is converted to estrogen. The estrogen, now sequestered from inactivation by peripheral influences, accumulates in relatively high concentrations in hypothalamic cells bearing estrogen receptor molecules and then exerts its effects by interactions with the chromosomes of hypothalamic cells (Fig. 1).

Attractive as this hypothesis is, it must be borne in mind that the issue is probably more complicated than the scheme suggests. Factors other than α-fetoprotein (e.g., progesterone) may act as protective agents against estro-

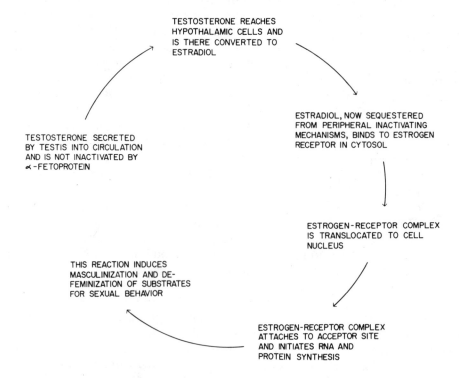

Figure 1. A metabolic sequence whereby estrogen derived from testicular androgen may influence sexual differentiation of the central nervous system.

gens or androgens (Dorfman, 1967). In guinea pigs, α-fetoprotein has not been demonstrated in blood (Savu *et al.*, 1974; Plapinger *et al.*, 1977). No conclusive evidence demonstrates that testosterone is unable to act in its own right as a major factor influencing sexual differentiation of the brain (Sheridan *et al.*, 1974b).

In summary, at this point it is uncertain whether testosterone or a metabolite of it is the major hormonal factor influencing neural differentiation. Even if the aromatization hypothesis should be validated for the rat, hormones other than estrogens may be significant factors in other species.

G. Do Perinatal Hormones Influence Noncopulatory as Well as Copulatory Behavior?

The prediction by Phoenix *et al.* (1959) that noncopulatory behavior might be influenced by the hormonal milieu at the time of neural differentiation has been amply fulfilled. The following is a partial catalog of effects of perinatal hormones on noncopulatory behaviors. More complete discussions can be found in reviews by Gorski (1971) and Goy and Goldfoot (1973).

It has been demonstrated that neonatally androgenized female mice and rats given androgen in adulthood attack other mice or rats more readily than females given no neonatal androgens (Edwards, 1968; Bronson and Desjardins, 1970). Conversely, male mice castrated neonatally and given androgen replacement in adulthood do not fight as readily as male mice that were not castrated at the maximally susceptible period (Edwards, 1969). Neonatally androgenized female hamsters display increased fighting behavior in adulthood, and these effects are manifested even before hormone replacement therapy is initiated in adulthood (Carter and Landauer, 1975). Early androgenization of female mice leads to production of a pheromone that stimulates aggression against the female by males (Lee and Griffo, 1973).

Neonatally castrated male rats given androgen replacement in adulthood did not engage in pup-killing behavior as frequently as males castrated later in life (Rosenberg and Sherman, 1975).

Some aspects of maternal behavior in rats were also influenced by perinatal hormone manipulation. For example, neonatally castrated rats were more likely to retrieve pups than males castrated later in life. Neonatally androgenized females, on the other hand, were, as adults, less likely to retrieve pups than neonatally untreated females (Quadagno and Rockwell, 1972; Bridges *et al.*, 1973). Prenatally androgen-treated female rabbits exhibited less nest-building behavior than controls when both groups were given estrogen–progesterone in adulthood (Anderson *et al.*, 1970).

Neonatal injections of androgen have been reported to influence food intake (Bell and Zucker, 1971), saccharin preference (Wade and Zucker, 1969), and spontaneous salt and water intake (Kreček *et al.*, 1975) in adult female rats. However, in these cases as well as in some other experiments dealing with noncopulatory behavior, it is difficult to decide whether the neonatal androgen acted directly on neural tissues or whether it acted by altering adult patterns of ovarian secretion.

Open-field behavior, maze performance, and escape–avoidance conditioning are also sexually dimorphic characteristics that are altered in a masculine direction by administration of androgen to neonatal female rodents (Swanson, 1967; Gray *et al.*, 1969; Beatty and Beatty, 1970; Stewart *et al.*, 1975). Of particular interest is the finding that this masculinization of open-field behavior and of emergence behavior is not dependent on the presence of gonadal tissue or exogenous gonadal steroids in adulthood (Pfaff and Zigmond, 1971; Blizard *et al.*, 1975).

Territorial scent-marking behavior in the Mongolian gerbil is exhibited more frequently by adult males than by adult females (Thiessen *et al.*, 1970), and the behavior is dependent on the presence of androgen in adulthood (Thiessen *et al.*, 1968). Turner (1975) demonstrated that early neonatal castration of males decreases, and early neonatal androgenization of females increases, territorial marking in response to administration of testosterone in adulthood.

Female dogs treated with androgen before birth and during infancy assume the masculine type of urination stance in adulthood (Beach, 1971). The sexually dimorphic patterning of micturition posture in dogs is apparently not dependent on activating effects of hormones in adulthood (Martins and Valle, 1948).

From the foregoing account, it is apparent that perinatal hormones influence a variety of noncopulatory behaviors. Sometimes they do so by altering estrogen–progesterone responsiveness in adulthood (e.g., for nest-building behavior in rabbits), sometimes by influencing androgen-responsive systems in adulthood (e.g., territorial marking in gerbils), and sometimes by influencing sexually dimorphic behavior patterns that are independent of the effects of hormones of adulthood (e.g., micturition behavior in dogs). The variety of behaviors affected by perinatal hormones and the variety of mechanisms by which these effects are achieved seem to suggest multiple sites of action for the perinatal hormones. The fact that perinatal hormones influence hormone-independent adult behavioral patterns is at variance with the view that perinatal hormones are merely chemical sensitizers that alter neural responsiveness to hormones of adulthood. In agreement with these thoughts, Pfaff and Zigmond (1971) suggested that alterations in uptake or retention of gonadal hormones induced by perinatal hormone treatments would be insufficient to account for all the behavioral consequences of such treatments.

H. Do Prenatal Hormones Influence Behavior of Primates?

After their work on the effects of prenatal androgens on the behavior of adult guinea pigs, Young *et al.* (1964) initiated a study of the consequences of prenatal androgenization of female rhesus macaques. Pregnant rhesus monkeys were given injections of testosterone propionate from days 40 to 90 of a 168-day pregnancy, and the behavior of female offspring was assessed prior to their attainment of puberty. The results of behavioral tests indicated that the pseudohermaphrodites were intermediate between control females and control males in frequency of display of behaviors such as rough and tumble play, sham threat, chasing, mounting, and play initiation (Fig. 2).

The results again suggest, as in the case of some nonprimates, that prenatal hormones influence the display of noncopulatory behaviors that do not require activating effects of gonadal steroids (Goy, 1970). However, a number of questions regarding the primate work remains to be answered. For example, is intracerebral aromatization of prenatal androgens a requirement for masculinization of any or all aspects of behavior? Do masculinizing effects of prenatal androgenization persist beyond puberty and into adulthood? On this point, some positive evidence already exists. For example, an adult pseudohermaphrodite displayed the complete pattern of male copulatory behavior when given androgen in adulthood (Goy and Resko, 1972). Is it conceivable that the increased frequency of masculine behavior in the pseudohermaphrodites is not the result of direct effects of prenatal androgen on central neural tissues? An effect on behavior might be mediated by other, more indirect mechanisms. For example, the prenatal androgen treatment may have caused increases in body size or muscle development. Or a subtle difference between the way a pseudohermaphrodite is reared and perceived by its mother and its peers and the way these developmental interactions proceed in normal females may account for masculinization of behavior in the pseudohermaphrodite.

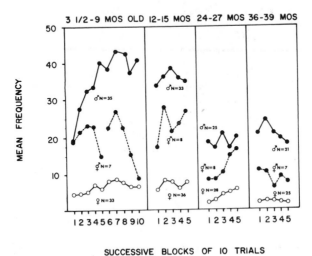

Figure 2. Frequency of play initiation in juveniles is increased by prenatal androgenization of female rhesus macaques. (Reproduced with permission from Goy and Resko, 1972.)

The role of prenatal hormones in the differentiation of sex-related behavioral characteristics in humans has been the subject of much conjecture. Androgenization of human female fetuses has occurred through the agency of excessive production of adrenal androgens (andrenogenital syndrome) and through the administration of antiabortion steroids with androgenic properties. In both types of cases, evidence has been presented that prepubertal behaviors are masculinized (e.g., increased tomboyishness) even though the individuals affected are raised as females (Money and Ehrhardt, 1972a). However, it would be unwise to conclude that our culturally grounded assumptions as to what constitutes "masculine" or "feminine" behaviors are necessarily reflections of biological processes (Bermant and Davidson, 1974). Certainly, some of the effects associated with exposure to prenatal androgens (e.g., choice of clothing style, emphasis on having a career) have lost much of their "masculine" connotation as a result of recent social changes (Money and Ehrhardt, 1972b).

A syndrome in which a genotypic human male is insensitive to the prenatal and postnatal actions of androgens (testicular feminization) has also been described (Hauser, 1963). In these cases, individuals have a female appearance and are raised as females. Their behavior is indistinguishable from normal females. The combined data on prenatal androgenization and on prenatal androgen insensitivity are not inconsistent with the basic principle that the presence of excessive androgen prenatally is associated with "masculinization" and the absence of adequate prenatal androgenic stimulation is associated with "feminization" of behavior. It is difficult to assign relative weights to each of the factors that might influence psychosexuality in humans. Undoubtedly, the major factor influencing gender identity is the sex of rearing. However, factors such as genetic sex, gonadal sex, hormonal sex, and sex of the internal and external genitalia may act prenatally to set a sexual bias by the time of birth. In this view, each individual at birth is sexually bipotential but not sexually neutral at birth (Fig. 3; Diamond, 1965).

In conclusion, there may be influences of prenatal hormones on psychosexuality in primates, including humans, but such influences are extremely difficult to assess because of the overriding significance of social factors. In a broad sense, primates can be said to have become relatively "emancipated" not only from the activating influences of hormones on behavior (Beach, 1947; but see also Nadler, 1975) but also from their organizing influences.

IV. SUMMARY

In this chapter the role of perinatal hormones in the differentiation of copulatory and noncopulatory behaviors was discussed. In rodents, hormones of testicular origin act perinatally both to defeminize (suppress lordosis behavior in response to estrogen–progesterone therapy in adulthood) and to masculinize (enhance male-like copulatory responses to androgen therapy in

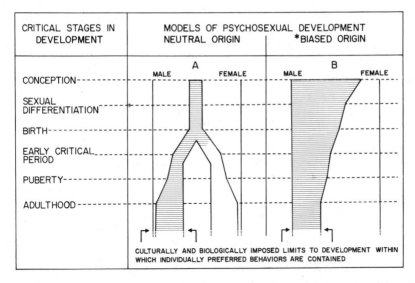

Figure 3. Two possible models of psychosexual differentiation of humans. (Reproduced with permission from Diamond, 1965.) *To avoid complications within the graph, only the development along a masculine direction is shown. Development of a female would be similar but on the opposite side.

adulthood). Evidence that these processes are independent and are, at least partially, mediated by CNS mechanisms was presented. Perinatal androgens also influence a wide range of noncopulatory sexually dimorphic patterns of behaviors, some of which do not require hormones for their activation in adulthood. Prenatal androgens or their metabolites may also influence neural circuits mediating experiential effects in primates, including humans.

ACKNOWLEDGMENTS. I am fortunate to have had the helpful comments of Dr. Frank A. Beach on this manuscript. His unique blend of brilliance, warmth, and cantankerousness has inspired and provoked all workers in the field of hormones and behavior ever since he founded the field with Dr. W. C. Young. Auri Naggar and Christina Williams also read the manuscript and offered invaluable suggestions to clarify it. I thank Ms. Winona Cunningham for typing the manuscript and Ms. Cindy Banas for preparing the graphics. The author is supported by Research Grant NIH-HD-04467 and Research Scientist Development Award NIMH-K2-29006. Contribution Number 300 of the Institute of Animal Behavior.

REFERENCES

Anderson, C. O., Zarrow, M. X., and Denenberg, V. H., 1970, Maternal behavior in the rabbit: Effects of androgen treatment during gestation upon the nest-building behavior of the mother and her offspring, *Horm. Behav.* 1:337.

Arén-Engelbrektsson, B., Larsson, K., Södersten, P., and Wilhelmsson, M., 1970, The female lordosis pattern induced in male rats by estrogen, *Horm. Behav.* **1**:181.

Attal, J., 1969, Levels of testosterone, androstenedione, estrone and estradiol-17β in the testes of fetal sheep, *Endocrinology* **85**:280.

Ball, J., 1937, Sex activity of castrated male rats increased by estrin administration, *J. Comp. Psychol.* **24**:135.

Barraclough, C. A., and Gorski, R. A., 1961, Evidence that the hypothalamus is responsible for androgen-induced sterility in the female rat, *Endocrinology* **68**:68.

Barraclough, C. A., and Gorski, R. A., 1962, Studies on mating behaviour in the androgen-sterilized female rat in relation to the hypothalamic regulation of sexual behaviour, *J. Endocrinol.* **25**:175.

Beach, F. A., 1945, Hormonal induction of mating responses in a rat with congenital absence of gonadal tissue, *Anat. Rec.* **92**:289.

Beach, F. A., 1947, Evolutionary changes in the physiological control of mating behavior in mammals, *Psychol. Rev.* **54**:297.

Beach, F. A., 1948, *Hormones and Behavior*, Paul B. Hoeber, New York.

Beach, F. A., 1971, Hormonal factors controlling the differentiation, development, and display of copulatory behavior in the ramstergig and related species, in: *The Biopsychology of Development* (E. Tobach, L. R. Aronson, and E. Shaw, eds.), pp. 249–295, Academic Press, New York.

Beach, F. A., and Holz, A. M., 1946, Mating behavior in male rats castrated at various ages and injected with androgen, *J. Exp. Zool.* **101**:91.

Beach, F. A., and Kuehn, R. E., 1970, Coital behavior in dogs. X. Effects of androgenic stimulation during development on feminine mating responses in females and males, *Horm. Behav.* **1**:347.

Beach, F. A., and Rasquin, P., 1942, Masculine copulatory behavior in intact and castrated female rats, *Endocrinology* **31**:393.

Beach, F. A., Noble, R. G., and Orndoff, R. K., 1969, Effects of perinatal androgen treatment on responses of male rats to gonadal hormones in adulthood, *J. Comp. Physiol. Psychol.* **68**:490.

Beatty, W. A., and Beatty, P. A., 1970, Hormonal determinants of sex differences in avoidance behavior and reactivity to electric shock in the rat, *J. Comp. Physiol. Psychol.* **73**:446.

Bell, D. D., and Zucker, I., 1971, Sex differences in body weight and eating: Organization and activation by gonadal hormones in the rat, *Physiol Behav.* **7**:27.

Bermant, G., and Davidson, J. M., 1974, *Biological Bases of Sexual Behavior*, Harper & Row, New York.

Black, M., 1962, *Models and Metaphors. Studies in Language and Philosophy*, Cornell University Press, Ithaca.

Blizard, D. A., Lippman, H. R., and Chen, J. J., 1975, Sex differences in open-field behavior in the rat: The inductive and activational role of gonadal hormones, *Physiol. Behav.* **14**:601.

Bridges, R. S., Zarrow, M. X., and Denenberg, V. H., 1973, The role of neonatal androgen in the expression of hormonally induced maternal responsiveness in the adult rat, *Horm. Behav.* **4**:315.

Bronson, F. H., and Desjardins, C., 1970, Neonatal androgen administration and adult aggressiveness in female mice, *Gen. Comp. Endocrinol.* **15**:320.

Brown-Grant, K., 1974, On "critical periods" during the post-natal development of the rat, in: *Endocrinologie Sexuelle de la Période Périnatale* (M. G. Forest and J. Bertrand, eds.), pp. 357–375, INSERM, Paris.

Brown-Grant, K., 1975, A re-examination of the lordosis response in female rats given high doses of testosterone propionate or estradiol benzoate in the neonatal period, *Horm. Behav.* **6**:351.

Campbell, H. J., 1965, Effects of neonatal injection of hormones on sexual behaviour and reproduction in the rabbit, *J. Physiol. (Lond.)* **181**:568.

Carter, C. S., and Landauer, M. R., 1975, Neonatal hormone experience and adult lordosis and fighting in the golden hamster, *Physiol. Behav.* **14**:1.

Carter, C. S., Clemens, L. G., and Hoekema, D. J., 1972, Neonatal androgen and adult sexual behavior in the golden hamster, *Physiol. Behav.* **9**:89.

Christensen, L. W., and Gorski, R. A., 1975, Neonatal steroid implants and adult sexual behavior (abstr.), Eastern Conference on Reproductive Behavior (May, 1975), Nags Head, North Carolina.

Clayton, R. B., Kogura, J., and Kraemer, H. C., 1970, Sexual differentiation of the brain: Effects of testosterone on brain RNA metabolism in newborn female rats, *Nature* **226**:810.

Clemens, L. G., 1973, Development and behavior, in: *Comparative Psychology* (D. A. Dewsbury and D. A. Rethlingshafer, eds.), pp. 238–268, McGraw-Hill, New York.

Clemens, L. G., and Coniglio, L., 1971, Influence of prenatal litter composition on mounting behavior of female rats (abstr.), *Am. Zool.* **11**:617.

Clemens, L. G., Shryne, J., and Gorski, R. A., 1970, Androgen and development of progesterone responsiveness in male and female rats, *Physiol. Behav.* **5**:673.

Collingwood, R. G., 1958, *The Principles of Art,* Galaxy, New York.

Coniglio, L. P., Paup, D. C., and Clemens, L. G., 1973, Hormonal factors controlling the development of sexual behavior in the male golden hamster, *Physiol. Behav.* **10**:1087.

Dantchakoff, V., 1938a, Rôle des hormones dans la manifestation des instincts sexuels, *C. R. Acad.[D] (Paris)* **206**:945.

Dantchakoff, V., 1938b, Sur les effets de l'hormone male dans une jeune cobaye femelle traité depuis un stade embryonnaire (inversions sexuelles), *C. R. Soc. Biol. (Paris)* **127**:1255.

Davidson, J. M., 1969, Effects of estrogen on the sexual behavior of male rats, *Endocrinology* **84**:1365.

Davidson, J. M., and Levine, S., 1969, Progesterone and heterotypical sexual behaviour in male rats, *J. Endocrinol.* **44**:129.

Denef, C., and De Moor, P., 1972, Sexual differentiation of steroid metabolizing enzymes in the rat liver. Further studies on predetermination by testosterone at birth, *Endocrinology* **91**:374.

Diamond, M., 1965, A critical evaluation of the ontogeny of human sexual behavior, *Q. Rev. Biol.* **40**:147.

Döhler, K. D., and Wuttke, W., 1975, Changes with age in levels of serum gonadotropins, prolactin, and gonadal steroids in prepubertal male and female rats, *Endocrinology* **97**:898.

Dorfman, R. I., 1967, The antiestrogenic and antiandrogenic activities of progesterone in the defense of a normal fetus, *Anat. Rec.* **157**:547.

Dörner, G., and Staudt, J., 1969, Structural changes in the hypothalamic ventromedial nucleus of the male rat, following neonatal castration and androgen treatment, *Neuroendocrinology* **4**:278.

Eaton, G., 1970, Effect of a single prepubertal injection of testosterone propionate on adult bisexual behavior of male hamsters castrated at birth, *Endocrinology* **87**:934.

Edwards, D. A., 1968, Mice: Fighting by neonatally androgenized females, *Science* **161**:1027.

Edwards, D. A., 1969, Early androgen stimulation and aggressive behavior in male and female mice, *Physiol. Behav.* **4**:333.

Edwards, D. A., 1970, Post-neonatal androgenization and adult aggressive behavior in female mice, *Physiol. Behav.* **5**:465.

Edwards, D. A., and Burge, K. G., 1971, Early androgen treatment and male and female sexual behavior in mice, *Horm. Behav.* **2**:49.

Emery, D. E., and Sachs, B. D., 1975, Ejaculatory pattern in female rats without androgen treatment, *Science* **190**:484.

Feder, H. H., 1967, Specificity of testosterone and estradiol in the differentiating neonatal rat, *Anat. Rec.* **157**:79.

Feder, H. H., and Whalen, R. E., 1965, Feminine behavior in neonatally castrated and estrogen-treated male rats, *Science* **147**:306.

Flerkó, B., Mess, B., and Illei-Donhoffer, A., 1969, On the mechanism of androgen sterilization, *Neuroendocrinology* **4**:164.

Fox, T. O., 1975, Oestradiol receptor of neonatal mouse brain, *Nature* **258**:441.

Gandelman, R., Vom Saal, F. S., and Reinisch, J. M., 1977, Contiguity to male foetuses affects morphology and behaviour of female mice, *Nature* **266**:722.

Gerall, A. A., and Kenny, A. McM., 1970, Neonatally androgenized female's responsiveness to estrogen and progesterone, *Endocrinology* **87**:560.

Gerall, A. A., and Ward, I. L., 1966, Effects of prenatal exogenous androgen on the sexual behavior of the female albino rat, *J. Comp. Physiol. Psychol.* **62**:370.

Gerall, A. A., Dunlap, J. L., and Wagner, J. W., 1976, Effects of dihydrotestosterone and gonado-tropins on the development of female behavior, *Physiol. Behav.* **17**:121.

Goldfoot, D. A., Feder, H. H., and Goy, R. W., 1969, Development of bisexuality in the male rat treated neonatally with androstenedione, *J. Comp. Physiol. Psychol.* **67**:41.

Goodale, H. D., 1918, Feminized male birds, *Genetics* **3**:276.

Gorski, R. A., 1971, Gonadal hormones and the perinatal development of neuroendocrine func-tion, in: *Frontiers in Neuroendocrinology* (L. Martini and W. F. Ganong, eds.), pp. 237–290, Oxford University Press, New York.

Gorski, R. A., and Barraclough, C. A., 1963, Effects of low dosages of androgen on the differentia-tion of hypothalamic regulatory control of ovulation in the rat, *Endocrinology* **73**:210.

Goy, R. W., 1970, Experimental control of psychosexuality, *Phil. Trans. R. Soc. Lond.* [B] **259**: 149.

Goy, R. W., and Goldfoot, D. A., 1973, Hormonal influences on sexually dimorphic behavior, in: *Handbook of Physiology*, Sect. 7, Vol. 2, Part 1 (R. O. Greep, ed.), pp. 169–186, American Physiological Society, Washington.

Goy, R. W., and Resko, J. A, 1972, Gonadal hormones and behavior of normal pseudo-hermaphroditic nonhuman female primates, *Recent Prog. Horm. Res.* **28**:707.

Goy, R. W., Bridson, W. E., and Young, W. C., 1964, Period of maximal susceptibility of the prenatal female guinea pig to masculinizing actions of testosterone propionate, *J. Comp. Physiol. Psychol.* **57**:166.

Goy, R. W., Phoenix, C. H., and Meidinger, R., 1967, Postnatal development of sensitivity to estrogen and androgen in male, female and pseudohermaphroditic guinea pigs, *Anat. Rec.* **157**:87.

Grady, K. L., Phoenix, C. H., and Young, W. C., 1965, Role of the developing rat testis in differentiation of the neural tissues mediating mating behavior, *J. Comp. Physiol. Psychol.* **59**:176.

Gray, J. A., Lean, J., and Keynes, A., 1969, Infant androgen treatment and adult open-field behavior: Direct effects and effects of injections to siblings, *Physiol. Behav.* **4**:177.

Green, R., Luttge, W. G., and Whalen, R. E., 1969, Uptake and retention of tritiated estradiol in brain and peripheral tissues of male, female, and neonatally androgenized female rats, *Endocrinology* **85**:373.

Harris, G. W., and Levine, S., 1965, Sexual differentiation of the brain and its experimental control, *J. Physiol. (Lond.)* **181**:379.

Hart, B. L., 1968, Neonatal castration: Influence on neural organization of sexual reflexes in male rats, *Science* **160**:1135.

Hart, B. L., 1972, Manipulation of neonatal androgen: Effects on sexual responses and penile development in male rats, *Physiol. Behav.* **8**:841.

Hauser, G. A., 1963, Testicular feminization, in: *Intersexuality* (C. Overzier, ed.), pp. 255–276, Academic Press, New York.

Hitt, J. C., Hendricks, S. E., Ginsberg, S. I., and Lewis, J. H., 1970, Disruption of male but not female sexual behavior in rats by medial forebrain bundle lesions, *J. Comp. Physiol. Psychol.* **73**:377.

Jakubczak, L. F., 1964, The effects of testosterone propionate on age differences in mating behavior, *J. Gerontol.* **19**:458.

Kraulis, I., and Clayton, R. B., 1968, Sexual differentiation of testosterone metabolism exemplified by the accumulation of 3β, 17α-dihydroxy-5α-androstane-3-sulfate as a metabolite of testo-sterone in the castrated rat, *J. Biol. Chem.* **243**:3546.

Kreček, J., Pánek, M., Salátová, J., and Zicha, J., 1975, The pineal gland and the effect of neonatal administration of androgen upon the development of spontaneous salt and water intake in female rats, *Neuroendocrinology* **18**:137.

Ladosky, W., and Gaziri, L. C. J., 1970, Brain serotonin and sexual differentiation of the nervous system, *Neuroendocrinology* **6**:168.

Leathem, J. H., 1961, Nutritional effects on endocrine secretions, in: *Sex and Internal Secretions*, Third Edition (W. C. Young, ed.), pp. 666–704, Williams & Wilkins, Baltimore.

Lee, C. T., and Griffo, W., 1973, Early androgenization and aggression pheromone in inbred mice, *Horm. Behav.* **4**:181.

Levine, S., and Mullins, R., Jr., 1964, Estrogen administered neonatally affects adult sexual behavior in male and female rats, *Science* **144**:185.

Lieberburg, I., and McEwen, B. S., 1975, Estradiol-17β: A metabolite of testosterone recovered in cell nuclei from limbic areas of neonatal rat brains, *Brain Res.* **85**:165.

Litteria, M., 1973, Inhibitory action of neonatal androgenization on the incorporation of (^{3}H)-lysine in specific hypothalamic nuclei of the adult female rat, *Exp. Neurol.* **41**:395.

Litteria, M., and Thorner, M. W., 1974, Inhibition in the incorporation of ^{3}H-lysine in the Purkinje cells of the adult female rat after neonatal androgenization, *Brain Res.* **69**:170.

Luttge, W. G., and Hall, N. R., 1973, Differential effectiveness of testosterone and its metabolites in the induction of male sexual behavior in two strains of albino mice, *Horm. Behav.* **4**:31.

MacKinnon, P. C. B., 1970, A comparison of protein synthesis in the brains of mice before and after puberty, *J. Physiol. (Lond.)* **210**:10P.

Martins, T., and Valle, J. R., 1948, Hormonal regulation of the micturition behavior of the dog, *J. Comp. Physiol. Psychol.* **41**:301.

Maurer, R., and Woolley, D., 1971, Distribution of ^{3}H-estradiol in clomiphene treated and neonatally androgenized rats, *Endocrinology* **88**:1281.

McDonald, P. G., and Doughty, C., 1972, Inhibition of androgen-sterilization in the female rat by administration of an anti-oestrogen, *J. Endocrinol.* **55**:455.

McEwen, B. S., and Pfaff, D. W., 1970, Factors influencing sex hormone uptake by rat brain regions. I. Effects of neonatal treatment, hypophysectomy, and competing steroids, *Brain Res.* **21**:1.

McGill, T. E., and Haynes, C. M., 1973, Heterozygosity and retention of ejaculatory reflex after castration in male mice, *J. Comp. Physiol. Psychol.* **84**:423.

McGuire, J. L., and Lisk, R. D., 1969, Oestrogen receptors in androgen or oestrogen sterilized female rats, *Nature* **221**:1068.

Meijs-Roelofs, H. M. A., Uilenbroek, J. T. J., de Jong, F. H., and Welschen, R., 1973, Plasma oestradiol-17β and its relationship to serum follicle-stimulating hormone in immature female rats, *J. Endocrinol.* **59**:295.

Money, J., and Ehrhardt, A. A., 1972a, *Man and Woman Boy and Girl*, Johns Hopkins University Press, Baltimore.

Money, J., and Ehrhardt, A. A., 1972b, Gender dimorphic behavior and fetal sex hormones, *Recent Prog. Horm. Res.* **28**:735.

Nadler, R. D., 1968, Masculinization of female rats by intracranial implantation of androgen in infancy, *J. Comp. Physiol. Psychol.* **66**:157.

Nadler, R. D., 1975, Sexual cyclicity in captive lowland gorillas, *Science* **189**:813.

Naftolin, F., Morishita, H., Davies, I. J., Todd, R., Ryan, K. J., and Fishman, J., 1975, 2-Hydroxyestrone induced rise in serum luteinizing hormone in the immature male rat, *Biochem. Biophys. Res. Commun.* **64**:905.

Noumura, T., Weisz, J., and Lloyd, C. W., 1966, *In vitro* conversion of 7-^{3}H-progesterone to androgens by the rat testis during the second half of fetal life, *Endocrinology* **78**:245.

Nunez, E., Engelmann, F., Benassayag, C., and Jayle, M.-F., 1971, Identification et purification préliminaire de la foeto-protéine liant les oestrogenes dans le serum de rats nouveau-nés, *C. R. Acad. Sci. [D] (Paris)* **273**:831.

Paup, D. C., Coniglio, L. P., and Clemens, L. G., 1972, Masculinization of the female golden hamster by neonatal treatment with androgen or estrogen, *Horm. Behav.* **3**:123.

Pfaff, D. W., 1966, Morphological changes in the brains of adult male rats after neonatal castration, *J. Endocrinol.* **36**:415.

Pfaff, D., 1970, Nature of sex hormone effects on rat sex behavior: Specificity of effects and individual patterns of response, *J. Comp. Physiol. Psychol.* **73**:349.

Pfaff, D. W., and Zigmond, R. E., 1971, Neonatal androgen effects on sexual and nonsexual behavior of adult rats tested under various hormone regimes, *Neuroendocrinology* **7**:129.

Phoenix, C. H., Goy, R. W., Gerall, A. A., and Young, W. C., 1959, Organizing action of prenatally administered testosterone propionate on the tissues mediating mating behavior in the female guinea pig, *Endocrinology* **65**:369.

Plapinger, L., McEwen, B. S., and Clemens, L. E., 1973, Ontogeny of estradiol-binding sites in rat brain. II. Characteristics of a neonatal binding macromolecule, *Endocrinology* **93**:1129.

Plapinger, L., Landau, I. T., McEwen, B. S., and Feder, H. H., 1977, Characteristics of estradiol-binding macromolecules in fetal and adult guinea pig brain cytosols, *Biol. Reprod.* **16**:586.

Quadagno, D. M., and Rockwell, J., 1972, The effect of gonadal hormones in infancy on maternal behavior in the adult rat, *Horm. Behav.* **3**:55.

Raisman, G., and Field, P. M., 1973, Sexual dimorphism in the neuropil of the preoptic area of the rat and its dependence on neonatal androgen, *Brain Res.* **54**:1.

Raynaud, J.-P, Mercier, B. C., and Baulieu, E. E., 1971, Rat estradiol binding plasma protein (EBP), *Steroids* **18**:767.

Reddy, V. V. R., Naftolin, F., and Ryan, K. J., 1974, Conversion of androstenedione to estrone by neural tissues from fetal and neonatal rats, *Endocrinology* **94**:117.

Resko, J. A., 1970, Androgen secretion by the fetal and neonatal rhesus monkey, *Endocrinology* **87**:680.

Resko, J. A., Feder, H. H., and Goy, R. W., 1968, Androgen concentration in plasma and testis of developing rats, *J. Endocrinol.* **40**:485.

Revesz, C., Kernaghan, D., and Bindra, D., 1963, Sexual drive of female rats "masculinized" by testosterone during gestation, *J. Endocrinol.* **25**:549.

Rosenberg, K. M., and Sherman, G. F., 1975, The role of testosterone in the organization, maintenance and activation of pup-killing behavior in the male rat, *Horm. Behav.* **6**:173.

Rosenblatt, J. S., and Aronson, L. R., 1958, The decline of sexual behavior in male cats after castration with special reference to the role of prior sexual experience, *Behaviour* **12**:285.

Sand, K., 1919, Experiments on the internal secretion of the sexual glands, especially on experimental hermaphroditism, *J. Physiol. (Lond.)* **53**:257.

Savu, L., Vallette, G., Nunez, E., Azrai, M., and Jayle, M.-F., 1974, Etude comparative de la liason entre les proteines ceiques a les oestrogenes libre au cours du développement de diverse especes animales, in: *L'Alphafoetoproteine* (R. Masseyeff, ed.), pp. 75–83, INSERM, Paris.

Sheridan, P. J., Sar, M., and Stumpf, W. E., 1974a, Autoradiographic localization of ^{3}H-estradiol or its metabolites in the central nervous system of the developing rat, *Endocrinology* **94**:1386.

Sheridan, P. J., Sar, M., and Stumpf, W. E., 1974b, Interaction of exogenous steroids in the developing rat brain, *Endocrinology* **95**:1749.

Shimada, H., and Gorbman, A., 1970, Long lasting changes in RNA synthesis in the forebrains of female rats treated with testosterone soon after birth, *Biochem. Biophys. Res. Commun.* **38**:423.

Short, R. V., 1974, Sexual differentiation of the brain of the sheep, in: *Endocrinologie Sexuelle de la Période Périnatale* (M. G. Forest and J. Bertrand, eds.), pp. 121–142, INSERM, Paris.

Singer, J. J., 1968, Control of male and female sexual behavior in the female rat, *J. Comp. Physiol. Psychol.* **66**:738.

Södersten, P., and Larsson, K., 1974, Lordosis behavior in castrated male rats treated with estradiol benzoate or testosterone propionate in combination with an estrogen antagonist, MER-25, and in intact male rats, *Horm. Behav.* **5**:13.

Spemann, H., 1938, *Embryonic Development and Induction*, Yale University Press, New Haven.

Steinach, E., 1940, *Sex and Life*, Viking Press, New York.

Stern, J. J., 1969, Neonatal castration, androstenedione, and the mating behavior of the male rat. *J. Comp. Physiol. Psychol.* **69**:608.

Stewart, J., Skvarenina, A., and Pottier, J., 1975, Effects of neonatal androgens on open-field behavior and maze learning in the prepubescent and adult rat, *Physiol. Behav.* **14**:291.

Swanson, H. H., 1967, Alteration of sex-typical behavior of hamsters in open-field and emergence tests by neonatal administration of androgen or oestrogen, *Anim. Behav.* **15**:209.

Swanson, H. H., 1971, The origin of sex differences in behaviour in the golden hamster, *Brain Res.* **34**:9.

Thiessen, D. D., Friend, H. C., and Lindzey, G., 1968, Androgen control of territorial marking in the Mongolian gerbil, *Science* **160**:432.

Thiessen, D. D., Blum, S. L., and Lindzey, G., 1970, A scent marking response associated with the ventral sebaceous gland in the Mongolian gerbil (*Meriones unguiculatus*), *Anim. Behav.* **18**:26.

Tiefer, L., 1970, Gonadal hormones and mating behavior in the adult golden hamster, *Horm. Behav.* **1**:189.

Toran-Allerand, C. D., 1975, Sex hormones and the development of long-term cultures of the newborn mouse hypothalamic/preoptic region (abstr.), The Endocrine Society Program, 57th Meeting, p. 55, The Endocrine Society, Bethesda, Maryland.

Turner, J. W., Jr., 1975, Influence of neonatal androgen on the display of territorial marking behavior in the gerbil, *Physiol. Behav.* **15**:265.

Valenstein, E. S., Riss, W., and Young, W. C., 1955, Experiential and genetic factors in the organization of sexual behavior in male guinea pigs, *J. Comp. Physiol. Psychol.* **48**:397.

Velasco, M. E., and Taleisnik, S., 1969, Release of gonadotropins induced by amygdaloid stimulation in the rat, *Endocrinology* **84**:132.

Vertes, M., and King, R. J. B., 1971, The mechanism of oestradiol binding in rat hypothalamus: Effect of androgenization, *J. Endocrinol.* **51**:271.

Wade, G. N., and Feder, H. H., 1972, 1,2-^{3}H-Progesterone uptake by guinea pig brain and uterus: Differential localization, time-course of uptake and metabolism and effects of age, sex, estrogen-priming and competing steroids, *Brain Res.* **45**:525.

Wade, G. N., and Zucker, I., 1969, Taste preferences of female rats: Modification by neonatal hormones, food deprivation and prior experience, *Physiol. Behav.* **4**:935.

Ward, I. L., 1969, Differential effect of pre- and postnatal androgen on the sexual behavior of intact and spayed female rats, *Horm. Behav.* **1**:25.

Ward, I. L., 1972, Prenatal stress feminizes and demasculinizes the behavior of males, *Science* **175**:82.

Ward, I. L., and Renz, F. J., 1972, Consequences of perinatal hormone manipulation on the adult sexual behavior of female rats, *J. Comp. Physiol. Psychol.* **78**:349.

Ward, I. L., and Weisz, J., 1980, Maternal stress alters plasma testosterone in fetal males, *Science* **207**:328.

Weisz, J., and Gibbs, C., 1974, Metabolites of testosterone in the brain of the newborn female rat after an injection of tritiated testosterone, *Neuroendocrinology* **14**:72.

Weisz, J., and Gunsalus, P., 1973, Estrogen levels in immature female rats: True or spurious— ovarian or adrenal? *Endocrinology* **93**:1057.

Whalen, R. E., and Edwards, D. A., 1967, Hormonal determinants of the development of masculine and feminine behavior in male and female rats, *Anat. Rec.* **157**:173.

Whalen, R. E., and Luttge, W. G., 1971, Perinatal administration of dihydrotestosterone to female rats and the development of reproductive function, *Endocrinology* **89**:1320.

Whalen, R. E., and Massicci, J., 1975, Subcellular analysis of the accumulation of estrogen by the brain of male and female rats, *Brain Res.* **89**:255.

Whalen, R. E., and Nadler, R. D., 1963, Suppression of the development of female mating behavior by estrogen administration in infancy, *Science* **141**:273.

Whalen, R. E., and Rezek, D. L., 1974, Inhibition of lordosis in female rats by subcutaneous implants of testosterone, androstenedione, or dihydrotestosterone in infancy, *Horm. Behav.* **5**:125.

Wilson, J. G., 1943, Reproductive capacity of adult female rats treated prepuberally with estrogenic hormone, *Anat. Rec.* **86**:341.

Wilson, J. G., and Wilson, H. C., 1943, Reproductive capacity in adult male rats treated prepuberally with androgenic hormone, *Endocrinology* **33**:353.

Wilson, J. G., Hamilton, J. B., and Young, W. C., 1941, Influence of age and presence of the ovaries on reproductive function in rats injected with androgens, *Endocrinology* **29**:784.

Young, W. C., 1961, Hormones and mating behavior, in: *Sex and Internal Secretions*, Third Edition (W. C. Young, ed.), pp. 1173–1239, Williams & Wilkins, Baltimore.

Young, W. C., Goy, R. W., and Phoenix, C. H., 1964. The hormones and sexual behavior. Broad relationships exist between the gonadal hormones and behavior, *Science* **143**:212.

Zucker, I., and Feder, H. H., 1966, The effect of neonatal reserpine treatment on female sex behaviour of rats, *J. Endocrinol.* **35**:423.

7

Early Organizational Effects of Hormones

An Evolutionary Perspective

ELIZABETH ADKINS-REGAN

I. INTRODUCTION

Sex differentiation offers one of the most striking examples of the realization of genetic differences by epigenetic means. "Indeed, especially in . . . [cold-blooded vertebrates] the environment assumes a greater part in fashioning the end-product than in almost any other genetically controlled process" (Dodd, 1960). In particular, behavioral sex differentiation provides a dramatic example of a permanent effect of sex steroids on brain function. There is also the possibility, already achieved in some species, of experimentally producing complete sex reversal.

The proliferation of sex differentiation as a field of study sometimes makes it difficult to integrate data and detect general organizing principles: the purpose of this chapter is to introduce the reader to the empirical data on zoological variations in the pattern of sex differentiation. Although most of the work on hormonal mechanisms controlling sex differentiation has been performed on laboratory rodents (see Chapters 5 and 6), the addition of a broad comparative perspective should both increase our understanding of major evolutionary and adaptive trends and also provide information about basic constraints and mechanisms of sexual differentiation in general.

ELIZABETH ADKINS-REGAN • Department of Psychology and Section of Neurobiology and Behavior, Cornell University, Ithaca, New York 14853.

This chapter will cover differentiation of gonads, other sex structures, and behavior (or, in physiological terms, differentiation of the neural substrate underlying behavior) chiefly in animals other than mammals. (Differentiation in mammals is treated in Chapters 1, 2, 5, 6, 8, 9, 10.) To some extent, the contents of this chapter were dictated by the amount of information available. Thus, while a good deal is known about morphological differentiation in bony fish, amphibians, and birds and about behavioral differentiation in birds, almost nothing is known about other topics such as differentiation in cartilaginous fish and reptiles and behavioral differentiation in fish, amphibians, and reptiles. Furthermore, differentiation of the physiological control of ovulation is still almost exclusively a mammalian research topic.

Since morphological sex differentiation has been reviewed frequently in the past, information in these reviews will be briefly summarized and greater detail will be reserved for experiments conducted more recently and for experiments with a behavioral emphasis.

A. Definitions and a Note on Taxonomy

A few definitions will help to prevent confusion. A hermaphrodite is an animal that produces both male and female germ cells, either simultaneously or successively. This is a normal condition in some species. An intersex has both male and female characters but produces only one kind of germ cell, if any (Bacci, 1965). In some species this also occurs in nature (e.g., toads) but usually occurs spontaneously only in a few aberrant individuals. The neutral (anhormonal) sex is the phenotype that results from differentiation in the absence of gonads. The homogametic sex is the sex with two similar sex chromosomes (e.g., XX). The homogametic sex can be either the male or the female, depending on the species. The heterogametic sex is the sex with two dissimilar sex chromosomes (e.g., XY). The dominant gonad refers to the fact that if two differentiating opposite-sexed gonads are cultured together *in vitro*, or if two differentiating opposite-sexed individuals are joined in parabiosis, or if a gonad is grafted into a differentiating individual of the opposite sex, the gonad of one sex will be altered by the gonad of the other sex. The gonad that alters, rather than is altered, is dominant. Homologous sex hormones are hormones that are characteristic of the sex (androgens in males and estrogens in females). Heterologous hormones are estrogens in males and androgens in females. Although both sexes produce both kinds of steroids, males generally produce more androgens than do females and are more sensitive to them than are females; conversely, females produce more estrogens than do males and are more sensitive to these hormones. Male behavioral and physical characteristics are often androgen-dependent; female characteristics are often estrogen-dependent.

A firm grasp of the taxonomic status of the vertebrate species covered will be necessary, and so this information is given in Table 1, along with identification of all vertebrates mentioned in the chapter.

In many of the experiments to be described, one or more of the sex structures of an individual is altered or even completely sex-reversed (i.e., a

Table 1. Taxonomic Guide to the Vertebrates Discussed in the Text

Class, order, and family	Scientific name	Common name
Osteichthyes (bony fish)		
Clupeiformes		
Salmonidae	*Salmo salar*	Atlantic salmon
Cypriniformes		
Cyprinidae	*Carassius auratus*	Goldfish
Cyprinodontiformes		
Cyprinodontidae	*Oryzias latipes*	Medaka
Poeciliidae	*Poecilia reticulata*	Guppy
	Xiphophorus maculatus	Platyfish
	Xiphophorus helleri	Swordtail
	Gambusia holbrookii	Mosquito fish
Synbranchiformes		
Synbranchidae	*Monopterus albus*	Rice eel
Perciformes		
Cichlidae	*Aequidens latifrons*	Blue acara
	Tilapia mossambica	Mozambique mouth-breeder
	Hemihaplochromis multicolor	Egyptian mouth-breeder
	Hemichromis bimaculatus	Jewel cichlid
Embiotocidae	*Cymatogaster aggregata*	Shiner perch
Belontiidae	*Macropodus opercularis*	Paradise fish
(Anabantidae)	*Betta splendens*	Siamese fighting fish
	Trichogaster trichopterus	Blue (three-spot) gourami
Gobiidae	*Bathygobius soporator*	Frillfin goby
Serranidae	*Anthias squamipinnis*	—
Amphibia		
Urodela		
Hynobiidae	*Hynobius nebulosus*	(Asiatic salamander)
	Hynobius retardatus	(Asiatic salamander)
Ambystomidae	*Ambystoma mexicanum*	Axolotl
Salamandridae	*Pleurodeles waltlii*	Ribbed salamander
	Triturus helveticus	Palmate newt
Anura		
Discoglossidae	*Discoglossus pictus*	Painted frog
Pipidae	*Xenopus laevis*	African clawed frog
Bufonidae	*Bufo bufo*	Common toad
	Bufo arenarum	Argentine toad
Hylidae	*Pseudocris nigrita*	Southern chorus frog
Ranidae	*Rana esculenta*	Edible frog
	Rana temporia	Common frog
	Rana japonica	(Japanese frog)
	Rana pipiens	Leopard frog
	Rana sylvatica	Wood frog

(Continued)

Table 1. (*Continued*)

Class, order, and family	Scientific name	Common name
Reptilia		
Testudines		
Testudinidae	*Emys orbicularis*	European pond terrapin
	Emys leprosa	Pond terrapin
	Testudo graeca	Iberian land tortoise
	Malaclemmys centrata	Diamondback terrapin
	Chrysemys marginata	Painted turtle
Crocodylia		
Alligatoridae	*Alligator mississippiensis*	American alligator
Crocodylidae	*Crocodylus niloticus*	Nile crocodile
Squamata		
Iguanidae	*Anolis carolinensis*	Carolina anole
	Sceloporus sp.	Spiny lizards
Lacertidae	*Lacerta vivipara*	Common lizard
	Lacerta viridis	Green lizard
Anguidae	*Anguis fragilis*	Blindworm
Colubridae	*Thamnophis sirtalis*	Garter snake
Aves		
Anseriformes		
Anatidae	*Anas platyrhynchos*	(Domestic mallard) duck
Galliformes		
Phasianidae	*Coturnix coturnix*	(Domestic) quail
	Phasianus colchicus	Ring-necked pheasant
	Gallus gallus	(Domestic) fowl
Meleagrididae	*Meleagris gallopavo*	(Domestic) turkey
Gruiformes		
Rallidae	*Fulica atra*	European coot
Turnicidae	*Turnix* spp.	Hemipodes
Charadriiformes		
Rostratulidae	*Rostratula* spp.	Painted snipes
Phalaropodidae	*Steganopus tricolor*	Wilson's phalarope
	Lobipes lobatus	Northern phalarope
Laridae	*Larus argentatus*	Herring gull
Columbiformes		
Columbidae	*Streptopelia* sp.	Ring dove
	Columba livia	Rock dove (domestic pigeon)
Passeriformes		
Ploceidae	*Passer domesticus*	House sparrow
	Serinus canarius	Canary
	Poephila guttata	Zebra finch
Mammalia		
Marsupialia		
Didelphidae	*Didelphis marsupialis*	Virginia opossum
Artiodactyla		
Bovidae	*Bos taurus*	(Domestic) cattle
Rodentia		
Muridae	*Rattus norvegicus*	Norway (laboratory) rat

testis becomes an ovary or vice versa). The basis of such reversal is the morphological bisexuality of the embryos of all vertebrates. The basis for behavioral sex reversal is similar in that the nervous system is also potentially bisexual. Early in life, prior to the development of the sex organs, the two sexes are identical morphologically. In the case of the early gonaducts, each sex possesses both male and female primordia; in the case of external genitalia, a single set of primordia becomes either male or female genitalia. The gonads of vertebrates, with the possible exception of teleost fish (see Chan *et al.*, 1975), begin as sexually bipotential primordia located to each side of the midline (see Fig. 1).

The undifferentiated gonad consists of an outer region of cortical tissue and an inner region of medullary tissue. If the animal is a genetic female, the

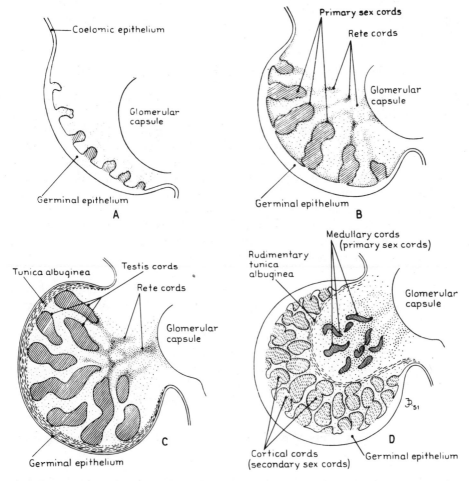

Figure 1. Gonadal differentiation in higher vertebrates. A, B, and C or D represent successive stages in development. At stage B the gonad is still in the indifferent stage. At C, a testis is differentiating. At D, an ovary is differentiating. (Reproduced with permission from Burns, 1961.)

cortical tissue proliferates and becomes the ovarian tissue, and the medullary tissue fails to proliferate. If the animal is a genetic male, the medullary tissue proliferates at the expense of the cortical tissue (Van Tienhoven, 1968). The primoridal germ cells (future oocytes and spermatocytes) migrate from the endoderm to the gonadal primordium prior to differentiation of the gonads and become associated with what will be the dominant portion of the gonad (Van Tienhoven, 1968). Gonadal sex differentiation is followed by differentiation of other sex structures into a male or female form.

B. Research Questions, Methods, and Strategies

A complete investigation of the role of hormones in the differentiation of a specific trait or character in one particular species would require answering at least the following questions.

1. Is the Substrate for the Trait Sexually Dimorphic in the Adult?

Answering this question requires more than just observing the animals, since sex differences in adults may result from differences in circulating hormones and not from differences in the soma. Recall that in mammals sex hormones have quite different actions in early and adult life (see Chapters 5 and 6 for further explanation). During the fetal or neonatal period, sex hormones have permanent organizational effects on sex structures and behavior, determining what form they will take. At puberty, sex hormones have activational effects on the substrates that were previously organized. Such activational effects are reversed if the hormones are removed. The gonads of adults are dimorphic, and any sex difference observed may be simply a result of the difference in circulating activational gonadal hormones. This is particularly true of behavioral characteristics. To demonstrate a sex difference in the neural substrate for behavior, it is necessary to remove the gonads of both males and females, inject or otherwise treat them with the same dosage of the appropriate sex steroid, and observe or test them under identical conditions. Even this procedure may not constitute adequate equalization of adult activational hormone exposure if sex differences in hormone half-life are also operating. Only if a sex difference in the neural substrate or other portion of the "soma" is apparent would it be worthwhile to investigate the role of embryonic gonadal secretions in producing the dimorphism.

2. What Are the Effects of Early Sex Hormone Removal on Subsequent Differentiation?

If the embryonic gonads are responsible for the observed adult sex difference through an organizational action, then removal of the gonads prior to differentiation should result in lack of differentiation in at least one sex; and both sexes should develop similarly. Thus determination of the neutral sex, the sex that results from differentiation in the absence of the gonads, is of great theoretical importance. (Experimentally, this is called the castrate or anhormonal sex.) An organizational role is indicated if gonadectomy prior to differentiation has different effects from gonadectomy after differentiation.

Embryonic gonadectomy presents challenging technical difficulties, particularly when differentiation occurs before hatching (some reptiles, some birds) or during internal gestation (some fish, some reptiles, some mammals). Although surgical castration is the traditional method for determining the neutral sex, because of the technical problems it presents, several investigators have developed alternative techniques. Raynaud (1963) has developed a procedure whereby reptile eggs undergo development *in vitro*. The culture medium consists of the albumen of hen eggs and Tyrode solution. Since the egg membrane is transparent, the developing embryo can be seen; X-irradiation is then used to destroy the appropriate portion of the embryo. Similarly, Wolff (1959) has gonadectomized avian embryos by destroying with localized X-rays the germinal ridges of 2- to 4-day embryos in the eggs. Unfortunately, such methods have not been compatible with survival to an age at which behavioral data can be obtained. Differentiation of sex organs in the absence of sex hormones can also be observed by removing the primordial organ tissue prior to differentiation and allowing it to develop *in vitro* (Burns, 1961; Wolff, 1959).

Where destruction of gonadal tissue is not possible, chemical antihormones provide an alternative method of insuring development uninfluenced by embryonic sex steroids.

3. What Are the Effects of Early Administration of Sex Hormones on Subsequent Differentiation?

Of greatest interest are permanent organizational effects occurring during a critical period. A variety of methods has been used to administer sex steroids. In fish and amphibians, where differentiation occurs in aquatic young after hatching, the steroids can simply be put in the water, thus eliminating injection damage and handling trauma. Yamamoto (1969) obtained complete sex reversal in the fry of the medaka (*Oryzias latipes*) by putting steroids in their food. In reptiles and birds, eggs containing developing embryos can be injected with steroids (Dantschakoff, 1938; Adkins, 1975). Avian embryos can also be treated by dipping the ends of the intact eggs for a few seconds in an alcohol solution of the steroid (the Seltzer technique; Pincus and Hopkins, 1958) or by spraying them with fuel oil as the vehicle (Wentworth *et al.*, 1968). Dipping and spraying suffer from the disadvantage that the hormone vehicles are fairly toxic. Sex organs developing *in vitro* can be treated by applying the steroid to the culture medium (Burns, 1961).

In choosing the particular androgen or estrogen to administer, most recent investigators have favored testosterone, often in the propionated form, and estradiol-17β, usually estradiol benzoate. Occasionally the nonsteroidal estrogen diethylstilbestrol (DES) has been used. This chemical is actually a more powerful estrogen than estradiol-17β, but caution should be exercised in using diethylstilbestrol for behavioral studies in species that have not been checked for DES activity. Cheng and Lehrman (1973) found that DES, unlike estradiol benzoate, did not reinstate receptivity in ovariectomized adult female ring doves, suggesting that neural tissue responds differently to these two estrogens.

If there is an effect of early hormone treatment, one must be sure that the mechanism of this effect is an organizational change of the soma and not a permanent modification of the hormone-secreting gonad. In the latter case, the embryonically affected gonad would have an altered pattern of secretion in adulthood; and although there would be an "organizational" effect, it would be on the gonad and not the brain. To accomplish this separation, it is necessary to gonadectomize both control and experimental subjects, preferably in adulthood, and to inject or otherwise treat both groups with the same quantity of exogenous sex steroid. The experimental subjects should have an altered threshold to the adult hormones. It is also necessary to expose the embryos or larvae to hormones for delimited periods of time that are varied systematically.

4 Are the Gonads of Either Sex Functional during the Time of Sex Differentiation

Even though it may be possible to alter sexual organization by early hormone manipulation, it is always possible that such manipulations are pharmacological and do not reflect the natural course of sexual development. Therefore, it is important to determine whether the gonads are producing hormones at the time that exogenous hormones are effective, what these hormones are (Are they steroids? Are they the same steroids produced by adult gonads?), and whether the secretions of embryonic or larval gonads are capable of organizing sex structures and behavior.

Several methods have been used to determine the functional capabilities of developing testes and ovaries. Gonads of different ages have been examined for histological or enzymatic evidence of steroid production. For example, histochemical demonstration of the presence of the enzyme Δ^5-3β-hydroxysteroid dehydrogenase has been taken as indirect evidence that steroid synthesis is occurring (Gallien, 1967). Another approach has been to culture embryonic gonads of different ages *in vitro*, administer radioactively labeled steroid precursors such as [^{14}C]progesterone, and assess the labeled products (Haffen, 1975). Finally, the secretions of embryonic gonads *in vivo* have been detected by performing standard steroid assays on extracts of the gonads, on amniotic fluid, or on the culture medium in which an organism has developed *in vitro*. Although considerable evidence of steroid production by embryonic gonads has been obtained, it has seldom been possible to conclusively identify the specific estrogen(s) or androgen(s) present (Ozon, 1972a,b).

The question of whether the organizing sex hormones are steroids is a difficult one to answer. So far the main approach has been to compare differentiation as it occurs in intact animals (or in animals with gonadal grafts) with differentiation in early castrates or intact embryos receiving exogenous sex steroids of known composition. There are well-known cases in which such comparison yields quite dissimilar results, for example, the effect of testosterone compared with testicular secretions on Müllerian duct differentiation in male mammals. But in none of these cases have the true differentiating substances been identified.

To show that the secretions of embryonic gonads are capable of modifying sex differentiation, investigators have traditionally used either parabiosis or gonad grafts (Burns, 1961; Wolff, 1959). If two opposite-sexed undifferentiated larvae or embryos are joined so that cross-circulation is established, the sexual development of one sex will be modified by the other (which sex is modified depends importantly on the species). If a gonad is removed from a young animal after gonadal differentiation has occurred and is implanted into an embryo or larva prior to sex differentiation, the graft may become attached and vascularized. Depending on the species and sex of the recipient and donor, the subsequent sex differentiation of the recipient may be modified. In some species, opposite-sexed twins occasionally occur in which enough cross-circulation takes place for the differentiation of one sex to be modified by the other—the freemartin effect. Such natural experiments are found, for example, in cattle (Burns, 1961) and in chickens and ducks (double-yolked eggs— Lutz and Lutz-Ostertag, 1975). A similar effect can even be seen in rats, which normally have large litters. Females show more masculine sexual behavior as adults if they come from litters containing males than if they come from all-female litters, and they are especially masculinized if they were surrounded on both sides by males *in utero* (Clemens, 1974).

5. Are Secretions of Embryonic Endocrine Glands Other Than Gonads Controlling Agents in Sex Differentiation?

Some obvious candidates would be the pituitary and the adrenal glands. The pituitary–gonadal axis is functional in embryos (Burns, 1961), but whether pituitary hormones have any direct role in sex differentiation, one not mediated by the gonads, is not known.

6. To What Extent Is Sex Differentiation Controlled by Nonhormonally Mediated Genetic Differences?

The induction of complete sex reversal with exogenous hormones would suggest that nonhormonally mediated genetic influences were minimal. A major difficulty with this type of experiment, however, is assessment of the true chromosomal sex of the individuals whose gonads have been altered. Furthermore, it cannot be assumed without evidence that normal females have XX

chromosomes (i.e., are homogametic) and normal males have XY chromosomes (i.e., are heterogametic). The chromosomal sex-determining mechanism varies from species to species in ways that appear to be importantly
related to the pattern of sex differentiation (this will be discussed in greater
detail in Section VII). For the moment, simply note that in mammals, some
reptiles and amphibians, and most fish, the female is XX (male XY), whereas in
birds and some reptiles and amphibians, the female is XY (male XX).

How, then, can one determine whether a phenotypic male is a true
chromosomal male or a chromosomal female whose phenotypic sex has been
reversed by the experimental treatment? Two commonly used sexing methods
are sex-linked color markers, such as occur in some fish, and analysis of the sex
ratio of the offspring of treated individuals. In the latter method, if the
experimenter suspects that some phenotypic males that had been given testosterone as larvae are actually sex-reversed genetic females, these "males" are
mated with known genetic females. If the "males" are really genetic females,
the sex ratio of the offspring will be either 0M : 1F (if it is a species in which the
female is XX and the male XY), 1M : 3F (if the female is XY, and YY individuals are viable), or 1M : 2F (if the female is XY, and YY individuals are inviable).
If the "males" are truly genetic males, the sex ratio of the offspring will of
course be 1M : 1F.

7. If Organizational Effects of Gonadal Hormones on Behavior Can Be Demonstrated, Are These Effects Occurring Peripherally or in the Central Nervous System?

If the hormones are acting on the brain, what specific actions do they have
on these neurons? It has been assumed in avian research that such effects are
central (e.g., Wilson and Glick, 1970), partly because of the lack of obvious
relevant peripheral structures (the chicken does not have a penis). One approach that has been used in rodents is to place hormone implants into the
brain (Nadler, 1973), but this would be technically difficult in animals that
differentiate before birth or hatching. The specific effects of early hormones
on the brains of chickens have been investigated, and the methods used will be
presented in the section on birds (Section VI). Gross neuroanatomical dimorphism has recently been found in brain centers controlling vocalization in
canaries (*Serinus canarius*) and zebra finches (*Poephila guttata*) (Nottebohm and
Arnold, 1976) and will provide an excellent opportunity to study the role of
early hormones in neural differentiation underlying behavior.

8. Do the Hormones of the Mother Influence the Differentation of Any of the Offspring, and If Not, Why Not?

Even in animals lacking internal gestation, such as birds, hormones (at
least, exogenously administered hormones) can pass from the female to her
eggs (Riddle and Dunham, 1942).

So it can be seen that a comprehensive study of sex differentiation is a multidisciplinary effort involving biochemistry, histology, embryology, genetics, endocrinology, neurobiology, and animal behavior. Additional strategies and methods are also possible, and certain species may well turn out to present special problems of their own.

A program of research on the sex differentiation of even a single species, as outlined above, takes years to complete, and so it is not surprising that few investigators have been able to include more than one or two species in their research programs. And, the reader may ask, why do we need to study more than one or two species anyway? In the remainder of this chapter, I hope to answer this question by showing that significant species differences exist in the process of sex differentiation and that a comparative approach to the subject reveals important unifying principles that otherwise go undetected. The major groups of animals that have been studied with respect to sex differentiation will be surveyed, beginning with invertebrates, and a final overview will pull together these comparative aspects and unifying principles.

II. DIFFERENTIATION OF REPRODUCTIVE FUNCTION IN INVERTEBRATES

Sex differentiation in invertebrates has not received nearly the attention it deserves, and most of what is known is confined to the phylum Arthropoda. Physical and behavioral sex dimorphism is extraordinarily pronounced in some invertebrates, and the mechanisms by which this dimorphism is achieved in development are still quite obscure for the most part. Invertebrate sexual endocrinology is quite different in several respects from that of vertebrates. Invertebrates possess endocrine and neuroendocrine organs not found in vertebrates, and vice versa. The combination of gametogenic and endocrine functions in the gonads is not a general rule in invertebrates as it is in vertebrates. The beach flea *Orchestia,* an amphipod crustacean, illustrates this point well (Gorbman and Bern, 1962). The androgenic gland, which secretes sex hormones, is attached to the sperm duct that leads from the gamete-producing testis to the surface of the body. In most cases the sex hormones of invertebrates have not been chemically identified and cannot be assumed to be related to vertebrate sex steroids. As in studies on lower vertebrates, the emphasis has more often been on reproductive physiology than on sexual behavior.

A. Coelenterates, Nemerteans, and Molluscs

Experiments with several species of *Hydra* (Coelenterata) strongly suggest that in the gonochoristic members of this genus (those in which the two kinds of gametes are in separate individuals, i.e., nonhermaphrodites), sex is determined epigenetically by some chemical inducer (Gallien, 1967). A female *H.*

fusca joined to a male in parabiosis will be masculinized, eventually to the point of producing sperm (Brien, 1962; Brien and Pirard, 1962; Tardent, 1975). In other words, testicular tissue is dominant over ovarian tissue in this preparation. Similar results are obtained with nemertine (proboscis) worms (Bierne, 1975). Since sex can be fully reversed in adulthood, it is not clear that there is any organizational period at all in the sense applied to mammals.

Research with molluscs indicates that in two species of hermaphroditic snails (Gastropoda), anhormonal differentiation of gonads is female, suggesting that an androgenic hormone is required for male gonadal differentiation (Joosse, 1975; Le Gall and Streiff, 1975).

B. Insects

In insects, the corpus allatum (a nonneural organ) secretes a juvenile hormone that inhibits growth and differentiation of the gonads until metamorphosis (Wigglesworth, 1970). In the adult, the corpora allata are gonadotropic, at least with respect to the ovary. In the male *Locusta* and in the female *Gomphocerus* (a grasshopper) and female *Drosophila*, the corpora allata are also behaviorally significant. Their removal in the first two cases eliminates sexual behavior, and their implantation into immature female *Gomphocerus* and *Drosophila* can induce precocious sexual receptivity (Girardie, 1966; Loher and Huber, 1966; Manning, 1966). Whether these effects are mediated by the gonads is not clear. Removal of the corpora allata has a much more minor effect on receptivity in cockroaches (Barth, 1968) and has no effect on the sexual behavior of male *Gomphocerus* (Loher and Huber, 1966).

Thus, the endocrine system has a role in the sexual physiology and behavior of some species of insects. Do the endocrine organs or gonads also have a role in sexual differentiation? In most insects that have been studied, surgical removal of the gonads, even in early stages of development, is not followed by changes in the reproductive tract or secondary sex characters (Gorbman and Bern, 1962), nor can sex differentiation be altered by sex hormones (Gallien, 1967). Apparently sex is determined more directly by the genes in the tissues, with some modification possible by environmental factors such as temperature (Wigglesworth, 1970).

In some insects, however, there are indications that hormones are involved in behavioral and physical sex differentiation. In the pea aphid *Megoura*, the sex ratio depends on the photoperiod: day lengths below 14 hr result in sexually reproducing males and females, whereas day lengths above 14 hr result only in parthenogenetic females (Wigglesworth, 1970). It is believed that photoperiod, which acts directly on the brain, causes hormonal secretion (neurosecretion?) that affects the development of the embryos in the ovary (Wigglesworth, 1970).

Some aspects of the pronounced sex dimorphism of the butterfly *Orgya antiqua*, in which the male has wings, but the female has only wing stumps, also appear to have a hormonal basis. Female wing stumps transplanted into males become male wings, and male wings transplanted into females also become male wings (Gallien, 1967). Thus, wing stumps can be organized to become male wings and, once formed, remain morphologically developed regardless of the host's hormonal milieu.

Genetic female midges (*Chironomus,* Diptera) whose larval ovaries are destroyed by a nematode parasite develop male internal and external sex organs, suggesting that differentiation of the genitalia is under hormonal control (Wigglesworth, 1970).

Sex differentiation in the glow-worm *Lampyris noctiluca* (Coleoptera) is known to be under hormonal control of a type strongly reminiscent of mammals (Gallien, 1967; Naisse, 1963, 1965, 1966). The gonads differentiate during the larval period. Tissue that apparently secretes an androgenic hormone develops at one end of the testis but not on the ovary. This apical tissue is well-developed at the time of sexual differentiation, then regresses and disappears. If a testis is implanted into a larval female after the apical tissue on the transplanted gonad has appeared, the female will be completely masculinized. As an adult, she will have testes and male sex structures, will behave as a male, and will be capable of fertilizing females. If testes are implanted after the apical tissue has regressed, no such masculinization will occur. An ovariectomized larval female will continue to develop as a female. If ovaries are implanted into a male during the time of sexual differentiation, the male will be unchanged, but the ovaries will be transformed into testes. Thus sex differentiation in *Lampyris* follows a system in which the female is the neutral (anhormonal) sex, the male genotype leads to testicular development, a testicular secretion organizes behavior and morphology into male patterns, and the testis is dominant over the ovary. Whether or not the embryonic gonad forms apical androgenic tissue appears to be determined by the neurosecretory activity of the corpora cardiaca and corpora allata. Larval males, but not older males, whose corpora cardiaca and corpora allata are removed become females.

C. Crustaceans

Organization of the male phenotype by androgenic tissue also occurs in another arthropod class, the Crustacea, in particular in the higher Crustacea (Malacostraca) such as Isopoda (pillbugs), Amphipoda (scuds), and Decapoda (crabs, lobsters, prawns, shrimps). This androgenic tissue can be a gland separate from the gamete-producing testes (the androgenic, or vas deferens, gland), as in Amphipoda, or can be partly in the testis, as in Isopoda (Gorbman and Bern, 1962). Crustacean sex differentiation is best understood in the beach flea *Orchestia*, an Amphipod (Carlisle, 1960; Charniaux-Cotton, 1965, 1975; Gallien, 1967). Removal of the gonads at any stage does not affect sex differentiation, but removal of the androgenic gland in a male results in either a nonsexual indeterminate form or in a female form with ovaries, depending on the species. Testes implanted into males lacking androgenic glands become ovaries. If an androgenic gland is implanted into a female, even if she has already laid eggs, she will become a functional male with male gonads, sex structures, and behavior. Since in the absence of androgenic hormone both sexes become females, the female is the neutral sex. Apparently the main difference between the male and female is in the genes controlling the development of the androgenic gland (Charniaux-Cotton, 1965). As in *Lampyris*, the system is reminiscent of mammalian sex differentiation.

The androgenic gland seems to have a similar role in Isopods: females implanted with androgenic glands become complete and functional males (Gallien, 1967).

The study of sex differentiation in Decapods has been greatly aided by two naturally occurring phenomena. First, in some "experiments of nature," parasites destroy the androgenic glands of males; such destruction is followed by the acquisition of female sex structures and the formation of oocytes in the gonads (Bacci, 1965). Second, a number of species of prawns and shrimps are normally successive hermaphrodites, that is, they change sex during their life cycle and produce male gametes at one stage in the cycle and female gametes at another stage. For example, the prawn *Lysmata* matures reproductively at about 1 year of age. The young prawns spend the first reproductive season (summer) as males, regress sexually the following winter, and function again as males during the early part of the next summer. Then the male organs regress, to be replaced by female gonads and other characters. The prawns complete the summer as females, spend the following summer as females, and then die (Charniaux-Cotton, 1975). Sex change in crustaceans is usually protandrous, that is, from male to female (Carlisle, 1960), and this spontaneous sex change is probably under hormonal control. In *Lysmata* the change from male to female is correlated with regression of the androgenic gland, and females implanted with an androgenic gland become males (Charniaux-Cotton, 1959). Carlisle (1960) hypothesized that sex reversal in prawns is caused by a combination of degeneration of the androgenic gland and a decrease in the secretion of ovary-inhibiting hormone from the eyestalk.

D. Summary

The overall picture of invertebrate sexual differentiation that emerges is as follows. In some species of coelenterates, nemertine worms, arthropods, and possibly molluscs, hormonal factors seem to be involved in the development of morphological and, in some cases, behavioral sex. The process resembles mammalian differentiation in that the female is the neutral sex and male hormones masculinize females. In contrast to the mammalian situation, differentiation in arthropods is controlled by nongonadal organs or tissues, and induction of sex by hormones is evidently not limited to any particular sensitive or critical period, suggesting that the concept of "organizational" effects may not even be appropriate for these creatures.

III. DIFFERENTIATION OF REPRODUCTIVE FUNCTION IN FISH (OSTEICHTHYES)

Of all the vertebrates, fish contain the richest material for the study of sex. The variety of reproductive phenomena in fish is simply astounding and includes oviparity, viviparity, unisexual species, hermaphroditism of every known type, even self-fertilization, parental care by the male, by the female, by both, all extremes of sexual dimorphism, and environmental influences on the sex ratio (Atz, 1964). Considerable variability can even be found within a single family, such as the Cichlidae (Fryer and Iles, 1972). Fish are abundant, both in terms of number of species and in terms of number of individuals in some species. The common freshwater aquarium species are inexpensive, prolific, easily maintained, and will readily display reproductive behavior in the laboratory. A sizable literature on fish endocrinology exists, stimulated in part by the economic importance of certain species. Given all these advantages, it is surprising and unfortunate that work on hormones and behavior is quite limited.

External sex dimorphism is marked in some species, and can include size, color, fin shape and size, shape and size of appendages, head shape, and external sex structures such as the gonopodia used for internal fertilization (Sadleir, 1973). Male characters are generally reduced or eliminated following castration and are restored with androgens, whereas female characters are reduced or eliminated by ovariectomy and restored by estrogens (Chester-Jones et al., 1972; Liley, 1969; Van Tienhoven, 1968; Yamamoto, 1969). Several of the sex steroids commonly found in mammals have also been identified in fish (Ozon, 1972a,b). Testes often contain considerable estrogen. In some species, 11-ketotestosterone, a hormone known to occur in flounder and salmon (Idler et al., 1976), is a more potent androgen than testosterone (Ozon, 1972a).

A. Morphology

The reproductive tracts of teleost fish are shown in Fig. 2 (for a comparison with mammals see Fig. 7). Morphological studies have been almost entirely confined to the gonads. Fish generally have paired gonads; but the females of a few species, such as the guppy (*Poecilia reticulata*) and medaka (*Oryzias latipes*), have only one ovary. According to some authors, the embryology of fish gonads differs significantly from that of other vertebrates in that instead of separate

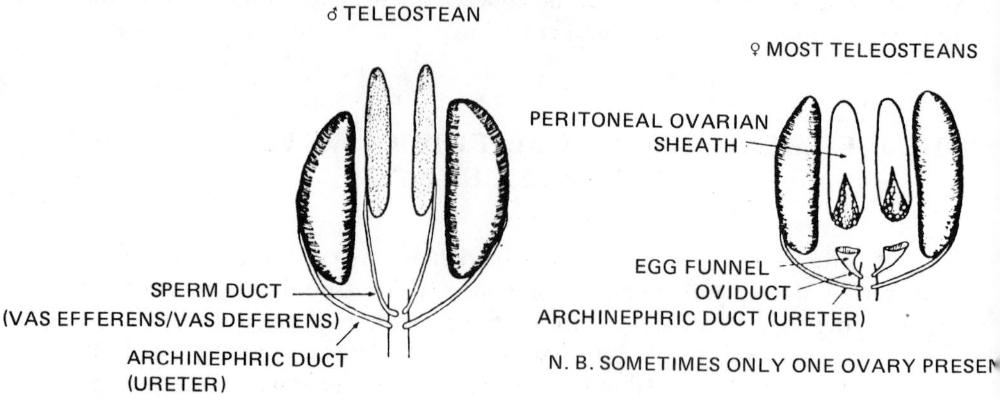

Figure 2. Gonads and gonaducts of teleost fish. (Reproduced with permission from Sadleir, 1973.)

cortical (future ovarian) and medullary (future testicular) tissue (see Fig. 1), only one type of tissue is present in the gonadal primordium which is said to resemble somewhat the ovarian cortex of other vertebrates (e.g., Atz, 1964). According to Chan *et al.* (1975), however, sufficient information is not yet available to determine whether teleosts have a dual induction system in a common gonadal substratum or a gonadal soma with dual embryonic origin (as in other vertebrates).

Grafting of gonads into adult fish and treatment of fish with exogenous sex hormones both alter the gonads, causing partial or complete sex reversal, depending on the species and the age at treatment. Satoh (1973) transplanted undifferentiated gonads of the fry of *Oryzias latipes* into the anterior chamber of the eye of adults. Genetic male grafts became testes, whereas genetic female grafts took on the sex of the host. Thus gonadal sex reversal from female to male can be accomplished by physiological levels of male sex hormones, but reversal from male to female cannot be accomplished by physiological levels of female sex hormones (Satoh and Egami, 1973).

Where gonadal sex differentiation occurs prior to birth or hatching, as in *Poecilia reticulata, Xiphophorus helleri,* or *Gambusia holbrookii,* treatment of fry with sex steroids produces only partial gonadal sex reversal (Atz, 1964; Liley, 1969; Yamamoto, 1969). Where differentiation occurs after birth or hatching, complete and functional gonadal sex reversal can be induced with sex steroids. The most famous example of this phenomenon is found in Yamamoto's work with the oviparous medaka (Yamamoto, 1962, 1968, 1969; Yamamoto and Matsuda, 1963). This species never shows spontaneous sex reversal or inter-sexuality. Sex-linked color markers make assessment of genetic sex possible in that colors produced by genes on the male sex chromosomes are expressed regardless of phenotypic sex. Gonadal differentiation takes place when the fry are 6 to 11 mm long. If the fry are fed diets containing sex steroids from hatching until 12-mm length is reached (a period of 10 weeks), complete sex reversal is achieved. Genetic females treated with androgens (including methyltestosterone and androstenedione) mature as males, produce sperm, and successfully fertilize normal females. Genetic males are reversed completely with estrogens (including estradiol, estrone, and diethylstilbestrol). Some quantitative aspects of this phenomenon are shown in Fig. 3. Treatment after primary sex differentiation has occurred never results in complete reversal, and thus a critical period exists for gonadal reversal. Reversal produced by treatment during the critical period is permanent.

Complete reversal can also be obtained in the guppy, provided hormone exposure occurs prenatally, prior to gonadal differentiation. The guppy also has sex-linked color markers that permit identification of genetic sex. Methyltestosterone given to gravid females for 24 hr results in all-male broods in which some of the males are genetic females (Dzwillo, 1962).

Complete reversal has been obtained in female *Tilapia mossambica* (Clemens and Inslee, 1968), male and female *Carassius auratus* (Yamamoto and Kajishima, 1968), male *Hemihaplochromis multicolor* (Hackman and Reinboth, 1974), and female *Xiphophorus helleri* (Baldwin and Goldin, 1939; Essenberg, 1926) (see Table 2). For a complete tabular summary of the many experiments on hormonal treatment and manipulation of sex, see Schreck (1974).

These experiments in which the sex of fish is completely reversed are fascinating, yet the relevance of the phenomena to normally occurring sex differentiation is not always clear. Little is known of the secretions of the gonads of fish fry. Yamamoto (1969) presented evidence that sex steroids similar to those used experimentally are the natural inducers that determine the course of gonadal differentiation, but Reinboth (1970) argued that this was not the case. In addition, there is a certain difficulty in concluding that sex

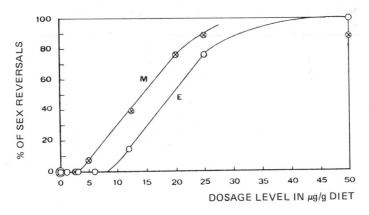

Figure 3. Percentage of sex reversals in the medaka, *Oryzias latipes*, as a function of hormone dosage. Curve M represents reversals in genetic females given methyltestosterone. Curve E represents reversals in genetic males given estrone. (Reproduced with permission from Yamamoto, 1959.)

Table 2. Summary of Experimentally Produced Sex Reversal in Bony Fish

Species	Age at treatment	Treatment	Result[a]
Oryzias latipes	Fry	Several sex steroids	F→M and M→F[b]
Tilapia mossambica	Fry	Methyltestosterone	F→M
Carassius auratus	Fry	Methyltestosterone or estrone	F→M and M→F
Hemihaplochromis multicolor	Fry	Several sex steroids	M→F
Xiphophorus helleri	Adult	Testosterone	F→M
Poecilia reticulata	Prenatal	Methyltestosterone	F→M
Betta splendens	Juvenile or adult	Ovariectomy	F→M
Macropodus opercularis	Juvenile	Ovariectomy	F→M
Monopterus albus[c]	Adult	Mammalian LH	F→M
Anthias squamipinnis[c]	Young adult	Testosterone	F→M

[a] F→M indicates that genetic females were completely masculinized, becoming phenotypic males with functional testes. M→F indicates that genetic males were completely feminized.
[b] Reversal from female to male can be accomplished with lower dosages than reversal from male to female.
[c] Protogynous successive hermaphrodites.

steroids are the inducers. How can these hormones determine gonadal sex if their production is dimorphic only after gonadal differentiation has begun? Or is it dimorphic before histological differentiation has begun?

Complete and functional sex reversal can occasionally be produced in adults. In *Betta splendens* and *Macropodus opercularis*, this is accomplished by ovariectomizing juvenile or adult females (Becker *et al.*, 1975). Lowe and Larkin (1975) found that, out of 160 operated *Betta* females that lived, 104 became completely male, physically and behaviorally, after about 70 days. Twenty-three of these "neomales" were mated to normal females and produced offspring. Castrated males do not reverse sex, nor are the ovaries of juvenile *Betta* masculinized by testosterone (Reinboth, 1970). *Betta* seems to be an exception to the rule that differentiated adults are difficult to reverse. It is notable that neither *Betta* nor *Macropodus* is known to undergo spontaneous reversal, either in the laboratory or in the field.

Complete functional reversal does occur spontaneously in adulthood in the successively hermaphroditic fish species. The physiological factors causing this sex change are not yet known for most species (Chan *et al.*, 1975). Tang *et al.* (1974) gave various androgens to female eels (*Monopterus albus*), a protogynous species (one that changes from female to male). The treated females did not undergo precocious reversal, even when endogenous estrogens were also removed. However, mammalian LH caused 70% of the females to commence active spermatogenesis, suggesting that pituitary changes may underlie sex reversal. Female *Anthias squamipinnis*, another protogynous species, become males when treated with testosterone (Fishelson, 1975). Once again, however, these experiments are difficult to interpret in that the same steroids would have to be both a cause and a result of reversal.

B. Behavior

The relationship between sex hormones and sexual behavior is quite variable in fish. In some species, courtship, copulation, and receptivity disappear following gonadectomy and are restored by treatment with the homologous sex steroid (e.g., *Cymatogaster aggregata*, *Xiphophorus maculatus*, female *Betta splendens*, *Xiphophorus helleri*, *Hemihaplochromis multicolor*, female *Hemichromis bimaculatus*, *Salmo salar*, *Tilapia mossambica*, *Oryzias latipes*, female *Poecilia reticulata*, *Trichogaster trichopterus*—Baggerman, 1968; Aronson, 1957; Liley, 1969; Reinboth, 1972; Van Tienhoven, 1968). In other species, gonadectomy does not reduce or eliminate sexual behavior (male *Hemichromis bimaculatus*, *Bathygobius soporator*, male *Betta splendens*. *Aequidens latifrons*—Baggerman, 1968; Aronson, 1957; Liley, 1969; Reinboth, 1972; Van Tienhoven, 1968). In some of these cases, it is possible that gonadectomy was not complete. In other cases, pituitary hormones may be involved: although castration does not eliminate sexual behavior in *Bathygobius soporator*, hypophysectomy does (Tavolga, 1955).

Androgens can activate considerable male behavior in the adult females of several species (*Hemihaplochromis multicolor*, *Xiphophorus maculatus*, *X. helleri*,

Oryzias latipes, Poecilia reticulata—Liley, 1969; Reinboth, 1972). The behavioral effects of estrogens in males do not appear to have been assessed.

Studies of sex differentiation in fish with behavior as the main emphasis have not yet appeared, and seldom have the behaviors of hormonally treated and normal fish been compared (Atz, 1964). However, it is clear from the studies described above in which the sex of fry or embryos is experimentally reversed that these fish grew up to be behaviorally reversed as well. The fact that the treated *Oryzias latipes* and *Hemihaplochromis multicolor* mated with other fish and produced offspring suggests that behavioral reversal was fairly complete.

Of the experimentally masculinized genetic female guppies studied by Clemens *et al.* (1966), 86% of those that sired young displayed courtship, and 50% displayed gonopodial thrusting (male copulatory behavior). Control males exhibited these behavior patterns even more frequently. However, only 25% of those sex-reversed females that failed to sire young displayed courtship, and 20% thrusted. It cannot be assumed, however, that these behavioral effects reflect organizational effects of sex steroids, because the capacity of the normal adults of these species to display heterotypical sexual behavior when treated with heterologous hormones is not known. In other words, the first question discussed in the introduction has not yet been answered. In *Betta splendens,* the period during which hormones can reverse behavior extends into adulthood: the females that were ovariectomized in adulthood and became functional males also displayed typically male threat, courtship, and mating behavior (Lowe and Larkin, 1975). Whether adult male *Bettas* are capable of exhibiting normal female receptivity is not known.

C. Summary

Overall, the research on hormones and sexual differentiation in fish indicates that the phenotypic and behavioral sex of the fry or adults of several species can be completely reversed by sex steroid treatment, suggesting that these steroids have an important role in the normal course of sexual differentiation. Table 2 summarizes the results of these experiments (they are compared with data from other vertebrate classes in Table 10). In most of the gonochoristic fish that have been studied, hormonally induced sex reversal can only be accomplished during a limited critical period. Whether behavioral sex reversal is similarly limited to a critical period remains to be determined. In some species (the successive hermaphrodites), sexual differentiation is not fixed at maturity, and spontaneous sex reversal may occur in adulthood. The mechanisms of this second period of sexual differentiation that occurs in adulthood are still obscure. In these hermaphroditic fish, it is not yet clear that there exists a specific period of time (or specific periods of time) to which organizational effects of hormones are limited.

IV. DIFFERENTIATION OF REPRODUCTIVE FUNCTION IN AMPHIBIANS

Amphibia have figured importantly in the study of sex differentiation, at least partly because of the extreme bipotentiality of their gonads and the resulting ease with which complete sex reversal can be accomplished experimentally (Foote, 1964). Sex differentiation occurs slowly and rather late in Amphibia (around the third week after hatching in *Xenopus laevis*, the African Clawed Frog—Witschi, 1971) and is therefore amenable to experimental intervention. As with fish, hormones can be administered by putting them in the water the larvae live in. The amphibia that will be dealt with here are divided into two major groups: the Anurans (frogs and toads) and Urodeles (newts and salamanders).

Amphibia possess a number of sexually dimorphic characters that make useful end points, such as body shape and size, color, cloacal morphology, courtship and mating, and, in Anurans, nuptial thumb pads, ear size and shape, vocal sac size, and calling. Male amphibians possess cloacal glands that are larger than the pelvic glands of the females. Sex structures typically are reduced following gonadectomy and are restored by treatment with the homologous sex steroid (Chester-Jones *et al.*, 1972; Gallien, 1955; Van Tienhoven, 1968).

A. Gonads

The reproductive tracts of amphibia are shown in Fig. 4 (for a comparison with mammals see Fig. 7). Amphibia possess paired internal gonads that generally differentiate in a manner typical of tetrapod vertebrates in that there is a dual primordium, with medullary tissue becoming testicular and cortical tissue becoming ovarian. A larger amount of the primordial tissue of the opposite sex gonad is retained, however, than is retained in the gonads of other vertebrates, and as a result, the potential for gonadal sex reversal is considerable (Foote, 1964). Both sexes of adult toads have Bidder's organs anterior to the gonads; these are derived from the cortical tissue and contain small oocytes (Burns, 1961).

Experiments in which differentiated gonads are grafted into hosts with undifferentiated gonads show that the testis is dominant over the ovary. A testis graft will cause the indifferent gonad of a female host to differentiate as a testis (Van Tienhoven, 1968). In *Xenopus laevis* and *Ambystoma mexicanum* (the axolotl), complete and functional sex reversal from female to male can be accomplished by this method (Witschi, 1971; Burns, 1961; Dodd, 1960; Foote, 1964; Gallien, 1967).

Experiments in which two undifferentiated larvae are joined in parabiosis

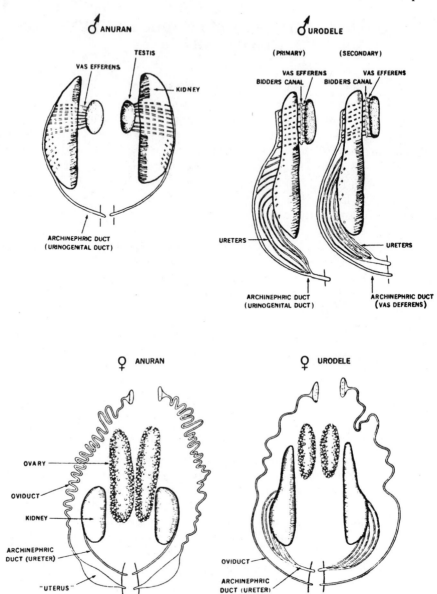

Figure 4. Gonads and gonaducts in amphibians. Anurans are frogs and toads. Urodeles are newts and salamanders. (Reproduced with permission from Sadleir, 1973.)

again demonstrate the dominance of the testis in both Anuran and Urodele amphibians. The ovaries of females are masculinized by a male parabiont, but the male's testes are unchanged (Burns, 1961; Dodd, 1960; Foote, 1964; Gallien, 1967).

Treatment of larval but not adult amphibian gonads with sex steroids can have quite striking effects and can even cause complete functional sex reversal

(Gallien, 1955). The type of reversal depends importantly on the taxonomic status and chromosomal sex determination mechanism of the subjects. Androgens administered to the larvae of higher Anurans (Ranidae and Hylidae) strongly masculinize the ovaries of females. Complete and permanent masculinization of larvae occurs in the tree frog *Pseudacris* and in *Rana temporia, R. japonica,* and *R. sylvatica* (Burns, 1961; Dodd, 1960; Gallien, 1965, 1967). Masculinized females assume a male appearance, produce sperm, and mate with normal females. The sex ratio of the progeny of these matings confirms that the "males" are genetic females that have undergone sex reversal. In these species, the females are XX. In *R. sylvatica,* as little as 1 ppm testosterone propionate in the water still produces complete masculinization of all females, and in *R. temporia* significant masculinization occurs even if treatment begins after metamorphosis (Gallien, 1955). In other species, such treatment either has no effect or causes only a temporary partial masculinization. Estrogens at low dosages cause some temporary feminization of gonads in higher Anurans, but at higher dosages cause masculinization in Ranidae, apparently by destroying the cortical tissue (Dodd, 1960; Gallien, 1955).

The effects of sex steroids on more primitive Anurans and on Urodeles are quite the opposite: estrogens strongly feminize the gonads of males, and androgens, instead of strongly masculinizing females, have weak feminizing or masculinizing effects. Complete functional permanent sex reversal of male larvae has been observed in *Ambystoma, Xenopus, Hynobius, Triturus helveticus,* and *Pleurodeles waltlii* (Foote, 1964; Gallien, 1955, 1965, 1967). In the latter species, 600 μg/liter of estradiol benzoate reverses all males. Again, the genetic sex of the treated animals was confirmed by breeding experiments; and, in contrast to the higher Anurans, the males are XX in those cases where conclusive information about sex determination is available. Androgens either cause feminization (high doses), apparently by destroying the medulla, or cause slight temporary masculinization (Dodd, 1960; Gallien, 1955). In other Urodeles, sex steroids either have no effect or have only a slight temporary effect. It is puzzling that exogenous androgenic steroids fail to strongly masculinize the gonads of primitive Anurans and Urodeles, yet the testes of these same species, like those of the higher Anurans, dominate ovaries in grafting or parabiotic experiments (more about this discrepancy below).

Permanent and complete feminization of *Xenopus* males by estrogen occurs only during a limited critical period (Witschi, 1971). In this species, the gonads differentiate during the third week after hatching. If estrogen is applied for a week or 10 days during this period, 100% females will be obtained. Treatment earlier or later does not have this effect. If treatment is of short duration, intersexual gonads rather than ovaries are found.

The ease with which some amphibian gonads can be reversed with sex steroids suggests that the gonadal sex inducers are sex steroids. In an attempt to test this hypothesis, Chieffi *et al.* (1974) put either testosterone, estradiol, cyproterone, cyproterone acetate, or ICI 46,474 in water containing *Rana esculenta* tadpoles. Cyproterone and cyproterone acetate function as antiandrogens, at least in adult frogs; ICI 46,474 [*trans*-1-(*pβ*-dimethylaminoethoxyphenyl)-1,2-diphenylbut-l-ene] is an antiestrogen. Testosterone, cyproterone, and cyproterone acetate masculinized gonads, estradiol feminized them, and ICI 46,474 had no effect. The authors concluded that the embryonic sex inducers are not similar to sex steroids on the grounds that, if the embryonic sex inducers are structurally similar to sex steroids, their effects on gonadal differentiation should be inhibited by antagonists that block sex steroids in adults. It is possible, however, that the inducers are sex steroids but that the sterioid receptors in the larval gonads differ from those in other target organs in adults, so that the question remains open. Huchon (1974) injected larvae of *Discoglossus pictus* with cyproterone acetate and found no effect on gonad differentiation. The fact that, in Urodeles, testosterone does not permanently reverse ovaries but testis implants do, also suggests that the inducer is not a sex steroid, or at least is not testosterone. One is forced to conclude that, as is the case for the other vertebrate classes, the chemical nature of the gonadal sex inducers remains unknown (see also Vannini *et al.*, 1975). Furthermore, as was pointed out in the discussion of fish gonads, any claim that sex steroids are the inducers of amphibian gonadal differentiation faces the difficulty of explaining how sex steroids can be both a cause and a result of differentiation.

Several experiments have been aimed at determining the onset of secretion by the embryonic gonads and identifying the secretions. Steroids are secreted as early as the third week by the larval gonads of *Rana pipiens* (Ozon, 1969). Δ^5-3β-Hydroxysteroid dehydrogenase (an enzyme important in steroid synthesis) is present in the larval testes of *Pleurodeles waltlii*, and the capacity for such synthesis, based on *in vitro* studies, is already present during metamorphosis (Ozon, 1969; Rao *et al.*, 1969). The gonadal medulla of *Xenopus* manufactures androstenedione by age 6 weeks in both sexes, but evidence of estrogen synthesis is not found before the end of metamorphosis (age 8 weeks).

In *Bufo*, treatment with exogenous steroids does not cause complete permanent sex reversal. However, removal of the testes of adult male *Bufo bufo* is followed by development of the Bidder's organs into functional ovaries, with ensuing complete functional feminization (Gallien, 1965).

See Table 3 for a summary of gonad differentiation in amphibians.

B. Other Sex Structures

Interest has chiefly centered around the gonaducts, cloacal glands, and nuptial thumb pads of Anurans. In females, the urinary and reproductive ducts are separate, and the embryonic Müllerian ducts develop into paired oviducts (see Fig. 4). In male Anurans and in primitive Urodeles, the ureter and sperm duct (Wolffian duct) are not separate. Wolffian ducts persist in female amphibians but in a nonsexual capacity as ureters. Müllerian ducts persist in some males as rudiments (Foote, 1964; Sadleir, 1973).

Table 3. Summary of Experiments on Sexual Differentiation in Amphibia

Species[a]	Age at treatment	Treatment	Effect on[b]			
			Gonads	Gonaducts	Other sex structures	Behavior
Several (U and A)	Larva	Parabiosis	F→M			F→M
Ambystoma mexicanum (U)	Larva	Gonad graft	F→M	F→M	F→M	
	Larva	Estrogens	M→F	M→F	M→F	M→F
Hynobius (2 spp.) (U)	Larva	Estrogens	M→F	M→F	M→F	M→F
Triturus helveticus (U)	Larva	Estrogens	M→F	M→F	M→F	M→F
Pleurodeles waltlii (U)	Larva	Estrogens	M→F	M→F	M→F	M→F
Xenopus laevis (A)	Larva	Gonad graft	F→M			M→F
	Larva	Estrogens	M→F	M→F	M→F	F→M
	Adult	Ovariectomy + androgens				F→M
Pseudocris nigrita (A)	Larva	Androgens	F→M	F→M	F→M	F→M
Rana (3 spp.) (A)	Larva	Androgens	F→M	F→M	F→M	F→M
Bufo bufo (A)	Adult	Castration of male	→F[c]			F→M

[a] (U) indicates urodeles; (A) indicates anurans.
[b] F→M indicates complete masculinization (sex reversal) of the character; M→F indicates complete feminization.
[c] I.e., ovaries developed.

The primordia for both sets of ducts are present in the embryos of both sexes (Foote, 1964). The Wolffian ducts develop first, prior to gonadal differentiation (Gallien, 1955). The Müllerian ducts develop later—after metamorphosis in Anurans, and during the larval stage in Urodeles (Foote, 1964; Gallien, 1955).

In both *Triturus* and *Xenopus*, male and female larvae castrated prior to sex differentiation develop identically with undifferentiated gonaducts. The Wolffian ducts remain as nephric ducts (Burns, 1961; Gallien, 1965). Müllerian ducts persist in male *Xenopus* only if castration is performed before age 7 months. Estrogens promote development of the Müllerian ducts in both sexes at any age (Burns, 1961; Van Tienhoven, 1968). Males that undergo complete sex reversal develop functional oviducts. The effect of androgens on the Müllerian ducts depends on age. If they are applied prior to duct differentiation, the ducts will be inhibited; if they are applied afterward, hypertrophy of the ducts may occur (Burns, 1961; Gallien, 1955; Van Tienhoven, 1968). The responses of males and females are identical, and gonadal grafts duplicate the effects of exogenous hormones (Burns, 1961; Gallien, 1955).

Since Wolffian ducts persist in both sexes and differentiate prior to gonadal differentiation, it is hardly surprising that they differentiate independently of sex steroids. Androgens cause hypertrophy of the Wolffian ducts in both sexes; the magnitude of the hypertrophy is independent of genetic sex. In sex-reversed females, the Wolffian ducts take on a sexual function (Burns, 1961; Gallien, 1955).

Thus, the neutral gonaduct form in Amphibia is undifferentiated, but closer to the female form than to the male form. Data are available for only a few species, however, and all are Urodeles or lower Anurans. It may be that this conclusion does not apply to the higher Anurans.

The cloacal glands, which are most pronounced in adult male Urodeles, and nuptial pads, characteristic of adult male Anurans, appear to differentiate under the influence of gonadal secretions. Gonadal sex change from male to female is accompanied by complete feminization of the cloacal glands (Burns, 1961; Gallien, 1955).

C. Behavior

Understanding the role of sex hormones in behavioral differentiation in amphibians is made difficult by the fact that the hormonal control of behavior in the adults is not well understood.

Most amphibians are oviparous. Fertilization is external in Anurans, and in mating the male clasps the female reflexively around the "waist" (the amplexus reflex). Courtship commonly involves vocalization. Fertilization is internal in Urodeles. The male deposits a spermatophore on the ground which the female picks up in her cloaca (Halliday, 1975). Courtship may include the secretion of special pheromones and postural displays (Sadleir, 1973).

Castration of *Bufo arenarum, Rana pipiens,* and *Xenopus laevis* abolishes the clasp reflex (Aronson, 1958; Kelley and Pfaff, 1976; Palka and Gorbman, 1973). Restoration of sexual behavior with sex hormone treatment has proved somewhat difficult. In *Bufo bufo* and *B. arenarum*, a combination of testosterone and gonadotropins will activate the clasp reflex. Clasping can be restored in castrated *Rana pipiens* with implants of testicular tissue from pituitary-treated frogs or with testosterone implants in the preoptic nucleus (Wada and Gorbman, 1977) but not by systematic injections of testosterone, dihydro-testosterone, estradiol, or other steroids (Palka and Gorbman, 1973). Clasping in castrated male *Xenopus* can be restored with pellets of testosterone or dihydro-testosterone (Kelley and Pfaff, 1976), and testosterone will also activate clasp-ing in castrated females.

The endocrinology of Urodele sexual behavior is virtually unexplored. Courtship can be activated in three *Triturus* species with prolactin (Grant, 1966). The endocrinology of female sexual behavior, in both Urodeles and Anurans, is unknown.

Clearly, hormonal manipulations early in life can have profound and permanent effects on amphibian behavior. In the experiments described in Section IV.A, hormonally treated larvae were functionally sex reversed to the point of mating and producing progeny with individuals of the same genetic sex. As was the case in fish, interpretation of these experiments in terms of organizational effects is risky, since sex differences in the ability to respond to activational hormones have not been assessed. Furthermore, most of the data do not allow one to tell whether the effects of sex hormones vary with age in a manner suggesting a critical period. Finally, the behavior of sex-reversed animals has not been studied in any detail.

D. Summary

Table 3 summarizes sexual differentiation in amphibians (these are con-trasted with other vertebrate classes in Table 10). It appears that higher anurans can readily be masculinized, both morphologically and behaviorally, by early hormone treatment, with complete functional sex reversal possible in some species. The neutral sex is as yet unknown. In *Xenopus* and Urodeles, in contrast, feminization is the usual result of early hormone treatment, and the female is the neutral sex (undifferentiated sex, to be more accurate). Except in the case of *Bufo*, where males castrated in adulthood become functional females, hormone treatments have strong sex-reversing effects only during the larval period, suggesting that true organizational effects confined to a limited critical period are occurring. Whether this conclusion can be extended to behavior will depend on the results of studies, yet to be done, in which animals of different ages are administered heterologous hormones.

V. DIFFERENTIATION OF REPRODUCTIVE FUNCTION IN REPTILES

Reptiles occupy an important position in vertebrate phylogeny, and a full understanding of their reproductive physiology and behavior is essential for comparative neuroendocrinology. It is especially unfortunate, therefore, that less is known about sex differentiation in reptiles than in any other vertebrate class. Reptiles do pose some special practical problems. The long period of time required to reach sexual maturity in most species combined with the difficulty of successfully rearing hatchlings in captivity make developmental research troublesome.

Small lizards are the most promising subjects. Among reptiles, lizards exhibit the most pronounced behavioral and physical dimorphism, including sex differences in cloacal morphology, coloration, throat flaps, dorsal crests, and size and shape. Male lizards possess two hemipenes and a hormone-dependent renal sex segment which varies in size seasonally (Sadleir, 1973).

The reproductive tracts of reptiles are shown in Fig. 5 (see Fig. 7 for a comparison with mammals). The secondary sex characters of adult reptiles respond to gonadectomy in a manner similar to that seen in higher vertebrates—they are reduced in size (Chester-Jones *et al.*, 1972; Miller, 1959; Van Tienhoven, 1968). The sex characters are restored by injections of testosterone in males and estrogen in females. Testosterone administered to adult females, either intact or castrated, stimulates the oviducts (Kehl and Combescot, 1955; Miller, 1959), feminizes the cloaca, and causes hypertrophy of the rudimentary male secondary sex characters (Forbes, 1964; Miller, 1959) and thus has both masculinizing and feminizing effects. Estrogen administered to adult males sometimes inhibits and sometimes stimulates the epididymides and may inhibit the hemipenes and renal sex segments and feminize the cloaca (Chester-Jones *et al.*, 1972; Forbes, 1964; Miller, 1959).

Sexual differentiation sometimes occurs slowly in reptiles and is not always complete at hatching. In snakes and lizards, the Wolffian ducts are often retained in adult females, and thus females have two sets of ducts. In some species, the Müllerian ducts may also be present in both sexes (Forbes, 1964). Occasionally, spontaneous intersexuality occurs in snakes and lizards (Kehl and Combescot, 1955).

A thorough description of the sexual embryology of the European lizard *Lacerta vivipara* has been provided by Dufaure (1966). In this species, the gonads, especially the testes, differentiate very rapidly with only a very short bipotential stage. A sex difference in the length of the Müllerian ducts appears as soon as the gonads differentiate, and by birth these ducts have degenerated in the male. At about the same time that this sex difference in the ducts begins,

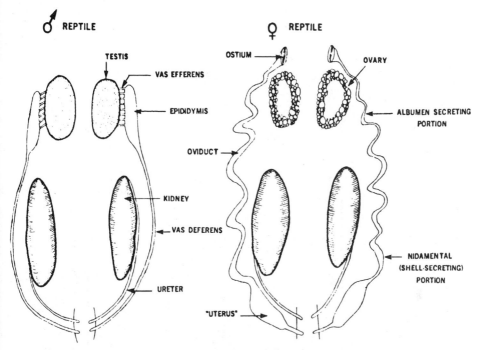

Figure 5. Gonads and gonaducts in reptiles. (Reproduced with permission from Sadleir, 1973.)

the genital tubercles of the male begin to grow, and those of the female begin to shrink. In the male, these tubercles go on to become the two hemipenes.

A. Gonads

Experimental treatment of embryonic reptilian gonads with sex steroids can modify their development, but such effects are not necessarily permanent.

In general estrogen feminizes embryonic gonads, and testosterone has a slight masculinizing effect (Dodd, 1960) (see Table 4). In both cases the degree of gonadal reversal is often slight. Pieau (1974) treated incubating turtle eggs (*Emys orbicularis*) with either estradiol benzoate or testosterone propionate at the beginning of the period of sexual differentiation of the gonads. Both treatments feminized gonads, but only partially, producing ovotestes. Dantschakoff (1937, 1938) injected estrone or folliculin into lizard eggs (*Lacerta* sp.) and found that both the cortical and medullary portions of female gonads were stimulated, whereas the medulla of male gonads was inhibited, and the cortex was stimulated, producing ovotestes. Thus, gonads of males were feminized, but gonads of females were neither feminized nor masculinized. In contrast, Dufaure (1966) found that neither estrogens, androgens, nor a mixture of the two resulted in gonadal intersexuality in *Lacerta vivipara*. Pituitary gonadotropins feminized gonads, but sex differentiation took place normally in decapitated (and therefore hypophysectomized) embryos, contraindicating

Table 4. Summary of Experiments on Sex Differentiation in Reptilia

Species	Age at treatment	Treatment	Effect on[a]		
			Gonads	Gonaducts	Other sex structures
Several	Embryos	Gonadectomy		M→F	
Several	Embryos	Estrogens	m→f		
Lacerta vivipara	Embryos	Gonadectomy		M→F	F→M
	Embryos	Parabiosis			M→F
	Embryos	Androgens			f→m
	Embryos	Estrogens	m→f	M→F	M→F
Anguis fragilis	Embryos	Testosterone		F→M	
Anolis carolinensis	Juveniles	Estrogen			M→F
Sceloporus sp.	Juveniles	Estrogen			M→F
Alligator mississippiensis	Juveniles	Testosterone		m→f	f→m
Crocodylus niloticus	Juveniles	Testosterone	f→m	m→f	
Thamnophis sirtalis	Embryos	Testosterone		m→f	
Malaclemmys centrata	Juveniles	Estradiol		m→f	f→m
	Juveniles	Testosterone	m→f		
Chrysemys marginata	Embryos	Testosterone	f→m		
Emys orbicularis	Embryos	Estradiol or testosterone	m→f		
Emys leprosa	Recently hatched	Androgens		m→f	f→m
	Recently hatched	Estrogen	m→f	m→f	
Testudo graeca	Embryos	Estradiol	m→f	m→f	

[a]F→M indicates extensive or complete masculinization of the character; M→F indicates extensive or complete feminization. f→m indicates slight or partial masculinization; m→f indicates slight or partial feminization.

a role for pituitary hormones in normal gonadal development. Raynaud (1962, 1963) studied development in embryos of the blindworm *Anguis fragilis* (a lizard) cultured *in vitro* that had been hypophysectomized either by localized X-irradiation or by decapitation and found that gonadal differentiation into testes or ovaries took place normally.

Little is known about the actual secretions of embryonic reptilian gonads, and in no case has a particular hormone been conclusively identified (Ozon, 1972a,b). Raynaud and Pieau (1971) observed an increase in Δ^5-3β-hydro-xysteroid dehydrogenase activity in the testes of *Lacerta viridis* embryos just before Müllerian duct growth becomes arrested, suggesting increased steroid synthesis at this time.

Ovaries of juvenile *Lacerta vivipara* will feminize embryonic chick testes when cultured *in vitro* with them (Lutz-Ostertag and Dufaure, 1961), suggesting that these ovaries are actively secreting an estrogenic hormone.

It is interesting to note that incubation temperature has a marked effect on gonadal differentiation in two species of turtles, *Emys orbicularis* and *Testudo graeca* (Pieau, 1975). At low temperatures, male phenotypes predominate, and at high temperatures, female phenotypes predominate.

B. Other Sex Structures

Differentiation of sex structures appears to be under hormonal control, perhaps by sex steroids (see Table 4). Castration of embryos prior to differentiation results in the retention of both sets of gonaducts in both sexes of reptiles (recall that the Wolffian ducts normally are retained in the female but that the Müllerian ducts commonly degenerate in the male) (Wolff, 1950). Early castration of *Lacerta vivipara* embryos results in retention of the genital tubercles in the female (Dufaure, 1966), and thus the neutral sex in this species (in which the male is homogametic) is female for gonaducts and male for the genital tubercle. It is not uncommon in vertebrates for the gonaducts to differentiate according to different rules than other morphological structures; this point will be discussed further in Section VII.

Treatment of lizard embryos with testosterone causes only slight masculinization of sex structures. Androgens stimulate the genital tubercles of female *Lacerta vivipara* embryos (Dufaure, 1966), but it is not clear whether this effect is permanent. Testosterone has its most pronounced effects on the Müllerian ducts, and it is possible that testosterone or some other testicular hormone is responsible for suppression of these ducts in male lizard embryos (Raynaud *et al.*, 1969). Exogenous testosterone inhibits the Müllerian ducts in developing *Anguis fragilis* embryos treated *in vivo* (Raynaud and Pieau, 1973), and in five species of reptiles, including three lizards, the earlier the differentiation of the testis, the earlier the arrest of the elongation of the Müllerian ducts (Raynaud *et al.*, 1970). However, Dufaure (1966), working with *Lacerta vivipara* embryos, found that androgens applied to females did not result in degeneration of the Müllerian ducts. Whether species differences underlie these contradictory results is not yet known.

In contrast to the rather weak effects of androgens on female lizard embryos, estrogens cause rather extensive feminization of male embryos. Dantschakoff (1938) removed eggs about to be laid from female lizards (*Lacerta* sp.) and injected them with folliculin, an estrogen. The lizards hatched after 6 weeks and were examined after hatching. In both sexes the Müllerian ducts were stimulated, and the Wolffian ducts were retained (as they are in a normal female). The cloaca and outer genital region were feminized in males and stimulated in females; both sexes then resembled a normal adult female in breeding condition.

Degeneration of the genital tubercles occurs in male *Lacerta vivipara* joined to female embryos by parabiosis (Dufaure, 1966). In the same series of experiments, nearly total sex reversal of the sex structures of male embryos was obtained by treating them first with pituitary gonadotropins, which caused persistence of the Müllerian ducts, and then later in development with estrogen, which stimulated further development of the ducts and caused regression of the genital tubercles. Estrogen caused marked feminization of the reproductive tract of posthatching *Anolis* or *Sceloporus* by stimulating female structures and inhibiting male tissues (Forbes, 1964).

The few experiments on sex differentiation in reptiles other than lizards again indicate that exogenous sex steroids administered early in life have more dramatic effects on accessory sex structures than on the gonads and that feminization is more readily obtained than masculinization. Forbes (1938, 1939) examined the effects of testosterone propionate in 3-month-old and 17-month-old *Alligator*. At hatching, both sexes normally have both sets of gonaducts and a phallus. Testosterone had a bisexual effect in females, stimulating the oviducts and the phallus. Such a bisexual effect also occurs when juvenile female *Crocodylus niloticus* are treated with testosterone. Ovaries are masculinized, Wolffian ducts regress, and Müllerian ducts hypertrophy (Godet, 1961). Hartley (1945) injected testosterone propionate into the amniotic cavities of developing embryos of the garter snake (*Thamnophis sirtalis*, a viviparous species) during the month of gestation. Such treatment inhibited ovarian development without stimulating medullary tissue and stimulated the Müllerian ducts.

Turtle embryos are also altered as a result of exposure to sex steroids. Testosterone propionate applied to juvenile diamondback terrapins (*Malaclemmys centrata*) caused development of the phallus in both sexes and of Müllerian ducts in females (Risley, 1941). Estradiol dipropionate feminized the gonads of males and stimulated Müllerian ducts. Risley (1940) applied testosterone propionate to *Chrysemys marginata* embryos and observed no effects in the single male subject, no effect on the gonaducts, and slight masculinization of the ovaries. Androgens administered to recently hatched *Emys leprosa* caused hypertrophy of the Müllerian ducts and phallus, whereas estrogen resulted in ovotestes and hypertrophied Müllerian ducts (Forbes, 1964). More recently,

Pieau (1970) gave estradiol benzoate to embryos of *Testudo graeca* before or after differentiation of the gonads. Feminization of gonads was very slight, and the phalli developed normally. Müllerian ducts were stimulated by the treatment at either time.

C. Behavior

Our knowledge of activational effects of sex hormones on adult reptile behavior is based on data from only two species—the Carolina anole (*Anolis carolinensis*) and the garter snake (*Thamnophis sirtalis*). Castration of males is followed by a complete absence of sexual activity, and sexual behavior is restored by treatment with testosterone. Receptivity in female *Anolis* is estrogen-dependent (Crews, 1974, 1976; Mason and Adkins, 1976; Noble and Greenberg, 1940, 1941). Castrated female *Anolis* treated with testosterone display considerable male behavior, courting and pursuing other females, whereas castrated males treated with estrogen appear to be relatively refractory to estrogen behaviorally (Mason and Adkins, 1976). Organizational effects of sex hormones on adult reptile behavior have not yet been investigated, but the foundations for such work have been laid in *Anolis carolinensis*.

D. Summary

In contrast to fish and amphibians, early hormone treatment of reptiles does not have dramatic effects, and permanent complete sex reversal with sex steroid treatment has not been obtained. The predominant effect of hormone treatment of embryos is feminization of gonads and external sex structures (see Table 4 and, for comparison with other vertebrate classes, Table 10). With respect to gonaducts, estrogens stimulate Müllerian (female) ducts, and androgens inhibit them. Organizational effects are a distinct possibility in that most of the treatments have been confined to embryos but cannot be safely assumed, since neither permanence nor limitation to a critical period has generally been demonstrated. Behavioral differentiation remains a topic for the future.

VI. DIFFERENTIATION OF REPRODUCTIVE FUNCTION IN BIRDS

The class Aves contains many species that are ideal for research on sex differentiation. Marked physical and behavioral dimorphism is common in birds. Domestic species are prolific and mature rapidly compared with poikilothermic vertebrates. Not surprisingly, then, there is a sizable and fascinating literature on hormones and sex differentiation in birds, stimulated also in part by the desire of poultrymen to be able to experimentally induce sex reversal and increase the proportion of hens hatching. Perhaps because of these economic considerations, most of this literature centers around only six of the approximately 8600 species of birds.

A. Gonads

The avian reproductive tracts are shown in Fig. 6 (see Fig. 7 for a comparison with mammals). In birds, the primordial germ cells migrate in greater numbers to the left than to the right side, and thus an asymmetry in the size of the gonads is established quite early and persists after hatching in most birds. Adult females have a functional ovary on the left side and only a gonadal rudiment on the right; males generally have a slightly larger testis on the left than on the right (Lofts and Murton, 1973; Taber, 1964). Initially, medullary tissue (testicular primordium) develops on both sides. In a genetic female, cortical tissue (ovarian primordium) then develops on the left gonad and to a slight degree on the right (Taber, 1964). Sex differentiation of the gonads occurs after about 6.5 days of incubation in the domestic chick (*Gallus gallus*) (incubation period 21 days), 8 days in the duck (*Anas platyrhynchos*) (28-day incubation period), and 5.5 days in the quail (*Coturnix coturnix*) (17- to 18-day incubation period) (Haffen, 1975). The left gonad of the female chick undergoes rapid growth from the ninth to the eleventh day of incubation (Mittwoch, 1973). The species studied are all precocial (well-developed at hatching).

Ovarian development on the right side is customary in some raptors

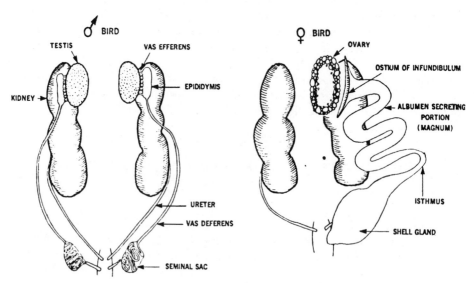

Figure 6. Gonads and gonaducts in birds. (Reproduced with permission from Sadleir, 1973.)

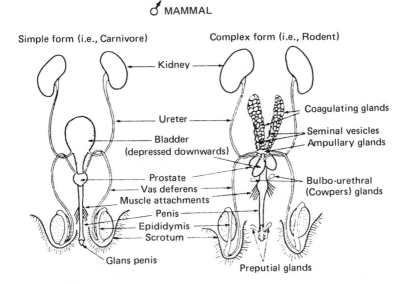

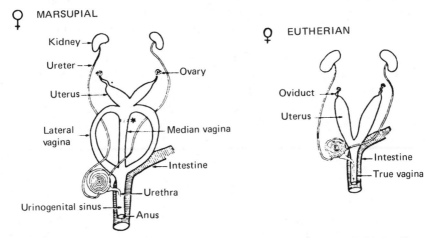

Figure 7. Reproductive systems of marsupial and eutherian mammals. (Reproduced with permission from Sadleir, 1973.)

(falcons, vultures, and accipitrine hawks) and occasionally occurs in pigeons, herring gulls, and chickens (Taber, 1964).

The ambisexual state (i.e., mixed medullary–cortical tissue) of the right gonad in females is believed to underlie the numerous cases of gonadal intersexuality that have been recorded. In chickens spontaneous intersexuality occurs most commonly in females. A normal hen stops laying eggs and begins to look and act like a male (Taber, 1964). Autopsy reveals that the right gonad has developed into a testis or ovotestis (a gonad with both ovarian and testicular tissue), occasionally one that produces sperm. This condition is often caused by inactivation of the left ovary by disease or tumors; this apparently releases the medullary tissue of the right gonad from estrogenic inhibition (Taber, 1964). This same kind of intersexuality can be produced by surgically removing the left ovary, especially in young chickens (Masui, 1967; Taber, 1964). The tendency to develop testicular tissue on the right side following sinistral ovariectomy varies from breed to breed in chickens, and in the most pronounced cases the testicular tissue produces sperm (Masui, 1967). Hybrids produced by crossing two avian species occasionally have intersexual gonads (Gomot, 1975).

Avian gonadal primordia can be cultured *in vitro* and allowed to differentiate independently of the rest of the embryo. In ducks, chickens, and quail, the result is normal testicular differentiation in males (Haffen, 1975). The left primordium of females becomes an ovary or an ovary with some medullary tissue, whereas the right primordium either regresses or becomes an ovotestis (Haffen, 1975; Gallien, 1967).

If pairs of embryonic gonads are cultured together, the ovary is dominant over the testis in chickens and ducks in that a testis is feminized by an ovary and does not masculinize the ovary (Jost, 1960; Wolff, 1959). This occurs even if both gonads are still at the indifferent stage at the beginning of the experiment and occurs even if a right ovary is used (Jost, 1960). Feminization of an embryonic testis by an ovary also occurs if a gonad from one individual is grafted into the body cavity of another individual (Jost, 1960; Wolff, 1959). Apparently the embryonic gonads are secreting hormones.

When embryonic gonads of quail, chickens, turkeys (*Meleagris gallopavo*), and herring gulls (*Larus argentatus*) are exposed to estrogens, either *in vivo* or *in vitro*, the result, if any, is almost invariably feminization of testes, occasionally permanently (Burns, 1961; Gallien, 1967; Taber, 1964; Witschi, 1961). In a classic study, Domm (1939) injected chicken eggs with estradiol on days 3 to 5 of incubation. As adults (age 2 years) some of the males had left gonads that were ovotestes with yolking follicles. Right gonads of males were testes. Van Tienhoven (1957) dipped chicken eggs prior to incubation in alcohol solutions of estradiol. On examination, the gonads of males were covered with cortical tissue which decreased with age. Functional ovaries were never seen in these males. Erickson and Pincus (1966) injected a variety of steroids into chicken eggs on the fourth day of incubation. Estrogens stimulated the cortex of the left gonad in males. A few males injected with diethylstilbestrol (a nonsteroidal estrogen) had ovarian follicles in the testis. Haffen (1965), working with quail, dipped eggs in a diethylstilbestrol solution on the fourth day of incubation and found extensive feminization of testes that persisted through maturity.

Ovotestes often revert back to testes by the end of the first year (Witschi, 1961). Testes that are not permanently feminized by early estrogen nonetheless are often permanently damaged to the point of being subfertile or sterile (Pantić and Kosanović, 1973; Wentworth *et al.*, 1968).

Several experiments have investigated the possibility that estrogens could pass from an ovulating female into the eggs and cause feminization. Fraps *et al.*

(1956) implanted pellets of diethylstilbestrol into 9-week-old chickens. Among the offspring there were more females than males. Since females suffer greater embryonic mortality than males (Bellairs, 1960), this result suggests that feminization of some males, rather than differential mortality, may have been responsible for the results. Pun (1958) obtained similar results using stilbestrol implants. Breeding experiments have shown, however, that the excess females are not sex-reversed males (Taber, 1964). Riddle and Dunham (1942) observed that in ring doves (*Streptopelia* sp.) there is normally an excess of females among newly-hatched squabs and that at hatching the left gonad of males has some ovarian cortex. They suggested that the female dove's own estrogen was responsible for these phenomena in her offspring. To see if a significant amount of estrogen could pass from a laying female to her eggs, they injected females with estradiol benzoate 26 to 34 hr before ovulation. Sex-linked color indicated the genetic sex. Twelve of 13 males killed within 26 days after hatching had left ovotestes, whereas females were unchanged. These researchers concluded that the cortex normally found in hatchling males' testes is probably caused by the mothers' estrogen.

In contrast to the effects of estrogens on embryonic testes, androgens have little or no effect on ovarian development (Taber, 1964) and have either no effect, a slight masculinizing effect, or a feminizing effect on testes (Jost, 1960; Burns, 1961; Erickson and Pincus, 1966; Riddle and Dunham, 1942). Six- and 7-day-old embryonic chick testes cultivated *in vitro* with testosterone, androstenedione, or dihydrotestosterone are feminized, becoming ovotestes (Weniger and Zeis, 1973).

Two main conclusions can be drawn from these experiments on avian gonadal differentiation (Table 5 summarizes the experiments). First, the results from experiments using different methods agree quite well (Burns, 1961); all indicate that ovarian secretions and sex steroids feminize testes but have little effect on ovaries and that ovaries are dominant over testes in that ovaries feminize testes, but testes do not masculinize ovaries. The feminizing actions of synthetic estrogens and androgens are quite similar to the actions of the embryonic gonads themselves (Gallien, 1967). Second, the feminizing effects of early sex steroid administration are not always permanent. The extent and duration of the feminization depends on the species. In order of decreasing sensitivity of the gonads, the species are herring gull > quail > chicken > duck (Jost, 1960). Feminization also depends on the genetic strain (Masui, 1967), the location of the gonad (whether left or right), the dose of hormone, the particular hormone used (diethylstilbestrol is the most powerful), the age at which the animal is examined, and the stage of development of the gonads at the time of treatment. The earlier the treatment, the better (Masui, 1967). Despite extensive experimentation, complete permanent functional sex reversal has not yet been produced in birds.

Several experiments described above strongly suggest that embryonic avian gonads are actively secreting sex hormones similar to those produced by adult gonads, but only recently has the endocrinology of the embryonic gonads

Table 5. Summary of Experiments on Sexual Differentiation in Birds

Species	Age at treatment	Treatment	Effect on[a]			
			Gonads	Gonaducts[b]	Other sex structures	Behavior
Anas platyrhynchos	Embryo	Gonad graft	M→F		F→M	
	Embryo	Gonadectomy		FM		
	Embryo	Estradiol			M→F	
Gallus gallus	Embryo	Gonad graft	M→F	F→M	F→M	
	Embryo	Gonadectomy		FM		
	Embryo	Estrogens	m→f	FM	M→F	M→F
	Embryo	Androgens	m→f	F→M		M→F
Coturnix coturnix	Embryo	Estrogen	M→F	FM	M→F	M→F
	Embryo	Androgen	M→F		m→f	M→F
	Embryo	Antiestrogen				f→m
Meleagris gallopavo	Embryo	Estrogens	m→f			
Larus argentatus	Embryo	Estrogens	M→F	FM		
Streptopelia sp.	Embryo	Estrogen	M→F	FM		
Columba livia	Squab	DES				m→f

[a] F→M indicates extensive (gonads) or complete (other variables) masculinization; M→F indicates extensive or complete feminization. f→m or m→f indicate incomplete masculinization or feminization.

[b] Here FM indicates that both Müllerian ducts were retained, a condition not seen in normal individuals of either sex. F→M indicates that Müllerian ducts were suppressed.

been investigated. The results of experiments with gonads cultured *in vitro* are summarized in Table 6. Avian gonads are capable of synthesizing steroids at least as soon as they have differentiated and sometimes earlier.

Our knowledge of *in vivo* steroid hormone production by embryonic avian gonads is much more limited. Ozon (1965), using spectrofluorimetry, assayed the blood and allantoic fluid of chick embryos for estrogens. The results are shown in Table 7 and indicate that female chick embryos actually produce more estrogen than do adult laying hens. Woods *et al.* (1975), using radio-immunoassay, found that testosterone is first present in chick embryos on day 5.5 and that from day 7.5 through 17.5, males produce more than females.

Thus, it appears that embryonic secretions of avian gonads are indeed sex steroids, at least in part, and that even at an early age ovaries probably produce more estrogen than do testes, whereas testes produce more androgens than do ovaries. That these secretions control the differentiation of the sex structures and probably behavior as well will become evident in the next sections.

B. Other Sex Structures

Of chief interest here will be the gonaducts, syrinx, and external sex organs (when present). Because the gonaducts differentiate somewhat differently from the other sex structures, they will be discussed separately.

1. Genital Tubercle, Syrinx, and Proctodeal Gland

Domestic ducks possess two structures showing marked dimorphism—the genital tubercle and the syrinx. The genital tubercle is the primordium from which the penis develops in male birds (in those few avian species that do have a penis) (Burns, 1961). It is present in both sexes prior to sexual differentiation and in adult males of most species, where it is typically rudimentary. In male ducks, it develops into a sizeable twisted organ capable of protruding from the cloaca (Taber, 1964). Even in the chicken, where it is rudimentary in the male, its presence can be detected at hatching and used for sexing. The syrinx of birds (a vocal organ) is a swelling at the point where the trachea and bronchial tubes join. It is sexually dimorphic in ducks, the European coot (*Fulica atra*), and some song birds (Nottebohm, 1975). In the female duck, it is small and symmetrical, whereas in the male it is large and asymmetrical. In ducks, there is no sex difference in the syrinx or genital tubercle until day 10 or 11 of incubation, at which time the genital tubercle of the female regresses, and the penis and syrinx grow in the male (the gonads differentiate on day 8) (Burns, 1961; Taber, 1964).

Differentiation of the genital tubercle and syrinx are controlled by the embryonic gonads, as shown by Wolff (1959), who has been able to castrate embryos *in vivo* prior to sex differentiation, on day 3 or 4, by X-irradiation of the gonadal primordium. The embryos were examined between the 17th and

Table 6. Steroid Hormone Production by Embryonic Avian Gonads[a]

Species	Gonad	Embryonic age (days)[b]	Method	Result[c]
Anas platyrhynchos	Ovary	12	Incubation with [Na-1-^{14}C]acetate	E_1 and E_2 produced
Gallus gallus	Ovary	7–9	Incubation with [Na-1-^{14}C]acetate	E_1 and E_2 produced
	Ovary	7.5 on	Incubation with [^{3}H]pregnenolone or [^{14}C]-P[d]	Estrogens and T produced
	Ovary	6–17	Incubation with [4-^{14}C]dehydroepiandrosterone	Estrogens but not T produced
	Indifferent	3.5–5.5	Immunofluorescence	Androgens detected
	Both	6.5 on	Immunofluorescence	Androgens detected
	Testis	7.5 on	Incubation with [^{3}H]pregnenolone or [^{14}C]-P[d]	Estrogens and T produced
	Testis	6–17	Incubation with [4-^{14}C]dehydroepiandrosterone	T but not estrogens produced
Coturnix coturnix	Ovary	10 and 15	Incubation with [4^{14}C]dehydroepiandrosterone	Estrogens but not T produced[e]
	Both	10 and 15	Incubation with [^{3}H]pregnenolone or [^{14}C]-P[d]	Estrogens and T produced[e]
	Testis	10 and 15	Incubation with [4-^{14}C]dehydroepiandrosterone	Estrogens and T produced[e]

[a] From Haffen (1975), Woods and Podczaski (1974), and Woods *et al.* (1975).
[b] Recall that the age of gonadal differentiation is 6.5 for *Gallus*, 8 for *Anas*, and 5.5 for *Coturnix*.
[c] E_1, [^{14}C]estrone; E_2, estradiol; T, testosterone.
[d] [^{14}C]progesterone.
[e] Ovaries produce more estrogen than testes do, and testes produce more T than ovaries do.

Table 7. Estrogen Production by Female Chickens Before and After Hatching[a]

	Adult	21-day female embyro	13-day female embryo	10-day female embyro
Source	60 ml blood	11 ml blood	244 ml allantoic fluid	12 ml allantoic fluid
Total estrogens (μg/100 ml)	2.2	6.6	0.2	4.9

[a] From Ozon (1965).

22nd day of incubation. In the absence of gonads both sexes of the duck develop a male-type genital tubercle and syrinx, and thus the male is the neutral (anhormonal) sex for these organs. Male differentiation is prevented and the female form is assumed if either ovary is spared. It is particularly interesting that the right rudimentary gonad of the female, acting alone, will cause feminization (Jost, 1960). These results are shown in Fig. 8. A natural equivalent to this experiment is the occasional occurrence of birds spontaneously lacking gonads. Gonadless pigeons, doves, ducks, and pheasants have a masculine phenotype (Taber, 1964).

Differentiation *in vitro* follows the same course as differentiation following early castration (Van Tienhoven, 1968). The genital tubercle and syrinx of the duck develop into the male type if explanted before gonadal differentiation (Wolff, 1959). If explanted after gonadal differentiation, they differentiate according to the gonadal sex. If these organs are cultured with an embryonic ovary or if estrodiol benzoate is put in the culture medium, they differentiate in a female manner.

Male embryos treated with estrogen are typically feminized, whereas female embryos treated similarly show no effect. Thus estradiol benzoate injected into incubating duck eggs causes the genital tubercle and syrinx of males to assume the female form; i.e., neither develop (Taber, 1964). The effects of hormones are the same on the chick's organs as on the duck's, except that the sex difference in the chick is always much smaller (Burns, 1961; Erickson and Pincus, 1966).

Androgens injected into incubating chicken eggs have little or no effect

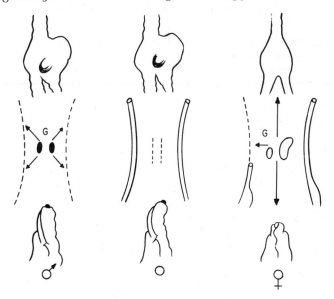

Figure 8. Differentiation of the syrinx (top row), Müllerian ducts (middle row), and genital tubercle (bottom row) of male (left), female (right), or anhormonal (center) ducks. Arrows represent actions of the embryonic gonads. (Reproduced with permission from Wolff, 1959.)

(Taber, 1964) aside from transient hypertrophy of the genital tubercle in the males (Erickson and Pincus, 1966). In the duck, testosterone stimulates the genital tubercle and syrinx, perhaps through suppression of endogenous ovarian estrogen (Taber, 1964). Large doses of testosterone inhibit the syrinx, a feminizing action (Burns, 1961).

The proctodeal gland of the quail (also called foam gland or cloacal gland) is also a convenient sexually dimorphic character with which to assess the results of early hormone administration. The proctodeal gland, which is externally visible, is androgen dependent (Sachs, 1967) and therefore is developed in the adult male but rudimentary in the female. A sex difference in the size of this gland persists even when adult birds are gonadectomized and given equal amounts of testosterone propionate (Adkins, 1975). Injection of either estradiol benzoate or testosterone propionate into eggs on the tenth day of incubation inhibits future proctodeal gland responsiveness to testosterone propionate in males such that, in the case of prenatal estrogen, the normal sex difference in gland responsiveness is eliminated (Adkins, 1975). Thus, the proctodeal gland is feminized by embryonic exposure to sex steroids.

2. Gonaducts

In birds the Wolffian ducts become the epididymides and vasa deferentia, whereas the Müllerian ducts become oviducts. These gonaducts in adult birds are highly responsive to androgen (male ducts) and estrogen (female ducts), become greatly enlarged at puberty, and, in seasonally breeding species, become enlarged during the breeding season (Lofts and Murton, 1973). In normal adult males, the Müllerian ducts are absent, and in normal adult females a well-developed oviduct is found only on the left side. The Wolffian ducts persist as rudiments in normal adult females (Taber, 1964). Prepubertally, the Wolffian ducts are only slightly dimorphic, and in some species (e.g., the house sparrow) the Wolffian ducts of females may enlarge during the breeding season (Witschi, 1961).

Embryologically, the Müllerian ducts initially develop in both sexes (Taber, 1964; Van Tienhoven, 1968). Beginning on about day 9 in the chicken, they begin to regress in the male and are gone by day 13. The right Müllerian duct of females also regresses during this period (Taber, 1964; Van Tienhoven, 1968).

As might be expected from the small degree of sex dimorphism in the Wolffian ducts, embryonic gonadal secretions play little role in their differentiation. Embryonic gonadectomy in either sex produces no change in the Wolffian ducts (Burns, 1961), nor does treatment of embryos with estrogen (Burns, 1961; Taber, 1964; Van Tienhoven, 1968). Treatment with androgens causes hypertrophy of these ducts (Burns, 1961; Erickson and Pincus, 1966; Taber, 1964), but it is not clear whether this effect is permanent (i.e., organizational).

In contrast, embryonic hormone manipulations have pronounced effects on the Müllerian ducts. Embryonic castration by X-irradiation early in incubation (third or fourth day) results in retention of both ducts by both sexes of the duck (Wolff, 1959), and thus the neutral sex, strictly speaking, is neither male nor female with respect to the Müllerian ducts. This phenomenon is shown in Fig. 8. Birds spontaneously lacking gonads also possess both Müllerian ducts. Müllerian ducts cultured *in vitro* develop in a similar manner. If the ducts are explanted from chicks prior to day 8, both survive from both sexes, but they will degenerate if cultured with an embryonic testis or with testosterone (Wolff, 1959). If cultured with estrogen, partial atrophy occurs (Wolff, 1959).

The experiments described above indicate that testicular androgens cause regression of the Müllerian ducts in the male, and that some ovarian secretion causes regression of the right Müllerian duct in females. Experiments in which exogenous steroids are administered to embryos are only partially consistent with these findings. Estrogens applied to incubating eggs by injection or dipping result in retention of both Müllerian ducts in both sexes of the chicken (Burns, 1961; Erickson and Pincus, 1966; Taber, 1964; Van Tienhoven, 1968; Kaufman, 1956), quail (Haffen, 1965), dove (Riddle and Dunham, 1942), and herring gull (Boss and Witschi, 1947), possibly because of inhibition of gonadal secretions (Taber, 1964). In the chicken, this effect is only obtained if the estrogen is applied before day 7 (Burns, 1961). Wentworth *et al.* (1968) sprayed quail eggs with mestranol (a steroidal estrogen) on day 0, 6, or 12 and found that all treated females retained the right oviduct and that many males had persisting Müllerian ducts. The effects of estrogens on oviducts are permanent (Boss and Witschi, 1947; Burns, 1961; Haffen, 1965; Riddle and Dunham, 1942).

Testosterone administered early enough in development appears to cause regression of both Müllerian ducts in the chicken (Burns, 1961; Erickson and Pincus, 1966); and embryonic testes grafted into the coelom of 2- or 3-day-old chicks cause regression of both Müllerian ducts (Wolff, 1959). Androsterone and dehydroandrosterone weakly masculinize female chicks (cause regression of the left Müllerian duct), but feminize males (cause persistence of both Müllerian ducts) (Burns, 1961; Taber, 1964).

Table 5 summarizes these experiments on gonaduct differentiation in birds. In two respects, the gonaducts appear to develop following rules slightly different from those that apply to other sex structures. First, anhormonal development results in two Wolffian and two Müllerian ducts, a condition not found in normal adults of either sex; thus, the neutral sex is neither male nor female. Second, some testicular secretion (which may not be a steroid—see below) seems to be required for regression of the Müllerian ducts in the male (Wolff, 1959). Wolff (1959) has shown that embryonic testes and synthetic androgens both have necrotic and autolytic actions on Müllerian duct tissues. Woods and Podczaski (1974) suggest that in the chick the androgens that are known to be produced by the testes and ovaries after day 6.5 are responsible for regression of the Müllerian ducts in the male and regression of the right duct in the female. More recently, Weniger *et al.* (1975) obtained evidence that the hormone responsible for regression of the Müllerian ducts is probably not a steroid.

C. Ovulation and Oviposition

In rodents, the permanent effects of early sex hormone administration on hypothalamic control of ovulation have received considerable attention. Such effects have received little attention in birds. Early exposure to sex hormones does definitely disturb egg production in birds, and this phenomenon will be briefly discussed, even though evidence that a central nervous system effect is involved is lacking.

An adult laying domestic hen ovulates and oviposits nearly every day. The sequence of events is as follows (Van Tienhoven, 1968). On a 14-hr-light : 10-hr-dark light cycle, three peaks of LH concentration occur, at 21, 13, and 8 hr prior to ovulation. Ovulation occurs within an hour after oviposition of the preceding egg, and both oviposition and ovulation begin in the morning and occur 2–4 hr later each day. When a point is reached at which oviposition would occur in the dark, it is delayed until the following morning, and the sequence begins again. In the quail, ovulation occurs 15 min–2 hr after oviposition, and successive ovipositions are between 24 and 25 hr apart (Opel, 1966). As in the chicken, a peak of LH occurs 6–8 hr prior to ovulation (Lofts and Murton, 1973). These LH peaks in birds are much smaller than those seen in rodents prior to ovulation (Lofts and Murton, 1973). As in rodents, the timing of the light–dark cycle importantly determines the exact timing of the ovulation (Nalbandov, 1959).

In both the chicken and the quail, hypothalamic regions appear to control LH release and ovulation (Lofts and Murton, 1973; Van Tienhoven, 1968). Lesions of the ventral preoptic area block both spontaneous and progesterone-induced ovulation in chickens, and electrical stimulation of the preoptic area causes ovulation. In the quail, lesions of the medial, ventral, or posterior infundibular nucleus block ovulation without causing changes in the ovary or oviduct (Stetson, 1972).

Embryonic exposure to sex hormones significantly lowers egg production in adult female chickens, sometimes inhibiting it altogether. Van Tienhoven (1957) observed lowered egg production in chickens hatched from eggs dipped in estrogen prior to incubation and found that at least some eggs had been ovulated but had gone into the body cavity. Glick (1961) dipped eggs in testosterone propionate on day 3 and obtained a 16% reduction in egg production. The eggs laid were infertile. This phenomenon has also been observed in quail following embryonic exposure to mestranol or estradiol benzoate (Adkins, 1975; Kincl et al., 1967; Wentworth et al., 1968).

The reason for the failure of these birds to produce eggs is not clear. The possibilities include: (a) failure of the ovary to produce yolked follicles; (b) failure of the hypothalamus or pituitary to secrete the proper releasing factors or hormones at the proper time (e.g., elimination of the daily LH peak); (c) failure of the ovary to respond properly to pituitary secretions; (d) failure of the ovulated eggs to reach the oviduct; and (e) oviduct abnormalities. Alternative (a) seems unlikely to be the major cause in view of the observations of

Wentworth *et al.* (1968) that oogenesis appeared normal. There are indications that (d) and (e) have occurred in some experiments. Domm and Davis (1948) found that some female chickens from estrogen-injected eggs failed to lay because of oviductal abnormalities. Kaufman (1956) observed that rutoestrol injected into chick eggs on day 1 or 2 resulted in females with pathological oviducts (thin-walled and fluid-filled). Erickson and Pincus (1966) found cystic oviducts in females injected with estrogens on day 4 of incubation and examined at 210 days posthatching. These cysts prevented oviposition. Adkins (1975) found that a number of female quail injected with testosterone propionate or estradiol benzoate on day 10 of incubation died at puberty because of difficulties in ovipositing. Possibility (b), suggested by the mammalian literature, has not been investigated. In addition, it is not known whether a sex difference exists in adult birds, as exists in rodents, in the ability of the hypothalamus to cause cyclic LH secretion.

D. Behavior

Activation of sexual behavior by sex hormones in adult birds constitutes the necessary background against which to evaluate organizational effects of hormones. Reviews of this material can be found in Chester-Jones *et al.* (1972), Lofts and Murton (1973), Van Tienhoven (1968), and Young (1961).

The male mating pattern generally includes grabbing the feathers of the female's head, standing on her back (mounting), sometimes with alternate stepping movements (treading), twisting the tail to bring the two cloacas into contact, and dismounting. A single brief contact is sufficient in some species. Associated with copulation may be strutting, courtship feeding, or other displays on the part of the male. Singing is not necessarily related to copulation, serving instead a territorial function (Welty, 1962), but the fact that sex differences in singing are common makes it of interest here.

Female sexual behavior may be preceded by displays and soliciting activities. Receptivity typically consists of squatting, holding still, and perhaps lifting the head and tail. A stereotyped posture similar to lordosis does not necessarily occur. Squatting may occur to the sight of the male or may occur as the male makes physical contact. The female turkey everts the lower portion of the oviduct during copulation and is unreceptive for a period of time after mating, ranging from minutes to days (Schein and Hale, 1965).

Gonadectomy eliminates copulation, receptivity, courtship, and dimorphic vocalizations in chickens, quail (Wilson and Bermant, 1972), pigeons, doves (Cheng, 1973), ducks, and turkeys. Gonadectomy results in a more complete absence of sexual behavior in birds than is commonly seen in mammals. In the quail, all sexual behavior ceases within 8 days of castration (Beach and Inman, 1965). The effects of castration are reversed in males by injections of testosterone. Copulation, but not courtship and vocalization, can also be restored in males with estradiol, and thus copulation is not strictly androgen dependent (Adkins and Adler, 1972; Young, 1961). Receptivity can be activated in females by injections of estradiol but is not stimulated by testosterone (Cheng, 1973; Cheng and Lehrman, 1975; Adkins and Adler, 1972).

Treatment of females, particularly ovariectomized females, with testosterone activates some male behavior, such as singing or crowing or courtship displays, but only rarely is the full copulatory pattern, complete with cloacal contact, activated (Young, 1961). In the juvenile and adult chicken and in the adult quail and dove, the female seems to be much less sensitive to androgen than the male; in the female, the neural mechanisms for copulation are relatively refractory to activation (Adkins and Adler, 1972; Cheng and Lehrman, 1975; Collias, 1950; Young, 1961).

In the quail and dove, estrogen stimulates receptivity in males (Adkins and Adler, 1972; Cheng and Lehrman, 1975). The male and female quail are equally sensitive to estradiol in terms of receptivity, and thus the normally observed dimorphism in the occurrence of receptivity in this species is the result of gonadal rather than neural dimorphism. An organizational role of early hormones in the development of receptivity is therefore not likely in the quail (see below for evidence that they have no such role).

The experiments just described in which adult gonadectomized birds are administered heterologous hormones show a pattern of results that is opposite to that in most mammals. In those birds that have been studied, males have a greater capacity for heterotypical (opposite-sex) sexual behavior than do females, and the sex difference in capacity for masculine copulatory behavior and in responsiveness to androgen is greater than the sex difference in capacity for receptivity and in responsiveness to estrogen. In most mammals that have been studied, the female has a greater capacity for heterotypical behavior, and the sex difference in receptivity and responsiveness to estrogen exceeds the sex difference in masculine copulatory behavior and responsiveness to androgen. In addition, it should be apparent by now that, at least for morphological characteristics, the neutral sex in birds is the male, and ovarian hormones are the organizing hormones, whereas in mammals, the neutral sex is the female, and testicular hormones are the organizers. Add to these contrasts the fact that the male bird is the homogametic (XX) sex, whereas the female mammal is homogametic, and there is a strong indication of important relationships between chromosomal sex, sex differentiation, and adult behavioral capacity. It would appear that the homogametic sex is the neutral sex and is the sex with the greatest capacity for heterotypical behavior in adulthood. This point will be discussed more fully in Section VII.

Sex hormones appear to stimulate sexual behavior in birds by acting centrally. Copulation and courtship can be activated in doves and chickens by androgen implants in the preoptic area of the hypothalamus (Barfield, 1969, 1971; Gardner and Fisher, 1968; Hutchison, 1971).

In addition to sexual behavior per se, many birds exhibit dimorphic behavior patterns such as fighting, nest building, and parental care, which are at least partially under hormonal control. These patterns would be interesting end points for studies on sexual differentiation of the brain, so it is unfortunate that little work of this sort has been done.

Administration of sex hormones to avian embryos can have dramatic effects on adult behavior. In one of the earlier experiments of this kind, Domm (1939) injected Brown Leghorn chicken eggs with 0.5–1 mg of each of several estrogens between the third and fifth days of incubation. The birds were divided into four classes based on the degree of feminization of the plumage, ranging from Class I (appearance of a normal male) to Class IV (nearly indistinguishable from a female) (Domm and Davis, 1948). The position of the males in a flock peck-order was highly correlated with the plumage type, with Class I males generally at the top, and Class IV males generally at the bottom with the females. In sex tests, Class IV males showed some waltzing or some components of waltzing (a male courtship pattern) but never progressed to pursuit of the female or copulation. Class I males waltzed, and four out of nine copulated. Inasmuch as the testes of these birds were feminized, it is possible that the reduction in male behavior resulted solely from insufficient testicular androgen in adulthood rather than from a true organizational effect of the early hormone treatment. In contrast to the abnormal behavior of the treated males, treated females behaved in a normal manner and some laid eggs regularly.

Kaufman (1956) injected 1.5 mg of rutoestrol into the air space of chicken eggs after 24 or 48 hr of incubation. No crowing or copulation was seen in birds observed at 4–7 months of age. Again, however, testes were also feminized, and a true organizational effect cannot be assumed.

Glick (1961) dipped day-3 eggs in solutions of testosterone propionate. The resulting two males both failed to produce offspring. In one male, the semen was normal and was fertile when used for artificial insemination, suggesting that the testes were reasonably normal. Nonetheless, this bird never mated. A later study of ten additional males treated similarly revealed that nine of the ten failed to mate, but semen samples from three out of four were fertile (Glick, 1965).

Male quail exposed to sex hormones as embryos also fail to mate. Wentworth *et al.* (1968) sprayed eggs with mestranol on day 0, 6, or 12 of incubation. Males hatched from treated eggs chased females, strutted, and copulated significantly less often than control males. Evidence of depressed androgen secretion at the time of testing was obtained.

Orcutt (1971) implanted subcutaneous pellets of DES into pigeon (*Columba livia*) squabs. When paired with females as adults, males implanted just after hatching with 2 mg DES showed significant reductions in nest-calling (a masculine behavior pattern), and near-significant reductions in bow-cooing (the male courtship pattern). Only DES-implanted males ever showed any female behavior patterns when paired with males.

None of the experiments described above can be said to show that early sex hormones have organizational effects on avian behavior. More recently, in both the chicken and the quail, evidence of organizational effects has been obtained that is unconfounded by the permanent and deleterious effect of the treatments on the gonads. Wilson and Glick (1970) dipped chicken eggs after 3 days of incubation in solutions of testosterone propionate or estradiol benzoate in ethyl alcohol or injected them at various times with oil solutions of these hormones. Males were to be observed at age 7 months, but most of them died before reaching this age. Thereafter birds were given exogenous testosterone propionate at 25 days of age, so that behavior would be activated precociously, and were tested at 41 days of age for 8 days. Frequencies of waltzing, attempted mating, and completed mating were recorded. The results for attempted matings are shown in Table 8. Treatment with either hormone prior to the 13th day of incubation greatly suppressed mating attempts. On or after day 13, treatment had no effect on mating attempts. This suppression was also seen in females. Results for waltzing and completed matings were similar but not as striking. When given exogenous estrogen (at an unspecified age), the males treated with either hormone before hatching became receptive. Treated females were receptive as adults. The authors concluded, first, that sex steroids induce behavioral sex differentiation in chickens (presumably estrogen feminizes embryos), second, that the effect of early sex hormone exposure is chiefly inhibition of the potential to display masculine behavior in response to exogenous testosterone, and third, that the critical period for this differentiation occurs prior to the 13th day of embryonic development.

A suggestion that behavior other than sexual behavior per se can be modified by early hormone treatment of chickens comes from an experiment by Mauldin *et al.* (1975). Eggs were dipped on the third day of incubation into solutions of testosterone propionate. Chicks were tested when 3 weeks old. Chicks treated with the higher of two dosages did not learn to move through a door to be near a group of other chicks as rapidly as control chicks learned the task.

The results of research with chickens suggest some alteration of central nervous system function as a result of early sex steroid exposure. Measurement of the cholesterol content of the cerebral hemispheres showed the greatest amounts in control chicks or chicks from eggs dipped in testosterone on day 18 and the lowest amounts in chicks from eggs dipped in testosterone on day 3, 6, or 12 (Wilson and Glick, 1970). These findings suggested to the authors that embryonic exposure to sex steroids prevents a high level of myelination of the brain that is needed for male but not female sexual behavior. In a later experiment (Kilgore and Glick, 1970), brains of chick embryos at various ages were analyzed for alkaline phosphatase. This enzyme was chosen for study because of evidence that differentiation of organs and onset of function are preceded by rapid rises in alkaline phosphatase levels in those organs. The activity of this enzyme decreased from day 9 to day 12, then increased from day 12 to day 21. Dipping eggs in a testosterone propionate (TP) solution reduced alkaline phosphatase activity in the brainstem on days 9, 12, 15, 18, and 21, suggesting that alkaline phosphatase activity is related to suppression of future copulatory potential and is involved in normal behavioral sex differentiation.

Table 8. Mean Number of Attempted Matings of Chickens Hatched from Eggs Treated during Incubation and Injected with 1 mg/day TP from 25 to 48 Days of Age[a]

Sex	Treatment[b]	Method of administration	Day (of incubation) of treatment						Untreated control
			3	11	12	13	14	15	
Males	TP	Dipping	2.4						34.6
Males	TP	Dipping	2.8						21.2
Males	TP	Injection	14.2		0.8				21.2
Males	TP	Injection			0.3			19.2	22.7
Males	TP	Injection		1.1	0.2	8.8c	7.7c	14.8c	15.2
Males	EB	Injection		0.0	1.3	6.3c	10.8c	12.5c	8.6
Females	TP	Injection		0.1	1.6	7.3c	12.2c	10.2c	8.6
Females	EB	Injection		0.4	0.2	3.6	13.4c	0.8	12.6

[a] From Wilson and Glick (1970).
[b] TP, testosterone propionate; EB, estradiol benzoate. Dosages were 1.28 g/100 ml for dipping and 1 mg for injection.
c Not different from untreated controls in that row.

Lesions of the red nuclei (midbrain structures) increased the mating behavior of normal male chickens but not of males from TP-treated eggs (Crawford and Glick, 1975). Thus, the depressant effect of early TP on mating is not just a reflection of hyperactivity of the inhibitory red nuclei (see also Haynes and Glick, 1974). An additional study of the effects of hormone implants in the preoptic area of normal males and males from TP-treated eggs is difficult to interpret because leakage from the brain implants into the general circulation occurred (Crawford and Glick, 1975).

Evidence that embryonic sex hormones may exert organizational effects on behavior has also been obtained in quail. Adkins (1975) injected eggs on the tenth day of incubation with 50 μg estradiol benzoate, 2.5 mg testosterone propionate, or oil vehicle. A fourth group of eggs was not treated. At sexual maturity, the birds were tested for both masculine and feminine behavior, then exposed to short days for 3 weeks (causing gonadal regression), injected for 9 to 11 days with either 2.5 mg/day testosterone propionate or 50 μg/day estradiol benzoate, and tested again. The masculine behavior shown by the males both before (phase I) and after (phase II) gonadal regression and testosterone replacement is shown in Table 9. In phase I, masculine behavior was greatly reduced by treatment of eggs with sex steroids. These deficits were still seen following gonadal regression and testosterone replacement. No males treated with estrogen ever copulated, strutted, or crowed. Sex steroids did not masculinize females; instead, they appeared to demasculinize them. However, because the control females showed very low levels of masculine behavior, the further reductions in the treated females were not significant. Neither estradiol nor testosterone changed the capacity of males or females to exhibit receptivity when given estrogen in adulthood.

In normal quail from eggs not treated with sex steroids, there is a pronounced sex difference in the capacity to respond to exogenous androgen in adulthood by displaying male behavior but little or no sex difference in the

Table 9. Percentage of Male Quail Exhibiting Masculine Behavior[a]

Egg treatment	Copulation	Strutting	Crowing
Phase I (intact and untreated)			
Nothing	65	55	35[b]
Oil	72	56	72
TP	20[b]	25	10[b]
EB	10[b]	5[b]	5[b]
Phase II (regressed gonads + testosterone propionate)			
Nothing	60	60	60
Oil	70	60	20
TP	10[b]	20	0
EB	0[b]	0[b]	0

[a] Data from Adkins (1975).
[b] Significantly different from oil-treated males.

capacity to respond to exogenous estrogen in adulthood by displaying receptivity (Adkins and Adler, 1972). Thus, the experimental manipulations produced results similar to those found in normal sexual development, i.e., estrogen demasculinized the embryos. As in Wilson and Glick's (1970) experiment with chickens, sex steroids feminized male quail by inhibiting the capacity for male behavior, thus eliminating the normal sex difference and making males like females. This demasculinizing effect of early estrogen exposure in quail has also been reported by Whitsett *et al.* (1977).

As in the chicken, demasculinization of quail by embryonic exposure to steroids only occurs during a limited period of time. Treatment with estradiol after day 12 of incubation is without effect (Adkins, 1979).

The embryonic quail brain is quite sensitive to estrogen—as little as $2 \mu g$ of estradiol-17β is sufficient to reduce masculine behavior significantly (Whitsett *et al.*, 1977). Much larger dosages of testosterone are required to produce such an effect (Adkins, 1979; Whitsett *et al.*, 1977). Demasculinization is readily produced with estriol, estrone, and diethylstilbestrol (Whitsett *et al.*, 1977), but not with dihydrotestosterone, regardless of dosage (Adkins, 1978). Since testosterone, but not dihydrotestosterone, can be converted to estrogen by several vertebrate species, these findings suggest that testosterone may mimic estrogen by being converted to an estrogen by the quail embryo.

All of these results, as well as those of Wilson and Glick (1970), suggest that in the quail and chicken, differentiation of the neural substrate underlying sexual behavior takes place in the masculine direction unless exposure to sex steroids takes place during the embryonic period. Presumably, during normal development, genetic females are feminized (altered from the neutral male pattern) by ovarian estrogen. Direct determination of the neutral sex for behavior is difficult, since embryos castrated prior to differentiation do not reach an age at which behavior can be tested. Chemical antihormones provide one possible alternative method for determining the neutral sex. Female quail treated with an antiestrogen prior to differentiation should be more masculine than controls and, unlike normal females, should be capable of copulating when given exogenous testosterone in adulthood.

Such an experiment was conducted by Adkins (1976). Eggs were injected on day 9 with 0.1 mg CI-628, a nonsteroidal antiestrogen, or with the distilled water vehicle. CI-628 (CN-55,945-27) is 1-[2-(p-[α-(p-methoxyphenyl)-β-nitrostyryl]phenoxy)ethyl]pyrrolidine monocitrate. At sexual maturity, the birds were exposed to short days for 3 weeks, which caused gonadal regression, injected with 1 mg/day testosterone propionate for 2 weeks, and tested with female partners.

The results are shown in Fig. 9. CI-628 increased the number of females attempting to copulate. Four of these females copulated in a manner identical to normal males, pursuing the females and achieving cloacal contact. No such behavior was seen in the control females, nor had copulation been seen in previous experiments in any of the females that had been given testosterone in adulthood (Adkins, 1975; Adkins and Adler, 1972). CI-628 had no effect on the males. Thus, it seems that endogenous estrogen in the developing female

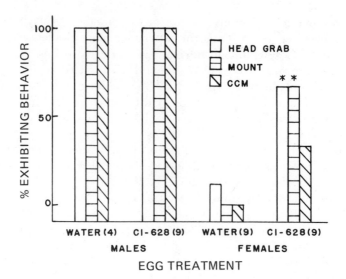

Figure 9. Masculine copulatory behavior of Japanese quail hatched from eggs injected with 0.1 mg CI-628 or with the water vehicle on day 9 of incubation. CCM, cloacal contact movement. The copulatory sequence is head grab–mount–CCM. Numbers in parentheses are Ns. *$P < .05$ compared with water-treated females.

quail embryo is responsible for the failure of normal females to copulate and that the male is the behavioral neutral sex.

As discussed previously, the embryonic ovaries of birds synthesize estrogens, and female chick embryos produce large quantities of estrogens. The brain of the chick embryo is known to take up estrogen in a manner suggesting that it is a target organ for this steroid. Martinez-Vargas *et al.* (1975) administered [^{3}H]estradiol-17β to chick embryos at various times during incubation. The embryos were sacrificed 1 hr later, and the brains subjected to autoradiography. Significant concentration of radioactivity was observed in the nuclei of cells in the hypothalamus (chiefly preoptic and ventromedial or nucleus hypothalmicus posterior) as early as day 10 of incubation (recall that the behavioral critical period ends on day 13).

Thus, there are strong suggestions that the brains of avian embryos are subject to hormonally controlled sexual differentiation. An excellent opportunity to examine this process has recently been provided by the work of Nottebohm and Arnold (1976) who showed that the vocal control nuclei of zebra finches and canaries are strikingly sexually dimorphic. Although this anatomical dimorphism could conceivably be under direct genetic control, it is more likely a consequence of differential embryonic hormone exposure—a superb preparation for studying the organization of the brain by sex hormones.

E. Summary

Our knowledge of sexual differentiation in birds is limited to a few species, but the results are remarkably consistent across species (see Table 5 for a summary and Table 10 for comparison with other vertebrate classes). Ovaries dominate testes (i.e., an ovary feminizes a testis, but a testis fails to masculinize an ovary), and steroids predominantly feminize gonads. Anhormonal development of gonaducts results in retention of both Müllerian ducts (a condition not seen in normal individuals of either sex), and gonadal hormones of an as yet unknown kind are required for regression of one or both ducts. Other sex structures such as the syrinx and genital tubercle are feminized by steroids, and the neutral sex for these organs is the male. Behavior differentiates according to a similar rule—embryonic exposure to steroids feminizes (more accurately, demasculinizes) behavior; the neutral sex is probably the male, and ovarian estrogen is likely to be the organizing hormone. All indications are that effects of early hormones on behavior are mediated by changes in the brain.

VII. OVERVIEW

A. Common Factors in Sex Differentiation (Including Mammalian)

It is possible to make a few general statements about sex differentiation in vertebrates, in spite of the obvious and striking species differences.

1. Sex differentiation of the gonads of vertebrates is directed by some kind(s) of hormone(s). The chemical nature of these inducers is not yet known. In fish, they may be sex steroids (Yamamoto, 1969). In mammals this is unlikely, because steroid treatment at any age does not cause sex reversal of gonads. In birds, gonads are capable of synthesizing steroids prior to sex differentiation, and so the inducers could be sex steroids. In several species of mammals, birds, and amphibians, the heterogametic sex (male mammal, female bird, male *Rana,* female *Xenopus*) produces an H-Y antigen that is a product of the primary sex-determining gene and is part of the chain of causal events leading to the differentiation of those gonads that will organize subsequent sexual development (Silvers and Wachtel, 1977). Regardless of what the actual inducers are, the fact that undifferentiated gonads of birds cultured *in vitro* autodifferentiate appropriately indicates that the necessary factor is present very early in development (Haffen, 1975). Usually gonadal sex reversal, either total or partial, occurs most readily during the period of gonadal sex differentiation.

2. The secretions of the embryonic, larval, or neonatal gonads control the differentiation of the sex structures through organizational actions. The chemical nature of these secretions is unknown in some species. In others, there is

evidence of sex steroid secretion during the period of differentiation of sex structures; and development, except of gonaducts (see especially Section VI.B), is probably controlled by hormones similar to those produced by adult gonads.

3. In those species in which behavioral effects of early hormone administration have been investigated (some fish, some amphibians, some birds and mammals), permanent effects on behavior have been noted. In a few birds and mammals, these effects have been shown to be organizational effects that occur only during limited critical periods.

4. Differentiation of the gonaducts follows different patterns than differentiation of the other sex structures. Early castration results in an ambisexual (mixed male–female) condition of the gonaducts (Witschi, 1959) rather than a clear male or female form. In birds, the female sex is organized by the embryonic ovary, and although the anhormonal form is male for most sex structures, some testicular secretion, as yet unknown, is required to suppress the Müllerian ducts in males. In mammals, males are organized by testicular secretions. Testicular sex steroids suppress the development of female characters, with the exception of the Müllerian ducts which seem to be suppressed by some nonsteroidal but as yet unknown testicular secretion. The fact that vertebrate gonaducts follow rules of their own is probably related to the fact that in the evolutionary past they had excretory (and therefore nonsexual) functions and were commonly retained in both sexes (Burns, 1961). This tendency can still be seen in female amphibians in which the Wolffian ducts persist as ureters and in snakes and lizards in which either sex may retain both sets of ducts.

5. When sex steroids are administered to embryos, larvae, or neonates, there is a marked tendency for androgens and estrogens to have similar effects. Paradoxical feminization by testosterone and masculinization by estradiol and estrone have been noted frequently in behavioral as well as morphological studies. The reasons for these paradoxical effects is generally obscure. Conversion of testosterone to estrogen is a distinct possibility, particularly in behavioral studies.

B. Species Differences

Table 10 summarizes vertebrate sexual differentiation and sex determination and draws attention to differences among taxa as well as to relationships among the different sexual endpoints. The table is organized in terms of classes, even though it is very risky to try to generalize about an entire class when the species sampling is so limited and so biased. The column headings should be interpreted as follows.

1. Homogametic Sex

The sex with the two similar sex chromosomes (e.g., XX) is referred to as the homogametic sex (as opposed to the heterogametic sex). These data are

Table 10. Sexuality in Vertebrates[a]

Class	Species	Homogametic sex	Dominant gonad	Embryonic sex most easily reversed	Neutral sex	Sex of greatest behavioral bipotentiality
Osteichthyes	*Carassius auratus*	F		Both		F?
	Oryzias latipes	F	M	F		F?
	Xiphophorus helleri	F		F		F?
	Poecilia reticulata	F		F		F?
	Hemihaplochromis multicolor	F		M?		
	Tilapia mossambica	F		F		
	Betta splendens	F				F?
	Macropodus opercularis	F				F?
Amphibia[b]	*Hynobius* (2 spp.) (U)	F?	M	M		
	Ambystoma mexicanum (U)	M	M	M		
	Pleurodeles waltlii (U)	M		M		
	Triturus helveticus (U)	M?	M	M		F?
	Xenopus laevis (A)	M	M	M		
	Pseudacris nigrita (A)	F		F		
	Rana (3 spp.) (A)	F	M	F		
Reptilia	*Lacerta vivipara*	M		M	M	
	Anolis carolinensis	F		M?		F
	Sceloporus sp.	F		M?		
	Alligator mississippiensis	?		F?		
	Crocodylus niloticus	?		F?		
	Malaclemmys centrata	?		M?		
	Chrysemys marginata	?		F?		
	Emys (2 spp.)	?		M		
	Testudo graeca	?		M?		
Aves	About 8 spp.	M	F	M	M	M
Mammalia	*Didelphis marsupialis*	F		M	F	
	Eutherians (about 11 spp.)	F	M	F	F	F

[a] See Section VII.B for fuller explanation of this summary table. Based in part on Van Tienhoven (1968, p. 4) and Witschi (1959, p. 373).
[b] U, Urodele; A, anuran.

drawn from Atz (1964), Beatty (1964, 1970), Dodd (1960), Gorman (1973), Morescalchi (1973), Reinboth (1975), and Yamamoto (1969).

2. Dominant Gonad

If two differentiating opposite-sexed gonads are cultured together, or if two differentiating opposite-sexed individuals are joined in parabiosis, or if gonads are grafted into differentiating animals of the opposite sex, typically the gonad of one sex will be altered by the gonad of the other sex. The sex of the gonad that alters, rather than is altered, is shown in Table 10. In the case of mammals (and to a lesser extent birds), bear in mind that these effects are generally weak.

3. Embryonic Sex Most Easily Reversed

If sex steroids are administered to embryos, larvae, or neonates, total or partial sex reversal will occur more readily in one direction than in the other. The information given in this column of the table combines gonadal reversal and reversal of other sex structures. For some fish and reptiles where data are limited, data showing that estrogens masculinized, rather than feminized, embryos were taken as evidence that masculinization is more easily accomplished, and data showing that androgens feminized, rather than masculinized, embryos were taken as evidence that feminization is more easily accomplished. Complete functional reversal of bird gonads has not been achieved experimentally, and therefore for birds, embryonic sex reversal means partial reversal of gonads and partial or complete reversal of other sex structures and of behavior. Embryonic gonads of mammals are notoriously resistant to permanent or extensive reversal by exogenous sex steroids; therefore, the entries for mammals should be interpreted as for birds. It is not clear why gonads of birds and mammals, in contrast to those of fish and reptiles, should be so resistant to steroid treatment, but one possibility is that the gonadal inducers are not steroids and that identification of the true inducers would permit experimental reversal. Question marks indicate that partial reversal of the sex indicated has been shown to occur but that no information is available as to whether reversal of the other sex can also be accomplished.

4. Neutral (Anhormonal) Sex

This is the phenotype that results from differentiation in the absence of gonads. For this table, gonaduct appearance has been excluded, since anhormonal gonaducts are ambisexual in most nonmammalian vertebrates (Witschi, 1959). (See Section VII.A, item 4 for more information on this point.)

5. Sex of Greatest Behavioral Bipotentiality

This indicates the sex in which, in adulthood, heterotypical sexual behavior can most readily be activated hormonally. A question mark indicates that considerable heterotypical behavior has been activated in the sex shown, but that it is not known whether heterotypical behavior could also be activated in the other sex.

6. Classes

A few comments about each class will be helpful prior to drawing conclusions from this table.

a. Osteichthyes

The species sampling problem is particularly acute in this class; most species studied are domesticated aquarium fish from only two orders. Many other fish also exhibit female homogamety but were not included in the table because nothing is known about their sexual differentiation (Mehl and Reinboth, 1975; Schreck, 1974; Thorgaard, 1977). In *Oryzias latipes*, both sexes can be reversed by steroid treatment, but Satoh's (1973) and Yamamoto's (1969) work suggest that reversal from female to male takes place at lower dosages than reversal from male to female. It is interesting to note that the majority of successive hermaphrodites are protogynous (change from female to male), but again the species sampling is quite biased (Choat and Robertson, 1975).

b. Amphibia

There is some disagreement over whether *Triturus* has male or female homogamety (Beatty, 1970). Recall that *Hynobius, Ambystoma, Pleurodeles,* and *Triturus* are urodeles, and *Xenopus, Pseudacris,* and *Rana* are anurans (*Xenopus* is considered primitive). The behavioral data on *Xenopus* are from Kelley and Pfaff (1976).

c. Reptilia

The sex-determining mechanism of turtles (Chelonia) and Crocodilia is unknown in spite of earlier claims to the contrary (Gorman, 1973). The behavioral data on *Anolis* came from Mason and Adkins (1976).

d. Mammalia

The relevant data are discussed in other chapters of this book and in Short (1972), Burns (1961), and Bruner-Lorand (1964). The behavioral entries are based on Arén-Engelbrektsson *et al.* (1970), McDonald *et al.* (1970), Pfaff (1970), and Young (1961). The hamster seems to be the major exception to the statement that the female is the behaviorally bipotential sex in mammals (Carter *et al.*, 1973).

Table 10 reveals that underlying the obvious species differences there is order in that the different indicators of sexuality are correlated (one must, however, remember the severe limitations on the species sampling). There is a distinct tendency for the homogametic sex to be the neutral sex, to be the embryonic sex most easily reversed, and to be the most behaviorally bipotential sex in adulthood. The gonad of the heterogametic sex tends to be the dominant gonad. Thus, in the fish that have been studied, the female is homogametic, is more easily reversed in early life, and displays considerable heterotypical behavior in adulthood when given heterologous hormones. Male homogamety is known to occur in only a few species of fish (whose sexual differentiation is unknown). The successive hermaphrodites fall outside the domain of Table 10, but it is interesting to note that several authors have hypothesized that protandry is derived from male homogamety and protogyny from female homogamety (e.g., Harrington, 1975). Amphibians are not uniform with respect to homogametic sex, but the correlations are still seen. In those with female homogamety (higher anurans in general?), the female is more easily reversed, and in those with male homogamety (urodeles and primitive anurans?), the male is more easily reversed. Reptiles, like amphibians, are not uniform with respect to homogametic sex, but again the correlations can be seen. In *Anolis* the female is homogametic and has a greater potential for heterotypical behavior in adulthood; in *Lacerta*, the male is homogametic, is the neutral sex, and is more easily reversed in embryonic life, and the female gonad is dominant.

These correlations are particularly evident when one compares birds and mammals. In birds the male is homogametic, is neutral (both behaviorally and morphologically), is more easily (partially) reversed in early life, and has more sexual bipotentiality in adulthood, whereas in mammals, the female fills all these roles. In birds, the female gonad is dominant and produces the principal organizing hormones; in mammals, the male gonad is dominant and produces the organizing hormones.

These facts about vertebrate sexuality, particularly avian and mammalian, can be summarized by saying that the homogametic sex is the neutral sex in ontogeny and is the most easily reversed, both morphologically (in early life) and behaviorally (in early life and in adulthood), and the heterogametic sex produces the organizing hormones.

These correlations have been noted by several authors with respect to sexual morphology (Burns, 1961; Foote, 1964; Gallien, 1965; Jost, 1960; Witschi, 1959); evidently they apply to sexual behavior as well. Furthermore, there is the intriguing possibility that invertebrates (at least those whose differentiation is controlled by sex hormones) might also be encompassed by this scheme. In *Orchestia*, the female is homogametic and is the neutral sex, and male hormones are the organizers (Charniaux-Cotton, 1975).

These correlations between sex chromosomes, anhormonal sex differentiation, and behavioral and physical sex reversal suggest causal relationships. Witschi (1959), however, considers that even one exception contraindicates causality. What are the major exceptions? The majority of them are those entries in Table 10 that are questionable (marked with "?") and that further research may invalidate. Exceptions backed by data include the following. (a) In urodele amphibians, the homogametic gonad is dominant, and yet the homogametic sex is still the most easily reversed. (b) In *Xenopus*, the adult female (who is XY) shows considerable masculine sexual behavior when treated with testosterone (Kelley and Pfaff, 1976); the male's capacity for feminine behavior is unknown, however, so it would be premature to state that the female is *more* sexually bipotential than the male. (c) Gonadal sex reversal in opossum (*Didelphis*) embryos occurs more readily in males, who are heterogametic, than in females (Burns, 1961).

C. Evolution of Sex Differentiation

One of the aims of a comparative approach is to be able to infer phylogenetic trends. Can any such trends be discerned in sex differentiation? The major difficulty, of course, is that none of the species in Table 10 are likely to be ancestral to any of the others (none of the fish discussed, for example, are in any sense primitive).

The universality or near universality in vertebrates of the control of sex differentiation by the secretions of the embryonic gonads suggests that this is an old mechanism phylogenetically. Just how old is unclear, since the more primitive vertebrates and chordates have been neglected. It is significant that in no case is morphological sex directly determined by sex genes or chromosomes. Rather, the internal physiological environment shapes tissue development, and thus the entire process is highly epigenetic. The universality of the epigenetic determination of sex suggests major advantages over direct genetic control which are still, however, obscure. It may be that less genetic information is needed to achieve sex differentiation in this manner. Recent studies suggest that a very small number of genes may be sufficient (Silvers and Wachtel, 1977). Epigenetic determination leaves some room for accidents, but the low frequency of spontaneous intersexes in wild individuals of bisexual (non-hermaphroditic) species suggests that the process seldom goes awry (Atz, 1964; Foote, 1964; Taber, 1964). And an important advantage of epigenetic determination, especially among fish, is that it makes successive hermaphroditism and control of sex by the physical or social environment possible.

Some invertebrates also achieve sex differentiation through sex hormones (not necessarily from the gonads). This similarity to vertebrate sex differentiation may well have appeared through convergent evolution rather than phylogenetic continuity. Is control of sex differentiation by sex hormones less frequent in invertebrates than in vertebrates? If so, is this because such control is evolutionarily recent, or is some more fundamental difference between invertebrate and vertebrate structure and function responsible?

Looking just at vertebrates, very few "trends" can be discerned aside from the relationships among sexual variables discussed above. Ease of experimental sex reversal is apparently not related to frequency of spontaneous intersexuality nor to degree of relatedness to hermaphroditic species (Atz, 1964). The apparent trend from fish to mammals toward increasing sexual stability and decreasing gonadal reversibility may be illusory. The gonads of many amphibians are as unresponsive to sex steroids as are mammalian gonads. Furthermore, the ease with which some fish and amphibian gonads can be reversed by sex steroids may actually reflect class differences in the chemical nature of the gonadal inducers. There is little evidence that teleost fish are not sexually stable (Atz, 1964), and *Xenopus*, in spite of the ease with which the gonads can be reversed, is as gonochoristic as any mammal. The existence of occasional hermaphroditic species does not indicate instability, for hermaphroditism involves sex change under highly specific conditions and is genetically programmed and adaptive.

There is a different sense in which sex can be said to have stabilized in the course of vertebrate evolution. In birds and mammals, sex and sex differentiation seem to be less variable among species (i.e., more constant within each class) than in amphibians or reptiles.

Any evolutionary trends in behavioral differentiation are elusive because of the lack of information on organizational hormonal actions in fish, amphibians, and reptiles. Only further research will reveal whether or not evolution has involved a progressive shortening of the critical period for behavioral sex reversal.

Witschi (1959) attempted to use the type of information given in Table 10 to infer the course of vertebrate evolution and the points at which various groups diverged. The data at that time indicated that the Reptilia uniformly had male homogamety as did birds. Based on the sexual characteristics of the various vertebrate groups, he suggested that salamanders are "rooted close to" the reptiles and birds, whereas frogs are "rooted close to" mammals. The fact that the opossum has mammalian-type sex chromosomes but nonmammalian-type gonad reversal was interpreted to mean that mammalian-type sex determination evolved prior to the mammalian type of gonadal "reaction pattern." More recent data on sex determination in reptiles force us to change this picture somewhat. Except for *Lacerta*, lizards commonly have female homogamety, and snakes have male homogamety (Gorman, 1973). Thus, fish, anuran amphibians, lizards, and mammals form one group, and urodele amphibians, snakes, and birds another. Unfortunately there are no definitive data for monotreme mammals.

Why do different animals possess different types of sex determination and differentiation? The uniformity within the classes Aves and Mammalia and vast difference between these two classes suggest considerable selective pressure operating, perhaps related to the fact that mammals have internal gestation. Burns (1961) reasoned that

> . . . explanation [of the fact that male hormones are the organizers in mammals] may be found in the special physiologic conditions incidental to the evolution of intrauterine development in mammals. A situation in which the female hormone has an active role in sex differentiation might present a serious difficulty with male embryos constantly exposed during development to the influence of the mother's hormones. . . . (p. 137)

This kind of hormone exposure would clearly have significant effects; even female rats exposed to the testicular secretions of their *in utero* male littermates are slightly masculinized behaviorally (Clemens, 1974). Short (1972) suggested that mammalian gonads have lost their plasticity as a result of the evolution of viviparity in order to protect male gonads against the feminizing influence of the maternal ovaries. Mittwoch (1971) noted that in birds, the embryonic ovaries, because of their task in sexual differentiation, undergo greater and earlier growth than do the testes, whereas this is reversed in mammals. She suggested that the task of sex differentiation is given to the testes of mammals so that they will be able to overcome any maternal hormones, and is given to the ovary of birds because ". . . extra growth at this stage might be of advantage in preparing it [the ovary] for its ultimately more demanding role of egg production . . ." (p. 433). She concludes that

> . . . it is understandable that in the early evolutionary period of sex chromosomes in vertebrates, two opposite systems, i.e., male and female heterogamety, were tried out. . . . Mammals had no choice but to adopt the system of male heterogamety. In order to develop a male phenotype, an embryo must counter the maternal sex hormones by secreting sufficient amounts of androgens at an early stage of development. Therefore, the function of the Y-chromosome may be to induce an early and rapid development of the embryonic gonad, thus enabling it to secrete male sex hormones before the embryo becomes feminized. By contrast, the avian embryo does not find itself in this predicament and so sex determination by female heterogamety is possible, where rapid growth leads to ovarian differentiation . . . (Mittwoch, 1975, p. 444).

This kind of constraint on sex differentiation would apply only to viviparous species in which the embryos are actually in contact with the mother's hormones. Furthermore, these sorts of explanations are not sufficient to account for the variation within the Amphibia, since all such species in Table 10 are oviparous.

In birds and mammals, the behavioral neutral sex is also the morphological neutral sex. Results from behavioral and anatomical investigations consistently agree, and the numerous parallels reinforce the idea that behavior (or the neural substrate underlying behavior) evolves and develops according to the same laws that govern peripheral morphological structures.

D. Areas for Future Research

One fruitful strategy would be to select species for study for which information on at least one of the variables in Table 10 is already available. Alternatively, one could select species quite unrelated to those that have been favored,
for example, a nongalliform bird or a noncichlid, noncyprinodont fish. Even
for those species that have been extensively studied, such as *Xenopus laevis*,
more systematic investigation of age at treatment, sex, and hormone dosage
variables is needed.

Some specific topics that could be especially promising include the following:

1. Detailed study of the behavior of animals capable of complete gonadal
   sex reversal, such as *Xenopus* and *Oryzias*, and comparison of the behavior of normal animals and sex-reversed animals. Parental and aggressive behavior could also be included.
2. Study of the effects of exogenous hormones in a species exhibiting both
   female homogamety and male homogamety, such as *Xiphophorus
   maculatus* (Kallman, 1973). If there is any causal relationship between
   chromosomal sex and other sex variables, differences in hormone
   responsiveness might be evident in comparisons of the two kinds of
   genetic populations.
3. Definitive work on sex differentiation in lizards is limited to species with
   male homogamety. Similar work with a species with female homogamety would be illuminating. *Anolis* would be a good choice because of
   the endocrine data already available.
4. Study of sex differentiation in viviparous snakes.
5. The study of behavioral sex differentiation in birds is progressing well,
   but is hampered by the fact that, in the species chosen so far, differentiation occurs before hatching. It seems likely that in some of the highly
   altricial species, behavioral differentiation would occur after hatching.
   Parental and aggressive behavior would be interesting dependent variables.
6. An intriguing topic would be sex differentiation in those avian species
   exhibiting reversed sex dimorphism. In the phalaropes, hemipodes,
   and painted snipes, the female is larger and more brightly colored (Van
   Tyne and Berger, 1959). Female phalaropes are more aggressive than
   males, do the courting, and do not assist in nest building or incubation
   (Jenni, 1974). In Wilson's phalarope (*Steganopus tricolor*) and the northern phalarope (*Lobipes lobatus*), data suggest that the adult female's
   ovary actually produces more testosterone than estrogen and produces
   more testosterone than do the adult male's testes (Höhn, 1970; Höhn
   and Cheng, 1967). Whether this creates special problems for sex differentiation is unknown, and the physiological basis of reversed sex
   dimorphism in the hemipodes and painted snipes is also unknown.

E. Conclusions

The basic mechanism of sex differentiation, control by embryonic gonadal secretions, is a fundamental theme of vertebrate organization. Some variations have been imposed on this theme for as yet unknown reasons in terms of which gonad, testis or ovary, has the major role in differentiation. Even though an understanding of sex differentiation in a wide variety of species still eludes us, it is already abundantly clear that a comparative approach to organizational effects of sex hormones can reveal otherwise undetectable relationships among genetic, gonadal, and behavioral sexuality, can suggest unifying principles, and can provide meaningful theoretical guidelines for the acquisition of new data.

ACKNOWLEDGMENTS. This chapter owes much to stimulating discussions with Frank Zemlan.

REFERENCES

Adkins, E. K., 1975, Hormonal basis of sexual differentiation in the Japanese quail, *J. Comp Physiol. Psychol.* **89**:61.

Adkins, E. K., 1976, Embryonic exposure to an antiestrogen masculinizes behavior of female quail, *Physiol Behav.* **17**:357.

Adkins, E. K., 1978, Sex steroids and the differentiation of avian reproductive behavior, *Am. Zool.* **18**:501.

Adkins, E. K., 1979, Effect of embryonic treatment with estradiol or testosterone on sexual differentiation of the quail brain: Critical period and dose–response relationships, *Neuroendocrinology* **29**:178.

Adkins, E. K., and Adler, N. T., 1972, Hormonal control of behavior in the Japanese quail, *J. Comp. Physiol. Psychol.* **81**:27.

Arén-Englebrektsson, B., Larsson, K., Södersten, P., and Wilhelmsson, M., 1970, The female lordosis pattern induced in male rats by estrogen, *Horm. Behav.* **1**:181.

Aronson, L. R., 1957, Reproductive and parental behavior, in: *The Physiology of Fishes* (M. E. Brown, ed.), pp. 271–304, Academic Press, New York.

Aronson, L. R., 1958, Hormones and reproductive behavior, in: *Comparative Endocrinology* (A. Gorman, ed.), pp. 98–120, Wiley, New York.

Atz, J., 1964, Intersexuality in fishes, in: *Intersexuality in Vertebrates Including Man* (C. N. Armstrong and A. J. Marshall, eds.), pp. 145–232, Academic Press, London.

Bacci, G., 1965, *Sex Determination*, Pergamon Press, Oxford.

Baggerman, B., 1968, Hormonal control of reproductive and parental behaviour in fishes, in: *Perspectives in Endocrinology: Hormones in the Lives of Lower Vertebrates* (E. J. W. Barrington and C. B. Jorgensen, eds.), pp. 351–404, Academic Press, London.

Baldwin, F. M., and Goldin, H. S., 1939, Effects of testosterone propionate on the female viviparous teleost, *Xiphophorus helleri* Heckel, *Proc. Soc. Exp. Biol. Med.* **42**:813.

Barfield, R. J., 1969, Activation of copulatory behavior by androgen implanted into the preoptic area of the male fowl, *Horm. Behav.* **1**:37.

Barfield, R. J., 1971, Activation of sexual and aggressive behavior by androgen implanted into the male ring dove brain, *Endocrinology* **89**:1470.

Barth, R. H., 1968, The comparative physiology of reproductive processes in cockroaches. I.

Mating behavior and its endocrine control, in: *Advances in Reproductive Physiology*, Vol. 3 (A. McLaren, ed.), pp. 167–207, Academic Press, New York.

Beach, F. A., and Inman, N. G., 1965, Effects of castration and androgen replacement on mating in male quail, *Proc. Natl. Acad. Sci. USA* **54**:1426.

Beatty, R. A., 1964, Chromosome deviations and sex in vertebrates, in: *Intersexuality in Vertebrates Including Man* (C. N. Armstrong and A. J. Marshall, eds.), pp. 17–144, Academic Press, London.

Beatty, R. A., 1970, Genetic basis for the determination of sex, *Phil. Trans. R. Soc. Lond.* [*Biol.*] **259**:3.

Becker, P., Roland, H., and Reinboth, R., 1975, An unusual approach to experimental sex inversion in the teleost fish, *Betta* and *Macropodus*, in: *Intersexuality in the Animal Kingdom* (R. Reinboth, ed.), Springer-Verlag, New York.

Bellairs, R., 1960, The development of birds, in: *Biology and Comparative Physiology of Birds* (A. J. Marshall, ed.), pp. 127–189, Academic Press, New York.

Bierne, J., 1975, Sex differentiation in regenerating male/female nemertine chimeras, in: *Intersexuality in the Animal Kingdom* (R. Reinboth, ed.), Springer-Verlag, New York.

Boss, W. R., and Witschi, E., 1947, The permanent effects of early stilbestrol injections on the sex organs of the herring gull *Larus argentatus, J. Exp. Zool.* **105**:61.

Brien, P., 1962, Induction gamétique chez les Hydres d'eau douce par la méthode des greffes en parabiose, *C. R. Acad. Sci.* [*D*] *(Paris)* **255**:1431.

Brien, P., and Pirard, É., 1962, Induction sexuelle et intersexualité chez une Hydre gonochorïque *(Hydra fusca)* par la méthode des greffes. *C. R. Acad. Sci.* [*D*]*(Paris)* **254**:2902.

Bruner-Lorand, J., 1964, Intersexuality in mammals, in: *Intersexuality in Vertebrates Including Man*, (C. N. Armstrong and A. J. Marshall, eds.), pp. 311–348, Academic Press, London.

Burns, R. K., 1961, Role of hormones in the differentiation of sex, in: *Sex and Internal Secretions* (W. C. Young, ed.), pp. 76–160, Williams & Wilkins, Baltimore.

Carlisle, D. B., 1960, Sexual differentiation in Crustacea Malacostraca, *Mem. Soc. Endocrinol.* **7**:9.

Carter, C. S., Michael, S. J., and Morris, A. H., 1973, Hormonal induction of female sexual behavior in male and female hamsters, *Horm. Behav.* **4**:129.

Chan, S. T. H., O, W.-S., and Hui, S. W. B., 1975, The gonadal and adenohypophyseal functions of natural sex reversal, in: *Intersexuality in the Animal Kingdom* (R. Reinboth, ed.), pp. 201–221, Springer-Verlag, New York.

Charniaux-Cotton, H., 1959, Masculinisation des femelles de la crevette à hermaphrodisme protérandrique *Lysmata seticaudata*, par greffe de glandes androgènes, *C. R. Acad. Sci.* [*D*] *(Paris)* **249**:1580.

Charniaux-Cotton, H., 1965, Contrôle endocrinien de la différenciation sexuelle chez les crustacés supérieurs, *Arch. Anat. Microsc. Morphol. Exp.* **54**:405.

Charniaux-Cotton, H., 1975, Hermaphroditism and gynandromorphism in malacostracan crustacea, in: *Intersexuality in the Animal Kingdom* (R. Reinboth, ed.), Springer-Verlag, New York.

Cheng, M.-F., 1973, Effect of estrogen on behavior of ovariectomized ring doves (*Streptopelia risoria*), *J. Comp. Physiol. Psychol.* **83**:234.

Cheng, M.-F., and Lehrman, D. S., 1973, Relative effectiveness of diethylstilbestrol and estradiol benzoate in inducing female behavior patterns of ovariectomized ring doves (*Streptopelia risoria*), *Horm. Behav.* **4**:123.

Cheng, M.-F., and Lehrman, D. S., 1975, Gonadal hormone specificity in the sexual behavior of ring doves, *Psychoneuroendocrinology* **1**:95.

Chester-Jones, I., Bellamy, D., Chan, D. K. O., Follett, B. K., Henderson, I. W., Phillips, J. G., and Snart, R. S., 1972, Biological actions of steroid hormones in nonmammalian vertebrates, in: *Steroids in Nonmammalian Vertebrates* (D. R. Idler, ed.), pp. 415–480, Academic Press, New York.

Chieffi, G., Iela, L., and Rastogi, R. K., 1974, Effect of cyproterone, cyproterone acetate and ICI 46,474 on gonadal sex differentiation in *Rana esculenta, Gen. Comp. Endocrinol.* **22**:532.

Choat, J. M., and Robertson, D. R., 1975, Protogynous hermaphroditism in fishes of the family

Scaridae, in: *Intersexuality in the Animal Kingdom* (R. Reinboth, ed.), pp. 263–283, Springer-Verlag, New York.

Clemens, H. P., and Inslee, T., 1968, The production of unisexual broods by *Tilapia mossambica* sex-reversed with methyl testosterone, *Trans. Am. Fish. Soc.* **97**:18.

Clemens, H. P., McDermitt, C., and Inslee, T., 1966, The effect of feeding methyl testosterone to guppies for sixty days after birth, *Copeia* **1966**:280.

Clemens, L. G., 1974, Neurohormonal control of male sexual behavior, in: *Reproductive Behavior* (W. Montagna and W. A. Sadler, eds), Plenum Press, New York.

Collias, N. E., 1950, Hormones and behavior with special reference to birds and the mechanisms of hormone action, in: *A Symposium on Steroid Hormones* (E. S. Gordon, ed.), pp. 277–326, University of Wisconsin Press, Madison.

Crawford, W. C., and Glick, B., 1975, The function of the preoptic, mammilaris lateralis and ruber nuclei in normal and sexually inactive male chickens, *Physiol. Behav.* **15**:171.

Crews, D., 1974, Castration and androgen replacement on male facilitation of ovarian activity in the lizard, *Anolis carolinensis, J. Comp. Physiol. Psychol.* **87**:963.

Crews, D., 1976, Hormonal control of male courtship behavior and female attractivity in the garter snake *(Thamnophis sirtalis sirtalis), Horm. Behav.* **7**:451.

Dantschakoff, V., 1937, Sur l'action de l'hormone sexuelle femelle chez les reptiles, *C. R. Acad. Sci.* [D] *(Paris)* **205**:424.

Dantschakoff, V., 1938, Über chemische Werkzeuge bei der Realisation normal bestimmter embryonaler geschlechtlicher Histogenese bei Reptilen, *Arch. Entwicklungsmech.* **138**:465.

Dodd, J. M., 1960, Genetic and environmental aspects of sex determination in cold-blooded vertebrates, *Mem. Soc. Endocrinol.* **7**:17.

Domm, L. V., 1939, Intersexuality in adult brown leghorn males as a result of estrogenic treatment during early embryonic life, *Proc. Soc. Exp. Biol. Med.* **42**:310.

Domm, L. V., and Davis, D. E., 1948, The sexual behavior of intersexual domestic fowl, *Physiol. Zool.* **21**:14.

Dufaure, J.-P., 1966, Recherches descriptives et expérimentales sur les modalités et facteurs du développement de l'appareil génital chez le lézard vivipare (*Lacerta vivipara* Jacquin), *Arch. Anat. Microsc. Morphol. Exp.* **55**:437.

Dzwillo, V. M., 1962, Über künstliche Erzeugung funktioneller Männchen weiblichen Genotyps bei *Lebistes reticulatus, Biol. Zentralb.* **81**:575.

Erickson, A. E., and Pincus, G., 1966, Modification of embryonic development of reproductive and lymphoid organs in the chick, *J. Embryol. Exp. Morphol.* **16**:211.

Essenberg, J. M., 1926, Complete sex reversal in the viviparous teleost, *Xiphophorus helleri, Biol. Bull.* **51**:98.

Fishelson, L., 1975, Ecology and physiology of sex reversal in *Anthias squamipinnis* (Peters), Teleostei: Anthiidae), in: *Intersexuality in the Animal Kingdom* (R. Reinboth, ed.), pp. 284–294. Springer-Verlag, New York.

Foote, C. L., 1964, Intersexuality in amphibians, in: *Intersexuality in Vertebrates Including Man* (C. N. Armstrong and A. J. Marshall, eds.), pp. 233–272, Academic Press, London.

Forbes, T. R., 1938, Studies on the reproductive system of the alligator II. The effects of prolonged injections of oestrone in the immature alligator, *J. Exp. zool.* **78**:335.

Forbes, T. R., 1939, Studies on the reproductive system of the alligator V. The effects of injections of testosterone propionate in immature alligators, *Anat. Rec.* **75**:51.

Forbes, T. R., 1964, Intersexuality in reptiles, in: *Intersexuality in Vertebrates including Man* (C. N. Armstrong, and A. J. Marshall, eds.), pp. 273–284, Academic Press, London.

Fraps, R. M., Sohn, H. A., and Olsen, M. W., 1956, Some effects of multiple pellet implants of diethylstilbestrol in 9 week old chickens, *Poult. Sci.* **35**:665.

Fryer, G., and Iles, T. D., 1972, *The Cichlid Fishes of the Great Lakes of Africa*, T. F. H. Publications, Neptune City, New Jersey.

Gallien, L., 1955, The action of sex hormones on the development of sex in amphibia, *Mem. Soc. Endocrinol.* **4**:188.

Gallien, L. G., 1965, Genetic control of sexual differentiation in vertebrates, in: *Organogenesis* (R. L. DeHaan and H. Ursprung, eds.), pp. 583–610, Holt, Rinehart and Winston, New York.

Gallien, L., 1967, Developments in sexual organogenesis, in: *Advances in Morphogenesis*, Vol. 6 (M. Abercrombie and J. Brachet, eds.), pp. 259–317, Academic Press, New York.

Gardner, J. E., and Fisher, A. E., 1968, Induction of mating in male chicks following preoptic implantation of androgen, *Physiol. Behav.* **3**:709.

Girardie, A., 1966, Controle de l'activité génitale chez *Locusta migratoria*. Mise en évidence d'un facteur gonadotrope et d'un facteur allatotrope dans la pars intercerebralis, *Bull. Soc. Zool. Fr.* **91**:423.

Glick, B., 1961, The reproductive performance of birds hatched from eggs dipped in male hormone solutions, *Poult. Sci.* **40**:1408.

Glick, B., 1965, Embryonic exposure to testosterone propionate will adversely influence future mating behavior in male chickens, *Fed. Proc.* **24**:700.

Godet, R., 1961, Action du propionate de testostérone sur des jeunes Crocodiles (*Crocodilus niloticus*) de sexe femelle, *C. R. Soc. Biol. (Paris)* **255**:394.

Gomot, L., 1975, Intersexuality in birds. Study of the effects of hybridization and postembryonic ovariectomy, in: *Intersexuality in the Animal Kingdom* (R. Reinboth, ed.), Springer-Verlag, New York.

Gorbman, A., and Bern, H. A., 1962, *A Textbook of Comparative Endocrinology*, Wiley, New York.

Gorman, G. C., 1973, The chromosomes of the reptilia, a cytotaxonomic interpretation, in: *Cytotaxonomy and Vertebrate Evolution* (A. B. Chiarelli and E. Capanna, eds.), pp. 349–424, Academic Press, London.

Grant, W. C., 1966, Endocrine induced courtship in three species of European newts, *Am. Zool.* **6**:585.

Hackman, E., and Reinboth, R., 1974, Delimitation of the critical stage of hormone-influenced sex differentiation in *Hemihaplochromis multicolor* (Hilgendorf) (Cichlidae), *Gen. Comp. Endocrinol.* **22**:42.

Haffen, K., 1965, Intersexualité chez la caille (*Coturnix coturnix*). Obtention d'un cas de ponte ovulaire par un mâle génétique, *C. R. Acad. Sci. [D] (Paris)* **261**:3876.

Haffen, K., 1975, Sex differentiation of avian gonads *in vitro*, *Am. Zool.* **15**:257.

Halliday, T. R., 1975, An observational and experimental study of sexual behavior in the smooth newt, *Triturus vulgaris* (Amphibia: Salamandridae), *Anim. Behav.* **23**:291.

Harrington, R. W., 1975, Sex determination and differentiation among uniparental homozygotes of the hermaphroditic fish *Rivulus marmoratus* (Cyprinodontidae: Atheriniformes), in: *Intersexuality in the Animal Kingdom* (R. Reinboth, ed.), Springer-Verlag, New York.

Hartley, R. T., Effects of sex hormones on the development of the urogenital system in the garter snake, *J. Morphol.* **76**:115.

Haynes, R. L., and Glick, B., 1974, Hypothalamic control of sexual behavior in the chicken, *Poult. Sci.* **53**:27.

Höhn, E. O., 1970, Gonadal hormone concentrations in northern phalaropes in relation to nuptial plumage, *Can. J. Zool.* **48**:400.

Höhn, E. O., and Cheng, S. C., 1967, Gonadal hormones in Wilson's phalarope (*Steganopus tricolor*) and other birds in relation to plumage and sex behavior, *Gen. Comp. Endocrinol.* **8**:1.

Huchon, D., 1974, Différenciation sexuelle en présence d'un antistéroïde anti-androgène, l'acétate de cyprotéron, chez *Discoglossus pictus* Otth (Amphibien Anoure, *Discoglossidae*), *C. R. Acad. Sci. [D] (Paris)* **278**:513.

Hutchison, J. B., 1971, Effects of hypothalamic implants of gonadal steroids on courtship behaviour in barbary doves (*Streptopelia risoria*), *J. Endocrinol.* **50**:97.

Idler, D. R., Reinboth, R., Walsh, J. M., and Truscott, B., 1976, A comparison of 11-hydroxytestosterone and 11-ketotestosterone in blood of ambisexual and gonochoristic teleosts, *Gen. Comp. Endocrinol.* **30**:517.

Jenni, D. A., 1974, Evolution of polyandry in birds. *Am. Zool.* **14**:129.

Joosse, J., 1975, Structural and endocrinological aspects of hermaphroditism in pulmonate snails, with particular reference to *Lymnaea stagnalis* (L.), in: *Intersexuality in the Animal Kingdom* (R. Reinboth, ed.), pp. 158–159, Springer-Verlag, New York.

Jost, A., 1960, Hormonal influences in the sex development of bird and mammalian embryos, *Mem. Soc. Endocrinol.* **7**:49.

Kallman, K. D., 1973, The sex-determining mechanism of the platyfish, *Xiphophorus maculatus*, in: *Genetics and Mutagenesis of Fish* (J. H. Schröder, ed.), pp. 19–28, Springer-Verlag, Berlin.

Kaufman, L., 1956, Experiments on sex modification in cocks during their embryonic development, *World's Poult. Sci. J.* **12**:41.

Kehl, R., and Combescot, C., 1955, Reproduction in the Reptilia, *Mem. Soc. Endocrinol.* **4**:57.

Kelley, D. B., and Pfaff, D. W., 1976, Hormone effects on male sex behavior in adult south African clawed frogs, *Xenopus laevis*, *Horm. Behav.* **7**:159.

Kilgore, L., and Glick, B., 1970, Testosterone's influence on brain enzymes in the developing chick, *Poult. Sci.* **49**:16.

Kincl, F. A., Sickles, J. S., and Henzl, M., 1967, Inhibition of sexual development in birds by treatment with steroid hormones during embryonic life or shortly thereafter, *Gen. Comp. Endocrinol.* **9**:401.

Le Gall, S., and Streiff, W., 1975, Protandric hermaphroditism in prosobranch gastropods, in: *Intersexuality in the Animal Kingdom* (R. Reinboth, ed.), pp. 170–178, Springer-Verlag, New York.

Liley, N. R., 1969, Hormones and reproductive behavior in fishes, in: *Fish Physiology*, Vol. III (W. S. Hoar and D. J. Randall, eds.), pp. 73–116, Academic Press, New York.

Lofts, B., and Murton, R. K., 1973, Reproduction in birds, in: *Avian Biology*, Vol. III (D. S. Farner and J. R. King, eds.), pp. 1–109, Academic Press, New York.

Loher, W., and Huber, F., 1966, Nervous and endocrine control of sexual behavior in a grasshopper (*Gomphocerus rufus* L., Acridinae), *Symp. Soc. Exp. Biol.* **20**:381.

Lowe, T. P., and Larkin, J. R., 1975, Sex reversal in *Betta splendens* Regan with emphasis on the problems of sex determination, *J. Exp. Zool.* **191**:25.

Lutz, H., and Lutz-Ostertag, Y., 1975, Intersexuality of the genital system and "free-martinism" in birds, in: *Intersexuality in the Animal Kingdom* (R. Reinboth, ed.), pp. 382–391, Springer-Verlag, New York.

Lutz-Ostertag, Y., and Dufaure, J. P., 1961, Association d'ovaire de Lézard vivipare et de testicule d'embryon de Poulet, *C. R. Soc. Biol. (Paris)* **127**:778.

Manning, A., 1966, Corpus allatum and sexual receptivity in female *Drosophila melanogaster*, *Nature* **211**:1321.

Martinez-Vargas, M. C., Gibson, D. B., Sar, M., and Stumpf, W. E., 1975, Estrogen target sites in the brain of the chick embryo, *Science* **190**:1307.

Mason, P., and Adkins, E. K., 1976, Hormones and social behavior in the lizard *Anolis carolinensis*, *Horm. Behav.* **7**:75.

Masui, K., 1967, *Sex Determination and Differentiation in the Fowl*, Iowa State University Press, Ames.

Mauldin, J. M., Wolfe, J. L., and Glick, B., 1975, The behavior of chickens following embryonic treatment with testosterone propionate, *Poult. Sci.* **54**:2133.

McDonald, P. G., Vidal, N., and Beyer, C., 1970, Sexual behavior in the ovariectomized rabbit after treatment with different amounts of gonadal hormones, *Horm. Behav.* **1**:161.

Mehl, J. A. P., and Reinboth, R., 1975, The possible significance of sex chromatin for the determination of genetic sex in ambisexual teleost fishes, in: *Intersexuality in the Animal Kingdom* (R. Reinboth, ed.), pp. 243–248, Springer-Verlag, New York.

Miller, M. R., 1959, The endocrine basis for reproductive adaptations in reptiles, in: *Comparative Endocrinology* (A. Gorbman, ed.), pp. 499–516, Wiley, New York.

Mittwoch, U., 1971, Sex determination in birds and mammals, *Nature* **231**:432.

Mittwoch, U., 1973, *Genetics of Sex Differentiation*, Academic Press, New York.

Mittwoch, U., 1975, Chromosomes and sex differentiation, in: *Intersexuality in the Animal Kingdom* (R. Reinboth, ed.), pp. 438–446, Springer-Verlag, New York.

Morescalchi, A., 1973, Amphibia, in: *Cytotaxonomy and Vertebrate Evolution* (A. B. Chiarelli and E. Capanna, eds,) pp. 233–348, Academic Press, London.

Nadler, R. D., 1973, Further evidence on the intrahypothalamic locus for androgenization of female rats, *Neuroendocrinology* **12**:110.

Naisse, J., 1963, Détermination sexuelle chez *Lampyris noctiluca* L. (Insecte Coléoptère Malacoderme), *C. R. Acad. Sci. [D] (Paris)* **256**:799.

Naisse, J., 1965, Contrôle endocrinien de la différenciation sexuelle chez les insectes, *Archiv. Anat. Microsc. Morphol. Exp.* **54**:417.

Naisse, J., 1966, Contrôle endocrinien de la différenciation sexuelle chez *Lampyris noctiluca* (Coléoptère Lampyride), *Gen. Comp. Endocrinol.* **7**:85.

Nalbandov, A. V., 1959, Neuroendocrine reflex mechanisms: Bird ovulation, in: *Comparative Endocrinology* (A. Gorbman, ed.), pp. 161–173, Wiley, New York.

Noble, G. K., and Greenberg, B., 1940, Testosterone propionate, a bisexual hormone in the American chameleon, *Proc. Soc. Exp. Biol. Med.* **44**:460.

Noble, G. K., and Greenberg, B., 1941, Effects of seasons, castration, and crystalline sex hormones upon the urogenital system and sexual behavior of the lizard *(Anolis carolinensis)*, *J. Exp. Zool.* **88**:451.

Nottebohm, F., 1975, Vocal behavior in birds, in: *Avian Biology*, Vol. V (D. S. Farner and J. R. King, eds.), pp. 284–332, Academic Press, New York.

Nottebohm, F., and Arnold, A. P., 1976, Sexual dimorphism in vocal control areas of the songbird brain, *Science* **194**:211.

Opel, H., 1966, The timing of oviposition and ovulation in the quail *(Coturnix coturnix japonica)*, *Br. Poult. Sci.* **7**:29.

Orcutt, F. S., 1971, Effects of oestrogen on the differentiation of some reproductive behaviours in male pigeons *(Columba livia)*, *Anim. Behav.* **19**:277.

Ozon, R., 1965, Mise en évidence d'hormones stéroïdes oestrogènes dans le sang de la poule adulte et chez l'embryon de poulet, *C. R. Acad. Sci. [D] (Paris)* **261**:5664.

Ozon, R., 1969, Steroid biosynthesis in larval and embryonic gonads of lower vertebrates, *Gen. Comp. Endocrinol. [Suppl.]* **2**:135.

Ozon, R., 1972a, Androgens in fishes, amphibians, reptiles, and birds, in: *Steroids in Nonmammalian Vertebrates* (D. R. Idler, ed.), pp. 329–389, Academic Press, New York.

Ozon, R., 1972b, Estrogens in fishes, amphibians, reptiles, and birds, in: *Steroids in Nonmammalian Vertebrates* (D. R. Idler, ed.), pp. 390–414, Academic Press, New York.

Palka, Y. S., and Gorbman, A., 1973, Pituitary and testicular influenced sexual behavior in male frogs, *Rana pipiens, Gen. Comp. Endocrinol.* **21**:148.

Pantić, V. R., and Kosanović, M. V., 1973, Testes of roosters treated with a single dose of estradiol dipropionate, *Gen. Comp. Endocrinol.* **21**:108.

Pfaff, D., 1970, Nature of sex hormone effects on rat sex behavior: Specificity of effects and individual patterns of response, *J. Comp. Physiol. Psychol.* **73**:349.

Pieau, C., 1970, Effets de l'oestradiol sur l'appareil génital de l'embryon de tortue Mauresque *(Testudo graeca* L.), *Arch. Anat. Microsc. Morphol. Exp.* **59**:295.

Pieau, C., 1974, Différenciation du sexe en fonction de la température chez les embryons d-*Emys orbicularis* L. (Chelonien), effets des hormones sexuelles. *Ann. Embryol. Morphol.* **7**:365.

Pieau, C., 1975, Temperature and sex differentiation in embryos of two chelonians, *Emys orbicularis* L. and *Testudo graeca* L., in: *Intersexuality in the Animal Kingdom* (R. Reinboth, ed.), pp. 332–339, Springer-Verlag, New York.

Pincus, G., and Hopkins, T. F., 1958, The effects of various estrogens and steroid substances on sex differentiation in the fowl, *Endocrinology* **62**:112.

Pun, C. F., 1958, The sex ratio in the progeny of oestrogen-treated parents in the brown leghorn, *Poult. Sci.* **37**:307.

Rao, G. S., Breuer, H., and Witschi, E., 1969, *In vitro* conversion of 17α-hydroxyprogesterone to androstenedione by mashed gonads from metamorphic stages of *Xenopus laevis, Gen. Comp. Endocrinol.* **12**:119.

Raynaud, A., 1962, Le développement de l'embryon d'Orvet *(Anguis fragilis* L.) décapité à un stade précoce, *C. R. Acad. Sci. [D] (Paris)* **255**:3041.

227

Raynaud, A., 1963, Hormones in development, in: *Techniques in Endocrine Research* (P. Eckstein and F. Knowles, eds.), pp. 261–288, Academic Press, London.

Raynaud, A., and Pieau, C., 1971, Evolution des canaux de Müller et activité enzymatique Δ⁵-3β-hydroxystéroïde déshydrogénasique dans les glandes génitales, chez les embryons de Lézard vert (*Lacerta viridis* Laur.), *C. R. Acad. Sci.* [D] (Paris) **273**:2335.

Raynaud, A., and Pieau, C., 1973, Nouvelles observations relatives à l'action de la testostérone sur les conduits génitaux, explantés *in vitro*, d'embryons de Reptiles, *C. R. Acad. Sci.* [D] (Paris) **277**:2545.

Raynaud, A., Pieau, C., and Raynaud, J., 1969, Aspects histologiques des processus de l'arrêt de développement des canaux de Müller, chez les embryons de Reptiles, *C. R. Acad. Sci.* [D](Paris) **268**:1619.

Raynaud, A., Pieau, C., and Raynaud, J., 1970, Étude histologique comparative de l'allongement des canaux de Müller, de l'arrêt de leur progression en direction caudale et de leur destruction, chez les embryons mâles de diverses espèces de Reptiles, *Ann. Embryol. Morphol.* **3**:21.

Reinboth, R., 1970, Intersexuality in fishes, *Mem. Soc. Endocrinol.* **18**:515.

Reinboth, R., 1972, Some remarks on secondary sex characters, sex, and sexual behavior in teleosts, *Gen. Comp. Endocrinol.* [Suppl.] **3**:565.

Reinboth, R. (ed.), 1975, *Intersexuality in the Animal Kingdom*, Springer-Verlag, New York.

Riddle, O., and Dunham, H. H., 1942, Transformation of males to intersexes by estrogen passed from blood of ring doves to their ovarian eggs, *Endocrinology* **30**:959.

Risley, P. L., 1940, Intersexual gonads of turtle embryos following injection of male sex hormone, *J. Morphol.* **67**:439.

Risley, P. L., 1941, A comparison of effects of gonadotropic and sex hormones on the urogenital systems of juvenile terrapins, *J. Exp. Zool.* **87**:477.

Sachs, B. D., 1967, Photoperiodic control of the cloacal gland of the Japanese quail, *Science* **157**:201.

Sadleir, R. M. F. S., 1973, *The Reproduction of Vertebrates*, Academic Press, New York.

Satoh, N., 1973, Sex differentiation of the gonad of fry transplanted into the anterior chamber of the adult eye in the teleost *Oryzias latipes*, *J. Embryol. Exp. Morphol.* **30**:345.

Satoh, N., and Egami, N., 1973, Preliminary report on sex differentiation in germ cells of normal and transplanted gonads in the fish, *Oryzias latipes*, in: *Genetics and Mutagenesis of Fish* (J. H. Schröder, ed.), pp. 29–32, Springer-Verlag, Berlin.

Schein, M. W., and Hale, E. B., 1965, Stimuli eliciting sexual behavior, in: *Sex and Behavior* (F. A. Beach, ed.), pp. 440–482, Wiley, New York.

Schreck, C. B., 1974, Hormonal treatment and sex manipulation in fishes, in: *Control of Sex in Fishes* (C. B. Schreck, ed.), Virginia Polytechnic Institute, Blacksburg.

Short, R. V., 1972, Sex determination and differentiation, in: *Reproduction in Mammals*, Book 2 (C. R. Austin and R. V. Short, eds.), pp. 43–71, Cambridge University Press, Cambridge.

Silvers, W. K., and Wachtel, S. S., 1977, H-Y antigen: Behavior and function, *Science* **195**:956.

Stetson, M. H., 1972, Hypothalamic regulation of gonadotropin release in female Japanese quail, *Z. Zellforsch. Mikrosk. Anat.* **130**:411.

Taber, E., 1964, Intersexuality in birds, in: *Intersexuality in Vertebrates Including Man* (C. N. Armstrong and A. J. Marshall, eds.), pp. 285–310, Academic Press, London.

Tang, F., Chan, S. T. H., and Lofts, B., 1974, Effect of steroid hormones on the process of natural sex reversal in the rice-field eel, *Monopterus albus* (Zuiew), *Gen. Comp. Endocrinol.* **24**:227.

Tardent, P., 1975, Sex and sex determination in Coelenterates, in: *Intersexuality in the Animal Kingdom* (R. Reinboth, ed.), pp. 1–13, Springer-Verlag, New York.

Tavolga, W. N., 1955, Effects of gonadectomy and hypophysectomy on prespawning behavior in males of the gobiid fish *Bathygobius soporator*, *Physiol. Zool.* **28**:218.

Thorgaard, G. H., 1977, Heteromorphic sex chromosomes in male rainbow trout, *Science* **196**:900.

Vannani, E., Stagni, A., and Zaccanti, F., 1975, Autoradiographic study on the mechanisms of testosterone-induced sex-reversal in *Rana* tadpoles, in: *Intersexuality in the Animal Kingdom*, (R. Reinboth, ed.), pp. 318–331, Springer-Verlag, New York.

Van Tienhoven, A., 1957, A method of "controlling sex" by dipping of eggs in hormone solutions, *Poult. Sci.* **36**:628.

Van Tienhoven, A., 1968, *Reproductive Physiology of Vertebrates*, Saunders, Philadelphia.

Van Tyne, J., and Berger, A. J., 1959, *Fundamentals of Ornithology*, Wiley, New York.

Wada, M., and Gorbman, A., 1977, Relation of mode of administration of testosterone to evocation of male sex behavior in frogs, *Horm. Behav.* **8**:310.

Welty, J. C., 1962, *The Life of Birds*, Saunders, Philadelphia.

Weniger, J.-P., and Zeis, A., 1973, Action féminisante des androgènes sur le testicule et le canal de Müller d'embryon de poulet *in vitro, Arch. Anat. Microsc. Morphol. Exp.* **62**:145.

Weniger, J.-P., Mack, G., and Holder, F., 1975, L'hormone responsable de la régression des canaux de Müller chez l'embryon de poulet mâle n'est pas un androgène, in: *Intersexuality in the Animal Kingdom* (R. Reinboth, ed.), Springer-Verlag, New York.

Wentworth, B. C., Hendricks, B. G., and Sturtevant, J., 1968, Sterility induced in Japanese quail by spray treatment of eggs with mestranol, *J. Wild. Manag.* **32**:879.

Whitsett, J. M., Irvin, E. W., Edens, F. W., and Thaxton, J. P., 1977, Demasculinization of male Japanese quail by prenatal estrogen treatment, *Horm. Behav.* **8**:254.

Wigglesworth, V. B., 1970, *Insect Hormones*, Freeman, San Francisco.

Wilson, J. A., and Glick, B., 1970, Ontogeny of mating behavior in the chicken, *Am. J. Physiol.* **218**:951.

Wilson, M. I., and Bermant, G., 1972, An analysis of social interactions in Japanese quail, *Coturnix coturnix japonica, Anim. Behav.* **20**:252.

Witschi, E., 1959, Age of sex-determining mechanisms in vertebrates, *Science* **130**:372.

Witschi, E., 1961, Sex and secondary sexual characters, in: *Biology and Comparative Physiology of Birds* (A. J. Marshall, ed.), pp. 115–168, Academic Press, New York.

Witschi, E., 1971, Mechanisms of sexual differentiation, in: *Hormones in Development* (M. Hamburgh and E. J. W. Barrington, eds.), pp. 601–618, Appleton-Century-Crofts, New York.

Wolff, E., 1950, Le rôle des hormones embryonnaires dans la différenciation sexuelle des oiseaux, *Arch. Anat. Microsc. Morphol. Exp.* **39**:426.

Wolff, E., 1959, Endocrine function of the gonad in developing vertebrates, in: *Comparative Endocrinology* (A. Gorbman, ed.), pp. 568–581, Wiley, New York.

Woods, J. E., and Podczaski, E. S., 1974, Androgen synthesis in the gonads of the chick embryo, *Gen. Comp. Endocrinol.* **24**:413.

Woods, J. E., Simpson, R. M., and Moore, P. L., 1975, Plasma testosterone levels in the chick embryo, *Gen. Comp. Endocrinol.* **27**:543.

Yamamoto, T.-O., 1959, The effect of estrone dosage level upon the percentage of sex-reversals in genetic male (XY) of the medaka *Oryzias latipes, J. Exp. Zool.* **141**:133.

Yamamoto, T.-O., 1962, Hormonic factors affecting gonadal sex differentiation in fish, *Gen. Comp. Endocr. [Suppl.]* **1**:341.

Yamamoto, T.-O., 1969, Sex differentiation, in: *Fish Physiology* (W. S. Hoar and D. J. Randall, eds.), differentiation in the medaka, *Oryzias latipes, Gen. Comp. Endocrinol.* **10**:8.

Yamamoto, T.-O., 1969, Sex differentiation, in: *Fish Physiology* (W. S. Hoar, and D. J. Randall, eds.), pp. 117–163, Academic Press, New York.

Yamamoto, T.-O., and Kajishima, T., 1968, Sex hormone induction of sex reversal in the goldfish and evidence for male heterogamety, *J. Exp. Zool.* **146**:163.

Yamamoto, T.-O., and Matsuda, N., 1963, Effects of estradiol, stilbestrol and some alkyl-carbonyl androstanes upon sex differentiation in the medaka, *Oryzias latipes, Gen. Comp. Endocrinol.* **3**:101.

Young, W. C., 1961, The hormones and mating behavior, in: *Sex and Internal Secretions,* Vol. 2 (W. C. Young, ed.), pp. 1173–1239, Williams & Wilkins, Baltimore.

8

Puberty

BRUCE D. GOLDMAN

I. INTRODUCTION

There is a lack of clear agreement among researchers as to the precise definition of the term "puberty." Perhaps it would be simplest to define puberty as that stage in its life history when an animal becomes fertile—i.e., when a male begins to produce mature sperm and when a female begins to ovulate. However, numerous other events normally occur at about the same time, and often these events are emphasized in studies of puberty. In humans, for example, puberty in the male is associated with a spurt of growth, the appearance of pubic and facial hair, deepening of the voice, and less well-defined psychological changes. In girls, puberty is accompanied by breast development, the appearance of pubic hair, and an increase in hip width. In nonprimates, too, several sex-related parameters show accelerated changes at the time of puberty.

A number of behavioral changes occur at puberty. The most widely studied of these are the increase in sexual behavior and, in some species, in aggressive behavior. Both of these behaviors appear to be altered quantitatively at puberty in response to the increasing levels of gonadal steroid hormones. Thus, both male and female rats can be induced to show sexual behaviors well before the time of puberty if they are treated with the appropriate sex hormones. Likewise, the tendency of male mice to display aggression toward conspecific males increases dramatically at about the time of the pubertal increase in blood androgen titers. These events occur somewhat before or after

BRUCE D. GOLDMAN • Department of Bio-Behavioral Sciences, University of Connecticut, Storrs, Connecticut 06268.

the achievement of fertility and do not necessarily all occur at the same time. For this reason, the author finds it convenient to view gonadal maturation as the central event in puberty. The rationale for this view is strengthened by the fact that most of the other pubertal changes are triggered largely by the changing titers of gonadal hormones.

II. NEUROENDOCRINE FOUNDATIONS OF THE PHYSIOLOGY OF PUBERTY

Puberty represents a time of transition from sexual immaturity to sexual maturity. Therefore, to understand this process, we must first review some important aspects of gonadal function as it occurs during adulthood. The gonads form part of a hormonal feedback system that operates as follows: The pituitary gonadotropic hormones (GTH)* stimulate growth and steroidogenesis in the gonads. Gonadal steroids (primarily testosterone, estradiol, and progesterone) inhibit the secretion of GTH by actions exerted both directly on the pituitary and also at the neural level. Thus, a closed feedback loop serves to regulate the levels of pituitary and gonadal activity. Estrogen and progesterone can also exert positive feedback effects with respect to their induction of the cyclical release of an ovulatory surge of GTH. Experimental evidence for the negative feedback effects of gonadal steroids stems mainly from observations of chronically elevated serum titers of gonadotropins following gonadectomy and from the ability of replacement with exogenous steroids (especially estrogen and androgen) to inhibit "castration hypersecretion" of gonadotropins. The positive feedback effect of estrogen can be demonstrated by injecting a large amount of estrogen during the follicular phase of the ovulatory cycle. Under certain conditions, such treatment may initiate a premature release of the preovulatory surge of LH, usually occurring approximately one day following the estrogen treatment (Ferin *et al.*, 1969; Labhsetwar, 1970; Norman, 1975).

Just as there are both positive and negative feedback effects of steroids on GTH, there are at least two brain nuclei of critical importance to the regulation of GTH secretion. The arcuate nucleus appears to control the tonic gonadotropin secretion. Tonic activity is the only pattern shown by the male and is also displayed in the female for the greater part of the ovulatory cycle. However, just before ovulation, there are a number of endocrine fluctuations. The preoptic area of the brain appears to regulate the cyclical release of large amounts of GTH in the female resulting in ovulation. Recent evidence indicates that the suprachiasmatic nuclei may be important in regulating the cyclical release in GTH. Thus, lesions of the suprachiasmatic nuclei prevent ovulation in the rat (Clemens *et al.*, 1976). In hamsters, the time of

*FSH and LH.

preovulatory LH release has been shown to be phase-related to the onset of physical activity (wheel-running) which has, in turn, been shown to be under control by the suprachiasmatic nuclei.

III. THE PROBLEM OF PUBERTY

Gonadal function in the immature organism obviously occurs at lower levels than in the adult. With the background given above, one can ask several pertinent questions regarding causal events in puberty.

1. To what extent is puberty the result of a decrease in pituitary or hypothalamic sensitivity to the negative feedback action of gonadal steroids, allowing for increased levels of GTH and a higher level of gonadal activity?
2. To what extent is puberty caused by an increase in gonadal sensitivity to GTH?
3. A third question, related to both 1 and 2, is that of which develops first—the ability to release an ovulatory surge of GTH or the ability to produce mature ovarian follicles?
4. Do physiological factors outside the hypothalamic–pituitary–gonadal axis (i.e., other hormones or neural centers) have an important role in initiating puberty?

A. Ovulatory Hormone Release

Female rats normally begin to ovulate at 35–45 days of age. However, immature females injected with pregnant mare serum gonadotropin (PMSG), a preparation with both FSH-like and LH-like activity, will ovulate 3 days after the injection. This effect has been observed even when the PMSG is administered as early as 20–21 days of age. Injections of PMSG are necessary but not sufficient to induce ovulation in these rats since hypophysectomy or administration of neural blocking drugs prevents the release of the ovulatory surge of GTH and subsequent ovulation. These observations have led to the conclusion that a potentially functional neural mechanism for the triggering of an ovulatory GTH surge is present as early as 23 days of age in this species. On the basis of this hypothesis, one could suggest that puberty is normally delayed until at least 2 weeks later because mature ovarian follicles are not present early in the animal's life. According to this scheme, PMSG acts to stimulate premature follicular maturation. There is one possible criticism of this interpretation. It may be that the ovulatory triggering mechanism is not yet mature at 21 days of age but matures rapidly either as a result of a direct effect of PMSG or as a result of the effects of ovarian steroids secreted by the developing follicles. Nevertheless, it does appear that, in the female rat, the capacity to produce mature ovarian follicles is the limiting factor in achieving puberty.

B. The Hypothalamus

Luteinizing hormone releasing factor (LRF) is present in the hypothalamus of the newborn rabbit. Also, neonatal rats release pituitary LH in response to treatment with LRF. Therefore, animals apparently make LRF and are able to respond to this hormone long before puberty. While it seems likely that LRF secretion begins at or before birth, direct proof for this in the form of measurements of LRF in blood is not available. Nevertheless, it would seem at this time that the ability to make LRF is not a limiting factor in reaching puberty. If LRF is involved, it is more likely that changes in the quantity and pattern of LRF secretion may be important in initiating reproductive function.

C. Steroid Feedback

Several investigators have obtained evidence that puberty is associated with, and perhaps initated by, a change in the set point of the so-called "hypothalamic gonadostat." The hypothesis is that the immature animal is highly sensitive to the negative feedback effects of gonadal steroids (especially estrogen and androgen) and that the blood levels of GTH are suppressed to a low level by this mechanism. At the time of puberty, a change in the set point of the "gonadostat" results in decreased sensitivity to these negative feedback effects. This would result in increased concentrations of GTH in blood and, consequently, increased gonadal activity. The main evidence supporting this hypothesis is as follows: Byrnes and Meyer (1951), using a parabiotic rat preparation, demonstrated that gonadotropin secretion could be inhibited in an ovariectomized, immature rat by doses of estrogen that were too low to directly stimulate uterine growth. In this study, two immature females were placed in parabiosis. One animal was ovariectomized; the other was hypophysectomized. Gonadotropins produced by the ovariectomized partner could be carried to the hypophysectomized female and stimulate her ovaries, resulting in uterine growth. When very small doses of estrogen were administered to the ovariectomized animal, uterine growth was blocked in the hypophysectomized parabiont. This observation was interpreted by Byrnes and Meyer to be the result of inhibition of pituitary gonadotropin secretion by the exogenous estrogen. The doses of estrogen used in the experiment were too low to stimulate the uteri of the animal receiving the injections.

Ramirez and McCann (1963) demonstrated that castrated immature rats of both sexes showed LH inhibition with smaller doses of exogenous estrogen and androgen than were required in castrated adults, even though doses were corrected for differences in body weight. This early work employed a bioassay to measure serum LH, but the results have recently been confirmed in male rats by using more sensitive and precise radioimmunoassay (RIA) techniques (Negro-Villar *et al.,* 1973). Furthermore, FSH secretion was also found to be more sensitive to androgen suppression in the prepubertal rat in the more recent studies.

If, indeed, puberty results from a decrease in the sensitivity of the negative feedback system resulting in a "release" of the pituitary gonadotropic cells to function at a higher level of activity, then one should find lower concentrations of GTH in the blood of prepubertal than of adult individuals. Such a relationship has been observed for humans of both sexes (Faiman and Winter, 1974). However, in the rat the situation is less clear. For example, in the male rat, serum LH levels do increase as the animal achieves puberty (Fig. 1), but the serum FSH concentrations are somewhat higher in prepubertal males as compared to adults (Fig. 2). However, the male rat may be a poor model for the study of the role of GTH in puberty. Male rats reach puberty at about 55–60 days of age. Approximately 40–45 days are required for complete maturation of spermatozoa from spermatogonia. Thus, the time required for completion

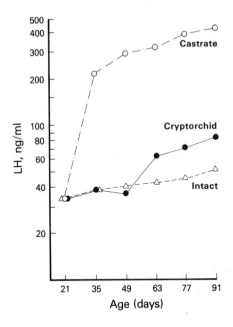

Figure 1. Serum LH in intact, cryptorchid and castrate rats. There was a small but progressive increase in serum LH with increasing age. No abrupt increase heralding sexual maturation was seen. Following cryptorchidism, serum LH was not increased until 63 days of age. Castration resulted in a prompt elevation of serum LH. (Reproduced with permission from Swerdlof *et al.,* 1971.)

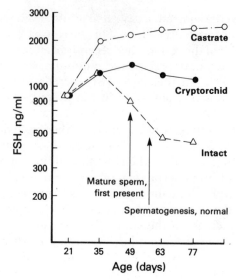

Figure 2. Serum FSH in intact, cryptorchid and castrate rats. In intact rats, serum FSH was high at 21 days of age when compared to adult levels (91 days). Serum FSH began to fall coincidentally with appearance of the first mature sperm (49 days), reaching adult levels at the time of completed spermatogenesis (63 days). In the cryptorchid rats, serum FSH was higher than in intact animals at 49 days of age (tubular atrophy) and did not fall to intact adult levels. (Reproduced with permission from Swerdloff *et al.*, 1971.)

of the spermatogenic cycle is probably an important factor in limiting the achievement of puberty in the male rat. Indeed, attempts to advance puberty in the male rat by treatment with GTH have not been successful. Nevertheless, even the female rat poses some problem for the "gonadostat" hypothesis, since serum GTH levels in the female reach a peak at around 13–17 days of age, and only after this time do the levels decline to rise once again at puberty (Figs. 3 and 4). The function, if any, of the very high levels of gonadotropins in 15-day-old female rats is not known. The pattern of gonadotropin secretion has not been very thoroughly studied in such young females of other species; however, female hamsters appear to have higher circulating levels of LH and FSH at 20–24 days of age as compared to the levels observed postpubertally (Bex, 1976). These observations in the female rat may not contradict the gonadostat hypothesis, since it may be that only very small amounts of ovarian hormones enter the brain during neonatal life in the female.

D. Gonadal Maturation

The difficulties in explaining certain observations within the framework of the gonadostat hypothesis have led some workers to propose an alternative but

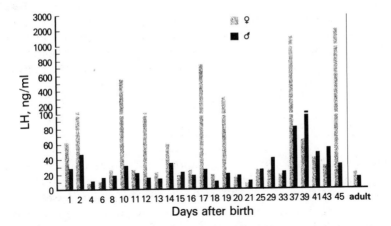

Figure 3. Serum LH levels in immature male and female rats. Note the higher values on days 1 and 2 in female newborn rats, although serum LH was increased in the males, too. Sporadic LH peaks are observed in female rats between days 10 and 20, whereas the males show only minor fluctuations. Preovulatory LH levels are seen on day 37. Day of vaginal opening = E_1. The following days of the estrous cycle are M_1, D_1, and P_2. The peripuberal time mark for male rats does not correspond to that of the females. Standard error of mean on top of each bar. (Reproduced with permission from Döhler and Wuttge, 1974.)

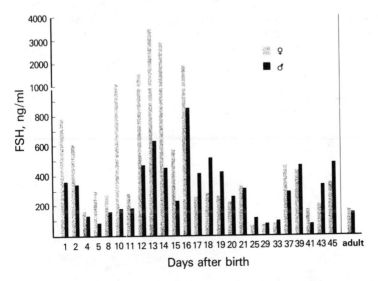

Figure 4. Serum FSH levels in immature male and female rats. Significantly higher values are found in the females during the first 2 postnatal days than in the males. Between days 10 and 20 serum FSH increases again in both sexes. The levels are significantly higher in females than in males. Note differences in time on abscissa at time after vaginal opening on day 37. Each day of the following estrous cycle is shown for the female rats. Values are given for alternate days from day 37, for male rats. Standard error of mean on top of each bar. (Reproduced with permission from Döhler and Wuttge, 1974.)

related model. It has been suggested that puberty may come about as a result of increased gonadal sensitivity to GTH. This model has received some support from the studies of Odell and Swerdloff (1974) who found that both the ovaries and the testes of the rat become more sensitive to GTH with increasing age.

E. Body Growth

It has often been noted that correlations exist between puberty and rate of body growth. In boys a considerable increase in the rate of growth occurs at about the time of puberty; girls show a similar increase but of lesser magnitude. These increases in growth rate have often been assumed to result at least partly from effects produced by the rising titers of gonadal sex hormones. More recently, it has also been suggested that a spurt of body growth may precede the achievement of puberty and that increased body size may somehow trigger physiological events leading to puberty. The average age at menarche (indicating puberty in girls) has steadily decreased in several European nations and in the United States since 1900 (Fig. 5). In the United States, for example, the average age at menarche was about 14 years in 1900 but was reduced to slightly less than 13 years by 1955 (Tanner, 1962). These historical changes may be partly related to diet and increasing growth rate of the human population, but obviously many other factors could be involved.

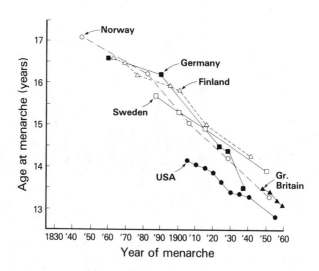

Figure 5. Change in the age of menarche in different countries. (Reproduced with permission from Tanner, 1962.)

F. Extrahypothalamic Structures Influencing Puberty

There is substantial evidence to suggest that areas of the brain lying outside the hypothalamic–pituitary complex may have a role in regulating the time of puberty. For example, complete or anterior deafferentation of the hypothalamus leads to precocious ovarian development and vaginal opening in the rat, although such animals are not able to respond to increased steroid titers by releasing an ovulatory surge of GTH. Electrolytic lesions of the medial amygdala induce true precocious puberty (with ovulation); in contrast, chronic electrical stimulation of the corticomedial amygdala delays vaginal opening. These findings suggest an inhibitory role of the amygdala in puberty. This seems paradoxical in that evidence exists that the amygdala may facilitate GTH secretion in the adult rat. Some evidence also exists for a possible role of the hippocampus in puberty; electrical stimulation of the hippocampus in 27-day-old rats advanced vaginal opening by 4–6 days (Gorski, 1974).

G. Role of Environmental Cues in Regulating the Onset of Puberty

The pineal gland has also been implicated in the regulation of puberty. Pinealectomy has resulted in advanced sexual maturation in rats of both sexes. This effect is consistent with the so-called "antigonadal" effects of the pineal. Furthermore, exposure to constant darkness delays puberty, whereas exposure to continuous illumination results in earlier vaginal opening in the rat. These effects may be mediated by the pineal. In the Siberian hamster (*Phodopus sungorus*), puberty is greatly delayed by exposure to a short photoperiod, and this effect is partially reversed by pinealectomy (Brackman and Hoffmann, 1977).

H. Pheromonal Influences

Several studies have indicated that pheromones may play an important role in determining the time of puberty in the mouse. When immature female mice are exposed to adult male conspecifics, the time of puberty is advanced by a few days. This effect is present even when the females are exposed only to male-urine-soaked shavings, suggesting that an odor cue is sufficient to influence the time of first ovulation. In these experiments there was a strong correlation between body weight of the females and susceptibility to the pheromonal influence; the larger females were much more likely to respond to the male odor. Recent evidence suggests that the initial effect of the pheromone may be to cause LH release from the pituitary (Bronson and Desjardins, 1974). Pheromonal cues may be important in population control; for example, it may be adaptive for young females to begin ovulating earlier when many adult males are present. The chemical nature of the puberty-accelerating pheromone has not yet been established.

I. Precocious Puberty and Pseudopuberty in Man

Precocious puberty may occur in humans. Sometimes this phenomenon appears to result from a brain lesion; in other cases (idiopathic) no causal factor is apparent. In any case, psychological problems are likely to ensue. Perhaps better understood is the phenomenon of precocious pseudopuberty which may occur in boys as a result of congenital adrenal hyperplasia or adrenal tumors. In either case, the adrenal produces excessive quantities of androgens, leading to premature stimulation of the external genital tissues as well as to other androgen-dependent pubertal changes. The condition is known as pseudo-puberty because the testes are not fully developed—only androgen target tissues are stimulated. Girls with congenital adrenal hyperplasia also produce considerable quantities of adrenal androgens, but in this case virilization generally results.

REFERENCES

Bex, F. J., 1976, Gonadotropic regulation of follicular development in the hamster and rat, Ph.D. Thesis, University of Connecticut.

Brackman, M., and Hoffmann, K., 1977, Pinealectomy and photoperiod influence testicular development in the Djungarian hamster, *Naturwissenschaften* **64**:431–432.

Bronson, F. H., and Desjardins, C., 1974, Circulating concentrations of FSH, LH, estradiol, and progesterone associated with acute, male-induced puberty in female mice, *Endocrinology* **94**:1658–1668.

Byrnes, W. W., and Meyer, R. K., 1951, The inhibition of gonadotrophic hormone secretion by physiological doses of estrogen, *Endocrinology* **48**:133–136.

Clemens, J. A., Smalstig, E. B., and Sawyer, B. D., 1976, Studies on the role of the preoptic area in the control of reproductive function in the rat, *Endocrinology* **99**:728–735.

Dohler, K. D., and Wultke, W., 1974, Serum LH, FSH, prolactin and progesterone from birth to puberty in female and male rats, *Endocrinology* **94**:1003–1008.

Faiman, C., and Winter, J. S. D., 1974, Gonadotropins and sex hormone patterns in puberty: Clinical data, in: *Control of the Onset of Puberty* (M. M. Grumbach, G. D. Grave, and F. E. Meyer, eds.), pp. 32–55, John Wiley and Sons, New York.

Ferin, M., Zimmering, P., and Vande Wiele, R. L., 1969, Effects of antibodies to estradiol-17 on PMS-induced ovulation in immature rats, *Endocrinology* **84**:893.

Gorski, R. A., 1974, Extrahypothalamic influences on gonadotropin regulation, in: *Control of the Onset of Puberty* (M. M. Grumbach, G. D. Grave, and F. E. Meyer, eds.), pp. 182–207, John Wiley and Sons, New York.

Labhsetwar, A. P., 1970, Role of estrogens in ovulation: A study using the estrogen-antagonist I.C.I. 46, 474, *Endocrinology* **87**:542–551.

Negro-Vilar, A., Ojeda, S. R., and McCann, S. M., 1974, Evidence for changes in sensitivity to testosterone negative feedback on gonadotropin release during sexual development in the male rat, *Endocrinology* **93**:729–735.

Norman, R. L., 1975, Estrogen and progesterone effects on the neural control of the preovulatory LH release in the golden hamster, *Biol. Reprod.* **13**:218–222.

Odell, W. D., and Swerdloff, R. S., 1974, The role of the gonads in sexual maturation, in: *Control of the Onset of Puberty* (M. M. Grumbach, G. D. Grave, and F. E. Meyer, eds.), pp. 313–332, John Wiley and Sons, New York.

Ramirez, V. D., and McCann, S. M., 1963, A comparison of the regulation of luteinizing hormone (LH) secretion in immature and adult rats, *Endocrinology* **72**:452–464.

Swerdloff, R. S., Walsh, P. C., Jacobs, H. S., and Odell, W. D., 1971, Serum LH and FSH during sexual maturation in the male rat: Effect of castration and cryptorchidism, *Endocrinology* **88**:120–128.

Tanner, J. M., 1962, *Growth at Adolescence,* 2nd edition, Blackwell Scientific Publications, Oxford.

III

Control of Reproduction on the Organismic and Physiological Levels of Organization

Experimental Analysis of Hormone Actions on the Hypothalamus, Anterior Pituitary, and Ovary

HARVEY H. FEDER

I. BRIEF HISTORY OF THE PROBLEM

The history of efforts to understand the factors that regulate cyclic gonadal function actually starts with research on a somewhat different problem. In the early 1900s, investigators such as Steinach (reviewed in Moore and Price, 1932) were interested in the problem of organ transplantation. Steinach attempted to transplant testes into intact female rats and ovaries into intact male rats. These transplants invariably failed to become functional or "take." However, when the host animal was gonadectomized, transplantation of the heterologous gonad was said to be more successful. Somewhat later, Lipschütz (1925) transplanted ovaries into intact male guinea pigs. He stated that the time required to stimulate male mammary growth was much greater than when the graft was made in castrated males. Furthermore, ovarian grafts that failed to "take" (in terms of stimulating mammary gland growth) did so almost immediately when the male's testes were removed. Lipschütz derived the idea that removal of the testes led to an "unbolting" of ovarian function.

The concept that there were antagonistic actions of the ovary and the testis flowed from these transplantation experiments. In 1926, Steinach and Kun extended this concept by claiming to demonstrate that the antagonistic actions

HARVEY H. FEDER • Institute of Animal Behavior, Rutgers University, Newark, New Jersey 07102.

of the gonads were exerted through their respective steroidal secretions. Moore and Price (1932) decided to thoroughly reexamine the question of direct antagonisms between the hormones secreted by the testes and the hormones produced by the ovaries. In the course of this reexamination, they came to the conclusion that failure of gonadal transplants to become functional in intact subjects had less to do with direct antagonisms between ovarian and testicular hormones than with suppression of pituitary activity by the transplanted gonads. After arriving at this conclusion, Moore and Price went on to hypothesize that gonadal secretion is regulated in normal animals by a reciprocal interaction between the gonads and the pituitary gland. The Moore–Price theory of the regulation of gonadal secretion has had, and continues to have, significant impact on the study of reproductive physiology. In its original form it consisted of four major principles.

1. Gonadal hormones stimulate homologous reproductive accessory tissues but are without effect on heterologous accessories. That is, androgen stimulates male, but not female, reproductive accessory tissues, whereas estrogen stimulates female, but not male, accessory tissues. Although this tenet is valid as a rough approximation, there is much evidence that demonstrates effects of androgens on uterus, vagina, oviduct, and breasts and effects of estrogens on seminal vesicles, prostate, epididymis, and coagulating, preputial, and Cowper's glands (Burrows, 1949).

2. Gonadal hormones have no direct effect on the gonads of either the same or the opposite sex. Although this, too, is not entirely true (Parkes and Deanesly, 1966a; Armstrong and Dorrington, 1976), the general principle was neatly demonstrated by Moore and Price (1932). They gave hypophysectomized male rats testosterone and showed that testosterone did not stimulate growth of the regressed testis.

3. Secretions of the hypophysis stimulate the gonads to function both in terms of germ cell production and in terms of hormone secretion. This had been demonstrated previously by Smith and Engle (1927) who performed hypophysectomies successfully.

4. Gonadal hormones of either sex exert a depressant effect on hypophyseal function, and this results in a diminished quantity of hypophyseal sex-stimulating factor available to the organism. This point was considered by Moore and Price to be the key to the problem of hormonal antagonism posed by the transplantation experiments of Steinach and Lipschütz. One experiment that Moore and Price performed to support this notion is outlined in Table 1.

The conclusion drawn from the experiment described in Table 1 was that "oestrin" (an estrogenic preparation that probably consisted primarily of estrone and estradiol) did not induce damage to testicular function as long as sufficient quantities of gonadotropic hormone (from implantation of multiple pituitaries) were present. Note that loss of testicular function occurred in

Table 1. Early Evidence That Steroid Hormones Exert a Depressant Effect on Pituitary Function in Rats[a]

Group	Treatment	Result
Normal males	Inject testosterone or oestrin	Loss of testicular function
Hypophysectomized males	—	Loss of testicular function
Hypophysectomized males	Reimplant excess pituitary tissue and inject oestrin	Testicular function regained

[a] The classic study of Moore and Price (1932).

normal males when either testosterone or estrogen was injected. Together, these data indicated that loss of gonadal activity was less a result of a direct antagonism between androgens and estrogens as proposed by Steinach and Lipschutz than the result of an excess of either androgen or estrogen that caused a diminution of pituitary function and a consequent loss of gonadal activity.

The Moore–Price description of the relationship between the steroid hormones and the pituitary hormones came to be known as the "push–pull" theory. It is quite well characterized in a quotation from George Corner (see Lamport, 1940):

> We are conjecturing a kind of see-saw effect. . . . The cycle is like a clockwork in which the pituitary is the driving force and the regulation is the reciprocal action of ovarian and pituitary hormones. The hypophysis starts the production of oestrin. . . . The rise in oestrin then checks the production of pituitary hormone, which begins to fall as oestrus occurs. The oestrin is used up or excreted, or both, and as it falls to a low ebb in the dioestrus interval, the hypophysis begins again to secrete its hormone.

This push–pull idea can be seen to have at least two implicit qualities. The idea supposes only an inhibitory relationship between gonadal steroids and pituitary hormones. That is, a rise in gonadal steroid concentration causes a drop in hypophyseal gonadotropin secretion. A drop in steroid secretion provokes a rise in gonadotropin output. The possibility of a stimulatory relationship, in which increases in steroid concentration cause increments in gonadotropin production, was not discussed. Probably, this was in great measure because of the dominance of the idea of homeostasis. It may not be coincidence that W.B. Cannon's influential book, *The Wisdom of the Body*, was published in 1932, the same year as the Moore and Price paper. In the context of the homeostatis concept, it may have been somewhat difficult to imagine a physiological role for stimulatory effects of steroids on gonadotropin secretion or to postulate a mechanism whereby such a system could slow itself down.

This difficulty is linked to a second implicit aspect of the push–pull idea. That is, the idea posits no role of external environmental factors in the regulation of gonadal function.

As Brown-Grant (1966) points out, the studies of F.H.A. Marshall had established, well before 1932, that exteroceptive factors play a role in initiating and sustaining sexual cycles. Yet Moore and Price in 1932 failed to appreciate the potential relevance of these exteroceptive factors to pituitary function. In fact, it was not until later that Marshall himself grasped the significance of the pituitary gland as a mediator of the effects of exteroceptive factors on sexual cycles. If the factor of external environmental influences had been incorporated by Moore and Price, it might have provided one theoretical basis for understanding how a mutual stimulation of the gonads and pituitary could be slowed down. However, the Moore–Price model of the pituitary–gonad loop was, in Corner's words, "like a clockwork: once wound up it could continue, in theory, to run in any surroundings. Given this bias, it is not surprising that the Moore and Price article makes no mention of the fact that certain animals are reflex ovulators and others show seasonal cycles of sexual activity. In these cases external factors surely must modify the running of the clock. Although it could be argued, by a proponent of the push–pull theory, that the pituitary or the ovary undergoes seasonal changes in sensitivity to hormones, an equally likely explanation of seasonal cyclicity is that the nervous system receives signals from the external environment that filter into the pituitary–ovarian system and regulate the activity of the two glands. With the latter perspective, it would not have required a great intuitive leap to guess that the nervous system could also receive signals from the internal environment and that these signals could feed into the pituitary–ovarian system in either a stimulatory or inhibitory manner.

Experimental tests of the validity of the Moore–Price model were not long in coming. As early as 1940, Lamport rejected the push–pull theory on mathematical grounds. He showed that the formula for harmonic motion used in physics described the push–pull theory of hormonal regulation. He compared the predictions generated by the formula for harmonic motion with the actual figures obtained when measurements of urinary estrogen excretion were placed in the formula. According to Lamport's data, the assumptions of the Moore–Price theory were inadequate to account for the periodicity of estrogen secretion in females.

Another line of inquiry that was to challenge the Moore–Price notion was initiated by Hohlweg and Junkmann (1932). These investigators transplanted pituitaries of rats into sites not adjacent to the hypothalamus. They noted that ovariectomy of the host animal did not lead to the appearance of so-called "castration cells" (enlarged gonadotrophs formed after ovariectomy) in the pituitary. Castration cells would have been apparent if the pituitary had been secreting large amounts of gonadotropin in response to lowered estrogen after ovariectomy. Because castration cells did not appear in the transplanted pituitaries, Hohlweg and Junkmann proposed the existence of a "sex center" in the hypothalamus that was responsive to estrogen and that regulated the function of the pituitary gland. This idea was supported by an experiment of Westman and Jacobsohn (1937a) in which it was demonstrated that electrical stimulation of the rabbit cerebrum ordinarily resulted in ovulation, but not when ·the pituitary stalk was destroyed prior to stimulation. This line of investigation continued in the laboratory of G. W. Harris and culminated in a series of brilliant experiments that clarified the nature of hypothalamic control of the pituitary. These experiments are reviewed in Harris' (1955) monograph.

Although his research group did not coin the term "releasing factor," the work of Harris and his colleagues made the existence of such factors evident. Releasing factors were hormones thought to be produced by neurons in the basal hypothalamus (in the "hypophysiotrophic area," Szentágothai et al., 1968) and carried to the pituitary by a hypophyseal portal vascular system (Fig. 1). When they reached the pituitary, these factors somehow caused release of the gonadotropins luteinizing hormone (LH) and follicle-stimulating hormone (FSH) as well as other trophic hormones. Therefore, the regulation of gonadal activity appeared to depend on three tissues (the gonads, the pituitary, and the diencephalic tissue overlying the pituitary), each of which had two properties. First, each tissue produced a blood-borne chemical that affected one or both of the other tissues. Second, each tissue possessed a monitoring system sensitive to the blood-borne chemicals of one or both of the other tissues. These components were thought to form a loop whose activity could account for the dramatic variations in ovarian hormone secretion seen during normal estrous or menstrual cycles.

However, experimentalists began to isolate environmental factors that interrupted the estrous cycle. The way in which the components of the diencephalic–hypophyseal–gonadal system were involved in some of these interruptions of estrous periodicity constitutes another story which began in 1922. In that year, Long and Evans (1922) found that when female rats with normal estrous cycles were mated with vasectomized males, estrous periodicity ceased for a time. Instead of regular estrous cyclicity, there was a prolonged period of diestrus, and the ovarian condition was marked by the presence of enlarged corpora lutea. This condition is known as pseudopregnancy, and it can be induced in rats not only by sterile mating but also by mechanical stimulation of the cervix with a glass rod. Cervical stimulation at an appropriate

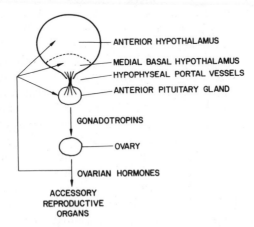

Figure 1. Schematic illustration of relationships among brain, pituitary, and ovary. (Reproduced with permission from Donovan and Harris, 1966.)

time in the estrous cycle could therefore produce a condition wherein corpora lutea are maintained over an extended period. The factors responsible for this "luteotropic" action were not known.

Selye and McKeown (1934) demonstrated that another stimulus, suckling by pups, also induced pseudopregnancy in rats, but the characteristics of the factors responsible for luteotropic action remained unknown. Considerable progress in the understanding of this problem resulted from the work of Desclin (1936) and Desclin and Grégoire (1937). Rats were ovariectomized at parturition, when new corpora lutea were just forming. In one group, suckling by pups was permitted. In this group (Group A), no castration cells appeared in the anterior pituitary glands. When animals in this group received transplants of immature ovaries under the kidney capsule, the ovarian grafts remained small, with no large follicles and no ovulation evident. Another group of rats (Group B), ovariectomized at parturition, was not exposed to the suckling stimulus. Castration cells appeared in the anterior pituitary glands of these animals, and subsequent ovarian transplants under the kidney capsule demonstrated follicular enlargement and ovulation. It was clear from these experiments that the pseudopregnant state (as in Group A) was inconsistent with the release of gonadotropins (LH and FSH) that are involved in ovarian follicular growth and rupture. The factor that maintained the corpora lutea of pseudopregnant animals seemed simultaneously to depress FSH and LH secretion.

E.B. Astwood (1941) concluded that the luteotropic factor could not be LH. Astwood reasoned that although LH induced ovulation and therefore the formation of new corpora lutea, LH did not maintain the corpora lutea once they were formed. As evidence, he cited the facts that the corpus luteum produced progesterone and that appropriately timed injections of progesterone prevented LH release and ovulation. Accordingly, an active corpus luteum should have the effect of diminishing LH secretion, and such a diminution seemed inconsistent with the conception of LH as a luteotropic substance. (Actually, later experiments were to show that LH is luteotropic in some species; see Greenwald, 1968; Ford and Yoshinaga, 1975). Astwood postulated the existence of a third trophic factor involved in reproduction and contended that this factor, in common with LH and FSH was produced by the adenohypophysis. An experiment supported this contention. Immature female rats were given pregnant's mare's serum (PMS), and they ovulated. Estrogen was injected into three groups of such females. The first group (Group A) was intact and showed mucification in the vaginal smear. The second group (Group B) was hypophysectomized and showed cornification of the vaginal smear. The third group (Group C) was hypophysectomized and given an extract of anterior pituitary. This group showed mucification of the vaginal smear. These data were interpreted as follows. In the absence of the pituitary (Group B), the exogenous estrogen acted unopposed and produced vaginal cornification. In the presence of the pituitary (Group A) or pituitary extract (Group C), progesterone of luteal origin antagonized the action of estrogen, and the vaginal smears were, as a consequence mucified, and not cornified.

If the luteotropic substance is of pituitary origin and is inversely related to FSH and LH activity, how is its secretion regulated? The first hint appeared in the work of Westman and Jacobsohn (1938). The pituitary stalk was sectioned in rats, and several hours later the cervix was stimulated. Pseudopregnancy ensued, and the authors concluded that release of hypophyseal hormone had been brought about by cervical stimulation despite previous stalk section. Desclin (1950) made further observations on pseudopregnant rats. Stilbestrol (a synthetic compound with high estrogenic activity) was shown to cause pseudopregnancy when given to normal rats at estrus, just after the formation of new corpora lutea. However, pseudopregnancy also occurred when the stilbestrol-treated rats underwent autotransplantation of the anterior pituitary gland under the kidney capsule. Desclin concluded that stilbestrol acted directly on the pituitary to induce it to secrete a luteotropic principle.

The full meaning of the work of Westman and Jacobsohn (1938) and of Desclin (1950) was not realized until the crucial studies of Everett (1954, 1956). The experiments were simple but the results and interpretation were of significance. Everett repeated the Desclin (1950) experiment with the exception that he did not treat his animals with stilbestrol or other estrogenic agents. Female rats were hypophysectomized, and the pituitary placed under the kidney capsule the day after ovulation. Three or 4 months later, the ovaries were removed. They contained very prominent, progesterone-secreting corpora lutea (indicating a luteotropic influence) and no large follicles (indicating diminished FSH and LH activity). The central concept that emerged from these experiments was that isolation of the anterior pituitary gland from the hypothalamus actually promotes release of luteotropin. The rat hypothalamus must therefore produce a factor that inhibits release of luteotropin. By removal of the anterior pituitary from the vicinity of the hypothalamus, by stalk section with an effective barrier (Nikitovitch-Winer, 1957, 1965), or by destruction of hypothalamic tissue (Nikitovitch-Winer, 1960; Chen *et al.*, 1970; Bishop *et al.*, 1971; MacLeod and Lehmeyer, 1972), this inhibition is dissipated, and the pituitary is freed to produce and secrete luteotropin.

In this brief overview, we have seen that the original proposal of a functional loop between the pituitary and the gonads (Moore and Price, 1932) suffered from certain deficiencies. The loop had to be expanded to include the hypothalamus when it was discovered that this area included neurons that produced releasing and inhibiting factors that regulate adenohypophyseal function. Further, discovery of the intimate functional relationship between the brain and the pituitary gland emphasized the potential for external environmental factors to influence the reproductive system. The introduction of the hypothalamus into the loop was such an important event in the history of endocrinology that it pushed the anterior pituitary gland (formerly known as "the master gland") into a rather subordinate position as a mere intermediary for transactions between the hypothalamus and the gonads. More recent studies have reemphasized that the pituitary has direct interactions with the gonads (see Section II.D of this chapter).

Even after addition of the hypothalamus to the ovarian regulatory loop, there were deficiencies in the basic concept of a simple push–pull relationship between the hypothalamo–hypophyseal unit and the gonads. The contribution of the hypothalamic factors to the system was, at first, thought to be primarily of a stimulatory nature. The existence of a variety of inhibitory factors (e.g., a factor that inhibits luteotropin release) of hypothalamic origin was established later. Conversely, increased levels of steroid hormones of gonadal origin were, at first, thought to exert exclusively inhibitory effects on release of gonadotropins mediated by the diencephalic–hypophyseal unit. The existence of stimulatory effects of increased steroid titers on release of gonadotropins was also demonstrated later on (see Section II.A). The potential of the diencephalic–hypophyseal unit and of the gonads to exert both inhibitory and stimulatory actions on each other complicates matters considerably. However, these additional complications help to adequately account for normal estrous or menstrual cyclicity in a way that the original push–pull model could not.

The intent of the next part of this chapter is to examine the stimulatory and inhibitory influences that exist within the functional system formed by the secretions of the diencephalon, the pituitary, and the gonads. This functional system is often referred to as the "long loop." Because of the complexity of the subject matter, we shall limit our attention primarily to diencephalic hormones that regulate only three of the pituitary hormones [LH, FSH, and luteotropic hormone (PRL*)] and to only two categories of ovarian steroid hormones (estrogens and progestins) in female mammals of reproductive age. No attempt will be made to cover, in entirety, the vast literature on this subject. Several reviews have appeared recently and should be consulted (Halász, 1972; Flerkó, 1974; Kawakami and Kimura, 1975; Sawyer, 1975; Yen *et al.*, 1975; MacLeod, 1976). Rather, attention will be focused on the strategies employed by endocrinologists to demonstrate stimulatory and inhibitory influences of blood-borne chemicals on each of the components of the long-loop system.

II. THE LONG-LOOP SYSTEM

A. General Orientation

There is ample evidence, gathered from a number of experimental paradigms, that steroid hormones suppress and stimulate the release of gonadotropic and luteotropic hormones from the pituitary. For example, the existence of inhibitory actions of steroid hormones on the release of gonadotropic hormones from the pituitary can be inferred from studies that show (a) that an increase in serum gonadotropins occurs after ovariectomy (Gay and Midgley, 1969; Brown-Grant, 1971), (b) that elevated serum gonadotropin levels in ovariectomized subjects are diminished by estrogen administration (Ramirez and McCann, 1963), (c) that appropriately timed dosages of proges-

*The discovery that "luteotropic hormone" also promoted milk secretion led to usage of the term "prolactin" for this hormone. The abbreviation of "prolactin," PRL, is now the commonly used and preferred notation for this hormone.

terone delay the occurrence of ovulation in intact, cyclic animals (Everett, 1948), and (d) that long-term administration of synthetic antiestrogens can lead to increased secretion of gonadotropins (Döcke, 1969).

The existence of stimulatory actions of steroids on gonadotropin release can be inferred from studies that show that (a) an increase in plasma estrogen levels precedes release of gonadotropic hormone necessary for ovulation in several species (Moore, et al., 1969, Corker et al., 1969; Naftolin et al., 1972; Baranczuk and Greenwald, 1973; Joshi et al., 1973; Schwartz, 1974; Shaikh and Shaikh, 1975), (b) that blockage of estrogen activity by antiestrogens or antisera to estrogen prevents the surge of gonadotropin required for ovulation (Shirley et al., 1968; Ferin et al., 1969; Labhsetwar, 1970), (c) that administration of estrogen in appropriate dosages and at appropriate times advances the onset of ovulation in mature females (Everett, 1948), (d) that appropriately timed doses of progesterone advance the occurrence of ovulation in cyclic females (Everett, 1948), and (e) that progesterone administration provokes ovulation in rats made anovulatory by exposure to continuous illumination (Everett, 1940; Mennin and Gorski, 1975).

Although these studies convincingly demonstrate the suppressive and stimulatory actions of steroids on release of pituitary hormones, they do not indicate where the steroids exert their effects. That at least some of these effects are exerted at the neural, rather than the pituitary level, was suggested by the finding that steroid effects on gonadotropin release could be suppressed by neural blocking agents (Sawyer et al., 1949; Everett and Sawyer, 1949). However, these experiments do not localize the sites of steroid action in the nervous system. In Sections II.B and II.C of this chapter, other types of experiments that are aimed at this problem will be considered. Experiments that show effects of steroids on the anterior hypothalamic–suprachiasmatic–preoptic region of the diencephalon will be discussed first (Section II.B). Next, studies that demonstrate effects of steroids on the medial basal hypothalamic area of the diencephalon will be examined (Section II.C). Finally, experiments that reconsider the possibility that gonadal steroids influence gonadotropin secretion by a direct action on the pituitary gland will be reviewed (Section II.D). These three potential targets of steroid action are depicted in Fig. 1, and the movement of the gonadal steroids to these targets may be thought of as the ascending part of the long-loop system. The descending components of the long loop may be thought of as including the actions of diencephalic hormones on the pituitary and the actions of the pituitary hormones on the gonads. These two relationships are also depicted in Fig. 1 and are described in Sections II.E and II.F, respectively.

B. Steroids Act on the Anterior Hypothalamic–Suprachiasmatic Nucleus and the Preoptic Area

The anterior hypothalamic–suprachiasmatic nucleus–preoptic area (AH–SCN–POA) of the diencephalon is not in intimate contact with the pituitary gland (Fig. 2). How, then, can steroidal influences on nerve cell bodies in

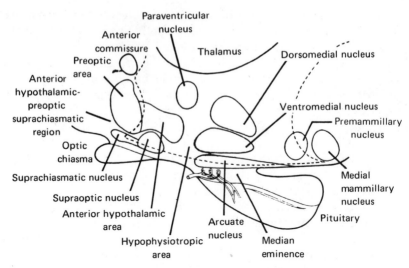

Paraventricular
nucleus

Anterior
commissure

Thalamus

Dorsomedial nucleus

Preoptic
area

Anterior
hypothalamic-
preoptic
suprachiasmatic
region

Ventromedial nucleus

Premammillary
nucleus

Optic
chiasma

Suprachiasmatic nucleus

Medial
mammillary
nucleus

Supraoptic nucleus

Anterior hypothalamic
area

Arcuate
nucleus

Pituitary

Hypophysiotropic
area

Median
eminence

Figure 2. Schematic diagram of hypothalamus. (Reproduced with permission from Levine, 1972.)

this area affect pituitary function? A reasonable hypothesis is that neurons from the AH–SCN–POA to the MBH in intact, cyclic animals. In rats, such disruption has been accomplished by knife cuts with the result that quantities of The projections may carry information relayed by neurotransmitter substances, but they may also release gonadotropin releasing hormone (GnRH, which causes release of LH and FSH) and other peptides. The sum of this information is then passed down to the pituitary where the peptidic releasing factors affect pituitary function.

A direct test of this hypothesis involves severing the neural projections from the AH–SCN–POA to the MBH in intact, cyclic animals. In rats, such disruption has been accomplished by knife cuts with the result that quantities of gonadotropin sufficient for ovulation were not released (Halász and Gorski, 1967; Kaasjager *et al.,* 1971; Blake *et al.,* 1972). Other variants of these experiments led to similar outcomes. Electrical or electrochemical stimulation of the medial POA provoked LH release in rats (Everett and Radford, 1961; Everett, 1964; Barraclough and Gorski, 1961; Cramer and Barraclough, 1971; Clemens *et al.,* 1971; Kalra *et al.,* 1971; Turgeon and Barraclough, 1973), but surgical interruption of the neural pathway from the POA to the MBH prevented this response to electrochemical stimulation (Tejasen and Everett, 1967). Lesions of the AH–SCN–POA resulted in anovulation, and estrogen treatment that stimulated a surge of LH release adequate for ovulation in intact controls failed to do so in the lesioned rats (Hillarp, 1949; Greer, 1953; Flerkó, 1954; Machida, 1971; Döcke, 1971; Bishop *et al.,* 1972a,b). A recent study suggested that electrolytic lesions limited to the medial POA did not prevent ovulation in uninjected rats, but that POA lesions that extended into the AH–SCN area prevented ovulation (Clemens *et al.,* 1976). Measurements of GnRH after a knife cut had severed the connections between AH–SCN–POA and MBH revealed a significant increment in concentration of this peptide hormone in the POA and a marked decrease of the peptide in the MBH of rats ovariectomized prior to the knife cut. These data suggest that POA neurons synthesize some GnRH and that transport of the peptide is blocked by the knife cut. Estrogen treatment of rats ovariectomized after the knife cut was made caused a pronounced increase in GnRH levels in the POA (Kalra, 1976). Araki *et al.* (1975) also demonstrated that GnRH concentration in the AH region varied as a function of estrogen secretion.

Other evidence also suggests that the AH–SCN–POA area is sensitive to steroids and helps to regulate pituitary function. Steroid sensitivity of the region is indicated by the presence of high-affinity receptors for estrogen (Pfaff and Keiner, 1973; McEwen and Pfaff, 1973; Stumpf *et al.*, 1975) and by neurophysiological recording studies that reveal a change in firing rate in the area after exposure to estrogen (Lincoln and Cross, 1967; Beyer and Sawyer, 1969; Cross, 1973; Yagi, 1973; Dufy *et al.*, 1976). Furthermore, estrogen implanted into the AH induced ovulation in immature rats (Döcke and Dörner, 1965), but the potential problem of hormone diffusion from the implant site must be kept in mind.

An additional technique to be considered here is that of measurement of thresholds to electrical stimulation in the AH–POA region in the presence of varying quantities of estrogen. For example, Quinn (1970) electrically stimulated the AH–POA region of intact, cyclic guinea pigs with biphasic pulse pairs. At a stimulating current of 1 mA, 0/10 animals at day 12 of the estrous cycle (presumably a stage of relatively low estrogen secretion) showed ovarian signs of increased gonadotropic secretion, whereas four-fifths showed such signs when 1 mA stimulation was applied at day 14 of the estrous cycle (when estrogen levels are presumably relatively high). All animals stimulated with 2 mA at days 12 and 14 of the cycle showed signs of increased gonadotropin release. Such data demonstrate that lowered thresholds to electrical stimulation in the AH–POA are consistent with elevated estradiol levels. But they do not show that estradiol caused a drop in threshold, because endogenous progesterone levels also change from the 12th to the 14th day of the guinea pig cycle. Somewhat similar types of experiments were performed by Kalra and Kalra (1974). These workers showed that electrochanical stimulation of the medial POA of 5-day cyclic rats did not elicit marked increases of LH secretion in rats during early diestrus day 3, but did elicit large increases in LH secretion on the afternoon of diestrus day 3. Because no significant change in serum progesterone levels occurred between the periods of early and later proestrus in this study, the change in responsiveness to stimulation of the medial POA probably reflected the amount of exposure to estrogen of this brain region. Spies *et al.* (1977) showed that estradiol pretreatment of ovariectomized rhesus monkeys resulted in a small, but unambiguous, facilitation of LH release (compared with ovariectomized, untreated controls) after electrical stimulation of the POA–SCN region. This study avoids the potentially confounding factor of variations in serum progesterone concentrations of ovarian origin (progesterone of adrenal origin was not ruled out) by its utilization of ovariectomized subjects.

Although the results of studies on rodents are consistent with the ideas that a neuronal system from the AH–SCN–POA region is sensitive to estrogen, converges on the MBH, and mediates release of ovulatory quotas of gonadotropins, species differences may exist. For example, controversy has been generated about the exact role of the AH–SCN–POA area in gonadotropin control in rhesus monkeys (Spies *et al.*, 1974; Knobil, 1974; Krey *et al.*, 1975).

The studies cited above are concerned primarily with actions of estrogen on the AH–SCN–POA that have consequences for release of quantities of LH adequate for ovulation. There are some studies that suggest the presence of an estrogen-sensitive system in the AH that regulates FSH secretion (Chappel and Barraclough, 1976). Knife cuts that separated the AH–SCN–POA area from the MBH suppressed FSH-dependent compensatory ovarian growth after unilateral ovariectomy in rats (Köves and Halász, 1969). Electrochemical stimulation of the POA (Clemens *et al.*, 1971) or the AH (Kalra *et al.*, 1971) caused elevation of FSH levels in rats.

Progesterone may also act on the AH–SCN–POA area, although it has been more difficult to demonstrate a progesterone uptake system than an estrogen uptake system in this region (Sar and Stumpf, 1973; Blaustein and Wade, 1978). Barraclough *et al.* (1964) showed that electrolytic lesions of the medial POA suppressed the ovulation-inducing action of progestone in rats. However, implantation of progesterone into the AH–POA failed to block ovulation in other experiments with rats (Döcke and Dörner, 1969). Ectors and Pasteels (1969) implanted progesterone into intact female rats and found that AH–POA implants caused pseudopregnancy (indicative of PRL release).

In summary, steroids have been shown to act on the AH–SCN–POA and thereby influence pituitary function.

C. Steroids Act on the Medial Basal Hypothalamus to Influence Pituitary Function

In the previous section, several experimental strategies were seen to be useful for demonstrating effects of steroids on the AH–SCN–POA region. These strategies include lesion techniques, implants of hormones in the brain, assays of GnRH, and analyses of the effects of pretreatment with steroids on electrical stimulation of the brain. The same types of methods have been used to show that steroids act on the MBH to influence pituitary function.

It had been noticed that at least some inhibitory effects of estrogen on gonadotropin release persisted after lesions of the AH–SCN–POA although stimulatory effects of estrogen were abolished (Taleisnik and McCann, 1961; Antunes-Rodrigues and McCann, 1967; Bishop *et al.*, 1972b). A logical next step was to place lesions in the MBH area caudal to the AH–SCN–POA to determine whether this would have the effect of abolishing inhibitory effects of estrogen on gonadotropin release. Bishop *et al.* (1972b) showed that such lesions of the MBH of rats prevented inhibitory actions of exogenous estrogens on gonadotropin release in ovariectomized females. However, the lesion strategy must be used with care in the MBH region. Tejasen and Everett (1967) found that bilateral cuts across the tuberal region of the MBH caused gonado-tropin release and ovulation in rats. Similarly, radiofrequency lesions of the arcuate nucleus area induced gonadotropin release, perhaps by causing abrupt release of GnRH from damaged neurons into the hypophyseal portal system (Bishop *et al.*, 1972a; Everett *et al.*, 1976; Everett and Tyrey, 1977). Thus, mechanical, or other nonspecific, damage to the MBH could conceivably lead to acute activation of the neighboring pituitary and thereby confound experi-ments designed to test the effects of steroids on the MBH region.

The closeness of the MBH to the pituitary gland also makes somewhat difficult the interpretation of steroid hormone implant studies. A number of such studies show that estrogen implants in the MBH suppressed LH and FSH release (Davidson and Sawyer, 1961; Kanematsu and Sawyer, 1964; Ramirez *et al.*, 1964; Chowers and McCann, 1967; Martini *et al.*, 1968) and stimulated PRL release (Nagasawa *et al.*, 1969). In support of these findings, receptors for estrogen (Pfaff and Keiner, 1973; McEwen and Pfaff, 1973; Stumpf *et al.*, 1975) have been found in the MBH.

Progesterone implants in the MBH have also been made in intact rats. In some studies, the implants provoked ovulation (Döcke and Dörner, 1969), whereas in others, they caused a blockade of ovulation (Dörner and Döcke, 1967). Schuiling *et al.* (1974) showed that the direction of the effect of proges-terone implanted in the MBH depends on the timing of the implant. When placed in the MBH at 1000 hr of proestrus, the progesterone provoked ovula-tion, but when placed at 1600 hr of the second day of diestrus, the progesterone blocked ovulation in rats. These authors, as well as Döcke and Dörner (1969), argue that the MBH, rather than the POA, is a crucial site of progesterone action. They consider that progesterone fails to affect secretion of gonadotro-pins in POA-lesioned rats (Barraclough *et al.*, 1964) not because the POA itself is progesterone sensitive, but because an intact POA is required to supply information to progesterone-sensitive neurons in the MBH. The issue cannot be decided by uptake studies, because progestin receptors that are saturable and translocatable to cell nuclei have been found in both the MBH area and the AH–SCN–POA of rats and guinea pigs (Sar and Stumpf, 1973; Blaustein and Wade, 1978).

A potential problem with interpretation of all of the MBH implant studies is that the implanted steroid may be carried by the hypophyseal portal system to the pituitary from the MBH and exert its effect directly on the pituitary. This problem will be considered in more detail in Section II.D of this chapter.

An effect of steroids on the MBH is also suggested, but not proven, by the fact that GnRH concentrations in this brain region fluctuate during the estrous cycle of rats (Araki *et al.*, 1975).

The effects of steroids on the outcome of electrical stimulation of the MBH have been studied. Gallo and Osland (1976) found that electrical stimulation of the arcuate nucleus of the MBH of ovariectomized rats caused inhibition of episodic LH release after electrical stimulation. On the other hand, LH release was increased in ovariectomized rhesus monkeys after electrical stimulation of the MBH, but estrogen pretreatment depressed LH release in response to electrical stimulation of the MBH (Spies *et al.*, 1977).

In summary, numerous experiments demonstrate that steroid hormones can act on the MBH region to influence gonadotropin release. The data are more convincing for estrogen than for progesterone. They generally indicate that estrogen in the MBH suppresses LH release, but there is also some evidence that estrogen implants in the MBH cause LH release (Palka *et al.*, 1966; Weick and Davidson, 1970) and that implants of antiestrogen in the MBH inhibit LH release (Billard and McDonald, 1973). Apparently, it is not only neural site but also dosage and timing factors that determine whether a steroid will have a stimulatory or an inhibitory action on pituitary hormone release.

D. Steroids Act Directly on the Anterior Pituitary

The Moore–Price (1932) theory of reproductive hormone regulation stated that gonadal hormones act on the anterior pituitary gland to regulate the activity of this gland. Although the discovery that steroid hormones of ovarian origin act on diencephalic tissues to stimulate and to inhibit release of anterior pituitary hormones did not logically rule out the possibility of direct gonadal influences on the hypophysis, this discovery, nevertheless, had the practical effect of distracting research attention from the pituitary as a site of action of ovarian hormones. Only after the role of the diencephalon in hypophyseal regulation was firmly established did investigators return their attentions to the actions of ovarian hormones on the pituitary. Among the first investigators to reassert the potential significance of gonadal effects on the pituitary were Rose and Nelson (1957) and Bogdanove (1963). These and other researchers (Chowers and McCann 1967; Ramirez *et al.*, 1964) used intrapituitary implants of estrogen to demonstrate an inhibitory effect of steroid on gonadotropins. At about the same time, Döcke and Dörner (1965) and Weick *et al.* (1971) showed that intrapituitary implants were more effective than intrahypothalamic implants of estrogen in stimulation of gonadotropin release in female rats. Implants of antiestrogen in the anterior pituitary gland were shown to inhibit gonadotropin release (Bainbridge and Labhsetwar, 1971; Billard and McDonald, 1973).

However, the proximity of the adenohypophysis to the hypothalamus made it difficult to assess whether implanted agents (a) were active at their site of implantation, (b) acted only at the level of the diencephalon to regulate release of peptide hormones that subsequently acted on the pituitary, or (c) traversed the pituitary stalk (in either direction) by diffusion and acted outside the implantation site. One aspect of the question of diffusion was addressed by Bogdanove (1964). He stated that the effects of neural implants may have been attributable to diffusion of steroids to the pituitary via the hypothalamo–hypophyseal portal system. Steroid from an implant located in the median eminence could be widely distributed by the portal vessels throughout the pituitary, whereas steroid from an intrapituitary implant might diffuse over a more limited region of the gland. The possibility that a hormone placed in the brain is actually a better "pituitary implant" than implantation of the hormone within the gland itself is known as the "implantation paradox." In view of the proximity of the hypothalamus to the pituitary, what strategies could be used to isolate the effects that steroids have directly on the pituitary?

The most obvious strategy is to incubate anterior pituitary tissue *in vitro* in the absence of hypothalamic tissue and to subject the incubates to steroid treatment. Measurements of the release of LH by pituitary implants exposed to estrogen have been made. Piacsek and Meites (1966) incubated rat pituitary tissue *in vitro* for 1 hr in the presence of estradiol and found a significant increase in LH released into the medium in the absence of hypothalamic tissue or exogenous GnRH. Schneider and McCann (1970) and Shally *et al.* (1973) also found that LH release was enhanced by estradiol pretreatment of incubated rat anterior pituitaries not exposed to GnRH. These data suggest a direct stimulatory action of estrogen on the release of LH that is independent of the action of GnRH. A direct effect of *in vivo* estrogen on LH synthesis by rat pituitaries *in vitro* has also been suggested by more recent work. Apparently, estrogen and GnRH can regulate LH synthesis by independent processes (Liu and Jackson, 1977).

Another strategy was used by McLean and Nikitovitch-Winer (1976). They showed an anatomical effect of estrogen directly on the pituitary after homografts of anterior pituitary tissue were made under the kidney capsule of hypophysectomized rats. Treatment of the rats with estrogen led to disappearance of "castration cells" in the grafts whether or not an extract that contained GnRH was administered along with the estrogen.

In addition to these studies, there is now evidence for another kind of effect of estrogen on anterior pituitary gland function. Many workers have noticed that the quantity of LH released by female rats (Cooper *et al.*, 1974a; Gordon and Reichlin, 1974; Martin *et al.*, 1974a), sheep (Reeves *et al.*, 1971a) and humans (Yen *et al.*, 1972) to a dose of GnRH is greater during late follicular than during early follicular phases of the estrous or menstrual cycle. Further examination of the problem revealed that diestrous or hypogonadal subjects released more LH in response to a given dose of exogenous GnRH when they were given appropriate estrogen treatment than when no estrogen was administered (Arimura and Schally, 1971; Reeves *et al.*, 1971b; Debeljuk *et al.*, 1972; Yen *et al.*, 1974; Martin *et al.*, 1974b; Young and Jaffe, 1976). These observations led to the supposition that estrogen acted on the anterior pituitary by increasing the sensitivity of the gland to the action of GnRH. An alternative hypothesis is that increased estrogen levels caused enhanced endogenous GnRH release and this, in turn, resulted in increased LH release. To decide whether estrogen increases sensitivity of anterior pituitary tissue to GnRH, Drouin *et al.* (1976) performed an *in vitro* experiment. They showed that preincubation of adenohypophyseal cells with 1×10^{-9} M estradiol for 10 hr decreased the concentration of GnRH required for half-maximal stimulation of LH release. Related work supports this finding (Libertun *et al.*, 1974a; Greeley *et al.*, 1975). The failure of other workers to obtain such stimulatory effects of estrogen (Schally *et al.*, 1973; Steinberger and Chowdhury, 1974; Tang and Spies, 1975) may have been the result of dosage and/or time factors in incubation. A lag period of about 10 hr occurs before an effect of estrogen on cultured pituitary cell sensitivity to GnRH is seen (Drouin *et al.*, 1976). Other factors such as age of the pituitary gland (Watkins *et al.*, 1975) and diurnal changes in pituitary responsiveness to GnRH (Debeljuk *et al.*, 1975) should also be borne in mind as potential confounding variables.

Reports of stimulatory effects of estrogen on pituitary sensitivity to GnRH and on LH release are accompanied by reports of inhibitory effects of estrogen on these parameters. For example, Negro-Vilar *et al.* (1973) found that after intravenous injection of estradiol, LH release was inhibited in ovariectomized rats for up to 4 hr after injection. Estradiol-injected, ovariectomized animals showed less pituitary responsiveness to GnRH than did controls. Other experiments demonstrated that estrogen, under specific conditions of dosage and timing, suppressed responsiveness of the rat pituitary to GnRH (Cooper *et al.*, 1974b; Schally *et al.*, 1973; Tang and Spies, 1975), and ovariectomy acutely increased responsiveness of the gland to GnRH (Cooper *et al.*, 1974c). Estrogen appears to have suppressive effects on pituitary sensitivity to GnRH in rhesus monkeys as well as rats (Spies and Norman, 1975). Some workers have brought attention to the fact that estrogen can cause either an increase or a decrease in pituitary sensitivity to GnRH in women, with the direction of effect dependent on timing and dosage factors (Yen *et al.*, 1974; Young and Jaffe, 1976). On the basis of work with the rat and human, it has been proposed that estrogen has a biphasic effect on LH release after GnRH exposure. That is, pituitary responsiveness to GnRH is at first blunted by estrogen, but after a sufficient time and appropriate dosage, pituitary responsiveness to GnRH is enhanced by estrogen (Libertun *et al.*, 1974b; Vilchez-Martinez *et al.*, 1974; Young and Jaffe, 1976).

The material presented above justifies the conclusion that estrogen is capable of exerting stimulatory and inhibitory actions directly on pituitary tissue involved in LH release. Many of the reports cited in support of this view also contain evidence that estrogen has direct actions on pituitary tissue involved in FSH release, and a few separate studies indicate such actions on the PRL system.

For the FSH system, it was noted that an extract that contained GnRH caused more FSH release *in vitro* from rat pituitaries taken at proestrus than from pituitaries taken at diestrus (Cooper *et al.*, 1974a). However, no cycle-dependent difference of this type was found for FSH *in vitro* in the same study. Intravenous injection of estrogen partially suppressed FSH responsiveness to GnRH *in vivo* at about 2 hr after injection but increased FSH in response to GnRH at 10 hr after estrogen injection. A biphasic action of estrogen at the pituitary level for the FSH system is suggested by these data (Libertun *et al.*,

1974b). In related studies with rats, it was found that ovariectomy acutely increased FSH response to GnRH *in vivo* and *in vitro* (Cooper *et al.,* 1974c) and that estrogen caused decreases in basal release of FSH and in FSH release in response to GnRH when explanted pituitaries were tested (Schally *et al.,* 1973).

In vitro experiments with ewe pituitaries showed that addition of low concentrations (10^{-11} to 10^{-9} M) of estradiol to the medium caused decreases in FSH production within 6 hr after treatment. Withdrawal of estrogen from the medium led to resumption of higher levels of FSH production, as in controls (Miller *et al.,* 1977). No stimulatory actions of estrogen on FSH synthesis were found in this study with ewe pituitaries.

In humans, there is some evidence for both stimulatory and inhibitory effects of estrogen on the FSH system at the pituitary level. For example, augmentation of FSH release was observed after estradiol benzoate treatment for 6 days, but the augmentation did not occur in the same dose-dependent fashion as for LH (Young and Jaffe, 1976). In another study with women, chronic administration of small doses of ethinyl estradiol blunted FSH release in response to a GnRH challenge (Yen *et al.,* 1974). Generally, the data on estrogen–FSH interrelationships at the pituitary as well as at the diencephalic level are less clear than corresponding data for estrogen–LH interrelationships.

For the PRL system, there is *in vivo* and *in vitro* evidence for direct estrogenic action at the pituitary level. Kanematsu and Sawyer (1963) implanted estrogen into the pituitary of intact rabbits. This procedure stimulated lactation and resulted in a slight decrease in pituitary PRL content. These effects were considered to demonstrate that estrogen acts on the pituitary to promote PRL release. In another *in vivo* experiment, Chen *et al.* (1970) ovariectomized and hypophysectomized female rats and placed pituitary transplants (ranging from no pituitaries to four pituitaries per transplant) under the kidney capsule. The animals were given estrogen treatment for 5 days, and PRL serum levels were measured. There was a positive correlation between amount of pituitary tissue transplanted and amount of PRL secreted under estrogen stimulation. These results were supported by the work of Desclin and Koulischer (1969). Although these *in vivo* experiments suggested an estrogenic action at the pituitary level, *in vitro* experiments gave more conclusive evidence on this point.

Nicoll and Meites (1962) were the first to show that explanted rat pituitaries responded to estradiol with an increase in production of PRL. More recently, Haug and Gautvik (1976) demonstrated that a clonal strain of pituitary tumor cells exposed to concentrations of estradiol in the physiological range displayed as much as a 300% increase in PRL production after 10 days of exposure. The increased PRL was caused by synthesis of new PRL because the clonal cells do not contain significant stores of PRL. Removal of estrogen from the incubation medium resulted in a decline in PRL production within 5 days. As the authors state, the results with a tumor cell line should be validated for normal pituitary tissue.

The finding that there are direct effects of estrogen on the anterior pituitary gland secretion of gonadotropins and PRL fits well with the observation that the pituitary contains an effective estrogen-concentrating system that is saturable and that is able to translocate estrogen to pituitary cell nuclei (Eisenfeld, 1970; Notides, 1970; McEwen, 1976).

An uptake system of equal magnitude does not appear to exist for progesterone in the anterior pituitary,* but progesterone is said to influence secretion of gonadotropins and PRL by action at the pituitary level. On the basis of *in vivo* experiments, progesterone has been claimed to act at the pituitary level to suppress responsiveness of the gland to GnRH (Spies *et al.,* 1969; Arimura and Schally, 1970; Hilliard *et al.,* 1971). For example. Hilliard *et al.* (1971) infused GnRH directly into the adenohypophyses of estrous rabbits. This resulted in LH release and, consequently, ovulation. When progesterone was administered 16–19 hr prior to GnRH, ovulation was blocked in 70% of cases. Higher doses of GnRH or an injection of estrogen ameliorated this suppressive effect of progesterone. The investigators concluded that progesterone inhibits anterior pituitary sensitivity to GnRH. Because an increased dosage of GnRH induced ovulation, they also concluded that the principal site of progesterone action on the LH release system was at the hypothalamic rather than the pituitary level. This type of experiment is difficult to interpret. The progesterone may have its suppressive effect at the level of the ovary rather than the pituitary. That is, progesterone may have inhibited ovarian estrogen secretion, with a resultant decrease in GnRH release, or it may have decreased ovarian responsiveness to LH. Progesterone may also have caused some change in peripheral metabolism of estrogen secreted by the ovary, with diminution of estrogenic activity as a consequence. Or the progesterone may have acted at the brain or pituitary level to antagonize some aspect of estrogen action in these areas. All of these alternative explanations are consistent with the finding of Hilliard *et al.* (1971) that injection of estrogen overrode the suppressive action of progesterone on LH release. This highlights a major exception to the principle proposed by Moore and Price (1932) that steroid–steroid interactions do not account for regulation of reproductive hormone secretion. Progesterone is a steroid hormone whose effects very much depend on how much, and for how long, hypothalamo–hypophyseal tissue has been exposed to estrogen. Thus, even if progesterone does have effects at the pituitary level, these effects may be indirect in the sense that they reflect blockade of the activity of estrogen-sensitive systems.

In vitro pituitary studies of the effects of progesterone on gonadotropins circumvent some, but not all of the objections, to the *in vivo* studies. Schally *et al.* (1973) found that high doses of progesterone in the absence of exogenous estrogen were required to partially inhibit LH and FSH release from pituitary explants in response to a GnRH challenge. Further studies suggested that

---

*Receptors for progesterone in the anterior pituitary have been demonstrated, however (Kato, J., and Onouchi, T., 1979, Nuclear progesterone receptors and characterization of cytosol receptors in the rat hypothalamus and anterior hypophysis, *J. Steroid Biochem.* **11**:845.

metabolic derivatives of progesterone, such as 20α-dihydroprogesterone, augment pituitary responsiveness to GnRH *in vitro* (Tang and Spies, 1975) and that 17α-hydroxyprogesterone and 5α-dihydroprogesterone were more effective suppressants of pituitary GnRH responsiveness *in vitro* than progesterone (Schally *et al.*, 1973). The potential importance of the 5α-dihydro derivative in neuroendocrine function has been emphasized by Karavolas and associates who have demonstrated the presence of 5α-reductase for progesterone in pituitary and the selective accumulation of 5α-dihydroprogesterone in anterior pituitary tissue (Karavolas and Nuti, 1976; Nuti and Karavolas, 1977).

Progesterone, or perhaps a metabolite of it, also causes a dose-related decrease in PRL production by rat pituitary cells in culture in the absence of exogenous estrogen and causes suppression of the stimulatory effect of estrogen on PRL production in the same preparation (Haug and Gautvik, 1976).

To summarize this section, there is evidence for direct stimulatory and inhibitory effects of estrogen and progesterone at the level of the pituitary.

E. Hypothalamic Hormones Affect Pituitary Hormones

The first part of the descending portion of the long-loop system (Fig. 1) that is to be considered is the effect of hypothalamic hormones on pituitary hormones. In view of the extensive treatment of hypothalamic hormones in the chapter by McCann (Chapter 13), only a cursory examination of some studies of this subject will be given here.

Hypothalamic hormones have two types of effects on pituitary hormones. They affect the release of pituitary hormones, and they affect the synthesis of pituitary hormones.

1. Actions of Hypothalamic Hormones on Release of Pituitary Hormones

Evidence that hypothalamic hormones affect the release of trophic hormones from the pituitary has been gathered by using *in vivo* and *in vitro* strategies. For example, Nikitovitch-Winer (1962) infused hypothalamic extracts that contained releasing hormone into the pituitaries of rats and observed gonadotropin release as reflected by the occurrence of ovulation. In more recent work, antiserum to GnRH suppressed discharge of LH in rodents (Koch *et al.*, 1973; Arimura *et al.*, 1974; Kerdelhué *et al.*, 1975; de la Cruz *et al.*, 1976) and monkeys (McCormack *et al.*, 1977). Infusion of GnRH into proestrous rats whose normal preovulatory surge of gonadotropic hormones had been blocked by a barbituate caused release of LH (Blake, 1976a) and FSH (Blake, 1976b).

This *in vivo* evidence is supported by *in vitro* work in which anterior pituitaries were subjected to the addition of various releasing hormone preparations to the medium. Thus, when Crighton *et al.* (1969) placed rat pituitaries *in vitro* and dosed them with GnRH, they found increased release of LH into the medium. In more recent studies, rat pituitary fragments superfused with pulses of GnRH released LH in a pulsatile manner (Serra and Midgley, 1970; Osland *et al.,* 1975). Synthetic antagonists of GnRH were shown to suppress release of LH by rat anterior pituitary glands *in vitro* (Labrie *et al.,* 1976a).

For the PRL system, there is also evidence that at least one hypothalamic hormone affects release of PRL. Nicoll (1971) summarized data that show significant release of PRL when the rodent pituitary is isolated *in vitro* and freed from the effects of a hypothalamic hormone that inhibits PRL secretion. When hypothalamic extract is placed *in vitro* with the anterior pituitary gland, a decrease in PRL released into the medium is observed (Pasteels, 1961; Talwalker *et al.,* 1963). Aside from the well-established and predominantly inhibitory effects of the hypothalamus on PRL secretion, there is some evidence for a hypothalamic factor that favors release of PRL from the pituitary in mammals (Nicoll, 1971; MacLeod, 1976). Interestingly, thyrotropin releasing hormone (TRH) is one factor that can induce PRL release (MacLeod, 1976).

2. Effects of Hypothalamic Hormones on Synthesis of Pituitary Hormones

Several lines of evidence suggest that hypothalamic hormones affect the synthesis of pituitary hormones. Among the paradigms that have been used to demonstrate this point are the following. The anterior pituitaries of intact female rats were explanted and dosed with GnRH over a period of 3 days. The finding that the total amount of LH in medium plus tissue was greater for GnRH-dosed pituitaries than for control pituitaries indicated that GnRH caused synthesis of LH (Mittler *et al.,* 1970). A second paradigm is illustrated by an experiment of Corbin and Daniels (1968). These investigators gave a single dose of crude hypothalamic extract to rats with lesions in the median eminence. The extract caused a depletion of pituitary FSH within 45 min because FSH was released from the pituitary. However, if a second injection of hypothalamic extract was then given, FSH levels in the pituitary returned to normal sooner than if a second injection were not administered. This suggests that synthesis of FSH was induced by the second injection of hypothalamic extract. A third approach to the problem of whether synthesis of gonadotropins was caused by hypothalamic hormones is illustrated by the work of Evans and Nikitovitch-Winer (1969). These authors noted that the pituitary loses functional capacity and undergoes cytological changes when it is transplanted to a site distant from the hypothalamus (e.g., under the kidney capsule). They reasoned that if a lack of hypothalamic hormone were responsible for the deterioration of the transplanted pituitary, it should be possible to reactivate transplanted pituitaries by continuously infusing them with hypothalamic extracts. When infusion was performed, pituitary function returned, as reflected by the presence of large ovarian follicles and secretion of estrogen in quantities sufficient to cause vaginal cornification. Apparently, the infused hypothalamic extract reinstated the ability of the transplanted pituitary to synthesize gonadotropins.

More recent work has emphasized that another potentially important action of GnRH is to sensitize the pituitary to subsequent exposure to GnRH. In these recent experiments, it has been shown that there is increased pituitary responsiveness to a second injection of GnRH given 1 hr after the first injection on the day of proestrus in rats (Aiyer *et al.*, 1973; Castro-Vasquez and McCann, 1975). It is conceivable that the first GnRH injection increases "the synthesis of a readily releasable pool of LH so that the response to the second injection is enhanced" (Castro-Vasquez and McCann, 1975).

In summary, there is evidence that hormones released from the hypothalamus influence both the synthesis and secretion of pituitary hormones. They may do so via the mediation of cyclic AMP (Labrie *et al.*, 1976b) and prostaglandins (McCann *et al.*, 1976).

F. Pituitary Hormones Act on Gonadal Tissue

Early evidence that the pituitary gland is important for the maintenance of the gonads was provided by the studies of Smith and Engle (1927) and Moore and Price (1932). More recent studies have used techniques such as intrafollicular injection or implants of pituitary hormones in ovarian bursae (Liao *et al.*, 1974) to demonstrate effects of these compounds on ovarian morphology. At least some of the morphological effects of gonadotropins (e.g., induction of follicular rupture) may be exerted through a mechanism that is independent of steroidogenesis (Bullock and Kappauf, 1973).

The nature of the interaction between pituitary hormones and the steroidogenic properties of the ovary has received attention from biochemists. Several studies have shown that follicular granulosa cells (Kammerman *et al.*, 1972) and luteal cells (Lunenfeld and Eshkol, 1967; Lee and Ryan, 1971; Han *et al.*, 1974) possess receptors on their plasma membranes that are specific for LH or human chorionic gonadotropin. FSH binds exclusively to granulosa cells (Rajaniemi and Vanha-Perttula, 1972). The concentration of LH and FSH receptors in rat ovaries is regulated, at least in part, by estrogens, LH, and FSH (Richards *et al.*, 1976). The manner in which steroidogenesis is induced by gonadotropins may be complex. Several authors have offered evidence from *in vitro* studies that LH stimulates the enzymatic steps between cholesterol and pregnenolone (Ichii *et al.*, 1963; Savard *et al.*, 1965; Koritz and Hall, 1965) and liberates cholesterol from its esters (Armstrong, 1968). However, other authors have evidence that gonadotropins also act at an earlier stage of steroidogenesis by stimulating conversion of acetyl-CoA to cholesterol (Morris and Gorski, 1973) and at a later stage of steroidogenesis by stimulating conversion of androgens to estrogens (Hollander and Hollander, 1958).

In addition to the stimulatory effects of gonadotropins on steroidogenesis, Katz and Armstrong (1976) and Hillensjö *et al.* (1976) have presented *in vivo* and *in vitro* evidence that exogenous LH inhibits the production of ovarian androgens and estrogens in rats. Similar findings were reported for sheep (Moor, 1974).

There may also be multiple sites of action of PRL in the steroid metabolic pathway. When pseudopregnant rats were hypophysectomized, the levels of enzymes involved in synthesis of cholesterol esters and in liberation of cholesterol from cholesterol esters fell. Prolactin treatment caused increased activity of these enzyme systems (Behrman *et al.*, 1970). But PRL may have another important site of action on ovarian luteal cells. Armstrong *et al.* (1970) showed that PRL inhibited the conversion of luteal progesterone to the relatively inactive metabolite, 20α-dihydroprogesterone. From their *in vitro* data, these authors were able to conclude that although total progestin synthesis in pseudopregnant rats does not depend on PRL, this trophic hormone plays a role in suppressing the conversion of progesterone to less active metabolites.

The manner in which the pituitary hormones signal the ovary to alter its steroid production has been the subject of much recent research. There now seems little question that LH and FSH stimulate the production of cyclic AMP in ovarian tissue (Marsh *et al.*, 1972; Kolena and Channing, 1972; Ling and Marsh, 1977). Luteinizing hormone or human chorionic gonadotropin also stimulate the production of prostaglandins in ovarian tissue (Chasalow and Pharriss, 1972; LeMaire *et al.*, 1973). Furthermore, in the absence of LH, steroidogenesis can be induced in gonadal tissue by cyclic AMP (Dorrington and Kilpatrick, 1969) or by prostaglandin (Speroff and Ramwell, 1970). These data have led to the idea that cyclic AMP (Ling and Marsh, 1977) and prostaglandin (Kuehl *et al.*, 1970) are essential intermediaries in the stimulation of steroidogenesis by gonadotropins. The data appear to be stronger for cyclic AMP than for prostaglandin (Kolena and Channing, 1972).

With this discussion of pituitary hormone effects on the ovary, we complete consideration of the long-loop system. However, it should be emphasized that there are several interactions in the long-loop system that we have not even touched on. For example, androgens of ovarian origin undoubtedly play a role in this loop (Gay and Tomacari, 1974). Nonsteroidal compounds of ovarian origin ("inhibin-like factors") may affect gonadotropins (Welschen *et al.*, 1977). Steroids of adrenal origin (Parkes and Deanesly, 1966b) as well as thyroidal hormones (Brown-Grant, 1956) are capable of affecting ovarian and hypophyseal function. Extrahypothalamic neural tissues are affected by steroid hormones and help to modulate gonadotropin discharge (Donovan, 1971; Taleisnik and Beltramino, 1975). There is a minute-to-minute regulation of pituitary hormone release by ovarian steroids (Naftolin and McInnes, 1977), and these short-term interactions are building blocks for long-term regulation of estrous and menstrual cyclicity. These issues, as well as the nature of the long-loop system for reproduction in males, require extensive treatment in future chapters. Until this point, the present chapter has attempted only to illustrate some of the experimental strategies and paradigms that endocrinologists have utilized to demonstrate the existence of a long-loop system that regulates cyclicity in female mammals.

The remaining sections of this chapter will deal with other control systems that are of potential value as regulators of female reproductivie cyclicity. These include regulation of hypothalamic secretions by hypophyseal hormones (short-loop system) and autoregulation of hypothalamic secretions and of ovarian activity (ultrashort systems).

III. PITUITARY HORMONES AFFECT PITUITARY HORMONE SECRETION—THE SHORT-LOOP SYSTEM

Fairly recent research suggests that the pituitary hormones are capable of regulating pituitary function. The technique that is used to demonstrate this potential control mechanism consists of implanting gonadotropic hormones in the brain and measuring gonadotropin concentrations in the pituitary or blood plasma. For example, implants of LH in the median eminence caused a 33% decrease in pituitary LH of ovariectomized rats and a 51% decrease in intact rats. Implants of other trophic hormones such as ACTH in the median eminence did not suppress pituitary LH concentrations (Corbin, 1966; Corbin and Cohen, 1966).

Similar types of studies have been carried out with FSH. Implantation of FSH in the median eminence reduced pituitary FSH concentrations (Corbin and Story, 1967; Arai and Gorski, 1968; Fraschini *et al.*, 1968; Motta *et al.*, 1969) and also reduced FSH-RH activity in the hypothalamus of adult rats (Corbin *et al.*, 1970). There is some indirect evidence that in immature female rats, implantation of FSH in the MBH results in an increase of FSH secretion (Ojeda and Ramirez, 1969).

Prolactin may also participate in the regulation of its own secretion. Injection of PRL into intact rats or transplantation of additional pituitary glands into ectopic sites in intact rats led to decreases in pituitary PRL content (Chen *et al.*, 1967; Mena *et al.*, 1968; Sinha and Tucker, 1968). Implants of PRL into the median eminence or the MBH caused a decrease in PRL secretion and a cessation of PRL-dependent processes such as pseudopregnancy and lactation in rats (Clemens and Meites, 1968; Voogt and Meites, 1971).

It is presumed that trophic hormones influence their own secretion by a short-loop mechanism. That is, trophic hormones produced by the pituitary reach the MBH and somehow signal the MBH to alter its synthesis or release of the peptide hormone that corresponds to the trophic hormone. The way in which hormone from the pituitary reaches the MBH may be by traveling upward towards the hypothalamus (Török, 1964; Bergland *et al.*, 1977; Oliver *et al.*, 1977) even though the major direction of flow in this system is downward.

The physiological significance of this type of control system for secretion of pituitary hormones has not been accurately evaluated. Despite the many experimental demonstrations of a short-loop control system, it is not known whether the threshold for operation of such a system is so far in excess of the threshold for operation of the long-loop control system as to render the short-loop system virtually inoperative during the course of a normal estrous or menstrual cycle.

IV. RELEASING FACTORS AFFECT RELEASING FACTOR PRODUCTION—THE ULTRASHORT LOOP

In order to demonstrate an effect of releasing factors on their own synthesis and/or release, it is necessary to remove the gonads and pituitary of the experimental subject. After this surgery, the long loop and short loop are no longer existent, and all that remains is a potential "ultrashort" loop. That is, releasing factor produced in the hypothalamus may act on this same tissue to inhibit further production of the factor. Martini and colleagues have shown that castrated, hypophysectomized rats injected systemically with a hypothalamic extract containing FSH-releasing properties showed significant decrements in their hypothalamic contents of GnRH (Fraschini *et al.*, 1968).

If there is uncertainty about the physiological significance of a short-loop system between the pituitary and the hypothalamus that controls releasing factor activity, at least the same doubt should be expressed about the physiological significance of an ultrashort control system within the hypothalamus. The ability of exogenous, excess quantities of releasing factor to inhibit further synthesis of the same releasing factor demonstrates only that the potential for an ultrashort control system exists. Proof of the value of an ultrashort control system to a normal animal requires that the system be shown to be operative within the limits of normal secretion of releasing factors. It should be noted that there is evidence for the ability of the hypothalamus to selectively concentrate and metabolize GnRH (Vaala and Knigge, 1974; Griffiths *et al.*, 1974; Corbin and Beattie, 1976).

V. OVARIAN HORMONES AFFECT THE OVARY

Despite the emphasis of Moore and Price (1932) on the principle that gonadal hormones do not affect the gonads in a direct fashion, there are several studies, some of them quite old, that indicate the existence of such direct effects.

One approach that demonstrated direct effects of ovarian hormones on ovarian function consisted of direct application of estrogen to one ovary of the immature rat. Such unilateral treatment led to increased ovarian weight, formation of corpora lutea, and increased sensitivity to gonadotropins in the ovary to which estrogen was applied locally as compared with the contralateral ovary (Bradbury, 1961).

Another approach to the problem is typified by studies that used hypophysectomized animals injected with estrogenic agents. Hypophysectomy deprives the animals of LH, FSH, and PRL and erases the influence of the hypothalamic peptide hormones that regulate secretion of these three trophic hormones. It has been found that estrogens act on the follicles and tend to prevent some of the regressive changes in the ovary that otherwise set in after hypophysectomy (Williams, 1945; Desclin, 1949). Interestingly, these effects of estrogen were negated when androgen was given simultaneously with estrogen to hypophysectomized rats (Payne *et al.*, 1956). This result is reminiscent of the ideas about direct estrogen–androgen antagonisms expressed by Steinach and Lipschütz at the turn of the century.

In hypophysectomized, pseudopregnant rabbits, there is evidence that estrogen acts to prolong the life of the corpora lutea (Robson, 1937; Westman and Jacobsohn, 1937b).

These data on direct effects of ovarian steroids on ovarian function are supported by the finding that the ovary contains receptors for estrogen (Stumpf, 1969; Richards, 1974, 1975). In a sense, these direct effects represent another ultrashort-loop system. There is no simple statement that can be made about the relative importance of this system in the control of reproduction because this would probably vary according to compartment of the ovary (follicles, corpora lutea, interstitial tissue) and according to species. Thus, direct effects of estrogens on follicular growth in hypophysectomized rats are overshadowed by the effects of pituitary hormones in intact rats. On the other hand, estrogenic stimulation of corpus luteum activity in rabbits may be a normal feature of reproductive function in this species (Keyes and Nalbandov, 1967).

VI. CONCLUSIONS

A long-loop regulatory system that consists of monitoring and secretory components in the diencephalon, anterior pituitary, and ovary appears to be primarily responsible for cyclic reproductive changes in female mammals. These components exert both stimulatory and inhibitory actions on each other. Shorter regulatory loops may also contribute to the modulation of reproductive function. There are mechanisms for regulation between the pituitary and the hypothalamus (short-loop system) and within the hypothalamus (ultrashort-loop system).

The primary purpose of this chapter has been to introduce the reader to a variety of strategies that can be used to demonstrate reactions to hormonal stimuli within individual components of the hypothalamo–hypophyseal–ovarian axis. Several authors have used concepts derived from cybernetics and control system theory to gain an integrated picture of how these individual reactions are interrelated during the course of normal female reproductive cycles (see Brown-Grant, 1976, for references). The next chapter will deal with these and other attempts at synthesis. For this reason, the jargon of control system theory (e.g., "negative and positive feedback") has been avoided as much as possible in the present discussion (see Davidson, 1969, for a discussion of the appropriateness of the use of engineering terms in biology).

ACKNOWLEDGMENTS. I thank Dr. J. W. Everett for his careful reading of the manuscript and his expert criticisms. Dr. B. L. Nock and Dr. C. Williams also read and commented on the manuscript, and their suggestions were very helpful. I am grateful to Ms. M. B. Grabon, W. Cunningham, and C. Banas for preparation of the manuscript. The author receives support from NIH Research Grant HD-04467 and NIMH Research Scientist Development Award K2-29006. Contribution Number 298 of the Institute of Animal Behavior.

REFERENCES

Aiyer, M. S., Chiappa, S. A., Fink, G., and Greig, F., 1973, A priming effect of luteinizing hormone releasing factor on the anterior pituitary gland in the female rat, *J. Physiol. (Lond.)* **234**:81P.

Antunes-Rodrigues, J., and McCann, S. M., 1967, Effect of suprachiasmatic lesions on the regulation of luteinizing hormone secretion in the female rat, *Endocrinology* **81**:666.

Arai, Y., and Gorski, R. A., 1968, Inhibition of ovarian compensatory hypertrophy by hypothalamic implantation of gonadotrophin in androgen-sterilized rats: Evidence for internal feedback, *Endrocrinology* **82**:871.

Araki, S., Ferin, M., Zimmerman, E. A., and Vande Wiele, R. L., 1975, Ovarian modulation of immunoreactive gonadotropin-releasing hormone (Gn-RH) in the rat brain: Evidence for a differential effect on the anterior and mid-hypothalamus, *Endocrinology* **96**:644.

Arimura, A., and Schally, A. V., 1970, Progesterone suppression of LH-releasing hormone-induced stimulation of LH-release in rats, *Endocrinology* **87**:653.

Arimura, A., and Schally, A. V., 1971, Augmentation of pituitary responsiveness to LH-releasing hormone (LH-RH) by estrogen, *Proc. Soc. Exp. Biol. Med.* **136**:290.

Arimura, A., Debeljuk, L., and Schally, A. V., 1974, Blockade of the preovulatory surge of LH and FSH and of ovulation by anti-LH-RH serum in rats, *Endocrinology* **95**:323.

Armstrong, D. T., 1968, Gonadotropins, ovarian metabolism, and steroid biosynthesis, *Recent Prog. Horm. Res.* **24**:255.

Armstrong, D. T., and Dorrington, J. H., 1976, Androgens augment FSH-induced progesterone secretion by cultured rat granulosa cells, *Endocrinology* **99**:1411.

Armstrong, D. T., Knudsen, K. A., and Miller, L. S., 1970, Effects of prolactin upon cholesterol metabolism and progesterone biosynthesis in corpora lutea of rats hypophysectomized during pseudopregnancy, *Endocrinology* **86**:634.

Astwood, E. B., 1941, The regulation of corpus luteum function by hypophyseal luteotrophin, *Endocrinology* **28**:309.

Bainbridge, J. G., and Labhsetwar, A. P., 1971, The role of oestrogens in spontaneous ovulation: Location of site of action of positive feedback of oestrogen by intracranial implantation of the anti-oestrogen ICI 46474, *J. Endocrinol.* **50**:321.

Baranczuk, R., and Greenwald, G. S., 1973, Peripheral levels of estrogen in the cyclic hamster, *Endocrinology* **92**:805.

Barraclough, C. A., and Gorski, R. A., 1961, Evidence that the hypothalamus is responsible for androgen-induced sterility in the female rat, *Endocrinology* **68**:68.

Barraclough, C. A., Yrarrazaval, S., and Hatton, R., 1964, A possible hypothalamic site of action of progesterone in the facilitation of ovulation in the rat, *Endocrinology* **75**:838.

Behrman, H. R., Orczyk, G. P., MacDonald, G. J., and Greep, R. O., 1970, Prolactin induction of enzymes controlling luteal cholesterol ester turnover, *Endocrinology* **87**:1251.

Bergland, R. M., Davis, S. L., and Page, R. B., 1977, Pituitary secretes to brain—Experiments in sheep, *Lancet* **2**:276.

Beyer, C., and Sawyer, C. H., 1969, Hypothalamic unit activity related to control of the pituitary gland, in: *Frontiers in Neuroendocrinology, 1969* (W. F. Ganong and L. Martini, eds.), pp. 255–288, Oxford University Press, New York.

Billard, R., and McDonald, P. G., 1973, Inhibition of ovulation in the rat by intrahypothalamic implants of an antioestrogen, *J. Endocrinol.* **56**:585.

Bishop, W., Krulich, L., Fawcett, C. P., and McCann, S. M., 1971, The effect of median eminence (ME) lesions on plasma levels of FSH, LH and prolactin in the rat, *Proc. Soc. Exp. Biol. Med.* **136**:925.

Bishop, W., Fawcett, C. P., Krulich, L., and McCann, S. M., 1972a, Acute and chronic effects of hypothalamic lesions on the release of FSH, LH and prolactin in intact and castrated rats, *Endocrinology* **91**:643.

Bishop, W., Kalra, P. S., Fawcett, C. P., Krulich, L., and McCann, S. M., 1972b, The effects of hypothalamic lesions on the release of gonadotropins and prolactin in response to estrogen and progesterone treatment in female rats, *Endocrinology,* **91**:1404.

Blake, C. A., 1976a, Simulation of the proestrous luteinizing hormone (LH) surge after infusion of LH-releasing hormone in phenobarbital-blocked rats, *Endocrinology* **98**:451.

Blake, C. A., 1976b, Simulation of the early phase of proestrous follicle-stimulating hormone rise after infusion of luteinizing hormone-releasing hormone in phenobarbital-blocked rats, *Endocrinology* **98**:461.

Blake, C. A., Weiner, R. I., and Sawyer, C. H., 1972, Pituitary prolactin secretion in female rats made persistently estrous or diestrous by hypothalamic deafferentation, *Endocrinology* **90**:862.

Blaustein, J. D., and Wade, G. N., 1978, Progestin binding by brain and pituitary cell nuclei and female rat sexual behavior, *Brain Res.* **140**:360.

Bogdanove, E. M., 1963, Direct gonad–pituitary feedback: An analysis of effects of intracranial estrogenic depots on gonadotrophin secretion, *Endocrinology* **73**:696.

Bogdanove, E. M., 1964, The role of the brain in the regulation of pituitary gonadotrophin secretion, *Vitam. Horm.* **22**:205.

Bradbury, J. T., 1961, Direct action of estrogen on the ovary of the immature rat, *Endocrinology* **68**:115.

Brown-Grant, K., 1956, Gonadal function and thyroid activity, *J. Physiol. (Lond.)* **131**:70.

Brown-Grant, K., 1966, Regulation and control in the endocrine system, in: *Regulation and Control in Living Systems* (H. Kalmus, ed.), pp. 176–255, John Wiley and Sons, New York.

Brown-Grant, K., 1971, The role of steroid hormones in the control of gonadotropin in adult female mammals, in: *Steroid Hormones and Brain Function* (C. H. Sawyer and R. A. Gorski, eds.), pp. 269–288, University of California Press, Berkeley.

Brown-Grant, K., 1976, Control of gonadotropin secretion, in: *Subcellular Mechanisms in Reproductive Neuroendocrinology* (F. Naftolin, K. J., Ryan, and I. J. Davies, eds.), pp. 485–502, Elsevier, Amsterdam.

Bullock, D. W., and Kappauf, B. H., 1973, Dissociation of gonadotropin-induced ovulation and steroidogenesis in immature rats, *Endocrinology,* **92**:1625.

Burrows, H., 1949, *Biological Actions of Sex Hormones, 2nd Edition,* Cambridge University Press, New York.

Cannon, W. B., 1932, *The Wisdom of the Body,* W. W. Norton, New York.

Castro-Vazquez, A., and McCann, S. M., 1975, Cyclic variations in the increased responsiveness of the pituitary to luteinizing hormone-releasing hormone (LHRH) induced by LHRH, *Endocrinology,* **97**:13.

Chappel, S. C., and Barraclough, C. A., 1976, Hypothalamic regulation of pituitary FSH secretion, *Endocrinology* **98**:927.

Chasalow, F. I., and Pharriss, B. B., 1972, Luteinizing hormone stimulation of ovarian prostaglandin biosynthesis, *Prostaglandins* **1**:107.

Chen, C. L., Minaguchi, H., and Meites, J., 1967, Effects of transplanted pituitary tumors on host pituitary prolactin secretion, *Proc. Soc. Exp. Biol. Med.* **126**:317.

Chen, C. L., Amenomori, Y., Lu, K. H., Voogt, J., and Meites, J., 1970, Serum prolactin levels in rats with pituitary implants or hypothalamic lesions, *Neuroendocrinology* **6**:220.

Chowers, I., and McCann, S. M., 1967, Comparisons of the effect of hypothalamic and pituitary implants of estrogen and testosterone on reproductive system and adrenal of female rats, *Proc. Soc. Exp. Biol. Med.* **124:**260.

Clemens, J. A., and Meites, J., 1968, Inhibition by hypothalamic prolactin implants of prolactin secretion, mammary growth and luteal function, *Endocrinology,* **82:**878.

Clemens, J. A., Shaar, C. J., Kleber, J. W., and Tandy, W. A., 1971, Areas of the brain stimulatory to LH and FSH secretion, *Endocrinology* **88:**180.

Clemens, J. A., Smalstig, E. B., and Sawyer, B. D., 1976, Studies on the role of the preoptic area in the control of reproductive function in the rat, *Endocrinology,* **99:**728.

Cooper, K. J., Fawcett, C. P., and McCann, S. M., 1974a, Variations in pituitary responsiveness to a luteinizing hormone/follicle stimulating hormone releasing factor (LH-RF/FSH-RF) preparation during the rat estrous cycle, *Endocrinology* **95:**1293.

Cooper, K. J., Fawcett, C. P., and McCann, S. M., 1974b, Inhibitory and facilitatory effects of estradiol-17β on pituitary responsiveness to a luteninizing hormone–follicle stimulating hormone releasing factor (LH-RF/FSH-RF) preparation in the ovariectomized rat, *Proc. Soc. Exp. Biol. Med.* **145:**1422.

Cooper, K. J., Fawcett, C. P., and McCann, S. M., 1974c, Augmentation of pituitary responsiveness to luteinizing hormone/follicle stimulating hormone-releasing factor (LH-RF) as a result of acute ovariectomy in the four-day cyclic rat, *Endocrinology* **96:**1123.

Corbin, A., 1966, Pituitary and plasma LH of ovariectomized rats with median eminence implants of LH, *Endocrinology* **78:**893.

Corbin, A., and Beattie, C. W., 1976, Effect of luteinizing hormone releasing hormone (LHRH) and an LHRH antagonist of hypothalamic and plasma LHRH of hypophysectomized rats, *Endocrinology* **98:**247.

Corbin, A., and Cohen, A. I., 1966, Effect of median eminence implants of LH on pituitary LH of female rats, *Endocrinology* **78:**41.

Corbin, A., and Daniels, E. L., 1968, Preliminary indications for the presence of a hypothalamic follicle stimulating hormone synthesizing factor. *Experientia* **24:**1260.

Corbin, A., and Story, J. C., 1967, "Internal" feedback mechanism: Response of pituitary FSH and of stalk–median eminence follicle stimulating hormone-releasing factor to median eminence implants of FSH, *Endocrinology* **80:**1006.

Corbin, A., Daniels, E. L., and Milmore, J. E., 1970, An "internal" feedback mechanism controlling follicle stimulating hormone releasing factor, *Endocrinology* **86:**735.

Corker, C. S., Naftolin, F., and Exley, D., 1969, Interrelationship between plasma luteinizing hormone and oestradiol in the human menstrual cycle, *Nature* **222:**1063.

Cramer, O. M., and Barraclough, C. A., 1971, Effect of electrical stimulation of the preoptic area on plasma LH concentrations in proestrous rats, *Endocrinology* **88:**1175.

Crighton, D. B., Schneider, H. P. G., and McCann, S. M., 1969, Possible interaction of luteinizing hormone-releasing factor with other hypothalamic releasing factors at the level of the adeno-hypophysis, *J. Endocrinol.* **44:**405.

Cross, B. A., 1973, Unit responses in the hypothalamus, in: *Frontiers in Neuroendocrinology, 1973* (L. Martini, and W. F. Ganong, eds.), pp. 133–172, Oxford University Press, New York.

Davidson, J. M., 1969, Feedback control of gonadotropin secretion, in: *Frontiers in Neuroendocrinology* (W. F. Ganong and L. Martini, eds.), pp. 343–388, Oxford University Press, New York.

Davidson, J. M., and Sawyer, C. H., 1961, Effects of localized intracerebral implantation of oestrogen on reproductive function in the female rabbit, *Acta Endocrinol. [Kbh.]* **37:**385.

Debeljuk, L., Arimura, A., and Schally, A. V., 1972, Effect of estradiol and progesterone on the LH release induced by LH-releasing hormone (LH-RH) in intact diestrous rats and anestrous ewes, *Proc. Soc. Exp. Biol. Med.* **139:**774.

Debeljuk, L., Rozados, R., Daskal, H., and Velez, C. V., 1975, Variation of the pituitary response to LH-releasing hormone (LH-RH) during a 24-hour period in male, diestrous female and androgenized female rats, *Neuroendocrinology* **17:**48.

de la Cruz, A., Arimura, A., de la Cruz, K. G., and Schally, A. V., 1976, Effect of administration of anti-serum to luteinizing hormone-releasing hormone on gonadal function during the estrous cycle in the hamster, *Endocrinology* **98:**490.

Desclin, L., 1936, A propos de l'influence de la lactation sur la structure du lobe antérieur de l'hypophyse du rat blanc, *C. R. Soc. Biol. (Paris)* **120**:526.

Desclin, L., 1949, Action des oestrogènes sur l'ovaire chez le rat normal et hypopysectomisé, *C. R. Soc. Biol. (Paris)* **143**:1004.

Desclin, L., 1950, A propos du méchanisme d'action des oestrogènes sur le lobe antérieur de l'hypophyse chez le rat, *Ann. Endocrinol.* **11**:656.

Desclin, L., and Grégoire, C., 1937, Influence de la lactation sur les fonctions gonadotropes du lobe antérieur de l'hypophyse chez le rat blanc, *C. R. Soc. Biol. (Paris)* **126**:250.

Desclin, L., and Koulischer, L., 1960, Action d'un traitement oestrogénique sur la teneur en prolactine de l'hypophyse greffée chez le rat, *C. R. Soc. Biol. (Paris)* **154**:1515.

Döcke, F., 1969, Ovulation-inducing action of clomiphene citrate in the rat, *J. Reprod. Fertil.* **18**:135.

Döcke, F., 1971, Studies on the anti-ovulatory and ovulation action of clomiphene citrate in the rat, *J. Reprod. Fertil.* **24**:45.

Döcke, F., and Dörner, G., 1965, The mechanism of the induction of ovulation by oestrogens, *J. Endocrinol.* **33**:491.

Döcke, F., and Dörner, G., 1969, A possible mechanism by which progesterone facilitates ovulation in the rat. *Neuroendocrinology* **4**:139.

Donovan, B. T., 1971, The extra-hypothalamic control of gonadotropin secretion, in: *Control of Gonadal Steroid Secretion* (D. T. Baird and J. A. Strong, eds.), pp. 1–14, Williams & Wilkins, Baltimore.

Donovan, B. T., and Harris, G. W., 1966, Neurohumoral mechanisms in reproduction, in: *Marshall's Physiology of Reproduction*, Vol. 3 (A. S. Parkes, ed), pp. 301–378, Longmans, Green, London.

Dörner, G., and Döcke, F., 1967, The influence of intrahypothalamic implantation of oestrogen or progestogen on gonadotrophin release, in: *International Congress Series No. 111*, p. 194, Excerpta Medica Foundation, Amsterdam.

Dorrington, J. H., and Kilpatrick, R., 1969, The synthesis of progestational steroids by the rabbit ovary, in: *The Gonads* (K. W. McKerns, ed.), pp. 27–54, Appleton-Century-Crofts, New York.

Drouin, J., Lagacé, L., and Labrie, F., 1976, Estradiol-induced increase of the LH responsiveness to LH releasing hormone (LHRH) in rat anterior pituitary cells in culture, *Endocrinology* **99**:1477.

Dufy, B., Partouche, C., Poulain, D., Dufy-Barbe, L., and Vincent, J. D., 1976, Effects of estrogen on the electrical activity of identified and unidentified hypothalamic units, *Neuroendocrinology* **22**:38.

Ectors, F., and Pasteels, J. L., 1969, Similitude d'action de l'estradiol et de progestagenes dur la même aire hypothalamique, *C. R. Acad. Sci. (Paris)* **269**:844.

Eisenfeld, A. J., 1970, ^{3}H-Estradiol—*In vitro* binding to macromolecules from the rat hypothalamus, anterior pituitary and uterus, *Endocrinology* **86**:1313.

Evans, J. S., and Nikitovitch-Winer, M. B., 1969, Functional reactivation and cytological restoration of pituitary grafts by continuous local intravascular infusion of median eminence extracts, *Neuroendocrinology* **4**:83.

Everett, J. W., 1940, The restoration of ovulatory cycles and corpus luteum formation in persistent-estrous rats by progesterone, *Endocrinology* **27**:681.

Everett, J. W., 1948, Progesterone and estrogen in the experimental control of ovulation time and other features of the estrous cycle in the rat, *Endocrinology* **43**:389.

Everett, J. W., 1954, Luteotrophic function of autografts of the rat hypophysis, *Endocrinology* **54**:685.

Everett, J. W., 1956, Functional corpora lutea maintained for months by autografts of rat hypophyses, *Endocrinology* **58**:786.

Everett, J. W., 1964, Preoptic stimulative lesions and ovulation in the rat: "Thresholds" and LH-release time in late diestrus and proestrus, in: *Major Problems in Neuroendocrinology* (E. Bajusz and G. Jasmin, eds.), pp. 346–366, S. Karger, New York.

Everett, J. W., and Radford, H. M., 1961, Irritative deposits from stainless steel electrodes in the preoptic rat brain causing release of pituitary gonadotropin, *Proc. Soc. Exp. Biol. Med.* **108**:604.

Everett, J. W., and Sawyer, C. H., 1949, A neural timing factor in the mechanism by which progesterone advances ovulation in the cyclic rat, *Endocrinology* **45**:581.

Everett, J. W., and Tyrey, L., 1977, Induction of LH release and ovulation in rats by radiofrequency lesions of the medial basal tuber cinereum, *Anat. Rec.* **187:**575.

Everett, J. W., Quinn, D. L., and Tyrey, L., 1976, Comparative effectiveness of preoptic and tuberal stimulation for luteinizing hormone release and ovulation in two strains of rats, *Endocrinology* **98:**1302.

Ferin, M., Tempone, A., Zimmering, P. E., and Vande Wiele, R. L., 1969, Effect of anti-bodies to 17β-estradiol and progesterone on the estrous cycle of the rat, *Endocrinology* **85:**1070.

Flerkó, B., 1974, Hypothalamic mediation of neuroendocrine regulation of hypophysial gonadotrophic functions, in: *MTP International Review of Science, Reproductive Physiology, Physiology, Series One,* Vol. 8 (R. O. Greep, ed.), pp. 1–32, Butterworths–University Park Press, Baltimore.

Ford, J. J., and Yoshinaga, K., 1975, The role of LH in the luteotrophic process of lactating rats, *Endocrinology* **96:**329.

Fraschini, F., Motta, M., and Martini, L., 1968, A "short" feedback mechanism controlling FSH secretion, *Experientia* **24:**270.

Gallo, R. V., and Osland, R. B., 1976, Electrical stimulation of the arcuate nucleus in ovariectomized rats inhibits episodic luteinizing hormone (LH) release but excites LH release after estrogen priming, *Endocrinology* **99:**659.

Gay, V. L., and Midgley, A. R., Jr., 1969, Response of the adult rat to orchidectomy and ovariectomy as determined by LH radioimmunoassay, *Endocrinology* **84:**1359.

Gay, V. L., and Tomacari, R. L., 1974, Follicle-stimulating hormone secretion in the female rat: Cyclic release is dependent on circulating androgen, *Science* **184:**75.

Gordon, J. H., and Reichlin, S., 1974, Changes in pituitary responsiveness to luteinizing hormone-releasing factor during the rat estrous cycle, *Endocrinology* **94:**974.

Greeley, G. H., Jr., Allen, M. B., Jr., and Mahesh, V. B., 1975, Potentiation of luteinizing hormone release by estradiol at the level of the pituitary, *Neuroendocrinology* **18:**233.

Greenwald, G. S., 1968, Evidence for a luteotropic complex in the hamster and other species, in: *Progress in Endocrinology,* Proceedings of the Third International Congress of Endocrinology, Mexico, June 30–July 5, 1968.

Greer, M. A., 1953, The effect of progesterone on persistent vaginal estrus produced by hypothalamic lesions in the rat, *Endocrinology* **53:**380.

Griffiths, E. C., Hooper, K. C., Jeffcoate, S. L., and Holland, D. T., 1974, The presence of peptidases in the rat hypothalamus inactivating luteinizing hormone-releasing hormone (LH-RH), *Acta Endocrinol. (Kbh.)* **77:**435.

Halász, B., 1972, Hypothalamic mechanisms controlling pituitary function, *Prog. Brain Res.* **38:**99.

Halász, B., and Gorski, R. A., 1967, Gonadotrophic hormone secretion in female rats after partial or total interruption of neural afferents to the medial basal hypothalamus, *Endocrinology* **80:**608.

Han, S. S., Rajaniemi, H. J., Cho, M. I., Hirshfield, A. N., and Midgley, A. R., Jr., 1974, Gonadotropin receptors in rat ovarian tissue. II. Subcellar localization of LH binding sites by electron microscopic radioautography, *Endocrinology* **95:**589.

Harris, G. W., 1955, *Neural Control of the Pituitary Gland,* Edward Arnold Ltd., London.

Haug, E., and Gautvik, K. M., 1976, Effects of sex steroids on prolactin secreting rat pituitary cells in culture, *Endocrinology* **99:**1482.

Hillarp, N. A., 1949, Studies on the localization of hypothalamic centres controlling the gonadotrophic function of the hypophysis, *Acta Endocrinol. (Kbh.)* **2:**11.

Hillensjö, T., Bauminger, S., and Ahren, K., 1976, Effect of luteinizing hormone on the pattern of steroid production by preovulatory follicles of pregnant mare's serum gonadotropin-injected immature rats. *Endocrinology* **99:**996.

Hilliard, J., Schally, A. V., and Sawyer, C. H., 1971, Progesterone blockade of the ovulatory response to intrapituitary infusion of LH-RH in rabbits, *Endocrinology* **88:**730.

Hohlweg, W., and Junkmann, K., 1932, Die hormonal-nervöse Regulierung der Funktion des Hypophysenvorderlappens, *Klin, Wochenschr.* **11:**321.

Hollander, N., and Hollander, V. P., 1958, The effect of follicle-stimulating hormone on the biosynthesis *in vitro* of estradiol-17β from acetate-1-C and testosterone-4-C, *J. Biol. Chem.* **233:**1097.

Ichii, S., Forchielli, E., and Dorfman, R. I., 1963, *In vitro* effect of gonadotrophins on the soluble cholesterol side-chain cleaving enzyme system of bovine corpus luteum, *Steroids* **2:**631.

Joshi, H. S., Watson, D. J., and Labhsetwar, A. P., 1973, Ovarian secretion of oestradiol, oestrone, 20-dihydroprogesterone and progesterone during the oestrous cycle of the guinea-pig, *J. Reprod. Fertil.* **35:**177.

Kaasjager, W. A., Woodbury, D. M., van Dieten, J. A. M., and van Rees, G. P., 1971, The role played by the preoptic region and the hypothalamus in spontaneous ovulation and ovulation induced by progesterone, *Neuroendocrinology* **7:**54.

Kalra, S., 1976, Tissue levels of luteinizing hormone-releasing hormone in the preoptic area and hypothalamus, and serum concentrations of gonadotropins following anterior hypothalamic deafferentation and estrogen treatment of the female rat, *Endocrinology* **99:**101.

Kalra, S. P., and Kalra, P. S., 1974, Effects of circulating estradiol during rat estrous cycle on LH release following electrochemical stimulation of preoptic brain or administration of synthetic LRF, *Endocrinology* **94:**845.

Kalra, S. P., Ajika, K., Krulich, L., Fawcett, C. P., Quijada, M., and McCann, S, M., 1971, Effects of hypothalamic and preoptic electrochemical stimulation on gonadotropin and prolactin release in proestrous rats, *Endocrinology* **88:**1150.

Kammerman, S., Canfield, R. E., Kolena, J., and Channing, C. P., 1972, The binding of iodinated HCG to porcine granulosa cells, *Endocrinology* **91:**65.

Kanematsu, S., and Sawyer, C. H., 1963, Effects of intrahypothalamic and intrahypophysial estrogen implants on pituitary prolactin and lactation in the rabbit, *Endocrinology* **72:**243.

Kanematsu, S., and Sawyer, C. H., 1964, Effects of hypothalamic and hypophysial estrogen implants on pituitary and plasma LH in ovariectomized rabbits, *Endocrinology* **75:**579.

Karavolas, H. J., and Nuti, K. M., 1976, Progesterone metabolism by neuroendocrine tissues, in: *Subcellular Mechanisms in Reproductive Neuroendocrinology* (F. Naftolin, K. J. Ryan, and I. J. Davies, eds.), pp. 305–326, Elsevier, Amsterdam.

Katz, Y., and Armstrong, D. T., 1976, Inhibition of ovarian estradiol-17β secretion by luteinizing hormone in prepubertal, pregnant mare serum-treated rats, *Endocrinology* **99:**1442.

Kawakami, M., and Kimura, F., 1975, Possible roles of CNS estrogen–neuron systems in the control of gonadotrophin release, in: *Anatomical Neuroendocrinology* (W. E. Stumpf, and L. D. Grant, eds.), pp. 216–231, S. Karger, New York.

Kerdelhué, B., Catin, S., and Jutisz, M., 1975, Short- and long-term effects of anti-LH-RH serum administration of gonadotropic regulation of the female rat, in: *Hypothalamic Hormones* (M. Motta, P. G. Crosignani, and L. Martini, eds.), pp. 43–56, Academic Press, London.

Keyes, P. L., and Nalbandov, A. V., 1967, Maintenance and function of corpora lutea in rabbits depend on estrogen, *Endocrinology* **80:**938.

Knobil, E., 1974, On the control of gonadotropin secretion in the rhesus monkey, *Recent Prog. Horm. Res.* **30:**1.

Koch, Y., Chobsieng, P., Zor, U., Fridkin, M., and Lindner, H. R., 1973, Suppression of gonadotropin secretion and prevention of ovulation in the rat by antiserum to synthetic gonadotropin-releasing hormone, *Biochem. Biophys. Res. Commun.* **55:**623.

Kolena, J., and Channing, C. P., 1972, Stimulatory effects of LH, FSH, and prostaglandins upon cyclic 3′,5′-AMP levels in porcine granulosa cells, *Endocrinology* **90:**1543.

Koritz, S. B., and Hall, P. F., 1965, Further studies on the locus of action of interstitial cell-stimulating hormone on the biosynthesis of progesterone by bovine corpus luteum, *Biochemistry* **4:**2740.

Köves, K., and Halász, B., 1969, Data on the location of the neural structures indispensable for the occurrence of ovarian compensatory hypertrophy, *Neuroendocrinology* **4:**1.

Krey, L. C., Butler, W. R., and Knobil, E., 1975, Surgical disconnection of the medial basal hypothalamus and pituitary function in the rhesus monkey. I. Gonadotropin secretion, *Endocrinology* **96:**1073.

Kuehl, F. A., Humes, J. L., Tarnoff, J., Cirillo, V. J., and Ham, E. A., 1970, Prostaglandin receptor site: Evidence for an essential role in the action of luteinizing hormone, *Science* **169**:883.

Labhsetwar, A. P., 1970, Role of oestrogen in spontaneous ovulation demonstrated by use of an antagonist of oestrogen, ICI 46, 474, *Nature* **225**:80.

Labrie, F., Savary, M., Coy, D. H., Coy, E. J., and Schally, A. V., 1976a, Inhibition of luteinizing hormone release by analogs of luteinizing hormone-releasing hormone (LHRH) *in vitro*, *Endocrinology* **98**:289.

Labrie, F., Borgeat, P., Barden, N., Beaulieu, M., Ferland, L., Drouin, J., Delean, A., and Morin, O., 1976b, Role of cyclic AMP in neuroendocrine control, in: *Subcellular Mechanisms in Reproductive Neuroendocrinology*, (F. Naftolin, K. J. Ryan, and I. J. Davies, eds.), pp. 391–406, Elsevier, Amsterdam.

Lamport, H., 1940, Periodic changes in blood estrogen, *Endocrinology* **27**:673.

Lee, C. Y., and Ryan, R. J., 1971, The uptake of human luteinizing hormone (hLH) by slices of luteinized rat ovaries, *Endocrinology* **89**:1515.

LeMaire, W. J., Yang, N. S. T., Behrman, H. H., and Marsh, L. M., 1973, Preovulatory changes in the concentration of prostaglandins in rabbit Graafian follicles, *Prostaglandins* **3**:367.

Levine, S., 1972, *Hormones and Behavior,* Academic Press, New York.

Liao, T. F., Pattison, M. L., and Chen, C. L., 1974, Prolongation of pseudopregnancy of rats by gonadotropins implanted in the ovarian bursae, *Endocrinology* **95**:1234.

Libertun, C., Cooper, K. J., Fawcett, C. P., and McCann, S. M., 1974a, Effects of ovariectomy and steroid treatment on hypophyseal sensitivity to purified LH-releasing factor (LRF), *Endocrinology* **94**:518.

Libertun, C., Orias, R., and McCann, S. M., 1974b, Biphasic effect of estrogen on the sensitivity of the pituitary to luteinizing hormone-releasing factor (LRF), *Endocrinology* **94**:1094.

Lincoln, D. W., and Cross, B. A., 1967, Effect of oestrogen on the responsiveness of neurones in the hypothalamus, septum and preoptic area of rats with light-induced persistent oestrus, *J. Endocrinol.* **37**:191.

Ling, W. Y., and Marsh, J. M., 1977, Reevaluation of the role of cyclic adenosine 3′,5′-monophosphate and protein kinase in the stimulation of steroidogenesis by luteinizing hormone in bovine corpus luteum slices. *Endocrinology* **100**:571.

Lipschütz, A., 1925, Is there an antagonism between the male and female sex-endocrine gland?, *Endocrinology* **9**:1.

Liu, T.-C., and Jackson, G. L., 1977, Effect of *in vivo* treatment with estrogen on luteinizing hormone synthesis and release by rat pituitaries *in vitro*, *Endocrinology* **100**:1294.

Long, J. A., and Evans, H. M., 1922, The oestrous cycle in the rat and its associated phenomena, *Mem. Univ. California* **6**:1.

Lunenfeld, B., and Eshkol, A., 1967, Immunology of human chorionic gonadotropin (HCG), *Vitam. Horm.* **25**:137.

Machida, T., 1971, Luteinization of ovaries under stressful conditions in persistent-estrous rats bearing hypothalamic lesions, *Endocrinol. Jpn.* **18**:427.

MacLeod, R. M., 1976, Regulation of prolactin secretion, in: *Frontiers of Neuroendocrinology*, Vol. 4 (L. Martini, and W. F. Ganong, eds.), pp. 169–194, Raven Press, New York.

MacLeod, R. M., and Lehmeyer, J. E., 1972, Regulation of the synthesis and release of prolactin, in: *Lactogenic Hormones*, (G. E. W. Wolstenholme and J. Knight, eds.), pp. 53–82, Churchill Livingstone, London.

Marsh, J. M., Mills, T. M., and LeMaire, J., 1972, Cyclic AMP synthesis in rabbit Graafian follicles and the effect of luteinizing hormone, *Biochim. Biophys. Acta* **273**:389.

Martin, J. E., Tyrey, L., Everett, J. W., and Fellows, R. E., 1974a, Variation in responsiveness to synthetic LH-releasing factor (LRF) in proestrous and diestrous—3 rats, *Endocrinology* **94**:556.

Martin, J. E., Tyrey, L., Everett, J. W., and Fellows, R. E., 1974b, Estrogen and progesterone modulation of the pituitary response to LRF in the cyclic rat, *Endocrinology* **95**:1664.

Martini, L., Fraschini, F., and Motta, M., 1968, Neural control of anterior pituitary function, *Recent Prog. Horm. Res.* **24**:439.

McCann, S. M., Ojeda, S. R., Harms, P. G., Wheaton, J. E., Sundberg, D. K., and Fawcett, C. P., 1976, Control of adenohypophyseal hormone secretion by prostaglandins, in: *Subcellular*

Mechanisms in Reproductive Neuroendocrinology (F. Naftolin, K. J. Ryan, and I. J. Davies, eds.), pp. 407–422, Elsevier, Amsterdam.

McCormack, J. T., Plant, T. M., Hess, D. L., and Knobil, E., 1977, The effect of luteinizing hormone releasing hormone (LHRH) antiserum administration on gonadotropin secretion in the rhesus monkey, *Endocrinology* **100**:663.

McEwen, B. S., 1976, Steroid receptors in neuroendocrine tissues: Topography, subcellular distribution, and functional implications, in: *Subcellular Mechanisms in Reproductive Neuroendocrinology* (F. Naftolin, K. J. Ryan, and I. J., Davies, eds.), pp. 277–304, Elsevier, Amsterdam.

McEwen, B. S., and Pfaff, D. W., 1973, Chemical and physiological approaches to neuroendocrine mechanisms: Attempts at integration, in: *Frontiers in Neuroendocrinology, 1973* (W. F. Ganong, and L. Martini, eds.), pp. 267–336, Oxford University Press, New York.

McLean, B. K., and Nikitovitch-Winer, M. B., 1976, Direct effects of estradiol and progesterone on pituitary graft gonadotrophs and their differential response to median eminence extract, *Neuroendocrinology* **20**:1.

Mena, F., Maiweg, H., and Grosvenor, C. E., 1968, Effect of ectopic pituitary glands upon prolactin concentration of the *in situ* pituitary of the lactating rat, *Endocrinology* **83**:1359.

Mennin, S. P., and Gorski, R. A., 1975, Effects of ovarian steroids on plasma LH in normal and persistent estrous adult female rats, *Endocrinology* **96**:486.

Miller, W. L., Knight, M. M., Grimek, H. J., and Gorski, J., 1977, Estrogen regulation of follicle stimulating hormone in cell cultures of sheep pituitaries, *Endocrinology* **100**:1306.

Mittler, J. C., Arimura, A., and Schally, A. V., 1970, Release and synthesis of luteinizing hormone and follicle-stimulating hormone in pituitary cultures in response to hypothalamic preparations, *Proc. Soc. Exp. Biol. Med.* **133**:1321.

Moor, R. M., 1974, The ovarian follicle of the sheep: Inhibition of oestrogen secretion by luteinizing hormone, *J. Endocrinol.* **61**:455.

Moore, C. R., and Price, D., 1932, Gonad hormone functions, and the reciprocal influence between gonads and the hypophysis, with its bearing on the problem of sex-hormone antagonism, *Am. J. Anat.* **50**:13.

Moore, N. W., Barrett, S., Brown, J. B., Schindler, I., Smith, M. A., and Smyth, B., 1969, Oestrogen and progesterone content of ovarian vein blood of the ewe during the oestrous cycle, *J. Endocrinol.* **44**:55.

Morris, P. W., and Gorski, J., 1973, Control of steroidogenesis of preovulatory cells. Luteinizing hormone stimulation of [^{14}C]acetate incorporation into sterols, *J. Biol. Chem.* **248**:6920.

Motta, M., Fraschini, F., and Martini, L., 1969, "Short" feedback mechanisms in the control of anterior pituitary function, in: *Frontiers in Neuroendocrinology, 1969* (W. F. Ganong and L. Martini, eds.), pp. 211–253, Oxford University Press, New York.

Naftolin, F., and McInnes, R., 1977, Neuroendocrine control of gonadotrophin secretion, in: International Society of Psychoneuroendocrinology, VIIIth International Congress, May 8–12, Emory University, Atlanta, Georgia.

Naftolin, F., Brown-Grant, K., and Corker, C. S., 1972, Plasma and pituitary luteinizing hormone and peripheral plasma oestradiol concentrations in the normal oestrous cycle of the rat and after experimental manipulation of the cycle, *J. Endocrinol.* **53**:17.

Nagasawa, H., Chen, C. L., and Meites, J., 1969, Effects of estrogen implant in median eminence on serum and pituitary prolactin levels in the rat, *Proc. Soc. Exp. Biol. Med.* **132**:859.

Negro-Vilar, A., Orias, R., and McCann, S. M., 1973, Evidence for a pituitary site of action for the acute inhibition of LH release by estrogen in the rat, *Endocrinology*, **92**:1680.

Nicoll, C. S., 1971, Aspects of the neural control of prolactin secretion, in: *Frontiers in Neuroendocrinology, 1971* (L. Martini and W. F. Ganong, eds.), pp. 291–330, Oxford University Press, New York.

Nicoll, C. S., and Meites, J., 1962, Estrogen stimulation of prolactin production by rat adenohypophysis *in vitro*, *Endocrinology* **70**:272.

Nikitovitch-Winer, M. B., 1957, Humoral influence of the hypothalamus on gonadotropin secretions, Doctoral dissertation, Duke University, Durham.

Nikitovitch-Winer, M. B., 1960, The influence of the hypothalamus on luteotrophin secretion in the rat, *Mem. Soc. Endocrinol.* **9**:70.

Nikitovitch-Winer, M. B., 1962, Induction of ovulation in rats by direct intrapituitary infusion of median eminence, *Endocrinology* **70**:350.

Nikitovitch-Winer, M. B., 1965, Effect of hypophysial stalk transection on luteotropic hormone secretion in the rat, *Endocrinology* **77**:658.

Notides, A. C., 1970, Binding affinity and specificity of the estrogen receptor of the rat uterus and anterior pituitary, *Endocrinology* **87**:987.

Nuti, K. M., and Karavolas, H. J., 1977, Effect of progesterone and its 5α-reduced metabolites on gonadotropin levels in estrogen-primed ovariectomized rats, *Endocrinology* **100**:777.

Ojeda, S. R., and Ramirez, V. D., 1969, Automatic control of LH and FSH secretion by short feedback circuits in immature rats, *Endocrinology* **84**:786.

Oliver, C., Mical, R. S., and Porter, J. C., 1977, Hypothalamic–pituitary vasculature: Evidence for retrograde blood flow in the pituitary stalk, *Endocrinology* **101**:598.

Osland, R. B., Gallo, R. V., and Williams, J. A., 1975, *In vitro* release of luteinizing hormone from anterior pituitary fragments superfused with constant or pulsatile amounts of luteinizing hormone-releasing factor, *Endocrinology* **96**:1210.

Palka, Y. S., Ramirez, V. D., and Sawyer, C. H., 1966, Distribution and biological effects of tritiated estradiol implanted in the hypothalamo–hypophysial region of female rats, *Endocrinology* **78**:487.

Parkes, A. S., and Deanesly, R., 1966a, The ovarian hormones, in: *Marshall's Physiology of Reproduction*, 3rd Edition, Vol. 3 (A. S. Parkes, ed.), pp. 570–828, Longmans Green and Co., London.

Parkes, A. S., and Deanesly, R., 1966b, Relation between the gonads and the adrenal glands, in: *Marshall's Physiology of Reproduction*, 3rd Edition, Vol. 3 (A. S. Parkes, ed.), pp. 1064–1111, Longmans Green and Co., London.

Pasteels, J. L., 1961, Sécrétion de prolactine par l'hypophyse en culture de tissus, *C. R. Acad. Sci.* [*D*] (*Paris*) **253**:2140.

Payne, R. W., Hellbaum, A. A., and Owens, J. N., Jr., 1956, The effect of androgens on the ovaries and uterus of the estrogen-treated hypophysectomized immature rat, *Endocrinology* **59**:306.

Pfaff, D., and Keiner, M., 1973, Atlas of estradiol-concentrating cells in the central nervous system of the female rat, *J. Comp. Neurol.* **151**:121.

Piacsek, B. E., and Meites, J., 1966, Effects of castration and gonadal hormones on hypothalamic content of luteinizing hormone releasing factor (LRF), *Endocrinology* **79**:432.

Quinn, D. L., 1970, Hypothalamic mechanisms involved in the control of gonadotropic hormone secretion in the guinea pig: Evidence of elevated brain thresholds to electrical stimulation in the medial–preoptic–anterior hypothalamus region during "early" diestrus, *Endocrinology* **87**:343.

Rajaniemi, H., and Vanha-Perttula, T., 1972, Specific receptor for LH in the ovary: Evidence by autoradiography and tissue fractionation, *Endocrinology* **90**:1.

Ramirez, V. D., and McCann, S. M., 1963, Comparison of the regulation of luteinizing hormone (LH) secretion in immature and adult rats, *Endocrinology* **72**:452.

Ramirez, V. D., Abrams, R. M., and McCann, S. M., 1964, Effect of estradiol implants in the hypothalamo–hypophysial region of the rat on the secretion of luteinizing hormone, *Endocrinology* **75**:243.

Reeves, J. R., Arimura, A., and Schally, A. V., 1971a, Pituitary responsiveness to purified luteinizing hormone-releasing hormone (LH-RH) at various stages of the estrous cycle in sheep, *J. Anim. Sci.* **32**:123.

Reeves, J. R., Arimura, A., and Schally, A. V., 1971b, Changes in pituitary responsiveness to luteinizing hormone-releasing hormone (LH-RH) in anestrous ewes pretreated with estradiol benzoate, *Biol. Reprod.* **4**:88.

Richards, J. S., 1974, Estradiol binding to rat corpora lutea during pregnancy, *Endocrinology* **95**:1046.

Richards, J. S., 1975, Estradiol receptor content in rat granulosa cells during follicular development: Modification by estradiol and gonadotropins, *Endocrinology* **97**:1174.

Richards, J. S., Ireland, J. J., Rao, M. C., Bernath, G. A., Midgley, A. R., Jr., and Reichert, L. E., Jr., 1976, Ovarian follicular development in the rat: Hormone receptor regulation by estradiol, follicle stimulating hormone and luteinizing hormone, *Endocrinology* **99**:1562.

Robson, J. M., 1937, Maintenance by oestrin of the luteal function in hypophysectomized rabbits, *J. Physiol. (Lond.)* **90**:435.

Rose, S., and Nelson, J. F., 1957, The direct effect of oestradiol on the pars distalis, *Aust. J. Exp. Biol. Med. Sci,* **35**:605.

Sar, M., and Stumpf, W. E., 1973, Neurons of the hypothalamus concentrate (^{3}H)progesterone or its metabolites, *Science* **182**:1266.

Savard, K., Marsh, J. M., and Rice, B. F., 1965, Gonadotropins and ovarian steroidogenesis, *Recent Prog. Horm. Res.* **21**:285.

Sawyer, C. H., 1975, Some recent developments in brain–pituitary–ovarian physiology, *Neuroendocrinology* **17**:97.

Saywer, C. H., Everett, J. W., and Markee, J. E., 1949, A neural factor in the mechanism by which estrogen induces the release of luteinizing hormone, *Endocrinology* **44**:218.

Schally, A. V., Redding, T. W., and Arimura, A., 1973, Effect of sex steroids on pituitary responses to LH- and FSH-releasing hormone *in vitro, Endocrinology* **93**:893.

Schneider, H. P. G., and McCann, S. M., 1970, Estradiol and the neuroendocrine control of LH release *in vitro, Endocrinology* **87**:330.

Schuiling, G. A., van Dieten, J. A. M. J., and van Rees, G. R., 1974, Induction and inhibition of ovulation in the rat by intracerebral progesterone implants, *Neuroendocrinology* **15**:38.

Schwartz, N. B., 1974, The role of FSH and LH and of their antibodies on follicle growth and on ovulation, *Biol. Reprod.* **10**:236.

Selye, H., and McKeown, T., 1934, Studies on pseudopregnancy, *Am. J. Physiol.* **109**:96.

Serra, G. B., and Midgley, A. R., Jr., 1970, The *in vitro* release of LH during continuous superfusion of single rat anterior pituitary glands, *Proc. Soc. Exp. Biol. Med.* **133**:1370.

Shaikh, A. A., and Shaikh, S. A., 1975, Adrenal and ovarian steroid secretion in the rat estrous cycle temporally related to gonadotropins and steroid levels found in peripheral plasma, *Endocrinology* **96**:37.

Shirley, B., Wolinsky, J., and Schwartz, N. B., 1968, Effects of a single injection of an estrogen antagonist on the estrous cycle of the rat, *Endocrinology* **82**:959.

Sinha, Y. N., and Tucker, H. A., 1968, Pituitary prolactin content and mammary development after chronic administration of prolactin, *Proc. Soc. Exp. Biol. Med.* **128**:84.

Smith, P. E., and Engle, E. T., 1927, Experimental evidence regarding the rôle of the anterior pituitary in the development and regulation of the genital system, *Am. J. Anat.* **40**:159.

Speroff, L., and Ramwell, P. W., 1970, Prostaglandin stimulation of *in vitro* progesterone synthesis, *J. Clin. Endocrinol. Metab.* **30**:345.

Spies, H. G., and Norman, R. L., 1975, Interaction of estradiol and LHRH on LH release in rhesus females: Evidence for a neural site of action, *Endocrinology* **97**:685.

Spies, H. G., Stevens, K. R., Hilliard, J., and Sawyer, C. H., 1969, The pituitary as a site of progesterone and chlormadinone blockade of ovulation in the rabbit, *Endocrinology* **84**:277.

Spies, H., Resko, J. A., and Norman, R. L., 1974, Evidence of preoptic hypothalamic influence on ovulation in the rhesus monkey, *Fed. Proc.* **33**:222.

Spies, H. G., Norman, R. L., Quadri, S. K., and Clifton, D. K., 1977, Effects of estradiol-17β on the induction of gonadotropin release by electrical stimulation of the hypothalamus in rhesus monkeys, *Endocrinology* **100**:314.

Steinach, E., and Kun, H., 1926, Antagonistische Wirkungen der Keimdrusenhormon, *Biol. Gen.* **2**:815.

Steinberger, A., and Chowdhury, M., 1974, Effect of testosterone and estradiol on the basal and LRF-stimulated secretion of gonadotropins in pituitary cell culture, *Endocrinol. Res. Commun,* **1**:389.

Stumpf, W. E., 1969, Nuclear concentration of ^{3}H-estradiol in target tissues. Dry-mount autoradiography of vagina, oviduct, ovary, testis, mammary tumor, liver and adrenal, *Endocrinology* **85**:31.

Stumpf, W. E., Sar, M., and Keefer, D. A., 1975, Atlas of estrogen target cells in rat brain, in: *Anatomical Neuroendocrinology* (W. E. Stumpf and L. D. Grant, eds.), pp. 104–119, S. Karger, New York.

Szentágothai, J., Flerkó, B., Mess, B., and Halász, B., 1968, *Hypothalamic Control of the Anterior Pituitary* 3rd Edition, Akadémiai Kiadó, Budapest.

Taleisnik, S., and Beltramino, C., 1975, Extrahypothalamic structures involved in regulation of gonadotropin secretion, in: *Anatomical Neuroendocrinology* (W. E. Stumpf and L. D. Grant, eds.), pp. 208–215, S. Karger, New York.

Taleisnik, S., and McCann, S. M., 1961, Effects of hypothalamic lesions on the secretion and storage of hypophysial luteinizing hormone, *Endocrinology* **68**:263.

Talwalker, P. K., Ratner, A., and Meites, J., 1963, *In vitro* inhibition of pituitary prolactin synthesis and release by hypothalamic extracts, *Am. J. Physiol.* **205**:213.

Tang, L. K. L., and Spies, H. G., 1975, Effects of gonadal steroids on the basal and LRF-induced gonadotropin secretion by cultures of rat pituitary, *Endocrinology* **96**:349.

Tejasen, T., and Everett, J. W., 1967, Surgical analysis of the preoptico–tuberal pathway controlling ovulatory release of gonadotropins in the rat, *Endocrinology* **81**:1387.

Török, B., 1964, Structure of the vasular connections of the hypothalamo–hypophysial region, *Acta Anat. (Basel)* **59**:84.

Turgeon, J., and Barraclough, C. A., 1973, Temporal patterns of LH release following graded preoptic electrochemical stimulation in proestrus rats, *Endocrinology* **92**:755.

Vaala, S. S., and Knigge, K. M., 1974, Transport capacity of median eminence: *In vitro* uptake of ³H-LRF, *Neuroendocrinology* **15**:147.

Vilchez-Martinez, J. A., Arimura, A., Debeljuk, L., and Schally, A. V., 1974, Biphasic effect of estradiol benzoate on the pituitary responsiveness to LH-RH, *Endocrinology* **94**:1300.

Voogt, J. J., and Meites, J., 1971, Effects of an implant of prolactin in median eminence of pseudopregnant rats on serum and pituitary LH, FSH, and prolactin, *Endocrinology* **88**:286.

Watkins, B. E., Meites, J., and Riegle, G. D., 1975, Age-related changes in pituitary responsiveness to LHRH in the female rat, *Endocrinology* **97**:543.

Weick, R. F., and Davidson, J. M., 1970, Localization of the stimulatory feedback effect of estrogen on ovulation in the rat, *Endocrinology* **87**:693.

Weick, R. F., Smith, E. R., Dominguez, R., Dhariwal, A. P., and Davidson, J. M., 1971, Mechanism of stimulatory feedback effect of estradiol benzoate on the pituitary, *Endocrinology* **88**:293.

Welschen, R., Hermans, W. P., Dullaart, J., and de Jong, F. H., 1977, Effects of an inhibin-like factor present in bovine and porcine follicular fluid on gonadotrophin levels in ovariectomized rats, *J. Reprod. Fertil.* **50**:129.

Westman, A., and Jacobsohn, D., 1937a, Experimentelle Untersuchungen über die Bedeutung des Hypophysen–Zwischenhirnsystems für die Produktion gonadotroper Hormone des Hypophysenvorderlappens, *Acta Obstet. Gynecol. Scand.* **17**:235.

Westman, A., and Jacobsohn, D., 1937b, Über Oestrinwirkungen auf die Corpus luteum-Funktion, *Acta Obstet. Gynecol. Scand.* **17**:13.

Westman, A., and Jacobsohn, D., 1938, Endokrinologische Untersuchungen an Ratten mit durchtrenntem Hypophysenstiel 6. Mitteiling: Produktion und Abgabe der Gonadotropin Hormone, *Acta Pathol. Microbiol. Scan.* **15**:445.

Williams, P. C., 1945, Ovarian stimulation by oestrogens: Stimulation in the absence of hypophysis, uterus, and adrenal glands, *J. Endocrinol.* **4**:125.

Yagi, K., 1973, Changes in firing rates of single preoptic and hypothalamic units following an intravenous administration of estrogen in the castrated male rat, *Brain Res.* **53**:343.

Yen, S. S. C., Vandenberg, G., Rebar, R., and Ehara, Y., 1972, Variation of pituitary responsiveness to synthetic LRF during different phases of the menstrual cycle, *J. Clin. Endocrinol. Metab.* **35**:931.

Yen, S. S. C., Vandenberg, G., and Siler, T. M., 1974, Modulation of pituitary responsiveness to LRF by estrogen, *J. Clin. Endocrinol. Metab.* **39**:170.

Yen, S. S. C., Lasley, B. L., Wang, C. F., LeBlanc, H., and Siler, T. M., 1975, The operating characteristics of the hypothalamic–pituitary system during the menstrual cycle and observations of biological action of somatostatin, *Recent Prog. Horm. Res.* **31**:321.

Young, J. R., and Jaffe, R. B., 1976, Strength–duration characteristics of estrogen effects on gonadotropin response to gonadotropin-releasing hormone in women. II. Effects of varying concentrations of estradiol, *J. Clin. Endocrinol. Metab.* **42**:432.

10

Estrous Cyclicity in Mammals

HARVEY H. FEDER

I. INTRODUCTION

In the previous chapter, several experimental manipulations designed to demonstrate that the secretions of the hypothalamus, the anterior pituitary, and the ovary can have stimulatory and inhibitory effects on one another were discussed. These experimental approaches were basically analytic. They served to dissect the effects of a particular hormone on one tissue from its effects on another tissue. From this analytic approach, an appreciation was gained of the range of potential reactions to hormonal stimuli of individual components of the hypothalamo–hypophyseal–ovarian axis. However, the analytic approach does not indicate which of the potential reactions are actually utilized during the course of normal reproductive cycles. Nor does the analytic method deal with the question of how the various stimulatory and inhibitory actions of hormones become linked together to form a repeatable endocrine pattern with a consistent periodicity. To resolve these problems, one must adopt a more synthetic outlook.

The object of this chapter is to introduce some of the sequences of events that occur during normal reproductive cycles in an extensively studied laboratory animal, the rat. An attempt will be made to show how the reactions of individual components of the rat hypothalamo–hypophyseal–ovarian axis, as revealed by the analytic approach, are synthesized and orchestrated to contribute to reproductive cyclicity in this animal. Much of what has been learned of the reproductive cyclicity of rats can be applied to other species. But there are

HARVEY H. FEDER • Institute of Animal Behavior, Rutgers University, Newark, New Jersey 07102.

also some interesting species differences. In order to illustrate some of these differences, selected aspects of reproductive cyclicity in hamsters, guinea pigs, ewes, dogs, rhesus monkeys, rabbits, and cats will be presented.

Complete female mammalian reproductive cycles consist of a chain of events that includes courtship, mating, ovulation, pregnancy, parturition, and care of young (Everett, 1961). Rather than attempt to synthesize all of the hormonal events involved in this chain, I will choose one link in the chain, ovulation, and use this as the key event around which to build a sequence of hormonal changes in the ovary, pituitary, and brain.

II. RAT ESTROUS CYCLES—OVARIAN ASPECT

The first sections of this chapter follow this general sequence: (a) ovarian hormones released during the estrous cycle—indirect and direct means used to determine the pattern and concentration of these hormones; (b) pituitary hormones released during the estrous cycle—indirect and direct means of measurement; (c) releasing factors released during the estrous cycle—indirect and direct means of measurement; (d) functional interrelationships among (a), (b), and (c) during the course of the estrous cycle.

A. Indirect Assessments of Cyclic Release of Ovarian Hormones

1. Cyclic Changes in Some Target Tissues for Ovarian Hormones

The story of attempts to arrive at an integrated picture of the hormonal events involved in ovulation began well before chemical assay methods for hormones in blood were available. Early endocrinologists sought and found indicators of changes in ovarian activity that did not require chemical assay procedures. These early workers noted that unmated laboratory rats exhibited cyclic changes in female sexual behavior (estrous behavior; the term comes from the Latin *oestrus*, possessed by the gadfly, in a frenzy) and cyclic changes in vaginal cytology. The term "estrous cycle" was used to describe the recurrent nature of these changes. Confidence that these changes in behavior and vaginal cytology were biological indicators of fluctuations in release of ovarian hormones was warranted because ovariectomy caused an immediate cessation of cyclic fluctuations of sex behavior and vaginal cytology (see reviews by Nalbandov, 1958; Schwartz, 1969). These biological indicators of ovarian hormone release were not only reliable, they were also very convenient. Variations in sexual behavior and vaginal cytology could be determined repeatedly in the same animal, and no surgical intervention was necessary.

The technique for assessment of changes in vaginal cytology is simple and rapid (Stockard and Papanicolaou, 1917). It consists of swabbing the vaginal lumen and examining, under a microscope, the cells obtained. This vaginal smear method revealed cyclic changes in the cellular content of the vaginal lumen. In most nonpregnant laboratory rats, a complete cycle of such changes occurred every 4 or 5 days (Long and Evans, 1922). For the sake of simplicity let us consider first only those animals that showed 4-day cycles. Let us also arbitrarily consider that the first stage of the cycle is the one in which cornified epithelial cells are present in the vaginal lumen (vaginal estrus: duration *ca.* 36 hr). This is followed by a period in which the cornified cells become less numerous and leucocytes are present (vaginal diestrus: duration *ca.* 48 hr). The next phase is characterized by the presence of many nucleated epithelial cells (vaginal proestrus: duration *ca.* 12 hr), some of which had already appeared in late diestrus. These changes in the vaginal smear picture are depicted in Fig. 1A.

Behavioral observations are made by placing a female rat with a male and noting the frequency of lordosis responses by the female after she is mounted by the male. Other motor patterns characteristic of behavioral estrus or "heat" include hopping, darting, and ear-quivering by the female. Lordosis and associated behaviors could also be assessed in the absence of a male rat. The experimenter could elicit these responses by manually stimulating the flanks and perineal region of the female rat. By these methods, it was found that lordosis and associated behaviors occurred only when the vaginal smear was of the proestrous or early estrous type (i.e., every 4 or 5 days) (see review by Young, 1961). Although the female's sexual behavior was called "estrous behavior" it should be noted that "behavioral estrus" and "vaginal estrus" are not identical in their timing of onset. Behavioral estrus begins and is most intense while the vaginal smear is still predominantly proestrous and ends when the vaginal smear is estrous. The relationship between vaginal smears and female sexual behavior in rats with 4-day cycles is shown in Fig. 1A,B. Data from the two nonsurgical techniques (vaginal smears and behavioral observations) suggested that in unmated laboratory rats, a cycle of ovarian activity takes 4 or 5 days. A third biological indicator of cyclic changes of ovarian hormone production is uterine weight and distension. Analysis of changes in uterine weight, which required surgery, also suggested an ovarian cycle of this length in rats (Astwood, 1939; Mandl, 1952; Schwartz, 1964). The total average weight (mg/100 g body wt.) of rat uteri varied from 242 at vaginal proestrus, to 172 at vaginal estrus, to 166 on the first day of diestrus, to 134 on the second day of diestrus (Astwood, 1939; Fig. 1C). Correlations among changes in sex behavior, vaginal cytology, and uterine weight could now be made. Without question, these changes were caused by changes in ovarian function: if the ovaries were removed, the fluctuations in sex behavior, vaginal cytology, and uterine weight disappeared (for exceptions see Parkes and Deanesly, 1966). The problem now was to determine precisely which ovarian changes caused cyclic changes in target tissues for ovarian hormones (e.g., neural substrate for behavior, vagina, uterus). In the absence of biochemical techniques for mea-

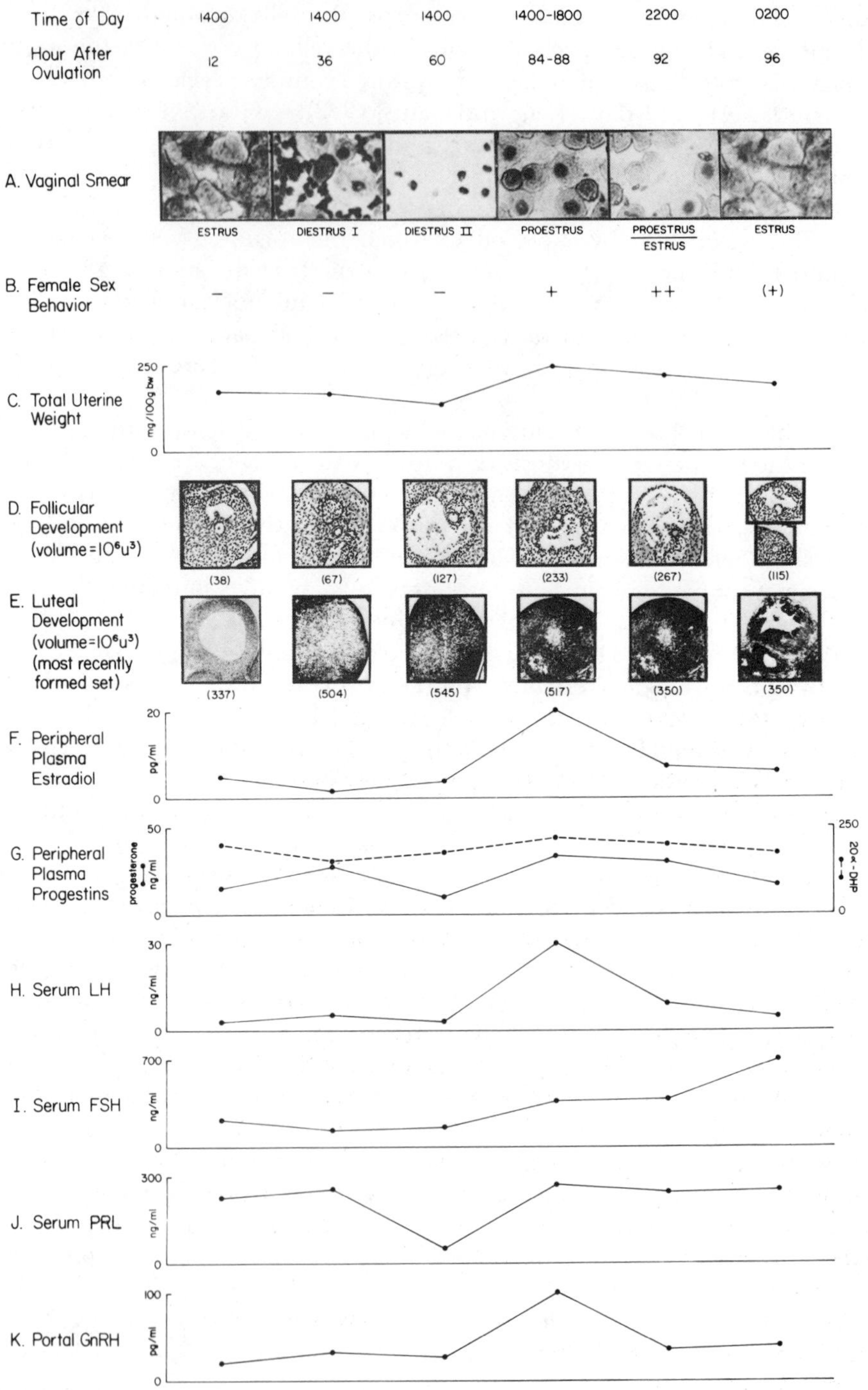

Time of Day
1400
1400
1400
1400-1800
2200
0200
Hour After Ovulation
12
36
60
84-88
92
96
A. Vaginal Smear
ESTRUS
DIESTRUS I
DIESTRUS II
PROESTRUS
PROESTRUS / ESTRUS
ESTRUS
B. Female Sex Behavior
–
–
–
+
++
(+)
C. Total Uterine Weight
mg/100g bw
250
0
D. Follicular Development (volume=10⁶u³)
(38)
(67)
(127)
(233)
(267)
(115)
E. Luteal Development (volume=10⁶u³) (most recently formed set)
(337)
(504)
(545)
(517)
(350)
(350)
F. Peripheral Plasma Estradiol
pg/ml
20
0
G. Peripheral Plasma Progestins
progesterone ng/ml
50
0
20α-DHP
250
0
H. Serum LH
ng/ml
30
0
I. Serum FSH
ng/ml
700
0
J. Serum PRL
ng/ml
300
0
K. Portal GnRH
pg/ml
100
0

surement of fluctuation in release of ovarian hormones, one answer to this problem lay in microscopic observations of cyclic changes of ovarian structure.

2. Cyclic Changes in Ovarian Structure

If the vaginal smear picture and estrous behavior could be temporally correlated with changes in ovarian structure in a reliable manner, this would allow some guesses to be made about the ovarian structural components involved in cyclic production of steroid hormones. To investigate these possible temporal correlations, rats with regular cycles of vaginal cytology were killed at various intervals after cessation of estrous behavior. Their ovaries and uteri were removed and examined. Not all of the variables we have mentioned (vaginal smear picture, sex behavior, ovarian appearance, uterine appearance) were considered in a single study, but the following discussion combines data from several studies (Long and Evans, 1922; Blandau *et al.*, 1941; Boling *et al.*, 1941; Boling, 1942; Mandl and Zuckerman, 1952). Because the ovary is a complex endocrine gland (Fig. 2), it is necessary to consider its various structural components one at a time. The first component to be considered is the ovarian follicle.

a. The Ovarian Follicle

The ovarian follicle (follicle = sac) surrounds the egg. The follicle forms from a flat layer of squamous epithelial cells that encapsulates the primary oocyte (primordial follicle stage). These epithelial cells enlarge to form a simple columnar epithelium (primary follicle stage) and then divide to form a stratified cuboidal epithelium, or granulosa (secondary follicle stage). The graulosa cells induce the surrounding connective tissue of the ovary to differentiate into the theca interna (theca = sheath). In turn, the connective tissue that surrounds the theca interna forms a thin layer of spindle-shaped cells (the theca externa). As the follicle continues to develop, a clear liquid (liquid folliculi) accumulates between the granulosa cells surrounding the oocyte and the granulosa cells on the wall of the follicle. The granulosa cells surrounding the oocyte form a hillock called the cumulus oophorus. The cumulus oophorus is attached to one side of the follicular wall. The granulosa cells that constitute the follicular wall are called mural granulosa cells. Eventually, so much liquor folliculi accumulates that the space between cumulus granulosa cells and mural granulosa cells coalesces and forms a single antrum (antrum = cavity) within the follicle (tertiary follicle stage) (see Mossman and Duke, 1973, for review). It

---

Figure 1. Sequence of events in the 4-day estrous cycle of the rat. The term Diestrus 1 is synonymous with what many authors term "metestrus." From Zarrow (1964) (vaginal smears); Feder *et al.* (1968a) (sex behavior); Astwood (1939) (uterine weight); Boling *et al.* (1941) (follicular development); Boling (1942) (luteal development); Brown-Grant *et al.* (1970) (estradiol); Nequin *et al.* (1975) (FSH, PRL, progestins); Naftolin *et al.* (1972) (LH); and Sarkar *et al.* (1976) (GnRH).

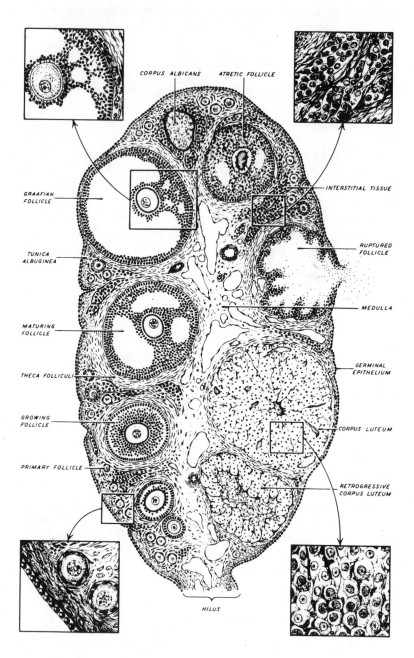

CORPUS ALBICANS

ATRETIC FOLLICLE

INTERSTITIAL TISSUE

GRAAFIAN
FOLLICLE

RUPTURED
FOLLICLE

TUNICA
ALBUGINEA

MEDULLA

MATURING
FOLLICLE

GERMINAL
EPITHELIUM

THECA FOLLICULI

GROWING
FOLLICLE

CORPUS LUTEUM

PRIMARY FOLLICLE

RETROGRESSIVE
CORPUS LUTEUM

HILUS

Figure 2. A composite mammalian ovary. Progressive stages in differentiation of a Graafian follicle are indicated on the left. The mature follicle may become atretic (top) or ovulate and undergo luteinization (right). From Turner (1966).

is at this point in the development of the follicle that one can begin reliably to correlate follicle growth with female sexual behavior, vaginal cytology, and uterine size. The following series of correlations has been made assuming a 4-day cycle (the follicle volumes are taken from Boling *et al.*, 1941 and the uterine weights from Astwood, 1939). (See Fig. 1D.)

Twelve Hours after Cessation of Estrous Behavior. Vaginal smear = estrus; total uterine weight (mg/100 g bw) = 172.2. The largest tertiary follicles have a mean volume of $38.3 \times 10^6 \mu m^3$. The antrum of each follicle is small, the granulosa is several layers thick, and there is a distinct theca interna.

Thirty-Six Hours after Cessation of Estrous Behavior. Vaginal smear = diestrus; total uterine weight = 166.0. The largest tertiary follicles have a mean volume of $67.1 \times 10^6 \ \mu m^3$. Mitoses are frequent in the granulosa cells, and the antra have increased in size.

Sixty Hours after Cessation of Estrous Behavior. Vaginal smear = diestrus; total uterine weight = 134.4. The tertiary follicles have enlarged (larger antra) and are called Graafian follicles. The mean volume of the Graafian follicles is $127 \times 10^6 \ \mu m^3$. Some follicles of various sizes begin to show signs of atresia (degeneration). Mitoses in the granulosa are less numerous.

Eighty-Four Hours after Cessation of Last Period of Estrous Behavior. A new period of female sexual behavior is about to begin. Vaginal smear = proestrus; total uterine weight = 242.2. A tremendously accelerated increase in volume of some follicles occurs at this point. This departure from linear growth is known as the preovulatory swelling. The preovulatory follicles have a mean volume of $233 \times 10^6 \ \mu m^3$. Their antra have become larger, and their mural granulosa thinner. The cumulus granulosa cells begin to be separated by fluid-filled spaces. The theca interna of the preovulatory follicles has thickened. Atresia is seen in some follicles of all sizes, but not in the follicles that are destined to ovulate.

Ninety-Two-Hours after Cessation of Last Period of Estrous Behavior. This is a few hours into the new period of female sexual behavior. Vaginal smear = proestrus/estrus; total uterine weight = 215.9. The mean volume of the preovulatory follicles is about $267 \times 10^6 \ \mu m^3$. The cumulus granulosa cells are widely separated. The theca interna is thicker except at the point where the preovulatory follicles will rupture. At this rupture point, the theca interna is very thin.

Ninety-Six Hours after Cessation of Last Period of Estrous Behavior. This is the approximate time of cessation of the current period of female sexual behavior. Vaginal smear = estrus; total uterine weight = 193.2. The preovulatory follicles rupture (ovulation). Immediately after ovulation, the walls of the follicle collapse, and the point of rupture is visible microscopically. The collapsed follicles have a mean volume of $115 \times 10^6 \ \mu m^3$. A new generation of tertiary follicles with mean volumes of $26.9 \times 10^6 \ \mu m^3$ and small antra can be seen. It is not clear whether these fresh tertiary follicles begin to develop from primary follicles at hour 84 (extension of the growth curve backward suggests this) or whether the growth of primary follicles does not always bear this predictable relation to the cycle.

b. The Corpus Luteum

Another important component of the ovary is the corpus luteum. The corpus luteum is a glandular structure that occupies the site of the ruptured follicle. The corpus luteum is formed by enlargement and multiplication of the follicular epithelium, supplemented by transformation of adjacent ovarian stromal cells into glandular cells (Mossman and Duke, 1973). In order to relate the growth of the corpus luteum to vaginal cytology, sex behavior, uterine weight, and ovarian follicular growth, the same times in the 4-day cycle that we used for follicular growth will be referred to (corpus luteum volumes are from Boling, 1942). (See Fig. 1E.)

Hour 12 after Ovulation and Cessation of Estrous Behavior. The point of rupture in the follicular wall is repaired, and a large, fluid-filled cavity is formed (mean volume = $337 \times 10^6 \ \mu m^3$). About the cavity is a wall of glandular luteal cells several layers thick.

Hour 36. The glandular luteal cells and their supporting vascular tissue fill up almost the entire cavity except for a small central region that contains some connective tissue. The mean volume of the corpora lutea is $504 \times 10^6 \ \mu m^3$.

Hour 60. Rapid growth of the corpus luteum continues, and a mean volume of $545 \times 10^6 \ \mu m^3$ is attained.

Hours 84 to 88. The glandular cells of the corpus luteum begin to regress, and the number of fibrocytes increases. The mean volume of the corpora lutea declines to $517 \times 10^6 \ \mu m^3$.

Hour 92 to Hour 96 or Hour 0. Regression of the corpus luteum continues, and a mean volume of $350 \times 10^6 \ \mu m^3$ is seen. At about this time, another group of preovulatory follicles ruptures, and a fresh set of corpora lutea is formed. The older set of corpora lutea continues to decline at a relatively slow rate. After several cycles, the corpora lutea are reduced to small masses of connective tissue (corpora albicantia) and eventually become indistinct from the ovarian stroma.

Unmated rats are said to have "nonfunctional" corpora lutea. That is, the freshly formed corpora lutea are unable to support a decidual reaction.* Rat corpora lutea are "functional" (i.e., able to support a decidual reaction) during pseudopregnancy or pregnancy. In other species, such as guinea pigs, sheep, rhesus monkeys, and humans, the corpora lutea formed even in the absence of mating are "functional" and support decidual reactions. As we shall see in Section II.B.2 of this chapter, the so-called "nonfunctional" corpus luteum of

---

*Decidual reaction: a reaction of the uterine endometrium to mechanical or chemical stimuli (e.g., injections of histamine dihydrochloride into uterine lumen) such that there is growth similar in appearance to the maternal placenta. During a normal rat estrous cycle, the corpora lutea produce insufficient progesterone to support a decidual reaction, but during a normal estrous cycle of a guinea pig, sufficient progesterone is produced by the corpora lutea to support a decidual reaction.

the unmated rat secretes significant quantities of steroid hormone, and this steroid production may play a role in regulation of estrus cycle length.

c. The Interstitial Gland

A third compartment of the ovary is the interstitial gland. Actually, interstitial gland cells are derived from several different ovarian sources. The most important source of interstitial gland cells in rats is the theca interna. Some interstitial gland cells are also derived from the ovarian stroma in rats. Interstitial gland cells normally go through recurring cycles of glandular differentiation.

In our study of the growth of ovarian follicles, we noted that many follicles undergo atresia (degeneration). In fact, about 95% of ovarian follicles undergo atresia, with the process most active during vaginal proestrus and vaginal estrus. It is the undifferentiated gland cells of the theca interna of atretic follicles that become transformed into interstitial gland cells in the rat. These interstitial gland cells are secretors of steroid hormones. Therefore, atresia is not just a way of getting rid of unfit or unnecessary eggs; it is also a means of producing a set of secretory cells.

In many species, the thecal type interstitial cell glands contain large vacuoles of fatty material that dissolve in the process of readying ovarian tissue for microscopic examination. This leaves a clear space in the cytoplasm, and the cells stain very lightly, distinguishing them from differentiated theca interna cells and corpus luteum cells. However, in rats, the distinction between thecal type interstitial gland cells and luteal cells is not very clear (Mossman and Duke, 1973). Burkl and Kellner (1954) have described the course of growth and degeneration of thecal type interstitial glands in rats.

If the data on biological indicators of ovarian activity and on fluctuations in ovarian structure throughout the rat estrous cycle are combined, the following salient features emerge:

1. The ovaries have a cycle of activity with a duration of 4 or 5 days.
2. The ovaries produce hormones that cause cyclical changes in vaginal cytology, uterine growth, and sexual receptivity.
3. Vaginal cornification starts to occur about 8 hr before the time of ovulation in 4-day cyclic rats.
4. The uterus reaches its maximum weight before the start of vaginal cornification, about 12–16 hr before ovulation.
5. Sexual receptivity starts a couple of hours after the beginning of vaginal cornification and 6–12 hr before ovulation in 4-day cyclic rats. The receptivity ends at about the time of ovulation.

Rats that have 5-day, rather than 4-day, cycles exhibit 3, rather than 2, days of diestrous vaginal smears. Vaginal cornification is prolonged in 5-day rats and begins about 30 hr prior to ovulation. The uterus reaches its maximum weight about 20 hr before ovulation, and sexual receptivity begins to be shown about 8–12 hr before ovulation (see review by Schwartz, 1969). As in the 4-day cyclic animals, there is, in the 5-day rats, linear growth of the follicles until shortly before ovulation, when a growth spurt occurs.

It is apparent that vaginal cornification, maximal uterine growth, and sexual receptivity all occur close to, but before the time of, follicular rupture in 4-day and 5-day cyclic rats. If we could determine which ovarian hormones are involved in vaginal cornification, uterine growth, and sexual behavior, we would have a fair idea of the nature of the ovarian hormones produced before ovulation. In the absence of biochemical assays for circulating steroid hormones, one way to determine which ovarian hormones favor vaginal cornification, uterine growth, and sexual receptivity is to ovariectomize experimental animals and institute replacement therapy with ovarian extracts or crystalline steroids manufactured in the laboratory.

3. Steroid Hormone Treatment of Ovariectomized Rats

a. Effects on Vagina

Although there are some exceptions (reviewed in Burrows, 1949; see Ohta and Iguchi, 1976, for an interesting example in mice), ovariectomy without steroid replacement therapy usually precludes the occurrence of vaginal cornification. Of the naturally occurring estrogens administered to ovariectomized rats, estradiol-17β appears to be the most potent for induction of the cornification reaction (Emmens, 1962; Beyer et al., 1971). However, this reaction is by no means an immediate one, even after estradiol* administration. The exact latency between time of estrogen administration and the appearance of cornified cells in the vagina varies according to route and vehicle of administration, type of estrogen given, and dosage of estrogen given. Nevertheless, it can be stated that it takes 48–72 hr for the vaginal epithelium to proliferate and then to become cornified after estrogen treatment (Young 1961; Emmens, 1962).

These data suggest that estradiol is the most significant estrogen of the normal estrous cycle and that an increase in estradiol secretion by the ovary occurs about 2 days before ovulation (the vaginal smear is cornified at ovulation). Furthermore, there is no indication from the hormone replacement experiments that steroids other than estrogens are required for the complete cornification reaction in rats.

b. Effects on Uterus

After ovariectomy, the rat's uterine horns become pale and slender. After injection of estradiol, a visible hyperemia occurs quickly, within 4 hr (Szego and Roberts, 1953), and for 6 hr after injection there is imbibition of water by the uterus (Astwood, 1938). In contrast to these rather rapid effects of estradiol, there is a slower increase in uterine growth, with dry weight of the uterus

---

*In the remaining parts of this chapter "estradiol" will refer to estradiol-17β.

continuing to increase for about 30 hr after subcutaneous estradiol injection (Astwood, 1939). When estradiol, estrone, and estriol are compared for their effects on the uterus, estradiol appears to be the most potent of the three (Emmens, 1962; 1969).

These experiments suggest that estradiol secretion inceases about 30 hr prior to vaginal proestrus (the time of maximal uterine weight during the estrous cycle) and about 42 hr prior to ovulation.

Another set of experiments concerned with steroid effects on the uterus indicates that progesterone might be produced a few hours prior to ovulation during a normal estrous cycle. In the normal estrous cycle, fluid accumulates in the uterine lumen, and this accumulation is attributable to estrogen action. However, there is a rapid loss of uterine luminal fluid about 8 hr after onset of vaginal estrus. This naturally occurring event, the loss of uterine luminal fluid, can be induced experimentally by administration of progesterone to estrogen-primed rats (Astwood, 1939; Armstrong, 1968). Thus, some time near the onset of vaginal estrus, and a few hours before ovulation, progesterone may be secreted by the ovary.

c. Effects on Estrous Behavior

Ovariectomized, untreated rats do not show estrous receptivity to males. When ovariectomized rats are given estradiol, estrone, or estriol, their estrous receptivity increases. Of these three forms of estrogen, estradiol appears to be the most potent (Beyer et al., 1971). Even after estradiol injection, estrous behavior does not become manifest until 16–24 hr after treatment (Green et al., 1970).

There seems little question that estrogen, by itself, can restore full estrous receptivity in rats that are adrenalectomized as well as ovariectomized (Davidson et al., 1968). However, early investigators noticed that progesterone given 24–48 hr after estrogen facilitated estrous receptivity in ovariectomized rats within a matter of a few hours (Boling and Blandau, 1939; see review by Feder and Marrone, 1977). In general, other progestins were less effective than progesterone in facilitation of lordosis in estrogen-primed, ovariectomized rats, but under certain circumstances, 20α-hydroxy-4-pregnen-3-one and 5α-pregnane-3,20-dione were also very potent (Meyerson, 1967, 1972; Langford and Hilliard, 1967; Zucker, 1967; Whalen and Gorzalka, 1972; Henrik and Gerall, 1976; Gorzalka and Whalen, 1977; Kubli-Garfias and Whalen, 1977). This led to the suggestion that in the normal estrous cycle, the ovary releases increased quantities of estrogen and then, about 1 or 2 days later, releases increased quantities of progesterone or related progestins. This idea was interesting because it implied that during the brief preovulatory phase the ovary was capable of secreting significant quantities of progesterone (recall that exhibition of estrous behavior precedes ovulation by several hours) in a normal estrous cycle. This idea was consistent with data that suggested that loss of uterine luminal fluid resulted from preovulatory secretion of progesterone (Astwood, 1939; Armstrong, 1968).

In summary, the implications about the normal estrous cycle drawn from work with steroid-treated, ovariectomized rats were: (a) estradiol is the most significant estrogen secreted during the cycle; (b) estradiol necessary for cyclic display of receptive behavior begins to be secreted at least 24 hr before the behavior is manifested and 36 hr before ovulation; and (c) an increase in progesterone secretion occurs about 4 hr before receptivity begins and about 8–12 hr before ovulation.

B. Direct Assessments of Cyclic Release of Ovarian Hormones

Consideration of the data obtained with ovariectomy and replacement therapy leads to the suppositions that during the course of the normal estrous cycle, estradiol secretion increases about 2 days before ovulation, and progesterone secretion increases about 8–12 hr before ovulation. Direct tests of these suppositions awaited the advent of sensitive techniques that could be used to measure estradiol and progesterone in the ovarian vein and in the peripheral circulation.

1. Estrogens

Early attempts at estimations of estrogens produced during the cycle involved examination of ovarian enzymes involved in the synthesis of these steroids (Pupkin *et al*., 1966; Kalvert and Bloch, 1968; Chatterton *et al*., 1969). More recently, estrogens have been measured in the ovarian vein and the peripheral plasma of 4- and 5-day cyclic rats. Hori *et al*. (1968) and Yoshinaga *et al*. (1969) used sensitive intravaginal bioassay tests for estrogens and concluded that estrogen in the ovarian vein of cyclic rats begins to increase at least 36 hr before ovulation. Maximum values of ovarian vein estrogen concentrations occur about 18 hr before ovulation, but a drastic decrease in concentrations of these steroids is seen about 6–12 hr before ovulation.

These data were soon confirmed by biochemical means. For example, Shaikh (1971) used a radioimmunoassay (RIA) procedure to demonstrate elevated ovarian vein estradiol levels on the morning of proestrus, with a significant drop by the evening of proestrus. At their peak, estradiol levels in ovarian vein were 2178 pg/ml plasma, whereas peak levels of estrone were only 416 pg/ml. Although estradiol and estrone showed a similar pattern of secretion, estradiol was secreted in much larger quantities than estrone. Competitive protein binding (Brown-Grant *et al.*, 1970) and RIA (Naftolin *et al.,* 1972) procedures were used to measure estradiol in peripheral plasma of cyclic rats. These methods revealed increased levels of the steroid about 30 hr prior to ovulation. Peak values were attained on the morning of proestrus (*ca.* 27 pg/ml peripheral plasma by competitive protein binding and *ca*.19 pg/ml by RIA).

Later work continued to demonstrate the same basic pattern of estrogen levels. Smith *et al.* (1975) measured peripheral plasma estradiol levels and obtained quite similar results. In the Smith *et al.* study, estradiol rose gradually from baseline concentrations of about 3–12 pg/ml plasma at vaginal estrus and the first day of diestrus (DiI) to about 30 pg/ml late in the second day of diestrus (DiII), then more steeply to over 40 pg/ml on the morning of proestrus. In late proestrus, there was a sharp decline, and baseline levels were present at the time of ovulation. Butcher *et al.* (1974) reported peak estradiol levels of about 80 pg/ml on the morning of proestrus, with baseline levels (*ca.* 20 pg/ml during vaginal estrus) beginning to rise as early as DiI. Horikoshi and Suzuki (1974) found peak levels of estradiol and estrone in peripheral plasma to be about 80 pg/ml for both steroids at proestrus, but variations in concentration were larger for estrone than for estradiol. Shaikh and Shaikh (1975) measured estrone and estradiol in ovarian and adrenal venous effluents and in peripheral plasma by RIA. Aside from the usual finding of increased estradiol concentrations in peripheral and ovarian vein plasma in DiII and early proestrus, these authors offered evidence of a significant secretion of estradiol (and to a lesser extent, estrone) by the adrenal gland. In fact, Shaikh and Shaikh (1975) found higher concentrations of "estradiol" in the adrenal venous effluent than in the ovarian venous effluent. The concentration of adrenal vein "estradiol" did not vary significantly over the cycle as the ovarian vein "estradiol" did. Further work should be conducted to determine whether the adrenal actually does produce such significant quantities of estradiol or whether the adrenals produce some other substances that crossreact with estradiol antiserum and cause overestimation of true estradiol values.

Finally, Schwartz and her colleagues (Schwartz, 1974; Nequin *et al.*, 1975) have also measured peripheral plasma estradiol throughout the estrous cycle. In the 1975 study, it was found that 4-day and 5-day cyclic rats had virtually identical levels of estradiol in the peripheral plasma during the first 3 days after ovulation (about 30 pg/ml, 60 pg/ml, and 110 pg/ml at 1, 2, and 3 days after ovulation, respectively). This finding suggests that differences between 4-day and 5-day cyclic rats in estradiol concentrations do not account for the difference in cyclic length.

These biochemical data confirm early suppositions about estrogen secretion based on experiments with estrogen-treated ovariectomized rats. To summarize: (a) estradiol is the major estrogen in the circulation, (b) estradiol concentrations in plasma begin to rise in DiII, about 36 hr before ovulation, and (c) estradiol concentrations in plasma reach a peak in early proestrus and decline sharply several hours before ovulation. The evidence for this pattern seems incontrovertible (see Fig. 1F for representative findings in 4-day cyclic rats). However, there are some disagreements about the absolute levels of estradiol in the peripheral circulation. These discrepancies may be caused by a number of factors including strain differences, methods of obtaining samples, anesthetics used, methods of assay, and relative contributions of ovarian and adrenal estradiol.

2. Progestins

By the late 1960s, several workers had determined concentrations of progesterone and related compounds within the ovary (Lindner and Zmigrod, 1967; Chatterton *et al.*, 1968) and in the ovarian vein plasma (Eto *et al.*, 1962; Telegdy and Endröczi, 1963; Uchida *et al.*, 1969a) during the course of rat estrous cycles of 4- and 5-day lengths. Several of these studies demonstrated a significant increase in progesterone concentration several hours before ovulation on the afternoon of proestrus. A smaller rise of progesterone concentration also occurred on the afternoon of DiI.

In the late 1960s, it became possible to measure progesterone and related steroids in the peripheral circulation. Gas–liquid chromatography (Feder *et al.*, 1968a; Barraclough *et al.*, 1971; Piacsek *et al.*, 1971), competitive protein-binding (Feder *et al.*, 1971; Butcher *et al.*, 1974) and RIA (Kalra and Kalra, 1974; Shaikh and Shaikh, 1975; Smith *et al.*, 1975; Nequin *et al.*, 1975) procedures all demonstrated a dramatic preovulatory increase in progesterone concentrations on the afternoon and evening of proestrus. By the time ovulation occurred, progesterone concentration had declined to baseline values. A smaller increase in progesterone concentration on DiI was also noted. The proestrus peak values were in the range of 25–50 ng/ml plasma, and the DiII and vaginal estrus values were in the range of 3–15 ng/ml plasma. Discrepancies among the studies are relatively minor. However, the contribution of the adrenal gland to the pool of circulating progesterone was found to be enormous, especially under conditions of stress (Feder *et al.*, 1968a; Barraclough *et al.*, 1971), and this factor, if not properly controlled for, could lead to major discrepancies in estimations of progesterone in peripheral plasma. Peripheral plasma progesterone also differed in 4-day and 5-day cyclic rats on day DiII. The 5-day cyclic rats had higher progesterone concentrations than the 4-day cyclic rats at this time (Nequin *et al.*, 1975). This may indicate that differences in concentration of progesterone of luteal origin account for differences in estrous cycle length.

Barraclough *et al.* (1971) measured plasma progestrone in the ovarian vein and in the peripheral circulation of 4-day cyclic rats. These authors noted a significant rise in peripheral plasma progesterone about 2–3 hr before a rise in ovarian vein plasma progesterone on the day of proestrus. This finding suggested an adrenal gland contribution to the proestrus peripheral plasma progesterone pool prior to an ovarian contribution to this pool. Other investigators who examined adrenal venous effluent for progesterone have conclusively demonstrated that the rat adrenal secretes considerable quantities of progesterone (Holzbauer *et al.*, 1969).

In many of the studies in which plasma progesterone was measured, another progestin, 20α-hydroxy-4-pregnen-3-one (20α-dihydroprogesterone, 20α-DHP), was also measured. Strangely, levels in ovarian vein and peripheral plasma were found to be far higher than those of progesterone (e.g., in Nequin *et al.*, 1975, peak progesterone concentrations in peripheral plasma were 40–60 ng/ml, whereas peak 20α-DHP levels were about 230 ng/ml). In the Nequin *et al.* (1975) study, the patterning of 20α-DHP levels was similar to that of progesterone in the sense that highest levels were attained at proestrus, somewhat lower levels at DiI, and lowest levels at DiII. However, the 20α-DHP did not drop as sharply at vaginal estrus as progesterone values (Nequin *et al.*, 1975), and 20α-DHP increased earlier in proestrus than did progesterone (Piacsek *et al.*, 1971). In a study by Horikoshi and Suzuki (1974), 20α-DHP was said to increase daily at 16.00–22.00 hours except on the day of proestrus. These data suggest that progesterone and 20α-DHP are secreted by different compartments of the ovary (Miyake, 1974).

Another progestin, 17α-hydroxyprogesterone, has been measured in ovarian vein and peripheral plasma of cyclic rats. Ovarian vein plasma concentrations of this steroid varied between 15–90 ng/ml plasma, adrenal vein concentrations between 120–200 ng/ml, and peripheral plasma between only 2–3 ng/ml.

Basically, the data on progestins in cyclic rats may be summarized as follows

1. There is a dramatic rise in progesterone concentration in the ovarian vein and in the peripheral circulation at the time of sexual receptivity, about 12 hr before ovulation. This finding is in total agreement with the prediction of the existence of a preovulatory surge of progesterone based on uterine and behavioral studies of ovariectomized, hormone-treated rats (Astwood, 1939; Boling and Blandau, 1939).

2. A smaller rise in progesterone concentration occurs during the first day of diestrus and probably indicates that the newly formed corpora lutea are functional in the sense that they produce progesterone.

3. 20α-DHP is present in much higher concentrations than progesterone in the plasma. Especially high levels of 20α-DHP are present during vaginal proestrus (Nequin *et al.*, 1975).

Representative data on progesterone and 20α-DHP in peripheral plasma of 4-day cyclic rats are illustrated in Fig. 1G.

III. RAT ESTROUS CYCLES—PITUITARY ASPECT

A. Indirect Assessments of Cyclic Release of Pituitary Hormones

Thus far, we have dealt with only the ovarian aspect of the long-loop system. We have seen that estradiol secretion begins to increase during diestrus and reaches a peak during proestrus; progesterone secretion increases dramatically about 8–12 hr before ovulation, declines sharply by the time of ovulation, and increases again, though less dramatically, during diestrus. The next problem we have to deal with is the changes that occur on the pituitary side of the long loop during the estrous cycle. Again, it was not until fairly recent times that sensitive biochemical techniques for measurements of circulating LH, FSH, and PRL became available. We shall briefly sketch the indirect means by which early workers estimated the timing of release of gonadotropic hormones during the estrous cycle and then give the results of the more recent biochemical measurements.

There is some early anatomical evidence for changes in pituitary cytology during the course of the rat estrous cycle. For example, Wolfe and Cleveland (1933) and Wolfe (1935) demonstrated cyclic variations in percentages of basophil cells (gonadotrophs and thyrotrophs are basophilic). The percentage of basophil cells with granules (presumably indicative of intracellular accumulation of gonadotropin) was highest at proestrus, intermediate at late diestrus, and lowest at early diestrus and (vaginal) estrus. Later, it was found that pituitary glycoprotein granules with a positive PAS reaction (probably representing gonadotropin accumulation) were most numerous in late diestrus (Catchpole, 1949). Purves and Griesbach (1954), using the PAS method, confirmed this result. Basically, these histological data suggested accumulation of gonadotropin in the pituitary beginning in late diestrus and release of gonadotropin from the pituitary prior to ovulation.

Histologically based guesses about the pattern of PRL secretion were harder to make. The PRL-releasing acidophils could not be distinguished from somatotropin-releasing acidophils, and changes in acidophils did not seem to bear a consistent relation to the estrous cycle (Self and Lloyd, 1966).

Other strategies were also used to estimate the pattern of cyclic release of hormones from the pituitary. One of these strategies involved the use of anovulatory animals such as immature rats or hypophysectomized rats. One could administer pituitary hormones to these anovulatory animals and determine which pituitary hormones induced ovulation, and with how long a latency. It was found that either LH or FSH, or combinations of these hormones administered to appropriately primed immature or hypophysectomized rats induced ovulation about 12 hr after administration (Rowlands and Williams, 1943; Lostroh and Johnson, 1966; Goldman and Mahesh, 1968).

An important advance in the understanding of estrous cyclicity was provided by the finding that ovulation in rats was dependent on environmental light/dark changes. When rats were kept in constant bright illumination, they became anovulatory (Browman, 1937; Hemmingsen and Krarup, 1937; Everett, 1961). Given the fact that the ovulatory process in the rat is sensitive to environmental light, it became imperative for investigators to keep rats under standardized conditions of light and dark. Everett (1961) used a regime of 14 hr light: 10 hr dark per day, with lights on at 0500 hours and off at 1900 hours. When rats were kept under these conditions, they ovulated at about 0100–0300 hours of the day of vaginal estrus. In all subsequent discussion, we shall use the Everett lighting schedule as our reference (one should bear in mind that some authors have used somewhat different schedules in their research (e.g., 12 : 12 light : dark).

If it takes about 12 hr for exogenous gonadotropin to induce ovulation in anovulatory rats, and if cyclic rats ovulate at about 0100–0300 hours of vaginal estrus, one would estimate that gonadotropin necessary for ovulation in cyclic rats would be released at about 1400–1500 hours of the day of vaginal proestrus. Experimental evidence that validated this estimate was reported. Everett (1956) hypophysectomized rats on the day of vaginal proestrus at 1445, 1515, or 1545 hours and determined whether ovulation occurred the next day. Ovulation was partially or completely blocked in 90% of the 1445-hours group, in 70% of the 1515-hours group, and in 33% of the 1545-hours group. Thus, by 1545 hours of vaginal proestrus, enough gonadotropin had already been released by the pituitary to provoke ovulation in a majority of animals.

The technique of surgical hypophysectomy tells us when the pituitary has released enough gonadotropin for ovulation but does not tell us when this release begins. To determine this, a procedure is required that will acutely and temporarily prevent hypophyseal release of gonadotropins. This sort of "functional hypophysectomy" can be performed by using "blocking drugs" (e.g., atropine, dibenamine, phenobarbital). These drugs apparently act by prevention of neurogenic stimulation of the pituitary (Everett, 1961). The drugs were effective in blocking ovulation the next day when given between 1300 and 1500 hours of the day of vaginal proestrus. If allowances are made for the time needed for the drug to exert its effects, these results indicate that ovulation is caused by a surge of gonadotropin release induced by a neurogenic stimulus that begins at 1400 hours and ends before 1600 hours of vaginal proestrus (this period is called the "critical period") (Everett *et al.*, 1949; Everett and Sawyer, 1950, 1953; Everett, 1956).

This rather remarkable feat of predicting, to the hour, the course of release of a hormone was accomplished in the absence of direct biochemical assays of gonadotropic hormone. Support for the prediction was provided by experiments in which antiserum to LH or to FSH was administered (this procedure blocks the effects of LH and FSH, respectively, but does not block release of these hormones from the pituitary) at 1300 hours of vaginal proestrus to cyclic rats. The antiserum to LH blocked ovulation, whereas the antiserum to FSH did not block ovulation (Schwartz, 1969). These data also indicated that even if LH and FSH are both released during the afternoon of proestrus, it is LH that is primarily responsible for the occurrence of ovulation.

The sum of these data strongly implies that gonadotropin is released on the afternoon of proestrus. Is this the only time in the cycle that gonadotropin is released? To find out, Lawton and Sawyer (1968) hypophysectomized rats during hours 0900–1800 of DiII. This procedure blocked ovulation, but it may have done so merely by precluding the release of gonadotropin at proestrus. However, the authors found that vaginal cornification and uterine growth occurred at the expected time of next estrus in rats hypophysectomized between 1500 and 1800 hours of DiII and not in rats hypophysectomized between 0900 and 1400 hours of DiII. This suggests that gonadotropin release important for estrogen production occurs between 0900 and 1400 hours of DiII. This release of gonadotropin is not sensitive to barbiturate blockade (Schwartz and Lawton, 1968; Brown-Grant, 1969).

B. Direct Assessments of Cyclic Release of Pituitary Hormones

Assessments of LH in the pituitary gland were made by means of the ovarian ascorbic acid depletion assay (OAAD). The results of Mills and Schwartz (1961), Schwartz and Bartosik (1962), and Schwartz and Caldarelli (1965) established that the pituitary content of LH in 4-day cyclic rats was higher at DiII and the morning of proestrus than at DiI or vaginal estrus. A drop in LH content of the pituitary occurred between the morning and evening of proestrus. No differences were noted between 4-day and 5-day cyclic rats in pituitary LH content.

Luteinizing hormone in the systemic circulation was measured by the OAAD method and by radioimmunoassay in 4-day and 5-day cyclic rats. The OAAD method generally yielded higher values than those obtained with radio-immunoassay (Bogdanove et al., 1971), but the two methods are in agreement with regard to the pattern of LH concentrations in serum. The data obtained in these studies unanimously support the prediction by Everett et al. (1949) of a dramatic increase in circulating LH concentration beginning at 1400 hours. Elevated levels of LH persist beyond the end of the critical period at 1600 hours until about 2000 hours of proestrus (McCann and Ramirez, 1964; Schwartz and Caldarelli, 1965; Monroe et al., 1969; Daane and Parlow, 1971; Linkie and Niswender, 1972; Kalra and Kalra, 1974; Butcher et al., 1974; Blake, 1974; Shaikh and Shaikh, 1975; Smith et al., 1975; and many others). Blake (1976a) has provided a detailed picture of the LH rise by taking blood samples at frequent (5-min) intervals between 1400 and 2000 hours of proestrus. He found a small but detectable rise in serum LH between 1400 and 1445 hours and a rapid linear increase starting at 1445–1650 hours and lasting for 20–50 min. Over the next 2 hr, there were relatively small erratic rises in serum LH and fluctuation around a plateau. A decline in serum LH concentration started at about 1800, this decline being interrupted by rapid transient increases in serum LH that were perhaps induced by pulses of GnRH (see Section IV of this chapter). At their proestrus peak, LH levels in serum are reported by recent RIA work to be of the order of 1500–2000 ng NIAMDD-ratLH-RP-1/ml (Blake, 1976a), but even the RIA data vary greatly from study to study. The important fact is that LH is present at very low baseline levels throughout the cycle (there may be small diurnal increases in serum LH during the cycle; Gay et al., 1970) except for a brief period on the day of proestrus, about 8–12 hr prior to ovulation. There seems to be little difference between 4-day and 5-day cyclic rats in LH release pattern, with peak levels perhaps somewhat higher in 5-day than in 4-day animals (Schwartz and Caldarelli, 1965; Nequin et al., 1975). Representative data for LH in serum of 4-day cyclic rats are shown in Fig. 1H.

Follicle-stimulating hormone content of the pituitary was measured by an ovarian weight augmentation test (Steelman–Pohley test) in several studies. Caligaris *et al.* (1967) used a mixture of 4-day and 5-day cyclic rats and found highest pituitary FSH concentrations on the morning of proestrus. By the afternoon of proestrus, there was a 67% drop in pituitary FSH content. Thereafter, there was a gradual increase in pituitary FSH content until the next period of proestrus. McClintock and Schwartz (1968) used 4-day cyclic rats and came to essentially the same conclusions. Other workers confirmed these results by use of the Steelman–Pohley test (Goldman and Mahesh, 1968) or RIA procedures (Taya and Igarashi, 1973).

The Steelman–Pohley test was used by McClintock and Schwartz (1968) to estimate FSH levels in the systemic circulation of 4-day cyclic rats. These investigators found an increase in serum FSH at 1500 hours of proestrus. However, the Steelman–Pohley assay was considered too insensitive to yield quantitatively reliable results for FSH in the systemic circulation. The more sensitive RIA methods were eventually utilized, and studies were carried out in 4-day and 5-day cyclic animals. There is good agreement among these studies (Daane and Parlow, 1971; Linkie and Niswender, 1972; Taya and Igarashi, 1973; Butcher *et al.*, 1974; Shaikh and Shaikh, 1975; Smith *et al.*, 1975; Blake, 1976b). They indicate that there are baseline levels of FSH during DiI and DiII (*ca*. 50–150 ng NIAMDD-rat FSH-RP-1/ml), with an increase on the afternoon of proestrus. This increase reaches a peak at about 1700–1900 hours of proestrus (*ca*.400–500 ng NIAMDD-rat FSH-RP-1/ml), about 4 hr after LH has attained its peak but several hours before ovulation. Follicle-stimulating hormone, in contrast to LH, does not decline precipitously. Rather, FSH levels remain close to peak levels for about 16 hr (i.e., into the morning of vaginal estrus and after ovulation) and then decline to about 200–250 ng NIAMDD-rat FSH-RP-1/ml on the afternoon of estrus. Although the peak values of FSH at proestrus were quite similar in 4- and 5-day cyclic rats, the 5-day animals appeared to exhibit a daily rhythmic increase (at 2400 hours) and decrease (at 1200 hours) that was not discernible in 4-day rats (Nequin *et al.*, 1975). Representative data for serum FSH in 4-day cyclic rats are shown in Fig. 11.

Early workers used a crop sac assay to measure pituitary content of PRL (Reece, 1939). Rats in proestrus and vaginal estrus were said to have a higher pituitary PRL content than rats in diestrus (Sar and Meites, 1967). More recent work suggests that there is a very significant decline in pituitary PRL on the afternoon of proestrus (Yokoyama *et al.*, 1971).

The crop sac assay was not sensitive enough to measure PRL in the systemic circulation of cyclic rats, and measurement of this hormone was delayed until the advent of RIA methods. Amenomori *et al.* (1970) found highest serum PRL (expressed in terms of a standard curve based on a purified rat PRL preparation) levels during vaginal estrus (68.5 ng/ml) and lowest levels during diestrus (27.6 ng/ml). However, more recent studies show that PRL in 4-day as well as 5-day cyclic rats reaches a peak in blood at 1200–2000 hours of proestrus. Attainment of this peak appears to be simultaneous with the LH peak prior to ovulation. The range of peak plasma values in the radioimmuno-assay studies is 70–250 ng/ml. Although the studies of Butcher *et al.* (1974) and Smith *et al.* (1975) suggest that PRL values decline to baseline by about 0600 hours of estrus, the data of Nequin *et al.* (1975) indicate a rather slower decline in PRL levels after the preovulatory peak. PRL baseline levels are of the order of < 20 ng/ml. The claim of some authors (e.g., Butcher *et al.*, 1974) that there is a second transient PRL peak on the afternoon of vaginal estrus is not accepted by some other workers. This second peak at estrus may have been the result of an artifact; rats may be particularly sensitive to stress at estrus, and stress may cause release of PRL (Neill, 1972; Smith *et al.*, 1975). Representative data for serum PRL in 4-day cyclic rats are represented in Fig. 1J.

IV. RAT ESTROUS CYCLES—HYPOTHALAMIC ASPECT

Evidence for the existence of GnRH was reviewed in the previous chapter (and in Guillemin, 1977; Schally *et al.*, 1978). Serious attempts at measurement of GnRH during the course of the estrous cycle began with bioassays of GnRH concentrations in brain tissues. The GnRH content of the hypothalamus was found, by OAAD, to drop abruptly during the afternoon of proestrus (Ramirez and Sawyer, 1965). Chowers and McCann (1965), also using the OAAD test, found that GnRH concentrations in hypothalamus peaked during DiII and declined significantly by the afternoon of proestrus. Kalra *et al.* (1973) found rhythmic increases and decreases in GnRH content of hypothalamus during proestrus. Araki *et al.* (1975) and Asai and Wakabayashi (1975) measured GnRH hypothalamic content by RIA rather than by bioassay. These workers found relatively high hypothalamic GnRH concentrations at 0800 hours, lower levels by 1000 hours, and increased levels again at 1700 hours of proestrus. Barr and Barraclough (1978), also using a RIA procedure, found basal levels of hypothalamic GnRH during estrus and diestrus, with rhythmic rises and falls during hours 1200–2100 of proestrus. These authors suggested that hypothalamic GnRH is released in a pulsatile fashion during proestrus.

There was general acceptance of the idea that increased quantities of GnRH are released into the hypophyseal portal vessels close to the time of the LH surge at proestrus. However, bioassay and RIA procedures (carried out after animals were anesthetized with urethane or sodium pentobarbitone) at first failed to detect increased portal vessel concentrations of GnRH at the expected time (Fink and Harris, 1970; Eskay *et al.*, 1975, 1977; Fink and Jamieson, 1976). Later experiments in which a different anesthetic was used (Althesin®, an anesthetic that apparently does not interfere with ovulation*) succeeded in detecting the expected rise in stalk GnRH concentrations. The data were based on a RIA technique that yielded GnRH levels of 20–35 pg/ml portal blood at DiI, DiII, and estrus, but GnRH levels of 50–150 pg/ml at various times of proestrus. The increase in GnRH began at 1500 hours of

*At least at certain dosages.

proestrus, or almost simultaneously with the beginning of the LH surge. Peak levels of stalk GnRH were attained at 1800 hours of proestrus. There was great interindividual variability, suggestive of pulsatile release of GnRH. By 2230 hours, stalk GnRH levels were back to baseline concentrations (Sarkar *et al.*, 1976; Fink *et al.*, 1976). Figure 1K shows stalk vessel concentrations of GnRH.

V. THE ESTROUS CYCLE—PUTTING IT ALL TOGETHER

The patterns of hormone production by the ovaries, pituitary, and hypothalamus during the course of the estrous cycle were reviewed in the foregoing sections. It is now time to attempt to see how these various secretions are orchestrated to produce recurrent estrous cycles of consistent duration. As in the preceding sections, we shall deal primarily with the 4-day cycle and relate the hormonal changes during the cycle to the occurrence of ovulation (at 0100 hours of vaginal estrus).

12 hr after Ovulation (1300 Hours of Vaginal Estrus). Estrogen, progesterone, LH and PRL levels in systemic plasma are low. Follicle-stimulating hormone levels in blood are declining, but have not yet returned to baseline. Apparently, testosterone secreted at proestrus (Dupon and Kim, 1973) is responsible for elevated FSH blood levels during the morning of vaginal estrus (Gay and Tomacari, 1974). It is probable that the ovaries are a source of the testosterone secreted at proestrus, with theca interna (Fortune and Armstrong, 1977) and interstitial cells likely to be the secretory elements involved (see reviews by Young, 1961; Parkes and Deanesly, 1966). One possible function of ovarian androgen is retardation of follicular development (Louvet *et al.*, 1975), perhaps contributing to the differential rate of growth among follicles.* The FSH produced during the evening of proestrus and the morning of vaginal estrus is thought to act on a fresh set of ovarian follicles and stimulate their growth (Welschen and Dullaart, 1976; review by Neill and Smith, 1974). Without gonadotropic stimulation (e.g., after hypophysectomy), follicles fail to grow beyond the preantral stage (Velardo, 1960; Lostroh and Johnson, 1966; Malven and Sawyer, 1966).

36 hr after Ovulation (1300 Hours of DiI). Estrogen, LH, FSH, and PRL systemic blood levels are low. However, LH and FSH act on the fresh set of follicles and cause a continued linear rate of growth. Under the influence of the gonadotropins, the size of the theca interna of growing follicles increases. The theca interna is thought to be the major source of ovarian estrogens, although interstitial gland cells and corpora lutea may also secrete estrogens (reviewed by Young, 1961; Parkes and Deanesly, 1966; see also Short, 1964; MacDonald *et al.*, 1966). Plasma progesterone levels are elevated, presumably because of

---

*For a recent summary of many aspects of follicular function see *Ovarian Follicular Development and Function* (A. R. Midgley, Jr. and W. A. Sadler, eds.), Raven Press, New York, 1979.

autonomous steroid secretion by the newest set of corpora lutea (Uchida *et al.*, 1969a).

56 hr after Ovulation (0900 Hours of DiII). Serum PRL levels remain low, as do serum concentrations of LH and FSH. The LH (and perhaps FSH) continues to act on the follicles, inducing a continued linear rate of growth and increased production of estradiol via increases in cyclic AMP and perhaps prostaglandins (see Chapter 9 and Labhsetwar, 1975). The follicular production of estrogen prevents follicular atresia (Harman *et al.*, 1975) and sensitizes the ovary to the action of gonadotropin by induction of LH receptors in the granulosa cells of the follicle (Richards and Midgley, 1976). Estrogen also increases the number of granulosa cells, thereby causing an increased binding of FSH to the fixed number of FSH receptors per granulosa cell (Louvet and Vaitukaitis, 1976). Thus, an intraovarian short-loop may be an important follicular growth regulator (Short, 1964). At this point, enough estrogen has been released into the circulation to cause, subsequently, at least partial vaginal cornification, but not enough estrogen has been released to cause maximal uterine ballooning, ovulation, or mating behavior (Kobayashi *et al.*, 1969a; Schwartz, 1969; Neill *et al.*, 1971).

Basal levels of LH may not only act to induce growth of the follicles, but may also exert a lytic effect on the corpora lutea, thereby decreasing the production of progesterone by this ovarian compartment (Rothchild, 1965). Rats that have 4-day cycles have less progesterone in the peripheral circulation (Nequin *et al.*, 1975) and in the ovarian vein (Roser and Bloch, 1971) on DiII than rats with 5-day cycles. Because elevated levels of progesterone slow the rate of follicular development (Buffler and Roser, 1974), it is reasonable to suppose that the longer secretory life of the corpus luteum is a primary causative factor in the generation of 5- rather than 4-day cycles. The effects of progesterone on the slowing of follicular growth may be accompanied by a slowing of estrogen secretion (Schwartz, 1969, but see Nequin *et al.*, 1975) or a retardation of estrogen priming of neural and anterior pituitary gland target tissues (Tapper *et al.*, 1974, reviewed by Feder and Marrone, 1977; Goodman, 1978a,b).

62 hr after Ovulation (1500 Hours of DiII). Estradiol levels continue to rise. At this point, pituitary stimulation of ovarian estradiol secretion is as complete as it need be (Schwartz, 1969). Serum gonadotropin levels remain low, perhaps because of inhibitory effects of estradiol on medial basal hypothalamic neurons (Brown-Grant, 1977). Progesterone concentrations in plasma are also low at this point in the cycle.

80-85 hr after Ovulation (0900–1400 Hours of Proestrus). Plasma LH, FSH, and PRL levels remain low, but plasma estradiol levels reach their maximum. A slight rise in peripheral plasma progesterone occurs, but this is apparently of adrenal rather than ovarian origin (Feder *et al.*, 1971; Barraclough *et al.*, 1971). The increase in adrenal release of progesterone may be attributable to estrogenic stimulation of ACTH (Barrett, 1960) or adrenocortical secretion (Kitay, 1963; Bartosik *et al.*, 1971). Some workers have suggested that progesterone of adrenal origin (Feder *et al.*, 1971; Nequin and Schwartz, 1971; Lawton, 1972; Mann and Barraclough, 1973a,b) or 20α-DHP of ovarian origin (Swerdloff *et al.*, 1972) released at this time facilitates the release or helps to regulate the timing of the impending surge of LH. However, these progestins are probably not required for LH release (Ferin *et al.*, 1969). Aside from its actions on the ovarian follicles and the adrenal, estradiol also acts on the pituitary and perhaps the diencephalon to increase the number of estrogen receptors in cell nuclei (Clark *et al.*, 1973; Menon and Gunaga, 1976; Sen and Menon, 1978) and on the diencephalon to cause release of GnRH into the hypophyseal portal system (Sarkar *et al.*, 1976; Fink *et al.*, 1976).

At this stage of the estrous cycle, enough estradiol has been secreted to cause, subsequently, maximal uterine ballooning and release of surges of LH, FSH, and PRL (Schwartz, 1969; Neill and Smith, 1974). The fact that estradiol is the causative factor in release of these three pituitary hormones has been established by experiments utilizing timed ovariectomies (Schwartz, 1964), or injections of progesterone (Everett and Sawyer, 1949; Zeilmaker, 1966; Brown-Grant, 1967; Kobayashi *et al.*, 1969b,c), synthetic antiestrogens (Callantine *et al.*, 1966; Shirley *et al.*, 1968; Labhsetwar, 1970a,b), or antisera to estradiol (Ferin *et al.*, 1969; Neill *et al.*, 1971). In some of the experiments with synthetic antiestrogens (Labhsetwar, 1970a) and antisera to estradiol (Neill *et al.*, 1971), the investigators administered estradiol or diethylstilbestrol (DES, an estrogenic compound that does not crossreact with antiserum to estradiol), respectively. All of these experiments demonstrated that deprivation of estradiol stimulation of the diencephalon [presumably the AH–SCN–POA area in particular (Brown-Grant, 1977)] and/or the pituitary by antiestrogen treatment, or treatment with antiserum to estradiol during the day before proestrus blocks the impending surge of LH on proestrus. Reversal of this blockade occurs if estradiol or DES is administered simultaneously with antiestrogen or antiserum to estradiol. Blockade does not occur if an estrogen deprivation procedure is initiated on the morning of proestrus. In other words, not enough estradiol has been produced by the morning of the day before proestrus to induce the LH surge, but enough estradiol has been secreted by noon of proestrus to induce the LH surge.

Ovariectomy at this stage of the estrous cycle does not permit subsequent display of lordosis behavior (Schwartz and Talley, 1965; Schwartz, 1969; Powers, 1970). This indicates that the threshold for activation of lordosis behavior by estradiol is higher than that for vaginal cornification, uterine ballooning, LH release, FSH release, and PRL release. The importance of this relatively elevated threshold for behavioral activation by estradiol will be discussed soon. Although insufficient estradiol has been produced for behavioral activation by this time in the cycle, estradiol is presumably priming the neural tissues that mediate lordosis behavior. According to recent work, the most sensitive of these tissues is the medial basal hypothalamus (Barfield and Chen, 1977), although other diencephalic regions may also be involved (Lisk, 1962; Dörner *et al.*, 1968; Rodgers and Law, 1968).

Eighty-Five to 89 Hours after Ovulation (1400–1800 Hours of Proestrus). Estradiol may stimulate release of a pulse of GnRH from the AH–SCN–POA region. This pulse may lower pituitary sensitivity to the tonic discharge of GnRH from the MBH (Brown-Grant, 1977). Alternatively, there may simply be an increased rate of GnRH release from the diencephalon (Blake, 1978). In any event, the result is a smooth, linear increase in serum LH at 1445–1650 hours that lasts for about 30 min (Gay *et al.*, 1970; Blake, 1976a). Sensitization of the pituitary gland to GnRH may occur not only because of a prior pulse of GnRH but also through a direct action of estradiol on the pituitary (Cooper *et al.*, 1974; Fink *et al.*, 1975; Sherwood *et al.*, 1976; Aiyer *et al.*, 1976). The surge of LH has multiple effects among which are:

1. Massive preovulatory swelling of follicles destined to ovulate (Boling *et al.*, 1941; Schwartz, 1969).
2. Atresia of antral follicles not destined to ovulate (Greep, 1961; Everett, 1967; Quinn and Everett, 1967; Louvet *et al.*, 1975).
3. Switching-over of preovulatory and degenerating follicles from estrogen production to progesterone production (Hori *et al.*, 1970).
4. Possibly, determination of the life-span of the corpora lutea to be formed after ovulation (Greig and Weisz, 1973). Some workers have noted that LH (and FSH and PRL) levels in serum at this time are higher in 5-day than in 4-day cyclic rats (Smith *et al.*, 1973). It is conceivable that such differences are factors in the determination of cycle length. In this connection, it is interesting to note that rats produce much more LH during the surge than they need for ovulation per se (Everett, 1956; Kobayashi *et al.*, 1968; Greig and Weisz, 1973; Gosden *et al.*, 1976).

That the sudden, dramatic rise in plasma progesterone concentration seen at this time point is a consequence of the LH surge has been shown in several studies. The release of LH always precedes the release of progesterone by the ovarian interstitial tissue (Hashimoto and Wiest, 1969) when data are analyzed for individual animals (Piacsek *et al.*, 1971; Barraclough *et al.*, 1971). Blockade of the LH surge by hypophysectomy (Uchida *et al.*, 1969b,c) or barbiturate treatment at 1300–1500 hours of proestrus blocks progesterone release (Barraclough *et al.*, 1971; Feder *et al.*, 1971; Ichikawa *et al.*, 1972). Injection of LH to barbiturate-blocked rats restores the preovulatory progesterone surge (Ichikawa *et al.*, 1972). The progesterone released during this preovulatory period has multiple effects among which are:

1. Completion of the final stages of follicular rupture by an action on the follicular wall (Takahashi *et al.*, 1974).
2. Facilitation of lordosis behavior (behavior commences at 1700–1800 hours; Schwartz, 1969; Feder *et al.*, 1971). As mentioned previously, the threshold for activation of sexual receptivity by estradiol appears to exceed the threshold for release of LH. In fact, during the estrous cycle, many animals do not produce enough estradiol to induce sexual recep-

tivity. They appear to require an additional "boost" that is provided by the preovulatory progesterone surge. This was demonstrated by Powers (1970) by means of timed ovariectomy experiments on the day of proestrus. The significance of this requirement for estrogen–progesterone synergy is that female rats will begin to display sexual receptivity after the surge of LH (which causes progesterone release), at a time when the ovulatory process has become inexorable. Thus, the differences in threshold to estradiol stimulation between sexual receptivity and LH release help to insure that the behavior will occur at an optimal time in relation to ovulation. Several investigators have indicated that the progesterone that gives the estrogen-primed behavioral system its final boost acts primarily on the midbrain reticular formation, with other brain areas perhaps also sensitive to progesterone action (Ross *et al.,* 1971; Powers, 1972; Ward *et al.,* 1975; Yanase and Gorski, 1976).* It may be mentioned that GnRH also facilitates estrogen-dependent lordosis (Moss and McCann, 1973, 1975; Pfaff, 1973), possibly via release of GnRH by prostaglandins (Hall *et al.,* 1975; Dudley and Moss, 1976). It is not yet known whether the behavior-facilitating actions of progesterone and GnRH are mediated by identical anatomical sites and identical biochemical mechanisms.

3. Relaxation of the cervical sphincter to permit release of intraluminal fluid from the uterus (Astwood, 1939; Armstrong, 1968; Ferin *et al.,* 1969). Estrogen-induced PRL secretion may play a role in relaxation of the cervical sphincter (Kennedy and Armstrong, 1972), perhaps through stimulation of progesterone release from the adrenal cortex by PRL (Piva *et al.,* 1973). Decreases in uterine weight later in proestrus may also be partially caused by decreases in ovarian estrogen secretion (Schwartz, 1964; Schwartz and Gold, 1967; Shirley *et al.,* 1968).

4. Blockade of daily surges of LH. Several workers have discovered that ovariectomized rats given particular regimens of estradiol injections display daily surges of LH release even after cessation of estradiol injections. These repeated estrogen-induced daily surges of LH do not occur if progesterone is given on the last day of estrogen injection (Neill and Smith, 1974). It has been proposed that preovulatory progesterone has a similar function during the course of the estrous cycle. It has been demonstrated that barbiturate-blocked rats given continuous progesterone from 1400 to 2400 hours of proestrus (Banks and Freeman, 1978) do not display daily surges of LH on subsequent days of the cycle, but blocked rats not given progesterone do exhibit daily LH surges (Freeman *et al.,* 1976). It is not clear how such daily surges of LH, if they did occur, would affect the estrous cycle.

---

*Unpublished work by B. Rubin and R. Barfield (personal communication) indicates that the primary site of the facilitative action of progesterone on lordosis behavior in the rat is the ventromedial nucleus of the hypothalamus.

Prolactin is released at about the same time as LH. Injection on the morning of DiII of antisera to estradiol (Neill *et al.*, 1971) or antisera to LH (recall that LH induces estrogen synthesis) (Freeman *et al.*, 1972) shows that estradiol secretion causes the preovulatory PRL surge. The release of PRL seems to have little or no influence on the estrous cycle (Neill and Smith, 1974). The PRL cannot act on existing first-generation corpora lutea to rescue them, because these corpora lutea have already been luteolyzed by LH during diestrus. The tranquilizer trifluoperazine (Stelazine ®), given during diestrus, permitted rescue of the corpora lutea by proestrous PRL. Presumably, trifluoperazine blocked LH release during diestrus (Schwartz, 1969). The preovulatory PRL surge is also not involved in ovulation per se, because PRL fails to induce preovulatory progesterone secretion or ovulation by itself or to synergize with LH in induction of progesterone secretion or ovulation in hormonally blocked, hypophysectomized, or barbiturate-blocked rats (Yoshinaga *et al.*, 1967; Uchida *et al.*, 1969b; Barraclough *et al.*, 1971). One possible purpose served by the PRL released during proestrus is to cause regression of corpora lutea from previous cycles (Wuttke and Meites, 1971). Another possible function is to cause more preovulatory progesterone secretion by action on the adrenal cortex (Piva *et al.*, 1973; Gelato *et al.*, 1976).

A significant increase in serum FSH occurs about 4 hr after the onset of LH, PRL, and progesterone surges at 1400 hours of proestrus. This initial portion of the FSH rise is probably mediated by estradiol (McClintock and Schwartz, 1968) and initiated by GnRH. The delay in FSH secretion relative to LH secretion may result from a slower action of GnRH on FSH than on LH release (Krulich *et al.*, 1974).* The fact that FSH begins to increase after plasma progesterone concentrations rise has suggested to some workers that progesterone may also influence the initial FSH surge (Caligaris *et al.*, 1967). Aside from its stimulation of a crop of fresh follicles, FSH may also synergize with LH in induction of ovulation. This kind of synergism has been demonstrated experimentally by treating hypophysectomized or pharmacologically blocked rats with combinations of FSH and LH (Harrington and Bex, 1970; Labhsetwar, 1970c, 1972a). However, this synergistic action of FSH seems not to be required for ovulation (Schwartz, 1969; Schwartz *et al.*, 1975).

Ninety-Two Hours after Ovulation (1200 Hours of Proestrus). Serum LH and PRL levels have declined to baseline values, but FSH concentrations in serum remain elevated. Gonadotropin-releasing hormone concentrations in the portal vessels have declined to baseline. Estradiol levels in plasma are low, but preovulatory progesterone concentrations are still above baseline. The decline in estradiol levels that began at 1400 hours of proestrus may have caused

---

*More recent evidence indicates that GnRH can stimulate selective FSH secretion depending upon the mode and rate of delivery of the releasing hormone to the anterior pituitary gland (Wise *et al.*, 1979). This supports the idea that there is a single GnRH for both LH and FSH. However, the possibility that separate releasing factors exist for the two gonadotropins is not excluded. Another possibility is that certain (as yet unidentified) hypothalamic substances modify the hypophyseal action of GnRH resulting in differential release of the two gonadotropins in particular circumstances (Yu *et al.*, 1978).

increased responsiveness of the pituitary to GnRH (Turgeon and Barraclough, 1977). Although the decline in estradiol concentrations is probably a significant causal factor in termination of estrous receptivity, there is some evidence that progesterone may serve to regulate duration of receptivity and to establish a temporary refractoriness to hormonal stimulation of lordosis behavior once receptivity has ended (Lisk, 1978; Marrone et al., 1979).

Ninety-Six Hours after Previous Ovulation or 0 Hours after New Ovulation (0100 Hours of Vaginal Estrus). Ovulation occurs. LH, PRL, estradiol, progesterone, and GnRH blood values are low. Only serum FSH* continues to be present at elevated levels. Recent work indicates that FSH is regulated not only by steroids but by an inhibin-like factor in follicular fluid (Marder *et al.,* 1977). Variations in this factor may account for some of the differences between patterns of FSH and LH secretion in rats.

VI. MODELING OF THE RAT ESTROUS CYCLE

We have already discussed the fact that laboratory rats have 4-day or 5-day estrous cycles. They do not have 4½-day estrous cycles. This implies that there is a 24-hr timing mechanism involved in the cycle. Many experiments have bolstered this idea. For example, administration of pentobarbital to a 4-day cyclic rat during the critical period on the day of proestrus delays ovulation by 24 hr (Everett and Sawyer, 1950). Similarly, appropriately timed injections of steroids to 4- or 5-day cyclic rats lengthens or shortens the duration of the cycle by 24 hr with the qualification that cycle length cannot be shortened to less than 4 days duration (Everett, 1948, 1961, 1969; Kobayashi *et al.,* 1971; Krey and Everett, 1973; Krey *et al.,* 1973). More recent experiments have shown that a daily LH surge occurs in ovariectomized rats treated with estradiol (Caligaris *et al.,* 1971; Legan and Karsch, 1975; Legan *et al.,* 1975). There is also a daily fluctuation in GnRH content of the POA and hypothalamus in ovariectomized rats, but this is not translated into surges of LH secretion unless sufficient estrogen is administered (Snabes *et al.,* 1977). A concept that arises from these findings is that a neural signal for release of a LH surge is emitted on each day of the rat's estrous cycle but that elevated circulating estradiol concentrations are required for the expression of this signal (Legan and Karsch, 1975).

In order to understand how this circadian rhythmicity interacts with changes in steroid hormone concentrations to generate repeatable estrous cycles of 4-day or 5-day duration, Schwartz (1968, 1969, 1970) has attempted to make a mathematical model of the estrous cycle. A diagram of one of the models developed is shown in Fig. 3. In this model, the follicular apparatus (see top right side of Fig. 3) consists of a population of follicles from which an

---

*FSH, and other pituitary hormones as well, may be pleomorphic. The various forms may have different intensities of biological activity, different clearance rates, and be differentially affected by steroids. This has obvious ramifications in the study of quantitative relationships between pituitary and gonadal hormones. For a review, see Bogdanove and Campbell (1975).

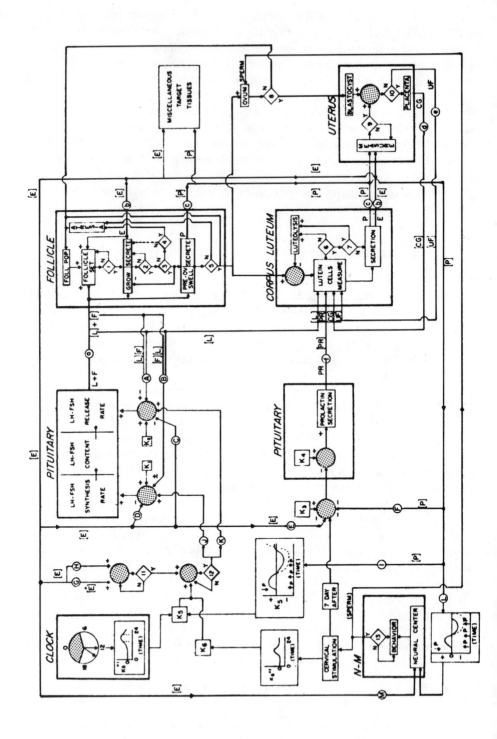

Figure 3. A model for control of the rat estrous cycle (from Schwartz, 1969). *Explanation of symbols in Fig. 3:*

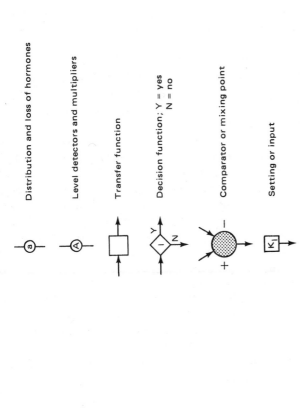

Distribution and loss of hormones

Level detectors and multipliers

Transfer function

Decision function; Y = yes
N = no

Comparator or mixing point

Setting or input

Explanation of decision functions: (1) Are LH and FSH both present? (2) Are follicles "ready" to ovulate? (3) Is (LH) rising rapidly? (4) Have 3 or more days passed since (2) was "yes"? (5) Has ovulation occurred? (6) Are prolactin and/or chorionic gonadotropin present? (7) Is LH or "uterine factor" (UF) present? (8) Has fertilization taken place? (9) Is the uterus "prepared" for implantation? (10) Did the blastocyst implant? (11) Are (E) and (E) in proper range? (12) Are (K₅) and/or (K₆) at threshold level? (13) Did mating occur? *Explanation of settings (inputs):* (K₁) Setting(s) for LH and FSH rate(s) of synthesis; (K₂) Setting(s) for LH and FSH rate(s) of release; (K₃) Setting for factor inhibiting prolactin release; (K₄) Setting (pituitary) for prolactin release; (K₅) Clock input (modifiable by progesterone) for LH surge release; (K₆) Cervical stimulation input for LH surge release. *Explanation of distribution and loss symbols:* (a) Volume of distribution and time constants for LH and FSH; (b) Volume and distribution and time constant of estrogen; (c) Volume of distribution and time constant for progesterone; (d) Volume of distribution and time constant for chorionic gonadotropin; (e) Volume of distribution (direct channel uterus to ovary?) and time constant for uterine luteolytic factor; (f) Volume of distribution and time constant for prolactin. *Explanation of detectors and multipliers:* (A) "internal feedback" receptors for LH and FSH on release rates of LH and FSH; (B) As in (A), but for LH and FSH synthesis; (E) rates; (C) Negative feedback receptor and feedback constant for estrogen levels on LH and FSH release; (D) As in (C), but for LH and FSH synthesis; (G) Receptor and differentiator for Feedback receptors for estrogen on prolactin release; (F) Feedback receptors for progesterone on prolactin release; (G) Receptor and differentiator for estrogen level for surge system; (H) Receptor for estrogen level for surge system; (I) Receptor for progesterone for effect on clock signal (K₅); (J) Multiplier for surge system signal for LH and FSH synthesis rates; (K) Multiplier for surge system signal for LH and FSH release rates; (L) Receptor for progesterone for mating behavior; (M) Receptor for estrogen for mating behavior.

ovulable set is recruited. Luteinizing hormone and FSH from the pituitary (central portion of Fig. 3) influence this set of follicles.

Timing factors involved in ovulation of this set of follicles include 2–3 days of linear growth needed for readying the follicle to ovulate and a 12-hr period between the LH surge and actual follicular rupture. After follicular rupture, the corpus luteum forms (see lower right side of Fig. 3). The duration of life of the corpus luteum depends on the presence of various hypophyseal factors (central portion of Fig. 3). The influence of the circadian clock (left side of Fig. 3) on pituitary and ultimately on ovarian function is also depicted. The model takes what is known about hormone levels, hormone clearance rates, timing factors, and anatomical compartmentalization and formalizes the inter-relationships among these factors. Tests of the validity of the formalization can then be made. If the formalization is inappropriate, experimental re-examination of the regulation of the estrous cycle can then be carried out in an orderly fashion. Schwartz (1969) tested one aspect of the model by computer simulation of the interactions among the follicles, LH, estrogen, and the circadian clock. The simulation used actual data on LH and estrogen rate loss constants and actual data on LH secretion rate. With this information, the computer generated a cycle of four times the length of the clock signal (i.e., a cycle of 4 days), and the timing of estrogen and LH surges during this cycle was also generated. Thus, the model appears to be valid for this aspect of the estrous cycle. Once this is established, the experimenter can environmentally, surgically, hormonally, or pharmacologically manipulate a particular point in the validated portion of the model and determine the effects of this manipulation. In this way, predictions can be evaluated within the context of the entire estrous cycle. Although this modeling approach is potentially powerful, its full impact on the study of reproductive endocrinology has yet to be felt. If such a computerized approach does become dominant in the years to come, it will be important that the more intuitive approach also be preserved, lest all of us become students of models of animal physiology rather than students of the physiology and behavior of living animals.

We have now completed a survey of the rat estrous cycle. In the next sections we shall discuss the sexual cycles of hamsters, guinea pigs, sheep, dogs, rhesus monkeys, rabbits, and cats. Discussion of these species will be less detailed than for the rat because less information is available. In general, aspects of sexual cyclicity that illustrate regulatory mechanisms different from those found in rats will be emphasized.

VII. HAMSTER ESTROUS CYCLES

The hamster, another rodent frequently studied in the laboratory, has an estrous cycle (4-day duration: one day of vaginal estrus, 2 days of diestrus, 1 day of proestrus) with many similarities to that of the rat. First, plasma estradiol begins to increase during late in the second day after ovulation (Labhsetwar *et al.*, 1973; Shaikh, 1972; Baranczuk and Greenwald, 1973). Plasma estradiol reaches its maximum between 0900 and 1500 hours of proestrus (187 pg/ml systemic plasma), whereas plasma estrone remains fairly constant throughout the cycle. The theca and granulosa cells of large preovulatory follicles apparently act synergistically to produce estradiol (Makris and Ryan, 1975, 1977). The increased plasma estradiol level is the causative agent in release of a surge of LH (Labhsetwar, 1972b). The LH surge is dependent on the integrity of the connection between the MPOA and MBH (Norman and Spies, 1974) and is greatly in excess of the quantity required for ovulation (de la Cruz *et al.*, 1976).

After the LH surge is initiated on the afternoon of proestrus (Bast and Greenwald, 1974; Stetson and Watson-Whitmyre, 1977), there is a sharp decline in plasma estradiol (Baranczuk and Greenwald, 1973) and a dramatic increase in preovulatory progesterone (Lukaszewska and Greenwald, 1970; Leavitt and Blaha, 1970; Ridley and Greenwald, 1975). The preovulatory progesterone is secreted primarily by the ovarian interstitium with perhaps some contribution by the follicles (Norman and Greenwald, 1971; Leavitt *et al.*, 1971). Preovulatory progesterone synergizes with the previously secreted estradiol to (a) facilitate sexual receptivity, (b) cause loss of uterine intraluminal fluid (Bosley and Leavitt, 1972), (c) block daily LH surges in response to estradiol (Norman *et al.*, 1973), and (d) prolong the single preovulatory surge of LH (Norman and Spies, 1974). The increase in plasma progesterone during the preovulatory period is accompanied by a significant increase in plasma testosterone (Saidapur and Greenwald, 1978), but the functional significance of this rise in androgen is not clear.

Follicle-stimulating hormone is also secreted in increased quantities (initiation of this increase occurs about an hour or so after the LH surge begins) during the preovulatory period (Bast and Greenwald, 1974). However, in contrast to LH, FSH is neither necessary nor sufficient for induction of follicular rupture (Greenwald, 1974; Rao *et al.*, 1974; Siegel *et al.*, 1976). A PRL surge also occurs during the preovulatory period, but its function during the cycle is not established (Bast and Greenwald, 1974). Ovulation occurs at 0100–0300 hours of vaginal estrus as a response to preovulatory LH. Corpora lutea are formed but are nonfunctional in terms of support of a decidual reaction. The corpora lutea produce progesterone until late in the evening of the second day after ovulation (DiI) (Terranova and Greenwald, 1978). At this point, the corpora lutea rapidly degenerate. As in the cyclic rat, this degeneration is not dependent on specific luteolytic factors from the uterus (Hilliard, 1973) (see Sections VIII and IX).

Despite these many similarities, estrous cycles of rats and hamsters differ in a number of ways. First, rats have a single, prolonged surge of serum FSH that extends from the evening of proestrus into the day of vaginal estrus. Hamsters have two major, separate FSH peaks, one during preovulatory proestrus, and the next on the day of vaginal estrus (Bast and Greenwald, 1974; Bex and Goldman, 1975). Chappel *et al.* (1977) have demonstrated that the first of these FSH peaks in the hamster requires an intact connection between the MPOA and MBH, but the second peak does not require integrity of this connection. It is conceivable that both peaks of FSH participate (along with LH) in induction of follicular maturation (Rani and Moudgal, 1977).

A second interesting species difference is that histological degeneration of corpora lutea of the cycle is much more rapid in hamsters than in rats. Three or more generations of corpora lutea can be discerned in ovaries from cyclic rats, but only one generation in ovaries from cyclic hamsters (Hilliard, 1973; Chatterjee and Greenwald, 1976). Terranova and Greenwald (1978) have made a detailed study of the demise of the hamster corpus luteum of the cycle and conclude that this compartment ceases to secrete progesterone between 2000 hours of DiI and 0400 hours of DiII. The decline in luteal progesterone secretion may contribute to enhancement of estrogen secretion by growing follicles.

A third species difference is that, although rat and hamster adrenal cortices are both capable of secretion of progesterone, the hamster normally produces less adrenal progesterone than the rat (Brown et al., 1976). This is probably related to the findings that (a) surgical stress on the morning of proestrus advances the timing of the LH surge in rats but not hamsters (Brom and Schwartz, 1968; Schwartz, 1969; Norman, 1975) and (b) there is a slight rise in systemic plasma progesterone (of adrenal origin) on the day of proestrus before the LH surge in rats (Feder et al., 1971; Barraclough et al., 1971) but not in hamsters (Lukaszewska and Greenwald, 1970).

A fourth difference is that rats exposed to continuous bright illumination soon stop exhibiting estrous cyclicity and go into a state of persistent vaginal estrus. Hamsters kept in continuous bright illumination are more resistant and show regular estrous cycles of slightly longer than 4 days' duration (Alleva et al., 1971). Stetson and Watson-Whitmyre (1977) postulate that this "circaquadridian" rhythm shown by hamsters in continuous bright light is based on the operation of a circadian clock that times release of gonadotropic hormones. It has been postulated that the suprachiasmatic nucleus is the site of this biological clock (Stetson and Watson-Whitmyre, 1976) and that estradiol is capable of influencing the clock (Morin et al., 1977a,b). See Fig. 4 for a summary of the hamster estrous cycle.

VIII. GUINEA PIG ESTROUS CYCLES

The guinea pig has a much longer estrous cycle (16–18 days) than other frequently studied rodents such as rats, hamsters, and mice. One factor that underlies this extended cycle length is the corpus luteum of the guinea pig. This species is unique among laboratory rodents in that it forms functional corpora lutea in the absence of mating (Brown-Grant, 1977). That the functional corpora lutea prolong the duration of the estrous cycle was dem-

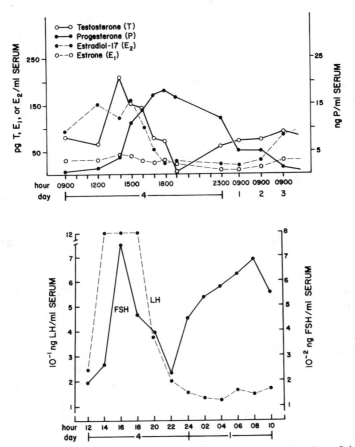

Figure 4. Steroids and gonadotropins during the estrous cycle of the hamster. From Saidapur and Greenwald (1978) and Siegel *et al.* (1976). LH and FSH experessed in terms of NIAMDD-rat LH-RP-1 and NIAMDD-rat FSH-RP-1, respectively.

onstrated by early workers who removed newly formed corpora lutea from the ovaries and caused shortening of estrous cycle duration (Loeb, 1911) and who injected progesterone into intact guinea pigs and prolonged estrous cycle length (Dempsey, 1937). Recent biochemical methods have enabled investigators to show that guinea pig corpora lutea produce progesterone at maximal levels from the 4th through 12th day after ovulation (Feder *et al.*, 1968b; Challis *et al.*, 1971; Blatchley *et al.*, 1976), an observation that fits well with older morphological studies of this ovarian compartment (Rowlands, 1956). The factors that maintain luteal function in guinea pigs are not known with certainty. Prolactin is apparently not luteotropic in guinea pigs (Rowlands, 1962), but LH and/or FSH may be (Choudary and Greenwald, 1969; Das and Benson, 1970). However, guinea pig corpora lutea maintain their histological integrity even when the pituitary gland is removed on or before midcycle (i.e., 8 days after ovulation). The factors that terminate corpus luteum function in guinea pigs are more clearly understood. In 1923 and 1927, Loeb found that removal

of the guinea pig bicornuate uterus a few days after ovulation led to a prolonged period of luteal function and a cessation of cyclic sexual activity and
ovulation. More recent work confirmed and extended these classic endocrinological studies (Fischer, 1967; Bland and Donovan, 1969; Butcher et al.,
1969) and led to the concept that the uterus produces a luteolytic factor.
Another line of evidence for this proposal emerged from studies in which the
uterus was irritated or distended by the introduction of glass beads into the
lumen (Donovan and Traczyk, 1962; Anderson et al., 1969). This manipulation, if carried out by the third day after ovulation, caused a shortening of the
estrous cycle, presumably by curtailing luteal activity. A series of in vivo and in
vitro studies subsequently showed that the luteolytic factor produced by the
uterus is prostaglandin $F_2\alpha$ (Poyser et al., 1971; Blatchley and Donovan, 1972;
Blatchley et al., 1972, 1975; reviewed in Hilliard, 1973). The concentration of
prostaglandin $F_2\alpha$ in the utero–ovarian vein increases on about day 10 after
ovulation, apparently in response to increasing secretion of estrogen by the
ovary (Joshi et al., 1973; Blatchley and Poyser, 1974). Here then is a short-loop
endocrine regulatory system that does not include the pituitary gland or brain.
The loop works as follows: the ovary produces increasing quantities of estrogen
beginning about day 10 after ovulation (Joshi et al., 1973), the estrogen acts on
the uterus, and the uterus responds by producing more prostaglandin $F_2\alpha$.
This substance then travels via the utero–ovarian vein and causes breakdown of
the corpus luteum. It may be mentioned here that hysterectomy causes no
change in estrous cyclicity of rats or hamsters, indicating that uterine luteolytic
factors do not play a significant role during the estrous cycle in these species
(Hilliard, 1973).

The formation of a functional corpus luteum is the most outstanding
feature that differentiates the guinea pig estrous cycle from that of the rat or
hamster. In several respects, the guinea pig cycle is similar to rat and hamster
estrous cycles. In guinea pigs, estradiol secretion begins to increase on about
day 10 postovulation and reaches a peak on day 15 or 16, the period of
proestrus (measurements of follicle growth: Myers et al., 1937; behavioral
evidence: Joslyn et al., 1971; ovarian vein measurements: Joshi et al., 1973;
systemic estradiol changes have been difficult to detect even by RIA methods:
Challis et al., 1971; Sasaki and Hanson, 1974; Croix and Franchimont, 1975).
The preovulatory LH surge is immediately followed by, and probably causes, a
transitory, but substantial release of preovulatory progesterone (Feder et al.,
1968b; Croix and Franchimont, 1975; Blatchley et al., 1976) from nonluteal
(i.e., interstitial or follicular) ovarian sources (Feder and Marrone, 1977). This
progesterone facilitates onset of sexual receptivity (Feder et al., 1968; Joslyn et
al., 1971), and the period of sexual receptivity terminates about 8–10 hr later,
almost simultaneously with ovulation (Young, 1969). In all of these respects,
there is no substantial difference among guinea pigs, rats, and hamsters.

However, RIA measurements have failed to detect an FSH peak in serum
during the preovulatory period (Croix and Franchimont, 1975; Blatchley et al.,
1976). Rather, serum FSH increases after ovulation and remains elevated for as
long as the 3rd through 11th day postovulation (Blatchley et al., 1976). Thus,

there seems to be a dissociation between LH and FSH secretion during the preovulatory phase of the estrous cycle in guinea pigs that is not apparent in rats and hamsters. This dissociation may be an artifact in that the RIAs being used may fail to measure biologically active but immunologically inactive species of FSH produced during the preovulatory period. In fact, Labhsetwar and Diamond (1965) report evidence for release of bioassayable FSH from guinea pig pituitaries prior to ovulation. This problem deserves further study, for it has potential implications for the study of effects of GnRH on LH and FSH secretion.

A few other interesting features of the guinea pig estrous cycle that set it apart from rat and/or hamster estrous cycles are: (a) although the timing of ovulation is somewhat influenced by environmental lighting, ovulation can occur at any time of day in guinea pigs (Donovan and Lockhart, 1972); (b) sterile mating does not delay onset of next ovulation in guinea pigs as it does in rats or hamsters (Hilliard, 1973); (c) the guinea pig, in contrast to the rat, produces little 20α-DHP, even when the corpora lutea are in regression (Feder *et al.*, 1968b; Joshi *et al.*, 1973); (d) during the diestrous, postovulatory period a connective tissue membrane forms over the vagina. The membrane dissolves some time around ovulation. Many workers have used rupture of the vaginal membrane as a marker for "estrus" and have related hormone measurements to this marker. However, the timing of rupture of the vaginal membrane is quite variable in relation to ovulation (Feder *et al.*, 1968b; Blatchley *et al.*, 1976) and is therefore a very poor marker. The most accurate and simplest external marker for ovulation is the occurrence of sexual receptivity, which invariably commences 7–9 hr prior to ovulation (Young, 1969). Finally, (e) like the hamster, but unlike the rat, the guinea pig adrenal secretes little progesterone unless stimulated by exogenous ACTH (Feder *et al.*, 1968b; Feder and Ruf, 1969). See Fig. 5 for a summary of the guinea pig estrous cycle.

IX. SHEEP ESTROUS CYCLES

In the previous sections of this chapter, we have reviewed evidence that the temporal sequence of events during the periovulatory period in several species of rodents is: (a) rise in estradiol secretion, (b) release of GnRH, (c) release of surges of LH and FSH, (d) massive, but transitory increase in progesterone secretion by the ovary, (e) onset of estrous behavior, and (f) ovulation. We shall now review evidence on the estrous cycle of sheep, for comparison with the rodent data.

A. Basic Patterns of Secretion of Ovarian and Pituitary Hormones

Robertson (1977) points out that the annual season of sexual activity of the ewe varies from a monoestrous condition of some wild species through a

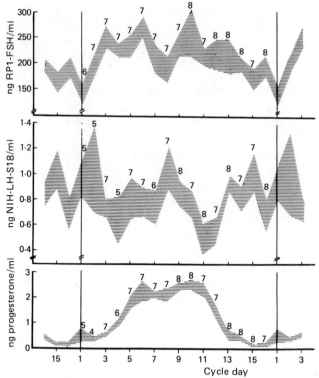

Figure 5. Mean plasma levels (± S.E.M.) of follicle-stimulating hormone (ng RP1-FSH/ml), luteinizing hormone (ng NIH-LH-S18/ml), and progesterone (ng/ml) in blood samples taken daily throughout an estrous cycle of guinea pigs with indwelling atrial catheters. The numbers of estimations for each hormone for each day of the cycle are indicated. The vertical lines denote the day of ovulation. The values for the first 3 and the last 3 days of the cycle are shown twice. From Blatchley *et al.* (1976).

seasonal polyestrous state in most domesticated breeds to certain tropical breeds that are able to reproduce at almost all times of year. In northern latitudes, the estrous season usually extends from September to February, with individual estrous cycles having a duration of 16.5 to 17.5 days. The onset of estrous behavior (usually defined as onset of the ewe's acceptance of mounting by a vasectomized ram) precedes spontaneous ovulation (only one or two ova shed per ovulation) by 24–27 hr, and estrous behavior has a duration of approximately 30 hr (Robertson, 1977). For a description of the sexual behavior of sheep, see Banks (1964).

Smeaton and Robertson (1971) studied ewes during the breeding season and found that only follicles that underwent growth surges at, or just before onset of behavioral estrus were destined to ovulate. Other sets of follicles underwent growth surges at days 3–4 and 6–9 (day 0 = day of ovulation), but these follicles did not persist throughout the cycle. Rather, they became atretic. Thus, there appear to be at least three waves of follicular growth (but note that follicles of all stages of development may occur at any time of the estrous cycle) during a single estrous cycle, with only the last wave culminating in ovulation. All three waves of follicular growth in the ewe are accompanied by increases in estradiol secretion, with the last wave providing maximal levels of estradiol secretion (Scaramuzzi *et al.*, 1970; Cox *et al.*, 1971; Mattner and Braden, 1972; Moor *et al.*, 1975; Hauger *et al.*, 1977). The existence of multiple waves of follicular growth within a single cycle has been established for the mouse (Peters and Levy, 1966), but apparently the problem has not received attention in other rodent species. Many investigators have assayed estradiol concentrations in the ovarian venous effluent and in systemic plasma throughout the estrous cycle (Moore *et al.*, 1969; Cox *et al.*, 1971; Yuthasastrakosol *et al.*, 1975; Baird *et al.*, 1976a; Pant *et al.*, 1977; Hauger *et al.*, 1977). These reports indicate that estradiol levels reach their maximum during the last wave of follicular growth about 12–24 hr before the onset of estrous behavior. A recent report by Pant *et al.* (1977) indicates that these peak values are of the order of 21 pg/ml systemic plasma. Apparently, this estradiol is produced exlusively by the theca interna of the Graafian follicle that is destined to ovulate (Moor *et al.*, 1971; Bjersing *et al.*, 1972. Hay and Moor, 1975). A major role of increased levels of estradiol on days 14–16 of the estrous cycle is undoubtedly stimulation of LH release. This is indicated by the facts that (a) increases in estrogen secretion always precede the preovulatory surge of LH in cyclic ewes (Scaramuzzi *et al.*, 1970; Chamley *et al.*, 1972), (b) passive immunization of ewes against estradiol prevents or diminishes a subsequent surge of LH (Scaramuzzi, 1975; Fairclough *et al.*, 1976), and (c) estradiol administration to properly primed ewes provokes release of a surge of LH (Pant, 1977; Legan *et al.*, 1977). As in rodents, the preovulatory LH surge terminates further estrogen secretion by the Graafian follicle (Moor, 1974).

Baird and his colleagues have noted that androstenedione secretion in ewes follows the same temporal pattern as estradiol (Baird *et al.*, 1976a,b). The preovulatory follicle, stroma, and corpus luteum are all potential sources of this androgen (Baird *et al.*, 1973; Baird and Scaramuzzi, 1976a).

Serum LH and FSH levels have been measured in a number of studies by radioimmunoassay procedures (Geschwind and Dewey, 1968; Niswender *et al.*, 1968; Pelletier *et al.*, 1968; Goding *et al.*, 1969; Wheatley and Radford, 1969; Scaramuzzi *et al.*, 1970; L'Hermite *et al.*, 1972; Salamonsen *et al.*, 1973; Cunningham *et al.*, 1975; Pant *et al.*, 1977). Simultaneous surges of the two gonadotropins begin about 9 hr (range 4–16) (Geschwind and Dewey, 1968) after onset of estrous behavior and 21–26 hr before ovulation (Cumming *et al.*, 1973). Pant *et al.* (1977) report that peak levels of serum LH are of the order of 75 ng/ml (expressed in terms of NIH-LH-S16), and peak levels of FSH are of the order of 170 ng/ml (expressed in terms of NIH-FSH-S9). As in the hamster, there is a second FSH peak (*ca.* 130 ng/ml serum) about 24 hr after the initial preovulatory rise (L'Hermite *et al.*, 1972; Salamonsen *et al.*, 1973; Pant *et al.*, 1977). As in rodents, GnRH stimulates the release of both FSH and LH (Jonas *et al.*, 1973; Hooley *et al.*, 1974), with maximal secretion of GnRH occurring shortly before onset of estrous behavior (Jackson *et al.*, 1971; Crighton *et al.*, 1973; Foster *et al.*, 1976) and maximal responsiveness of the pituitary to GnRH evident shortly after onset of estrous behavior (Foster and Crighton, 1976; Hooley *et al.*, 1974). The ewe is also similar to the rat in that prior exposure of the pituitary to GnRH may sensitize the gland to subsequent exposures to the peptide (Crighton and Foster, 1977).

Prolactin has been studied in ewes and has been found to reach maximal levels on the day prior to ovulation and the day of ovulation. These peak levels are of the order of 610 ng/ml (standard curve compared to bovine PRL NIH-B-3) serum (Polkowska *et al.*, 1976), but there is no evidence that PRL plays an important role in ovulation per se (Kann and Denamur, 1974).

About 3 or 4 days after induction of ovulation by LH, appreciable quantities of progesterone appear in the ovarian vein and systemic circulation (Thorburn *et al.*, 1969; Stabenfeldt *et al.*, 1969; Cunningham *et al.*, 1975; Hauger *et al.*, 1977; Pant *et al.*, 1977). The source of this progesterone is predominantly, if not exclusively, the newly formed corpus luteum (Short *et al.*, 1963). A midluteal peak of approximately 3.70 ng/ml systemic plasma has been recorded (Pant *et al.*, 1977). Progesterone levels then decline to about 1.86 ng/ml by day 13. This decline is well-correlated with the histological demise of the corpus luteum at day 12–13 (Deane *et al.*, 1966). The ewe and the guinea pig are similar in that both species have functional corpora lutea that produce progesterone in significant quantities for about 9 days of a 16-day cycle.

However, the ewe differs from the guinea pig, hamster, and rat in terms of progesterone secretion during the preovulatory period. The ovaries of ewes (and cows and pigs) do not have large proportions of interstitial tissue, because thecal cells dedifferentiate almost completely during the process of follicular atresia (Hansel *et al.*, 1973). Thus, a potential source of preovulatory progesterone is absent in ewes. Measurements of progesterone in systemic plasma of ewes reveal low levels (<0.5 ng/ml; Pant *et al.*, 1977) at the onset of estrous behavior. Even measurements of ovarian effluent reveal only a minor increase in progesterone during the preovulatory period (Wheeler *et al.*, 1975). Recall that a preovulatory surge in progesterone is an important feature of the estrous cycles of rats, hamsters, and guinea pigs because it helps to facilitate female sexual receptivity. In a later portion of this chapter, we shall see that luteal phase progesterone, rather than preovulatory phase progesterone, plays an important role in the sexual behavior of ewes.

To summarize, ewes are similar to rats and perhaps other rodents in having an intrinsic follicular cycle of about 4–5 days (recall that ewes have three to four waves of follicular development within a 16-day cycle) (Robertson, 1977). Ewes are also similar to rats, hamsters, and guinea pigs in that they show an increase in estrogen secretion that causes preovulatory release of LH. Ewes differ from these rodents because ewes lack a preovulatory surge of progesterone. Ewes and guinea pigs form a functional, long lived corpus luteum, but the corpora lutea of rats and hamsters have a shorter life-span. See Figs. 6 and 7 for a summary of the sheep estrous cycle.

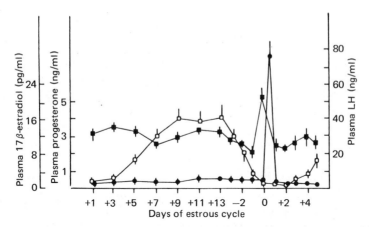

Figure 6. Mean concentration in jugular vein plasma of estradiol-17β (■), progesterone (□) and LH (●) in sex ewes during the estrous cycle. Day of oestrus is day 0. Each vertical line represents the standard error of the mean. From Pant *et al.* (1977).

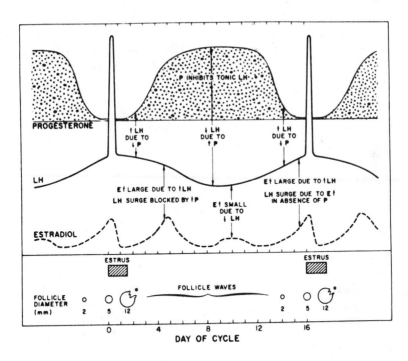

Figure 7. A model for hormonal control of the "typical" 16-day estrous cycle of the ewe. The upper box describes circulating hormones throughout the cycle and some of their controlling factors. P and E denote progesterone and estradiol, respectively. Short vertical arrows pointing up or down designate increases or decreases, respectively. The lower box describes the patterns of follicular development throughout the estrous cycle. From Hauger *et al.* (1977).

B. A More Detailed Look at Hormones a Few Days before and at the Periovulatory Period

Baird *et al.* (1976b) found that ewes produced pulses of LH about every 2 hr on days 12 and 14 of the estrous cycle. Within 5 min of each pulse of LH, estradiol secretion increased, but progesterone levels did not change as a result of the LH surges. These workers posited that the estradiol increases served to inhibit a massive surge of LH until about 9 hr after onset of estrous behavior on day 16. In a more recent study, Hauger *et al.* (1977) argued that estrogen is not the primary regulator of tonic LH levels and that progesterone plays a major role in this regulation. Part of their evidence was based on the finding that there was a consistent inverse relationship between serum LH and progesterone but not a consistent inverse relationship between serum estradiol levels and LH in the 3 or 4 days that precede massive release of LH. These combined data suggest roles for both estrogen and progesterone in maintenance of tonic levels of LH a few days prior to the LH surge.

In a very recent experiment, Baird (1978) examined the question of how estrogen levels rise in the 2 days prior to onset of estrous behavior. He found that on days 15 and 16 of the cycle, LH pulses increase in frequency (to more than once per hour) but have a smaller amplitude than during earlier stages of the cycle. Despite the smaller amplitude of LH pulses, more estradiol was secreted in response to each pulse than at earlier stages of the cycle. It is possible that the severe depression of progesterone levels at this time (Pant *et al.*, 1977) contributes to the increased stimulatory effect of LH on estradiol secretion. The data also suggest that the apparently smooth rise in plasma estrogen levels that begins about a day before estrous behavior is really composed of summated bursts of estradiol in response to repeated episodic pulses of LH that occur with increasing frequency.

At the onset of estrus, the LH pulses do not cause increases in estradiol. Shortly after this point, there is massive release of LH. This release may be prompted not only by a stimulatory action of estradiol (Legan *et al.*, 1977; Pant, 1977) but also by an appreciable drop in concentrations of progesterone (Radford *et al.*, 1969; Saba *et al.*, 1975; Pant, 1977). An interesting feature of estrogen-induced LH secretion in sheep is that there is a consistent interval (*ca.* 14 hr) between estrogen injection and onset of LH release regardless of the time of day of injection of the estrogen (Jackson and Thurmon, 1974; Jackson *et al.*, 1975). This situation appears to differ from that in rats which release LH in the late afternoon in response to constant levels of estrogen or estrogen injected at various times of day (Caligaris *et al.*, 1971; Burnet and MacKinnon, 1975; Legan *et al.*, 1975). These data imply that sheep do not possess the same type of neural timing mechanisms for cyclic surges of LH as rats.

C. A More Detailed Look at the Luteal Phase

The factors that are responsible for the formation and maintenance of the ovine corpus luteum are of pituitary origin (Kaltenbach, *et al.*, 1968a), but their nature is not established with certainty. Follicle stimulating hormone apparently plays no crucial role (Denamur, 1974). Prolactin is probably involved, but the degree of importance of this factor has been a subject of some debate (Kaltenbach *et al.*, 1968b; Schroff *et al.*, 1971; Karsch *et al.*, 1971; Denamur *et al.*, 1973). Prolactin can be reduced, by bromergocryptine, to negligible concentrations in the serum of cyclic ewes without effect on estrous cycle length, progesterone levels, or luteal regression (Niswender, 1974; Louw *et al.*, 1974). Several investigators claim a role for LH in luteal maintenance (Kaltenbach *et al.*, 1968a,b; Kann and Denamur, 1974; Denamur, 1974). Their view is supported by the finding that pulsatile GnRH administration elevates LH levels during the luteal phase and opposes the occurrence of luteolysis (Adams *et al.*, 1975). Furthermore, endogenous LH surges occur about once every 2 hr during the luteal phase (Baird *et al.*, 1976b). Although overall LH levels are quite low during the peak of luteal activity, it has been proposed that blood flow to the ovary with the corpus luteum is increased during the midluteal phase. This increase in blood flow may increase the exposure of the corpus luteum to LH and other luteotropic factors and thereby compensate for the generally low levels of LH in the circulation (Niswender *et al.*, 1975). The current reigning hypothesis is that LH and PRL are both luteotropic and may act in combination to maintain the corpus luteum of the cycle (Kann and Denamur, 1974; Denamur, 1974).

Although there was a spirited controversy about 15 years ago over the factors that cause demise of the corpus luteum (Nalbandov and Cook, 1968; Goding, 1974; Cumming, 1975), there now seems no doubt that uterine prostaglandin $F_2\alpha$ ($PGF_2\alpha$) produced under the influence of progesterone [estrogen causes further synthesis of $PGF_2\alpha$ in progesterone-primed subjects (Barcikowski *et al.*, 1974; Louis *et al.*, 1977)] is the luteolysin of the sheep estrous cycle (McCracken *et al.*, 1972; Goding, 1974; Horton and Poyser, 1976). A recent demonstration of this fact was reported by Scaramuzzi and Baird (1976). These authors found that neutralization of the biological activity of $PGF_2\alpha$ by active immunization against it resulted in failure of luteal regression and blockade of further ovulations. The various demonstrations of luteolytic activity of $PGF_2\alpha$ have been aided considerably by the use of utero–ovarian transplants to a subcutaenous skin loop in the neck (Fig. 8). This procedure results in the maintenance of normal estrous cycles and allows convenient collection of blood draining from the ovary and the uterus in conscious animals (Harrison *et al.*, 1968; McCracken *et al.*, 1970). Although $PGF_2\alpha$ is the major luteolysin of the sheep as well as guinea pig, it remains possible that intraovarian actions of estrogens may also be luteolytic (Cook *et al.*, 1974).

The functional role of the corpus luteum of the cycle has received attention with regard to regulation of sexual behavior and regulation of gonadotropins. Hauger *et al.*, (1977) and Karsch *et al.* (1977) provide evidence that luteal progesterone, acting in concert with estradiol, is a major regulator of tonic LH release during the cycle (see also Baird and Scaramuzzi, 1976b).

This interpretation of the role of luteal progesterone is strikingly similar to that proposed by Goodman (1978a) for rats. In sheep, there is evidence that

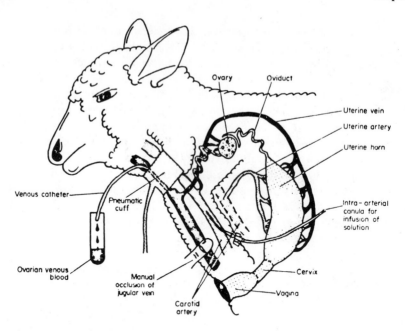

Figure 8. Diagram of utero–ovarian transplant in the ewe, showing anastomosis of the utero–ovarian vein and ovarian artery with vessels in a preformed jugulo–carotid loop and anastomosis of the uterine artery with the contralateral carotid artery. The technique for the continuous intraarterial infusion of the autotransplanted ovary and the periodic collection of utero–ovarian venous blood is also shown. From Cumming (1975).

progesterone secretion by the corpus luteum, followed by demise of the corpus luteum, is an important factor in sensitizing ewes to the facilitative effects of estrogen on sexual behavior and gonadotropin release (reviewed in Feder and Marrone, 1977). Thus, in sheep, it is the rise and fall of luteal progesterone rather than a rise in preovulatory progesterone that facilitates (with estrogen) sexually receptive behavior. Interestingly, sheep without recently active corpora lutea (e.g., pubertal sheep at first ovulation or sheep undergoing the first ovulation of a breeding season) often ovulate without manifesting estrous behavior. This "silent estrus" is presumably caused by a lack of progesterone priming of the neural tissues that mediate sex behavior (Robertson, 1977).

D. The Anestrous State

During the anestrous period, the ovaries are relatively, but not completely, quiescent. They secrete measurable quantities of estradiol and androstenedione (Martensz *et al.*, 1976) in response to endogenous pulses of LH that occur about once every 5 hr (Scaramuzzi and Baird, 1977). Mean serum LH levels are low during anestrus (Goding *et al.*, 1969), and ovarian estrogens apparently contribute to inhibition of LH release during anestrus (Roche *et al.*,

1974; Legan *et al.*, 1977). Anestrous females can respond to GnRH administration with increased LH and FSH secretion (Jonas *et al.*, 1973) and ovulation (Haresign *et al.*, 1975). However, the corpora lutea that are formed, at least after treatment with a single injection of GnRH, produce subnormal quantities of progesterone (Haresign *et al.*, 1975).

The transition between anestrous and breeding phases is regulated, at least in part, by a fall in the ratio of light to dark during a 24-hr period (Robertson, 1977). Legan *et al.* (1977) make the important observation that there is seasonal variation in the response of the hypothalamo–hypophyseal axis to the inhibitory effects of estradiol on LH release. Ovariectomy resulted in high serum LH at all times of year. When ovariectomized ewes were given silastic implants of estradiol at anestrus, serum LH levels were depressed, but the same implants failed to suppress serum LH levels during the breeding season. Thus, anestrous ewes appear to be more sensitive to inhibitory effects of estradiol on LH secretion than are ewes during the breeding season.

X. DOG ESTROUS CYCLES

In dogs, an estrous cycle can occur at any season of the year. Usually, the interval between estrous cycles is about 7–8 months. During the 7- to 8-month period, the following stages of reproductive activity may be observed:

1. Anestrus—about 125 days duration (range 15–265). This is a period of ovarian quiescence.
2. Proestrus—about 9 days duration (range 3–16). During this period the ovarian follicles grow, and the female does not accept the male. Vulval swelling and bleeding from the vagina occur at proestrus.
3. Estrus—about 9–10 days duration (range 4–12). Onset of estrus is marked by the female's acceptance of the male, and termination of estrus is marked by her refusal to copulate. Ovulation occurs during estrus.
4. Diestrus—about 75 days duration (range 51–82). Diestrus begins when the female refuses to copulate. During this period, functional corpora lutea persist (see review by Stabenfeldt and Shille, 1977).

In the past few years CPB and RIA techniques have been used to measure steroids and gonadotropins in the systemic circulation of beagle bitches (sometimes mongrels, labradors, and greyhounds have been used as well). There seems to be general agreement that immunoassayable estrogen begins to rise during proestrus (Jones *et al.*, 1973; Nett *et al.*, 1975; Concannon *et al.*, 1975; Hadley, 1975; Edqvist *et al.*, 1975; Austad *et al.*, 1976), although one group failed to find such an increase (Phemister *et al.*, 1973). A peak of estrogen is often seen 1 day before release of a surge of LH. The peak estrogen levels are of the order of 25–80 pg/ml. It is reasonable to assume that the rise in estrogen (probably, estradiol is the major estrogen involved; Austad, *et al.*, 1976) triggers the surge of LH. Maximum levels of LH occur on the first day of estrus (usually ±1 day) (Jones *et al.*, 1973; Phemister *et al.*, 1973; Smith and McDonald, 1974; Concannon *et al.*, 1975; Wildt *et al.*, 1978). The peak LH values are reported to be in the range of 7–45 ng/ml (using canine pituitary LH standard LER-1685-1) serum. An interesting feature of the LH surge in dogs is its prolonged nature. Serum LH remains elevated for 18–96 hr, with ovulation occurring about 24–72 hr after onset of the LH surge. The reason for this prolonged elevation of serum LH in dogs is not clear. After LH begins to be released, estrogen levels drop sharply, and progesterone levels rise gradually. Although progesterone levels did not appear to increase significantly prior to ovulation in some studies (Smith and McDonald, 1974), other studies demonstrate a clear preovulatory rise in plasma progesterone (Phemister *et al.*, 1973; Concannon *et al.*, 1975; Austad *et al.*, 1976). This preovulatory progesterone may have a facilitative effect on expression of female sexual behavior, as suggested by studies of ovariectomized dogs given estrogen plus progesterone replacement therapy (Beach and Merari, 1968). A truly puzzling finding is that sexual behavior persists for 8 or 9 days after ovulation. During this postovulatory period estrogen levels are low, and progesterone levels continue to increase as a result of growth of the newly formed corpora lutea.

Perhaps higher levels of progesterone, attained 10 days after ovulation, are required for inhibition of sexual behavior in dogs. In any event, corpus luteum function continues in unmated dogs for as long as 80 days. Peak levels of progesterone (*ca.* 30 ng/ml) are reached about 10–25 days after the LH surge (Smith and McDonald, 1974; Concannon *et al.*, 1975). After the peak is reached, progesterone levels stay at a plateau and then gradually decline to baseline by 75–80 days. It is rather remarkable that the life span of the corpora lutea of the unmated dog equals or even exceeds the life span of the corpora lutea of pregnant bitches. In this respect, the dog is similar to the blue fox, mink, and ferret (Paape *et al.*, 1975).

Aside from the questions of why bitches have prolonged periods of LH release and why they continue to display sexual behavior in the presence of elevated progesterone levels and decreased estrogen titers, there are several interesting endocrinological problems that do not appear to have been examined in bitches. For example, what is the pattern of FSH secretion? How is the corpus luteum maintained? What role does LH have during the estrous cycle? What environmental factors influence estrous cyclicity in dogs? See Fig. 9 for a summary of dog estrous cycles.

XI. RHESUS MENSTRUAL CYCLES

Whereas the cyclic nature of ovarian activity in spontaneously ovulating nonprimate mammals is reflected by relatively short cyclic intervals of estrous

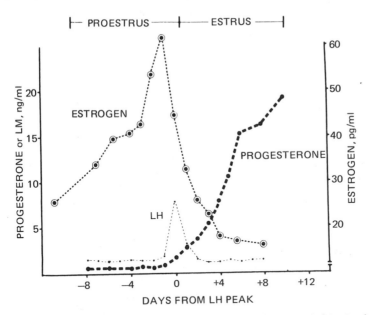

Figure 9. The endocrine and behavioral aspects of the periovulatory period in the dog. From Concannon *et al.* (1975).

behavior, the bleeding that accompanies periodic sloughing off of the uterine endometrium is the external manifestation that most clearly reveals the cyclic nature of ovarian function in primates. Because this chapter is meant to deal primarily with the physiology of estrous cycles in nonprimate mammals, the following remarks about the menstrual cycle of a primate (the rhesus macaque) will be brief.

The menstrual cycle of the rhesus macaque is about 28 days in duration, with ovulation occurring midway between menses (Knobil, 1974). The interval between menstruation and the occurrence of ovulation is the follicular phase. During this phase, estradiol (Hotchkiss *et al.*, 1971; Knobil, 1974; Czaja *et al.*, 1977) and testosterone (Hess and Resko, 1973) levels rise synchronously about 4 days before synchronous peaks of LH and FSH values are seen at midcycle (Boorman *et al.*, 1973; Yamaji *et al.*, 1973; Knobil, 1974; Faiman *et al.*, 1975; Hodgen *et al.*, 1976; Dufau *et al.*, 1977; Fig. 10). Experimental studies have demonstrated that the rise in estrogen levels causes the occurrence of the LH peak at midcycle (Ferin *et al.*, 1974). The source of this increase in estrogen during the follicular phase is the dominant follicle (Goodman *et al.*, 1977). The stimulatory effect of estrogen on LH secretion is accomplished, in part, by evoking an increase in hypothalamic GnRH secretion (Neill *et al.*, 1977). The timing of the initiation of the LH surge by estrogen is dependent on the concentration of estrogen in the circulation and is not synchronized with the light–dark cycle (Karsch *et al.*, 1973a).

About 6 hr after the release of LH has reached a peak, there is a slight, but measurable increase in plasma progesterone concentration (Johansson *et al.*,

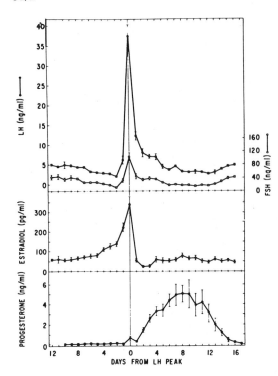

Figure 10. Plasma concentrations of luteinizing hormone (LH), follicle-stimulating hormone (FSH), estradiol, and progesterone throughout the normal rhesus monkey menstrual cycle normalized to the day of the midcycle LH peak (day 0). Each point represents the mean ±S.E. of 7 observations for FSH, 19 for LH, 11 for estradiol, and 7 for progesterone. From Knobil (1974).

1968; Kirton *et al.*, 1970; Weick *et al.*, 1973). The total duration of the LH (and FSH) rise above baseline is about 50 hr. As is the case for other mammals, the release of LH results in a decline of estradiol secretion, with a nadir in estradiol levels occurring 24 hr after the LH peak in rhesus monkeys (Weick *et al.*, 1973).

About 30 hr after the midcycle surge of LH, ovulation occurs, and the functional corpus luteum starts to form. This marks the beginning of the luteal phase of the menstrual cycle. By the time of ovulation, LH and FSH levels have declined considerably, but there is evidence that the basal levels of LH that persist during the luteal phase are luteotropic (Moudgal *et al.*, 1971; Mac-Donald and Greep, 1972; Knobil, 1973). Late in the luteal phase, there is a second smaller rise in FSH secretion (Yamaji *et al.*, 1973; Hodgen *et al.*, 1976) which is correlated with, but not caused by, a decline in progestin production by the waning corpus luteum (Resko *et al.*, 1974). The factor that appears to cause luteolysis is estrogen (Karsch *et al.*, 1973b), particularly estrone, which is produced in increased amounts by the corpus luteum during its late stages (Butler *et al.*, 1975a). Recent evidence indicates that estrogen has an intraovarian mechanism of luteolytic action (Karsch and Sutton, 1976) and diminishes the ability of late luteal cells *in vitro* to produce progesterone (Stouffer *et al.*, 1977). Thus, uterine prostaglandin, so important for luteolysis in guinea pigs and sheep, appears to have no significant role in luteolysis in rhesus monkeys.

Estrogen produced by the corpus luteum of primates may be important in another respect. Baird *et al.*, (1975) have argued that extrafollicular estrogen secreted by the corpus luteum of the primate suppresses the next wave of follicular development, making it necessary to initiate the growth of a new crop of small follicles. In contrast, animals such as sheep have no significant extra-follicular source of estrogen, and the next wave of follicular development proceeds throughout the luteal phase, rendering the ensuing follicular phase relatively brief compared to that in primates.

The role of PRL in cyclic rhesus monkeys is unclear. Interestingly, PRL levels do not rise at the time of maximal estradiol secretion, indicating that estrogen does not stimulate PRL secretion in monkeys as it does in rats (Butler *et al.*, 1975b). Quadri and Spies (1976) found no dramatic differences in PRL level throughout the menstrual cycle when daily samples were taken at 0800–0900 hours. However, at all stages of the cycle, PRL values were about twofold higher at night than during the day. This nyctohemeral rhythm of PRL is reminiscent of a similar rhythm in rats (Dunn *et al.*, 1972).

Mechanisms of control of gonadotropin release in primates are discussed in Chapter 9, in Hess *et al.* (1977), Nakai *et al.*, (1978), and Knobil and Plant (1978). A review of the relationship between hormones and behavior in primates has been published recently (Herbert, 1978).

XII. REFLEX OVULATORS—RABBITS

We have now discussed cyclic activity of the ovarian–hypophyseal–hypothalamic loop in a variety of "spontaneous" ovulators. In spontaneous ovulators, preovulatory maturation of follicles and ovulation can occur in the absence of males. However, there are many mammalian species in which preovulatory swelling of follicles and ovulation nearly always fail in the absence of the male (Everett, 1961). These species are termed "reflex ovulators." A strict dichotomy between spontaneous and reflex ovulators does not exist. Rather, they form a continuum. The estrous cycles of spontaneous ovulators are affected by environmental stimuli and, under certain conditions, copulation or other relevant stimuli can trigger reflex ovulation in a normally spontaneous ovulator (Zarrow and Clark, 1968). Conversely, hormone treatment can sometimes stimulate spontaneous ovulation in a species that normally ovulates reflexly (Sawyer, 1959). Conaway (1971) emphasizes that, among mammals, there are probably more species that fall into the reflex ovulator than into the spontaneous ovulator category.

The best studied of the reflex ovulators is the domestic rabbit. The rabbit will breed at any time of year and experiences irregular periods of persistent behavioral estrus. There is no estrous cycle in the strict sense (Asdell, 1964). The ovarian follicles develop in overlapping waves, so that as some follicles begin to degenerate, other have begun to mature (see Fig. 11). This arrangement favors a rather constant level of estrogen production and sexual receptivity during the breeding period. Although coitus provokes preovulatory growth

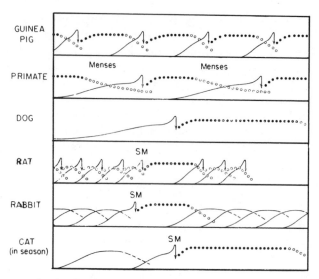

Figure 11. Diagrams of cycle of representative, familiar mammals. (———). The follicular phase, highly schematized and inaccurate in detail; (------), atresia; ↓, ovulation; ●, fully active corpora lutea; ○, corpora lutea regressing or otherwise not fully active. When sterile mating or equivalent stimulation (SM) is introduced, the cycles of the rat, rabbit, and cat become directly comparable with those of the other species. From Everett (1961).

of the follicles and ovulation, this stimulus is not an absolute requirement. Sometimes, ovulation occurs when one female mounts another or even when females are kept singly in cages (Fee and Parkes, 1930; Brooks, 1937).

Endocrinological studies have been carried out in estrous rabbits before coitus. These studies demonstrate that peripheral estradiol levels are of the order of 50 pg/ml (estrone concentrations are even higher than this) with testosterone levels of about the same magnitude. Peripheral plasma values of progesterone, 20α-DHP, and LH are low during estrus. When coitus occurs, there is neural activation within 1 min (Sawyer *et al.*, 1949) and then release of GnRH into the pituitary stalk. (This experiment was carried out in anesthetized rabbits given intravenous cupric acetate, a substance that mimics the effects of coitus, Tsou *et al.*, 1977.) The GnRH then stimulates release of LH from the pituitary (Amoss *et al.*, 1972; Kanematsu *et al.*, 1974).

Luteinizing hormone begins to be released in increased quantities by 30 min after coitus and by 90 min shows increases of as much as 100 times baseline values (Scaramuzzi *et al.*, 1972; Dufy-Barbe *et al.*, 1973). Early work in which rabbits were hypophysectomized at various times after copulation showed that enough gonadotropin has been released 1 hr after coitus to provoke ovulation (Fee and Parkes, 1929). LH levels remain elevated for about 6 hr after coitus (Hilliard *et al.*, 1964). Interestingly, no FSH surge accompanies LH release, at least during the initial 4 hr after coitus when measurements were made (Dufy-Barbe *et al.*, 1973). The most dramatic endocrine effect of the LH surge is induction of a substantial increase in progestin levels in ovarian vein peripheral plasma. This increase consists mostly of an elevation of 20α-DHP (a more modest increase in progesterone also occurs) which lasts until about 8 hr after coitus (Hilliard *et al.,* 1963, 1964; Wu *et al.,* 1977). The source of this newly synthesized progestin is the ovarian interstitium (Hilliard *et al.,* 1963, 1967). One study suggested that the preovulatory 20α-DHP helps to maintain the LH surge (Hilliard *et al.,* 1967), but more recent studies indicate that no ovarian steroids are required within 15 min after mating for a normal LH surge to occur (Goodman and Neill, 1976; Younglai, 1977). LH also binds rapidly to follicular receptors (Younglai, 1975) to induce increased preovulatory testosterone secretion (Wu *et al.,* 1977) from the interstitium and follicle (Hilliard *et al.,* 1974). The functional significance of increased testosterone secretion in females after coitus is not established. Luteinizing hormone release also results in an increased ovarian vein concentration of estradiol for about 3 hr (Hilliard and Eaton, 1971), although this increase may not be apparent in the peripheral circulation (Wu *et al.,* 1977). The transient elevation in estradiol may serve to enhance muscular activity of the oviduct during the ovulatory process (Hilliard and Eaton, 1971). Ovulation occurs about 10–12 hr after coitus, at which time steroid and LH levels have returned to basal levels.

XIII. REFLEX OVULATORS—CATS

Cats are usually considered to be seasonal breeders (but see Jemmett and Evans, 1977). In temperate zones, they undergo anestrus in fall and early winter. During the periods of sexual activity, there is a proestrous stage (1–3 days duration) followed by an estrous stage (usually 6–10 days duration, but there may be considerable variation). In unmated females there is usually an interval of 2–3 weeks between the multiple estrous periods during the breeding seasons (Stabenfeldt and Shille, 1977).

Verhage *et al.* (1976) measured estradiol and progesterone by RIA in four cats. They found peaks of estradiol (*ca.* 60 pg/ml plasma) at about 16-day intervals in unmated cats kept in a constant light : dark laboratory environment. During the troughs between these peaks, estradiol levels of about 8 pg/ml were found. Casual observations suggested that estrous behavior occurred during the times of peak estradiol levels. Progesterone was undetectable during this period of polyestrus. Experiments with ovariectomized cats had indicated that estrogen, without the addition of progesterone, is sufficient for sexual behavior to occur (Michael and Scott, 1957).

Because the cat is an induced ovulator, no ovulation occurs and no corpora lutea are formed unless there is coital stimulation (other factors such as olfactory stimuli do not appear to have been tested). If adequate coital stimulation occurs, progesterone remains undetectable for 2–3 days and then increases (Verhage *et al.,* 1976). Sterile mating increases the interestrual interval from 16 days to about 40 days (Paape *et al.,* 1975). Cats, like dogs, show a sharp decrease

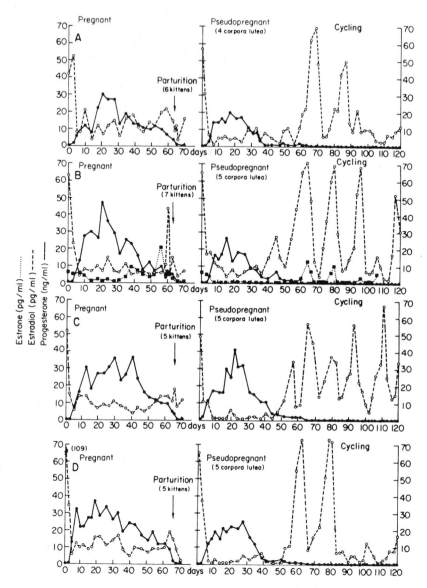

Figure 12. Profiles of plasma estradiol and progesterone in four individual cats and estrone in one cat (B) during pregnancy, pseudopregnancy, and polyestrus. From Verhage *et al.* (1976). The pregnant and pseudopregnant states are not discussed in the present chapter.

in estrogen levels and a gradual increase in progesterone immediately after ovulation and may continue to display sexual behavior during this post-ovulatory period (Paape *et al.*, 1975). The hormonal events surrounding ovulation are poorly understood in cats. Apparently, no measurements of LH, FSH, PRL, 20α-DHP, or androgen have been made during polyestrus in cats. Furthermore, no hormone measurements have been made in intact cats exposed to various environmental stimuli, even though stimuli such as light are known to affect reproduction in the cat (Scott and Lloyd, 1959). See Fig. 12 for a summary of changes in hormonal levels in cats during polyestrus.

XIV. SUMMARY

The estrous cycles of several mammalian species have been described and compared. In all of the spontaneously ovulating species described, an increase in plasma estradiol concentration was seen to be crucial for release of a surge of LH required for ovulation. In some species (e.g., rat and guinea pig) the surge of LH prior to ovulation caused significant release of progesterone from nonluteal compartments of the ovary during the preovulatory phase, whereas in other species (e.g., sheep) progesterone secretion during the preovulatory phase was not notable. Once ovulation occurred, the corpus luteum was maintained by various factors that differed among species. The demise of the corpus luteum of the cycle was caused by prostaglandins of uterine origin in some species (e.g., sheep, guinea pig) and by other factors in other species (e.g., intraovarian estrogen in rhesus monkeys). In any event, the steroids produced by the luteal compartment have important determining effects on the length of the estrous cycle across species.

ACKNOWLEDGMENTS. I thank Drs. Tina Williams and Bruce Nock for their helpful comments. To Marybeth Grabon, Jayashree Shah, Winona Cunningham, Nancy Jachim, and Cindy Banas I extend my thanks for preparation of the manuscript. Supported by NIH-HD-04467 and Research Scientist Development Award NIMH-29006. Contribution Number 317 of the Institute of Animal Behavior.

REFERENCES

Adams, T. E., Kinder, J. E., Chakraborty, P. K., Estergreen, V. L., and Reeves, J. J., 1975, Ewe luteal function influenced by pulsatile administration of synthetic LHRH/FSHRH, *Endocrinology* **97**:1460.

Aiyer, M. S., Sood, M. C., and Brown-Grant, K., 1976, The pituitary response to exogenous luteinizing hormone releasing factor in steroid-treated gonadectomized rats, *J. Endocrinol.* **69**:255.

Alleva, J. J., Waleski, M. V., and Alleva, F. R., 1971, A biological clock controlling the estrous cycle of the hamster, *Endocrinology* **88**:1368.

Amenomori, Y., Chen, C. L., and Meites, J., 1970, Serum prolactin levels in rats during different reproductive stages, *Endocrinology* **86**:506.

Amoss, M., Blackwell, R., and Guillemin R., 1972, Stimulation of ovulation in the rabbit triggered by synthetic LRF, *J. Clin. Endocrinol. Metab.* **34**:434.

Anderson, L. L., Bland, K. P., and Melampy, R. M., 1969, Comparative aspects of uterine–luteal relationships, *Recent Prog. Horm. Res.* **24**:255.

Araki, S., Ferin, M., Zimmerman, E., and Vande Wiele, R. L., 1975, Ovarian modulation of immunoreactive gonadotropins-releasing hormone (Gn-RH) in the rat brain: Evidence for a differential effect on the anterior and mid-hypothalamus, *Endocrinology* **96**:644.

Armstrong, D. T., 1968, Hormonal control of uterine lumen fluid retention in the rat, *Am. J. Physiol.* **214**:764.

Asai, T., and Wakabayashi, K., 1975, Changes of hypothalamic LH-RF content during the rat estrous cycle, *Endocrinol. Jpn.* **22**:319.

Asdell, S. A., 1964, *Patterns of Mammalian Reproduction*, Second Edition, Cornell University Press, Ithaca.

Astwood, E. B., 1938, A six-hour assay for the quantitative determination of estrogen, *Endocrinology* **23**:25.

Astwood, E. B., 1939, Changes in the weight and water content of the uterus of the normal adult rat, *Am. J. Physiol.* **126**:162.

Austad, R., Lunde, A., and Sjaastad, O. V., 1976, Peripheral plasma levels of oestradiol-17β and progesterone in the bitch during the oestrous cycle, in normal pregnancy and after dexamethasone treatment, *J. Reprod. Fertil.* **46**:129.

Baird, D. T., 1978, Pulsatile secretion of LH and ovarian estradiol during the follicular phase of the sheep estrous cycle, *Biol. Reprod.* **18**:359.

Baird, D. T., and Scaramuzzi, R. J., 1976a, The source of ovarian estradiol and androstenedione in the sheep during the luteal phase, *Acta Endocrinol. (Kbh.)* **83**:402.

Baird, D. T., and Scaramuzzi, R. J., 1976b, Changes in the secretion of ovarian steroids and pituitary luteinizing hormone in the periovulatory period in the ewe: The effect of progesterone, *J. Endocrinol.* **70**:237.

Baird, D. T., McCracken, J. A., and Goding, J. R., 1973, Studies in steroid synthesis and secretion with the autotransplanted sheep ovary and adrenal, in: *The Endocrinology of Pregnancy and Parturition* (C. G. Pierrepoint, ed.), pp. 5–16, Alpha Omega Alpha, Cardiff.

Baird, D. T., Baker, T. G., McNatty, K. P., and Neal, P., 1975, Relationship between the secretion of the corpus luteum and the length of the follicular phase of the ovarian cycle, *J. Reprod. Fertil.* **45**:611.

Baird, D. T., Land, R. B., Scaramuzzi, R. J., and Wheeler, A. G., 1976a, Endocrine changes associated with luteal regression in the ewe; the secretion of ovarian oestradiol, progesterone and androstenedione and uterine prostaglandin F$_2$α throughout the oestrous cycle, *J. Endocrinol.* **69**:275.

Baird, D. T., Swanston, I., and Scaramuzzi, R. J., 1976b, Pulsatile release of LH and secretion of ovarian steroids in sheep during the luteal phase of the estrous cycle, *Endocrinology* **98**:1490.

Banks, E., 1964, Some aspects of sexual behavior in domestic sheep, *Ovis aries, Behaviour* **23**:249.

Banks, J. A., and Freeman, M. E., 1978, The temporal requirement of progesterone on proestrus for extinction of the estrogen-induced daily signal controlling luteinizing hormone release in the rat, *Endocrinology* **102**:426.

Baranczuk, R., and Greenwald, G. S., 1973, Peripheral levels of estrogen in the cyclic hamster, *Endocrinology* **92**:805.

Barcikowski, B., Carlson, J. C., Wilson, L., and McCracken, J. A., 1974, The effect of endogenous and exogenous estradiol-17β on the release of prostaglandin F$_2$α from the ovine uterus, *Endocrinology* **95**:1340.

Barfield, R. J., and Chen, J. J., 1977, Activation of estrous behavior in ovariectomized rats by intracerebral implants of estradiol benzoate, *Endocrinology* **101**:1716.

Barr, G. D., and Barraclough, C. A., 1978, Temporal changes in medial basal hypothalamic LH-RH correlated with plasma LH during the rat estrous cycle and following electrochemical stimulation of the medial preoptic area in pentobarbital-treated proestrous rats, *Brain Res.* **148**:413.

Barraclough, C. A., Collu, R., Massa, R., and Martini, L., 1971. Temporal interrelationships between plasma LH, ovarian secretion rates and peripheral plasma progestin concentrations in the rat: Effects of Nembutal and exogenous gonadotropins, *Endocrinology* **88**:1437.

Barrett, A. M., 1960, Some factors affecting blood ACTH levels, *Acta Endocrinol. [Suppl.] (Kbh.)* **51**:421.

Bartosik, D., Szarowski, D. H., and Watson, D. J., 1971, Influence of functioning ovarian tissue on the secretion of progesterone by the adrenal glands of female rats, *Endocrinology* **88**:1425.

Bast, J. D., and Greenwald, G. S., 1974, Serum profiles of follicle-stimulating hormone, luteinizing hormone and prolactin during the estrous cycle of the hamster, *Endocrinology* **94**:1295.

Beach, F. A., and Merari, A., 1968, Coital behavior in dogs, IV. Effects of progesterone in the bitch, *Proc. Natl. Acad. Sci. USA* **61**:442.

Bex, F. J., and Goldman, B. D., 1975, Serum gonadotropins and follicular development in the Syrian hamster, *Endocrinology* **96**:928.

Beyer, C., Moralí, G., and Vargas, R., 1971, Effect of diverse estrogens on estrous behavior and genital tract development in ovariectomized rats, *Horm. Behav.* **2**:273.

Bjersing, L., Hay, M. F., Kann, G., Moor, R. M., Naftolin, F., Scaramuzzi, R. J., Short, R . V., and Younglai, E. V., 1972, Changes in gonadotrophins, ovarian steroids and follicular morphology in sheep at oestrus, *J. Endocrinol.* **52**:465.

Blake, C. A., 1974, Differentiation between the "critical period," the "activation period" and the "potential activation period" for neurohumoral stimulation of LH release in proestrous rats, *Endocrinology* **95**:572.

Blake, C. A., 1976a, A detailed characterization of the proestrous luteinizing hormone surge, *Endocrinology* **98**:445.

Blake, C. A., 1976b, Simulation of the early phase of the proestrous follicle-stimulating hormone rise after infusion of luteinizing hormone-releasing hormone in phenobarbital-blocked rats, *Endocrinology* **98**:461.

Blake, C. A., 1978, Changes in plasma luteinizing hormone-releasing hormone and gonadotropin concentrations during constant rate intravenous infusion of luteinizing hormone-releasing hormone in cyclic rats, *Endocrinology* **102**:1043.

Bland, K. P., and Donovan, B. T., 1969, Observations on the time of action and the pathway of the uterine luteolytic effect of the guinea pig, *J. Endocrinol.* **43**:259.

Blandau, R. J., Boling, J. L., and Young, W. C., 1941, Length of heat in albino rats as determined by copulatory response, *Anat. Rec.* **79**:453.

Blatchley, F. R., and Donovan, B. T., 1972, The effect of prostaglandin $F_2\alpha$ upon luteal function and ovulation in the guinea pig, *J. Endocrinol.* **53**:493.

Blatchley, F. R., and Poyser, N. L., 1974, The effect of oestrogen and progesterone on the release of prostaglandins from the uterus of the ovariectomized guinea-pig, *J. Reprod. Fertil.* **40**:205.

Blatchley, F. R., Donovan, B. T., Horton, E. W., and Poyser, N. L., 1972, The release of prostaglandins and progestin into the utero–ovarian venous blood of guinea-pigs during the oestrous cycle and following oestrogen treatment, *J. Physiol (Lond.)* **223**:69.

Blatchley, F. R., Donovan, B. T., and Poyser, N. L., 1975, Effect of intrauterine beads alone, or combined with oestrogen treatment, on utero–ovarian venous plasma prostaglandin $F_2\alpha$ and progesterone levels in the guinea-pig, *J. Endocrinol.* **68**:445.

Blatchley, F. R., Donovan, B. T., and ter Haar, M. B., 1976, Plasma progesterone and gonadotropin levels during the estrous cycle of the guinea pig, *Biol. Reprod.* **15**:29.

Bogdanove, E. M., and Campbell, G. T., 1975, Qualitative and quantitative gonad–pituitary feedback, *Recent Prog. Horm. Res.* **31**:567.

Bogdanove, E. M., Schwartz, N. B., Reichert, L. E., Jr., and Midgley, A. R., Jr., 1971, Comparisons of pituitary: Serum luteinizing hormone (LH) ratios in the castrated rat by radioimmunoassay and OAAD bioassay, *Endocrinology* **88**:644.

Boling, J. L., 1942, Growth and regression of corpora lutea during the normal estrous cycle of the rat, *Anat. Rec.* **82**:131.

Boling, J. L., and Blandau, R. J., 1939, The estrogen–progesterone induction of mating responses in the spayed female rat, *Endocrinology* **25**:359.

Boling, J. L., and Blandau, R. J., Soderwall, A. L., and Young, W. C., 1941, Growth of the Graafian follicle and the time of ovulation in the albino rat, *Anat. Rec.* **79**:313.

Boorman, G. A., Niswender, G. D., Gay, V. L., Reichert, L. E., Jr., and Midgley, A. R., Jr., 1973, Radioimmunoassay for follicle-stimulating hormone in the rhesus monkey using an anti-human FSH serum and rat FSH ^{131}I, *Endocrinology* **92**:618.

Bosley, C. G., and Leavitt, W. W., 1972, Dependence of preovulatory progesterone on critical period in the cyclic hamster, *Am. J. Physiol.* **222**:129.

Brom, G. M., and Schwartz, N. B., 1968, Acute changes in the estrous cycle following ovariectomy in the golden hamster, *Neuroendocrinology* **3**:366.

Brooks, C. M., 1937, The role of the cerebral cortex and of various sense organs in the excitation and execution of mating activity in the rabbit, *Am. J. Physiol.* **120**:544.

Browman, L. G., 1937, Light in its relation to activity and estrous rhythms in the albino rat, *J. Exp. Zool.* **75**:375.

Brown, G. P., Courtney, G. A., and Marotta, S. F., 1976, Progesterone secretion by adrenal glands of hamsters and comparison of ACTH influence in rats and hamsters, *Steroids* **28**:275.

Brown-Grant, K., 1967, The effects of a single injection of progesterone on the oestrous cycle, thyroid gland activity and uterus–plasma concentration ratio for radio-iodide in the rat, *J. Physiol. (Lond.)* **190**:101.

Brown-Grant, K., 1969, The effects of progesterone and of pentobarbitone administered at the dioestrous stage on the ovarian cycle of the rat, *J. Endocrinol.* **43**:539.

Brown-Grant, K., 1977, Physiological aspects of the steroid hormone–gonadotropin interrelationship, in: *International Review of Physiology, Reproductive Physiology II,* Vol. 13 (R. O. Greep, ed.), University Park Press, Baltimore.

Brown-Grant, K., Exley, D., and Naftolin, F., 1970, Peripheral plasma oestradiol and luteinizing hormone concentrations during the oestrous cycle of the rat, *J. Endocrinol.* **48**:295.

Buffler, G., and Roser, S., 1974, New data concerning the role played by progesterone in the control of follicular growth in the rat, *Acta Endocrinol. (Kbh.)* **75**:569.

Burkl, W., and Kellner, G., 1954, Über die Entstehung der Zwischenzellen im Rattenovar und ihre Bedeutung im Rahmen der Oestrogenproduktion, *Z. Zellforsch.* **40**:361.

Burnet, F. R., and MacKinnon, P. C. B., 1975. Restoration by oestradiol benzoate of a neural and hormonal rhythm in the ovariectomized rat, *J. Endocrinol.* **64**:27.

Burrows, H., 1949, *Biological Actions of Sex Hormones,* Second Edition, Cambridge University Press, New York.

Butcher, R. L., Barley, D. A., and Inskeep, E. K., 1969, Local relationship between the ovary and uterus of rats and guinea pigs, *Endocrinology* **84**:476.

Butcher, R. L., Collins, W. E., and Fugo, N. W., 1974, Plasma concentration of LH, FSH, prolactin, progesterone and estradiol-17β throughout the 4-day estrous cycle of the rat, *Endocrinology* **94**:1704.

Butler, W. R., Hotchkiss, J., and Knobil, E., 1975a, Functional luteolysis in the rhesus monkey: Ovarian estrogen and progesterone during the luteal phase of the menstrual cycle, *Endocrinology* **96**:1509.

Butler, W. R., Krey, L. C., Lu, K.-H., Peckham, W. D., and Knobil, E., 1975b, Surgical disconnection of the medial basal hypothalamus and pituitary function in the rhesus monkey. IV. Prolactin secretion, *Endocrinology* **96**:1099.

Caligaris, L., Astrada, J. J., and Taleisnik, S., 1967, Pituitary FSH concentrations in the rat during the estrous cycle, *Endocrinology* **81**:1261.

Caligaris, L., Astrada, J. J., and Taleisnik, S., 1971, Release of luteinizing hormone induced by estrogen injection into ovariectomized rats, *Endocrinology* **88**:810.

Callantine, M. R., Humphrey, R. R., Lee, S. L., Windsor, B. L., Schottin, M., and O'Brien, O. P., 1966, Action of an estrogen antagonist on reproductive mechanisms in the rat, *Endocrinology* **79**:153.

Catchpole, H. R., 1949, Distribution of glycoprotein hormones in the anterior pituitary gland of the rat, *J. Endocrinol.* **6**:218.

Challis, J. R., Heap, R. B., and Illingworth, O. V., 1971, Concentration of oestrogen and progesterone in the plasma of non-pregnant, pregnant and lactating guinea-pigs, *J. Endocrinol.* **51**:333.

Chamley, W. A., Buckmaster, J. U., Cain, M. D., Cerini, J., Cerini, M. E., Cumming, I. A., and Goding, J. R., 1972, The effect of prostaglandin F$_2\alpha$ on progesterone, oestradiol and luteinizing hormone secretion in sheep with ovarian transplants, *J. Endocrinol.* **55**:253.

Chappel, S. C., Norman, R. L., and Spies, H. G., 1977, Regulation of the second (estrous) release of follicle-stimulating hormone in hamsters by the medial basal hypothalamus, *Endocrinology* **101**:1339.

Chatterjee, S., and Greenwald, G. S., 1976, Biochemical changes in the corpus luteum of the cyclic hamster, *J. Endocrinol.* **68**:251.

Chatterton, R. T., Jr., MacDonald, G. J., and Greep, R. O., 1968, Biosynthesis of progesterone and 20α-hydroxypregn-4-en-3-one by the rat ovary during the estrous cycle and early pregnancy, *Endocrinology* **83**:1.

Chatterton, R. T., Jr., Chatterton, A. J., and Greep, R. O., 1969, In vitro biosynthesis of estrone and estradiol-17β by cycling rat ovaries. Effect of luteinizing hormone, *Endocrinology* **84**:252.

Choudary, J. B., and Greenwald, G. S., 1969, Reversal by gonadotrophins of the luteolytic effect of oestrogen in the cyclic guinea-pig, *J. Reprod. Fertil.* **19**:503.

Chowers, I., and McCann, S. M., 1965, Content of luteinizing hormone-releasing factor and luteinizing hormone during the estrous cycle and after changes in gonadal steroid titers, *Endocrinology* **76**:700.

Clark, J. H., Anderson, J. N., and Peck, E. J., Jr., 1973, Nuclear receptor–estrogen complexes in rat uteri: Concentration–time–response parameters, in: *Receptors and Reproductive Hormones. Advances in Experimental Medicine and Biology*, Vol. 36 (B. W. O'Malley and W. A. Means, eds.), pp. 15–53, Plenum Press, London.

Conaway, C. H., 1971, Ecological adaptation and mammalian reproduction, *Biol. Reprod.* **4**:239.

Concannon, P. W., Hansel, W., and Visek, W. J., 1975, The ovarian cycle of the bitch: Plasma estrogen, LH and progesterone, *Biol. Reprod.* **13**:112.

Cook, B., Karsch, F. J., Foster, D. L., and Nalbandov, A. V., 1974, Estrogen-induced luteolysis in the ewe: Possible sites of action, *Endocrinology* **94**:1197.

Cooper, K. J., Fawcett, C. P., and McCann, S. M., 1974, Variations in pituitary responsiveness to a luteinizing hormone/follicle stimulating hormone releasing factor (LH-RF/FSH-RF) preparation during the rat estrous cycle, *Endocrinology* **95**:1293.

Cox, R. I., Mattner, P. E., and Thorburn, G. D., 1971, Changes in ovarian secretion of oestradiol-17β around oestrus in the sheep, *J. Endocrinol.* **49**:345.

Crighton, D. B., and Foster, J. P., 1977, Luteinizing hormone release after two injections of synthetic luteinizing hormone releasing hormone in the ewe, *J. Endocrinol.* **72**:59.

Crighton, D. B., Hartley, B. M., and Lamming, G. E., 1973, Changes in the luteinizing hormone releasing activity of the hypothalamus, and in pituitary gland and plasma luteinizing hormone during the oestrous cycle of the sheep, *J. Endocrinol.* **58**:377.

Croix, D., and Franchimont, P., 1975, Changes in the serum levels of the gonadotrophins progesterone and estradiol during the estrous cycle of the guinea pig, *Neuroendocrinology* **19**:1.

Cumming, I. A., 1975, The ovine and bovine oestrous cycle, *J. Reprod. Fertil.* **43**:583.

Cumming, I. A., Buckmaster, J. M., Blockey, M. A. DeB., Goding, J. R., Winfield, C. G., and Baxter, R. W., 1973, Constancy of interval between luteinizing hormone release and ovulation in the ewe, *Biol. Reprod.* **9**:24.

Cunningham, N. F., Symons, A. M., and Saba, N., 1975, Levels of progesterone, LH and FSH in the plasma of sheep during the oestrous cycle, *J. Reprod. Fertil.* **45**:177.

Czaja, J. A., Robinson, J. A., Eisele, S. G., Scheffler, G., and Goy, R. W., 1977, Relationship between sexual skin colour of female rhesus monkeys and midcycle plasma levels of oestradiol and progesterone, *J. Reprod. Fertil.* **49**:147.

Daane, T. A., and Parlow, A. F., 1971, Periovulatory patterns of rat serum follicle stimulating hormone and luteinizing hormone during the normal estrous cycle: Effects of pentobarbital, *Endocrinology* **88**:653.

Das, R. M., and Benson, G. K., 1970, Effect of gonadotrophins on the oestrous cycle in the guinea-pig, *J. Endocrinol.* **47**:423.

Davidson, J. M., Rodgers, C. H., Smith, E. R., and Bloch, G. J., 1968, Stimulation of female sex behavior in adrenalectomized rats with estrogen alone, *Endocrinology* **82**:193.

Deane, H. W., Hay, M. F., Moor, R. M., Rowson, L. E. A., and Short, R. V., 1966, The corpus luteum of the sheep: Relationships between morphology and function during the oestrous cycle, *Acta Endocrinol. (Kbh.)* **51**:245.

de la Cruz, A., Arimura, A., de la Cruz, K. G., and Schally, A. V., 1976, Effect of administration of antiserum to luteinizing hormone-releasing hormone on gonadal function during the estrous cycle in the hamster, *Endocrinology* **98**:490.

Dempsey, E. W., 1937, Follicular growth rate and ovulation after various experimental procedures in the guinea pig, *Am. J. Physiol.* **120**:126.

Denamur, R., 1974, Luteotrophic factors in the sheep, *J. Reprod. Fertil.* **38**:251.

Denamur, R., Martinet, J., and Short, R. V., 1973, Pituitary control of the ovine corpus luteum, *J. Reprod. Fertil.* **32**:207.

Donovan, B. T., and Lockhart, A. N., 1972, Light and the timing of ovulation in the guinea-pig, *J. Reprod. Fertil.* **30**:207.

Donovan, B. T., and Traczyk, W., 1962, The effect of uterine distension on the oestrous cycle of the guinea-pig, *J. Physiol (Lond.)* **161**:227.

Dörner, G., Döcke, F., and Moustafa, S., 1968, Differential localization of a male and a female hypothalamic mating centre, *J. Reprod. Fertil.* **17**:583.

Dudley, C. A., and Moss, R. L., 1976, Facilitation of lordosis in the rat by prostaglandin E$_2$, *J. Endocrinol.* **71**:457.

Dufau, M. L., Hodgen, G. D., Goodman, A. L., and Catt, K. J., 1977, Bioassay of circulating luteinizing hormone in the rhesus monkey: Comparison with radioimmunoassay during physiological changes, *Endocrinology* **100**:1557.

Dufy-Barbe, L., Franchimont, P., and Faure, J. M. A., 1973, Time-courses of LH and FSH release after mating in the female rabbit, *Endocrinology* **92**:1318.

Dunn, J. D., Arimura, A. A., and Scheving, L. E., 1972, Effect of stress on circadian periodicity in serum LH and prolactin concentration, *Endocrinology* **90**:29.

Dupon, C., and Kim, M. H., 1973, Peripheral plasma levels of testosterone, androstenedione, and oestradiol during the rat oestrous cycle, *J. Endocrinol.* **59**:653.

Edqvist, L.-E., Johansson, E. D. B., Kasström, H., Olsson, S.-E., and Richkind, M., 1975, Blood plasma levels of progesterone and oestradiol in the dog during the oestrous cycle and pregnancy, *Acta Endocrinol. (Kbh.)* **78**:554.

Emmens, C. W., 1962, Estrogens, in: *Methods in Hormone Research,* Vol. 2 (R. I. Dorfman, ed.), pp. 59–112, Academic Press, New York.

Emmens, C. W., 1969, Estrogens, in: *Methods in Hormone Research,* Second Edition (R. I. Dorfman, ed.), pp. 61–120, Academic Press, New York.

Eskay, R. L., Oliver, C., Ben-Jonathan, N., and Porter, J. C., 1975, Hypothalamic hormones in portal and systemic blood, in: *Hypothalamic Hormones* (M. Motta, P. G. Crosignani, and L. Martini, eds.), pp. 125–137, Academic Press, New York.

Eskay, R. L., Mical, R. S., and Porter, J. C., 1977, Relationship between luteinizing hormone releasing hormone concentration in hypophysial portal blood and luteinizing hormone release in intact, castrated, and electrochemically-stimulated rats, *Endocrinology* **100**:263.

Eto, F., Masuda, H., Suzuki, Y., and Hasi, F., 1962, Progesterone and pregn-4-ene-20α-ol-3-one in rat ovarian venous blood at different stages in the reproductive cycle, *Jpn. J. Anim. Reprod.* **8**:34.

Everett, J. W., 1948, Progesterone and estrogen in the experimental control of ovulation time and other features of the estrous cycle in the rat, *Endocrinology* **43**:389.

Everett, J. W., 1956, The time of release of ovulating hormone from the rat hypophysis, *Endocrinology* **59**:580.

Everett, J. W., 1961, The mammalian female reproductive cycle and its controlling mechanisms, in: *Sex and Internal Secretions,* Third Edition, Vol. 1 (W. C. Young, ed.), pp. 497–555, Williams & Wilkins, Baltimore.

Everett, J. W., 1967, Provoked ovulation or long-delayed pseudopregnancy from coital stimuli in barbiturate-blocked rats, *Endocrinology* **80**:145.

Everett, J. W., 1969, Neuroendocrine aspects of mammalian reproduction, *Annu. Rev. Physiol.* **31**:383.

Everett, J. W., and Sawyer, C. H., 1949, A neural timing factor in the mechanism by which progesterone advances ovulation in the cyclic rat, *Endocrinology* **45**:581.

Everett, J. W., and Sawyer, C. H., 1950, A 24-hour periodicity in the "LH-release apparatus" of female rats disclosed by barbiturate sedation, *Endocrinology* **47**:198.

Everett, J. W., and Sawyer, C. H., 1953, Estimated duration of the spontaneous activation which causes release of ovulating hormones from the rat hypophysis, *Endocrinology* **52**:83.

Everett, J. W., Sawyer, C. H., and Markee, J. E., 1949, A neurogenic timing factor in control of the ovulatory discharge of luteinizing hormone in the cyclic rat, *Endocrinology* **44**:234.

Faiman, C., Stearns, E. L., Winter, J. S. D., Reyes, F. I., and Hobson, W. C., 1975, Radioimmunoassay for rhesus monkey gonadotropins, *Proc. Soc. Exp. Biol. Med.* **149**:670.

Fairclough, R. J., Smith, J. F., and Peterson, A. J., 1976, Passive immunization against oestradiol-17β and its effect on luteolysis, oestrus and ovulation in the ewe, *J. Reprod. Fertil.* **48**:169.

Feder, H. H., and Marrone, B. L., 1977, Progesterone: Its role in the central nervous system as a facilitator and inhibitor of sexual behavior and gonadotropin release, *Ann. N.Y. Acad. Sci.* **286**:331.

Feder, H. H., and Ruf, K. B., 1969, Stimulation of progesterone release and estrous behavior by ACTH in ovariectomized rodents, *Endocrinology* **69**:171.

Feder, H. H., Resko, J. A., and Goy, R. W., 1968a, Progesterone levels in the arterial plasma of pre-ovulatory and ovariectomized rats, *J. Endocrinol.* **41**:563.

Feder, H. H., Resko, J. A., and Goy, R. W., 1968b, Progesterone concentrations in the arterial plasma of guinea-pigs during the oestrous cycle, *J. Endocrinol.* **40**:505.

Feder, H. H., Brown-Grant, K., and Corker, C. S., 1971, Pre-ovulatory progesterone, the adrenal cortex and the "critical period" for luteinizing hormone release in rats, *J. Endocrinol.* **50**:29.

Fee, A. R., and Parkes, A. S., 1929, Studies on ovulation. I. The relation of the anterior pituitary body to ovulation in the rabbit, *J. Physiol. (Lond.)* **67**:383.

Fee, A. R., and Parkes, A. S., 1930, Studies on ovulation. III. Effect of vaginal anaesthesia on ovulation in the rabbit, *J. Physiol. (Lond.)* **70**:385.

Ferin, M., Tempone, A., Zimmering, P. E., and Vande Wiele, R. L., 1969, Effects of antibodies to 17β-estradiol and progesterone on the estrous cycle of the rat, *Endocrinology* **85**:1070.

Ferin, M., Dyrenfurth, I., Cowchock, S., Warren, M., and Vande Wiele, R. L., 1974, Active immunization to 17β-estradiol and its effects upon the reproductive cycle of the rhesus monkey, *Endocrinology* **94**:765.

Fink, G., and Harris, G. W., 1970, The luteinizing hormone releasing activity of extracts of blood from the hypophysial portal vessels of rats, *J. Physiol. (Lond.)* **208**:221.

Fink, G., and Jamieson, M. G., 1976, Immunoreactive luteinizing hormone releasing factor in rat pituitary stalk blood: Effects of electrical stimulation of the medial preoptic area, *J. Endocrinol.* **68**:71.

Fink, G., Aiyer, M. S., Jamieson, M. G., and Chiappa, S. A., 1975, Factors modulating the responsiveness of the anterior pituitary gland in the rat with special reference to gonadotrophin releasing hormone (GnRH), in: *Hypothalamic Hormones* (M. Motta, P. G. Crosignani, and L. Martini, eds.), pp. 139–160, Academic Press, London.

Fink, G., Chiappa, S. A., Pickering, A., and Sarkar, D., 1976, Control of rat oestrous cycle, in: *Excerpta Medica International Congress Series No. 402, Endocrinology Proceedings of the V International Congress of Endocrinology, Hamburg, July 18-24, 1976*, Vol. 1 (V. H. T. James, ed.), pp. 186–191, Excerpta Medica, Amsterdam.

Fischer, T. V., 1967, Local uterine regulation of the corpus luteum, *Am. J. Anat.* **121**:425.

Fortune, J. E., and Armstrong, D. T., 1977, Androgen production by theca and granulosa isolated from proestrous rat follicles, *Endocrinology* **100**:1341.

Foster, J. P., and Crighton, D. B., 1976, Pituitary responsiveness to a single injection of synthetic luteinizing hormone releasing hormone before and after the natural preovulatory plasma luteinizing hormone peak in the sheep, *J. Endocrinol.* **71**:269.

Foster, J. P., Jeffcoate, S. L., Crighton, D. B., and Holland, D. T., 1976, Luteinizing hormone and luteinizing hormone releasing hormone-like immunoreactivity in the jugular venous blood of sheep at various stages of the oestrous cycle, *J. Endocrinol.* **68**:409.

Freeman, M. E., Reichert, L. E., Jr., and Neill, J. D., 1972, Regulation of the proestrus surge of prolactin secretion by gonadotropin and estrogens in the rat, *Endocrinology* **90**:232.

Freeman, M. C., Dupke, K. C., and Croteau, C. M., 1976, Extinction of the estrogen-induced daily signal for LH release in the rat: A role for the proestrous surge of progesterone, *Endocrinology* **99**:223.

Gay, V. L., and Tomacari, R. L., 1974, Follicle-stimulating hormone secretion in the female rat: Cyclic release is dependent on circulating androgen, *Science* **184**:75.

Gay, V. L., Midgley, A. R., Jr., and Niswender, G. D., 1970, Patterns of gonadotrophin secretion associated with ovulation, *Fed. Proc.* **29**:1880.

Gelato, M., Dibbet, J., Marshall, S., Meites, J., and Wuttke, W., 1976, Prolactin–adrenal interactions in the immature female rat, *Ann. Biol. Anim. Biochim. Biophys.* **16**:395.

Geschwind, I. I., and Dewey, R., 1968, Dynamics of luteinizing hormone (LH) secretion in the cycling ewe: A radioimmunoassay study, *Proc. Soc. Exp. Biol. Med.* **129**:451.

Goding, J. R., 1974, The demonstration that $PGF_2\alpha$ is the uterine luteolysin in the ewe, *J. Reprod. Fertil.* **38**:261.

Goding, J. R., Catt, R. J., Brown, J. M., Kaltenbach, C. C., Cumming, I. A., and Mole, B. J., 1969, Radioimmunoassay for ovine luteinizing hormone. Secretion of luteinizing hormone during estrus and following estrogen administration in the sheep, *Endocrinology* **85**:133.

Goldman, B. D., and Mahesh, V. B., 1968, Fluctuations in pituitary FSH during the ovulatory cycle in the rat and a possible role of FSH in the induction of ovulation, *Endocrinology* **83**:97.

Goodman, A. L., and Neill, J. D., 1976, Ovarian regulation of postcoital gonadotropin release in the rabbit: Reexamination of a functional role for 20α-dihydroprogesterone, *Endocrinology* **99**:852.

Goodman, A. L., Nixon, W. E., Johnson, D. K., and Hodgen, G. D., 1977, Regulation of folliculogenesis in the cycling rhesus monkey: Selection of the dominant follicle, *Endocrinology* **100**:155.

Goodman, R. L., 1978a, A quantitative analysis of the physiological role of estradiol and progesterone in the control of tonic and surge secretion of luteinizing hormone in the rat, *Endocrinology* **102**:142.

Goodman, R. L., 1978b, The site of the positive feedback action of estradiol in the rat, *Endocrinology* **102**:151.

Gorzalka, B. B., and Whalen, R. E., 1977, The effects of progestins, mineralocorticoids, glucocorticoids, and steroid solubility on the induction of sexual receptivity in rats, *Horm. Behav.* **8**:94.

Gosden, R. G., Everett, J. W., and Tyrey, L., 1976, Luteinizing hormone requirements for ovulation in the pentobarbital-treated proestrous rat, *Endocrinology* **99**:1046.

Green, R., Luttge, W. G., and Whalen, R. E., 1970, Induction of receptivity in ovariectomized female rats by a single intravenous injection of estradiol-17β, *Physiol. Behav.* **5**:137.

Greenwald, G. S., 1974, Dissociation of ovulation and progesterone secretion following LH or FSH treatment of hypophysectomized proestrous hamsters, *Endocrinology* **95**:1282.

Greep, R. O., 1961, Physiology of the anterior hypophysis in relation to reproduction, in: *Sex and Internal Secretions*, Third Edition, Vol. 1 (W. C. Young, ed.), pp. 240–301, Williams & Wilkins, Baltimore.

Greig, F., and Weisz, J., 1973, Preovulatory levels of luteinizing hormone, the critical period and ovulation in rats, *J. Endocrinol.* **57**:235.

Guillemin, R., 1977, The expanding significance of hypothalamic peptides, or, is endocrinology a branch of neuroendocrinology?, *Recent Prog. Horm. Res.* **33**:1.

Hadley, J. C., 1975, Total unconjugated oestrogen and progesterone concentrations in peripheral blood during the oestrous cycle of the dog, *J. Reprod. Fertil.* **44**:445.

Hall, H. R., Luttge, W. G., and Berry, R. B., 1975, Intracerebral prostaglandin E_2: Effects upon sexual behavior, open field activity and body temperature in ovariectomized female rats, *Prostaglandins* **10**:177.

Hansel, W., Concannon, P. W., and Lukaszewska, J. H., 1973, Corpora lutea of the large domestic animals, *Biol. Reprod.* **8**:222.

Haresign, W., Foster, J. P., Haynes, N. B., Crighton, D. B., and Lamming, G. E., 1975, Progesterone levels following treatment of seasonally anoestrous ewes with synthetic LH-releasing hormone, *J. Reprod. Fertil.* **43**:269.

Harman, S. M., Louvet, J.-P., and Ross, G. T., 1975, Interaction of estrogen and gonadotrophins on follicular atresia, *Endocrinology* **96**:1145.

Harrington, F. E., and Bex, F. J., 1970, Ovulation in the rat as a result of synergism between follicle stimulating hormone and luteinizing hormone, *Endocrinol. Jpn.* **17**:387.

Harrison, F. A., Heap, R. B., and Linzell, J. L., 1968, Ovarian function in the sheep after autotransplantation of the ovary and uterus to the neck, *J. Endocrinol.* 40:xiii.

Hashimoto, I., and Wiest, W. G., 1969, Correlation of the secretion of ovarian steroids with function of a single generation of corpora lutea in the immature rat, *Endocrinology* 84:873.

Hauger, R. L., Karsch, F. J., and Foster, D. L., 1977, A new concept for control of the estrous cycle of the ewe based on the temporal relationships between luteinizing hormone, estradiol and progesterone in peripheral serum and evidence that progesterone inhibits tonic LH secretion, *Endocrinology* 101:807.

Hay, M. F., and Moor, R. M., 1975, Functional and structural relationships in the Graafian follicle population of the sheep ovary, *J. Reprod. Fertil.* 45:583.

Hemmingsen, A. M., and Krarup, N. B., 1937, Rhythmic diurnal variations in the oestrous phenomena of the rat and their susceptibility to light and dark, *Kgl. Danske Videnskab. Biol. Medd.* 13(7):1.

Henrik, E., and Gerall, A. A., 1976, Facilitation of receptivity in estrogen-primed rats during successive mating tests with progestins and methysergide, *J. Comp. Physiol. Psychol.* 20:590.

Herbert, J., 1978, Neurohormonal integration of sexual behaviour in female primates, in: *Biological Determinants of Sexual Behaviour* (J. B. Hutchison, ed.), pp. 465–491, John Wiley and Sons, New York.

Hess, D. L., and Resko, J. A., 1973, The effects of progesterone on the patterns of testosterone and estradiol concentrations in the systemic plasma of the female rhesus monkey during the intermenstrual period, *Endocrinology* 92:446.

Hess, D. L., Wilkins, R. H., Moossy, J., Chang, J. L., Plant, T. M., McCormack, J. T., Nakai, Y., and Knobil, E., 1977, Estrogen-induced gonadotropin surges in decerebrated female rhesus monkeys with medial basal hypothalamic peninsulae, *Endocrinology* 101:1264.

Hilliard, J., 1973, Corpus luteum function in guinea pigs, hamsters, rats, mice and rabbits, *Biol. Reprod.* 8:203.

Hilliard, J., and Eaton, L. W., Jr., 1971, Estradiol-17β, progesterone and 20α-hydroxpregn-4-en-3-one in rabbit ovarian venous plasma. II. From mating through implantation, *Endocrinology* 89:522.

Hilliard, J., Archibald, D., and Sawyer, C. H., 1963, Gonadotropic activation of preovulatory synthesis and release of progestin in the rabbit, *Endocrinology* 72:59.

Hilliard, J., Hayward, J. N., and Sawyer, C. H., 1964, Postcoital patterns of secretion of pituitary gonadotropin and ovarian progestin in the rabbit, *Endocrinology* 75:957.

Hilliard, J., Penardi, R., and Sawyer, C. H., 1967, A functional role for 20α-hydroxypregn-4-en-3-one in the rabbit, *Endocrinology* 80:901.

Hilliard, J., Scaramuzzi, R. J., Pang, C. N., Penardi, R., and Sawyer, C. H., 1974, Testosterone secretion by rabbit ovary *in vivo, Endocrinology* 94:267.

Hodgen, G. D., Wilks, J. W., Vaitukaitis, J. L., Chen, H.-C., Papkoff, H., and Ross, G. T., 1976, A new radioimmunoassay for follicle-stimulating hormone in macaques: Ovulatory menstrual cycles, *Endocrinology* 99:137.

Holzbauer, M., Newport, H. M., Birmingham, M. K., and Traikov, H., 1969, Secretion of pregn-4-ene-3,20-dione (progesterone) *in vivo* by the adrenal gland of the rat, *Nature* 221:572.

Hooley, R. D., Baxter, R. W., Chamley, W. A., Cumming, I. A., Jonas, H. A., and Findlay, J. K., 1974, FSH and LH response to gonadotropin-releasing hormone during the ovine estrous cycle and following progesterone administration, *Endocrinology* 95:937.

Hori, T., Ide, M., and Miyake, T., 1968, Ovarian estrogen secretion during estrous cycle and under the influence of exogenous gonadotropins in rats, *Endocrinol. Jpn.* 15:215.

Hori, T., Ide, M., Kato, G., and Miyake, T., 1970, Relation between estrogen secretion and follicular morphology in the rat ovary under the influence of ovulating hormone or exogenous gonadotropins, *Endocrinol. Jpn.* 17:489.

Horikoshi, H., and Suzuki, Y., 1974, On circulating sex steroids during the estrous cycle and the early pseudopregnancy in the rat with special reference to its luteal activation, *Endocrinol. Jpn.* 21:69.

Horton, E. W., and Poyser, N. L., 1976, Uterine luteolytic hormone: A physiological role for prostaglandin $F_2\alpha$, *Physiol. Rev.* 56:595.

Hotchkiss, J., Atkinson, L. E., and Knobil, E., 1971, Time course of serum estrogen and luteinizing hormone (LH) concentrations during the menstrual cycle of the rhesus monkey, *Endocrinology* **89**:177.

Ichikawa, S., Morioka, H., and Sawada, T., 1972, Acute effect of gonadotrophins on the secretion of progestins by the rat ovary, *Endocrinology* **90**:1356.

Jackson, G. L., and Thurmon, J., 1974, Absence of a critical period in estrogen-induced release of LH in the anestrous ewe, *Endocrinology* **94**:918.

Jackson, G. L., Roche, J. F., Foster, D. L., and Dziuk, P. J., 1971, Luteinizing hormone releasing activity in the hypothalamus of anestrous and cyclic ewes, *Biol. Reprod.* **5**:5.

Jackson, G. L., Thurmon, J., and Nelson, D., 1975, Estrogen-induced release of LH in the ovariectomized ewe: Independence of time of day, *Biol. Reprod.* **13**:358.

Jemmett, J. E., and Evans, J. M., 1977, A survey of sexual behavior and reproduction of female cats, *J. Small Anim. Pract.* **18**:31.

Johansson, E. D. B., Neill, J. D., and Knobil, E., 1968, Periovulatory progesterone concentration in the peripheral plasma of the rhesus monkey with a methodologic note on the detection of ovulation, *Endocrinology* **82**:143.

Jonas, H. A., Salamonsen, L. A., Burger, H. G., Chamley, W. A., Cumming, I. A., Findlay, J. K., and Goding, J. R., 1973, Release of FSH after administration of gonadotrophin-releasing hormone or estradiol to the anestrous ewe, *Endocrinology* **92**:862.

Jones, G. E., Boyns, A. R., Cameron, E. H. D., Bell, E. T., Christie, D. W., and Parkes, M. F., 1973, Plasma oestradiol, luteinizing hormone and progesterone during the oestrous cycle in the beagle bitch, *J. Endocrinol.* **57**:331.

Joshi, H. S., Watson, D. J., and Labhsetwar, A. P., 1973, Ovarian secretion of oestradiol, oestrone, 20-dihydroprogesterone and progesterone during the oestrous cycle of the guinea-pig, *J. Reprod. Fertil.* **35**:177.

Joslyn, W. D., Feder, H. H., and Goy, R. W., 1971, Estrogen conditioning and progesterone facilitation of lordosis in guinea pigs, *Physiol. Behav.* **7**:477.

Kalra, S. P., and Kalra, P. S., 1974, Temporal interrelationships among circulating levels of estradiol, progesterone and LH during the rat estrous cycle: Effects of exogenous progesterone, *Endocrinology* **95**:1711.

Kalra, S. P., Krulich, L., and McCann, S. M., 1973, Changes in gonadotropin-releasing factor content in rat hypothalamus following electrochemical stimulation of anterior hypothalamic area and during the estrous cycle, *Neuroendocrinology* **12**:321.

Kaltenbach, C. C., Graber, J. W., Niswender, G. D., and Nalbandov, A. V., 1968a, Effect of hypophysectomy on the formation and maintenance of corpora lutea in the ewe, *Endocrinology* **82**:753.

Kaltenbach, C. C., Graber, J. W., Niswender, G. D., and Nalbandov, A. V., 1968b, Luteotrophic properties of some pituitary hormones in nonpregnant or pregnant hypophysectomized ewes, *Endocrinology* **82**:818.

Kalvert, M., and Bloch, E., 1968, Conversion of 4-^{14}C-dehydroepiandrosterone to estrone and 17β-estradiol by the rat ovary with observations on variations during the estrous cycle, *Endocrinology* **82**:1021.

Kanematsu, S., Scaramuzzi, R. J., Hilliard, J., and Sawyer, C. H., 1974, Patterns of ovulation-inducing LH release following coitus, electrical stimulation and exogenous LHRH in the rabbit, *Endocrinology* **95**:247.

Kann, G., and Denamur, R., 1974, Possible role of prolactin during the oestrous cycle and gestation in the ewe, *J. Reprod. Fertil.* **39**:473.

Karsch, F. J., and Sutton, G. P., 1976, An intra-ovarian site for the luteolytic action of estrogen in the rhesus monkey, *Endocrinology* **98**:553.

Karsch, F. J., Cook, J. B., Ellicott, A. R., Foster, D. L., Jackson, G. L., and Nalbandov, A. V., 1971, Failure of infused prolactin to prolong the life span of the corpus luteum of the ewe, *Endocrinology* **89**:272.

Karsch, F. J., Weick, R. F., Butler, W. R., Dierschke, D. J., Krey, L. C., Weiss, G., Hotchkiss, J., Yamaji, T., and Knobil, E., 1973a, Induced LH surges in the rhesus monkey: Strength–duration characteristics of the estrogen stimulus, *Endocrinology* **92**:1740.

Karsch, F. J., Krey, L. C., Weick, R. F., Dierschke, D. J., and Knobil, E., 1973b, Functional luteolysis in the rhesus monkey: The role of estrogen, *Endocrinology* **92**:1148.

Karsch, F. J., Legan, S. J., Hauger, R. L., and Foster, D. L., 1977, Negative feedback action of progesterone on tonic luteinizing hormone secretion in the ewe: Dependence on the ovaries, *Endocrinology* **101**:800.

Kennedy, T. G., and Armstrong, D. T., 1972, Extra-ovarian action of prolactin in the regulation of uterine lumen fluid accumulation in rats, *Endocrinology* **90**:1503.

Kirton, K. T., Niswender, G. G., Midgley, A. R., Jr., Jaffe, R. B., and Forbes, A. D., 1970, Serum luteinizing hormone and progesterone concentration during the menstrual cycle of the rhesus monkey, *J. Clin. Endocrinol.* **30**:105.

Kitay, J. I., 1963, Pituitary–adrenal function in the rat after gonadectomy and gonadal hormone replacement, *Endocrinology* **73**:253.

Knobil, E., 1973, On the regulation of the primate corpus luteum, *Biol. Reprod.* **8**:246.

Knobil, E., 1974, On the control of gonadotropin secretion in the rhesus monkey, *Recent Prog. Horm. Res.* **30**:1.

Knobil, E., and Plant, T. M., 1978, Neuroendocrine control of gonadotropin secretion in the female rhesus monkey, in: *Frontiers in Neuroendocrinology*, Vol. 5 (L. Martini and W. F. Ganong, eds.), pp. 249–264, Raven Press, New York.

Kobayashi, K., Hara, K., and Miyake, T., 1968, Luteinizing hormone concentrations in pituitary and in blood plasma during the estrous cycle of the rat, *Endocrinol. Jpn.* **15**:313.

Kobayashi, F., Hara, K., and Miyake, T., 1969a, Causal relationship between luteinizing hormone release and estrogen secretion in the rat, *Endocrinol. Jpn.* **16**:261.

Kobayashi, F., Hara, K., and Miyake, T., 1969b, Effects of steroids on the release of luteinizing hormone in the rat, *Endocrinol. Jpn.* **16**:251.

Kobayashi, F., Hara, K., and Miyake, T., 1969c, Inhibitory and facilitatory effects of steroids on the release of luteinizing hormone in the rat, *Endocrinol. Jpn.* **16**:493.

Kobayashi, F., Hara, K., and Miyake, T., 1971, Induction of delayed or advanced ovulation by estrogen in 4-day cyclic rats, *Endocrinol. Jpn.* **18**:389.

Krey, L. C., and Everett, J. W., 1973, Multiple ovarian responses to single estrogen injections early in rat estrous cycles: Impaired growth, luteotropic stimulation and advanced ovulation, *Endocrinology* **93**:377.

Krey, L. C., Tyrey, L., and Everett, J. W., 1973, The estrogen-induced advance in the cyclic LH surge in the rat: Dependency on ovarian progesterone secretion, *Endocrinology* **93**:385.

Krulich, L., Hefco, E., Illner, P., and Read, C. B., 1974, The effects of acute stress on the secretion of LH, FSH, prolactin and GH in the normal male rat, with comments on their statistical evaluation, *Neuroendocrinology* **16**:293.

Kubli-Garfias, C., and Whalen, R. E., 1977, Induction of lordosis behavior in female rats by intravenous administration of progestins, *Horm. Behav.* **9**:380.

Labhsetwar, A. P., 1970a, Role of estrogens in ovulation: A study using the estrogen-antagonist, ICI 46,474, *Endocrinology* **87**:542.

Labhsetwar, A. P., 1970b, The role of oestrogens in spontaneous ovulation: Evidence for positive oestrogen feedback in the 4-day oestrous cycle, *J. Endocrinol.* **47**:481.

Labhsetwar, A. P., 1970c, Synergism between LH and FSH in the induction of ovulation, *J. Reprod. Fertil.* **23**:517.

Labhsetwar, A. P., 1972a, Further evidence for synergism between LH and FSH in the induction of ovulation in rats; lack of effects of prolactin, *J. Reprod. Fertil.* **29**:435.

Labhsetwar, A. P., 1972b, Role of estrogen in spontaneous ovulation: Evidence for positive feedback in hamsters, *Endocrinology* **90**:941.

Labhsetwar, A. P., 1975, Prostaglandins and studies related to reproduction in laboratory animals, in: *Prostaglandins and Reproduction* (S. M. M. Karim, ed.) pp. 242–270, University Park Press, Baltimore.

Labhsetwar, A. P., and Diamond, M., 1965, The influence of reproductive stage and gonadal hormones on pituitary FSH levels in the female guinea-pig, *Am. Zool.* **5**:219.

Labhsetwar, A. P., Joshi, H. S., and Watson, D., 1973, Temporal relationship between estradiol, estrone and progesterone secretion in the ovarian venous blood and LH in the peripheral plasma of cyclic hamsters, *Biol. Reprod.* **8**:321.

Langford, J., and Hilliard, J., 1967, Effect of 20α-hydroxypregn-4-en-3-one on mating behavior in spayed female rats, *Endocrinology* **80**:281.

Lawton, I. E., 1972, Facilitatory feedback effects of adrenal and ovarian hormones on LH secretion, *Endocrinology* **90**:575.

Lawton, I. E., and Sawyer, C. H., 1968, Timing of gonadotrophin and ovarian steroid secretion at diestrus in the rat, *Endocrinology* **82**:831.

Leavitt, W. W., and Blaha, G. C., 1970, Circulating progesterone levels in the golden hamster during the estrous cycle, pregnancy, and lactation, *Biol. Reprod.* **3**:353.

Leavitt, W. W., Bosley, C. G., and Blaha, G. C., 1971, Source of ovarian preovulatory progesterone, *Nature* [*New Biol.*] **234**:283.

Legan, S. J., and Karsch, F. J., 1975, A daily signal for the LH surge in the rat, *Endocrinology* **96**:57.

Legan, S. J., Coon, G. A., and Karsch, F. J., 1975, Role of estrogen as initiator of daily LH surges in the ovariectomized rat, *Endocrinology* **96**:50.

Legan, S. J., Karsch, F. J., and Foster, D. L., 1977, The endocrine control of seasonal reproductive function in the ewe: A marked change in response to the negative feedback action of estradiol on luteinizing hormone secretion, *Endocrinology* **101**:818.

L'Hermite, M., Niswender, G. D., Reichert, L. E., and Midgley, A. R., 1972, Serum follicle stimulating hormone in sheep as measured by radioimmunoassay, *Biol. Reprod.* **6**:325.

Lindner, H. R., and Zmigrod, A., 1967, Microdetermination of progestins in rat ovaries: Progesterone and 20α-hydroxy-pregn-4-en-3-one content during pro-oestrus, oestrus, and pseudopregnancy, *Acta Endocrinol. (Kbh.)* **56**:16.

Linkie, D. M., and Niswender, G. D., 1972, Serum levels of prolactin, luteinizing hormone, and follicle stimulating hormone during pregnancy in the rat, *Endocrinology* **90**:632.

Lisk, R. D., 1962, Diencephalic placement of estradiol and sexual receptivity in the female rat, *Am. J. Physiol.* **203**:493.

Lisk, R. D., 1978, The regulation of sexual "heat," in: *Biological Determinants of Sexual Behaviour* (J. B. Hutchison, ed.), pp. 425–466, John Wiley and Sons, New York.

Loeb, L., 1911, Über die Bedeutung des Corpus luteum für die Periodizität des sexuellen Zyklus beim weiblichen Säugetierorganismus, *Dtsch. Med. Wochenschr.* **37**:17.

Loeb, L., 1923, The effect of extirpation of the uterus on the life and function of the corpus luteum in the guinea-pig, *Proc. Soc. Exp. Biol. Med.* **20**:441.

Leob, L., 1927, The effects of hysterectomy on the system of sex organs and on the periodicity of the sexual cycle in the guinea-pig, *Am. J. Physiol.* **83**:202.

Long, J. A., and Evans, H. M., 1922, The oestrous cycle in the rat and its associated phenomena, *Mem. Univ. California* **6**:1.

Lostroh, A. J., and Johnson, R. E., 1966, Amounts of interstitial cell-stimulating hormone and follicle-stimulating hormone required for follicular development, uterine growth and ovulation in the hypophysectomized rat, *Endocrinology* **79**:991.

Louis, T. M., Parry, D. M., Robinson, J. S., Thorburn, G. D., and Challis, J. R. G., 1977, Effects of exogenous progesterone and oestradiol on prostaglandin F and 13,14-dihydro-15-oxo-prostaglandin $F_2α$ concentrations in uteri and plasma of ovariectomized ewes, *J. Endocrinol.* **73**:427.

Louvet, J.-P., and Vaitukaitis, J. L., 1976, Induction of follicle-stimulating hormone (FSH) receptors in rat ovaries by estrogen priming *Endocrinology* **99**:758.

Louvet, J.-P., Harman, S. M., Schreiber, J. R., and Ross, G. T., 1975, Evidence for a role of androgens in follicular maturation, *Endocrinology* **97**:366.

Louw, B. P., Lishman, A. W., Botha, W. A., and Baumgartner, J. P., 1974, Failure to demonstrate a role for the acute release of prolactin at oestrus in the ewe, *J. Reprod. Fertil.* **40**:455.

Lukaszewska, J. H., and Greenwald, G. S., 1970, Progesterone levels in the cyclic and pregnant hamster, *Endocrinology* **86**:1.

MacDonald, G. J., and Greep, R. O., 1972, Ability of luteinizing hormone (LH) to acutely increase serum progesterone levels during the secretory phase of the rhesus menstrual cycle, *Fertil. Steril.* **23**:466.

MacDonald, G. J., Armstrong, D. T., and Greep, R. O., 1966, Stimulation of estrogen secretion from normal rat corpora lutea by luteinizing hormone, *Endocrinology* **79**:289.

Makris, A., and Ryan, K. J., 1975, Progesterone, androstenedione, testosterone, estrone, and estradiol synthesis in hamster ovarian follicle cells, *Endocrinology* **96**:694.

Makris, A., and Ryan, K., 1977, Aromatase activity of isolated hamster granulosa cells and theca, *Steroids* **29**:65.

Malven, P. V., and Sawyer, C. H., 1966, Formation of new corpora lutea in mature hypophysectomized rats, *Endocrinology* **78**:1259.

Mandl, A. M., 1952, The phases of the oestrous cycle in the adult white rat, *J. Exp. Biol.* **28**:576.

Mandl, A. M., and Zuckerman, S., 1952, Cyclical changes in the number of medium and large follicles in the adult rat ovary, *J. Endocrinol.* **8**:341.

Mann, D. R., and Barraclough, C. A., 1973a, Changes in peripheral plasma progesterone during the rat 4-day estrous cycle: An adrenal diurnal rhythm, *Proc. Soc. Exp. Biol. Med.* **142**:1226.

Mann, D. R., and Barraclough, C. A., 1973b, Role of estrogen and progesterone in facilitating LH release in 4-day cyclic rats, *Endocrinology* **93**:694.

Marder, M. L., Channing, C. P., and Schwartz, N. B., 1977, Suppression of serum follicle stimulating hormone in intact and acutely ovariectomized rats by porcine follicular fluid, *Endocrinology* **101**:1639.

Marrone, B. L., Rodriguez-Sierra, J. F., and Feder, H. H., 1979, Intrahypothalamic implants of progesterone inhibit lordosis behavior in ovariectomized, estrogen-treated rats, *Neuroendocrinology* **28**:92.

Martensz, N. D., Baird, D. T., Scaramuzzi, R. J., and Van Look, P. F. A., 1976, Androstenedione and the control of luteinizing hormone in the ewe during anoestrus, *J. Endocrinol.* **69**:227.

Mattner, P. E., and Braden, A. W. H., 1972, Secretion of oestradiol-17β by the ovine ovary during the luteal phase of the oestrous cycle in relation to ovulation, *J. Reprod. Fertil.* **28**:136.

McCann, S. M., and Ramirez, V. D., 1964, The neuroendocrine regulation of hypophyseal luteinizing hormone secretion, *Recent Prog. Horm. Res.* **20**:131.

McClintock, J. A., and Schwartz, N. B., 1968, Changes in pituitary and plasma follicle stimulating hormone concentrations during the rat estrous cycle, *Endocrinology* **83**:433.

McCracken, J. A., Glew, M. E., and Levy, L. K., 1970, Regulation of corpus luteum function by gonadotrophins and related compounds, in: *Advances in the Biosciences*, Vol. 4 (G. Raspe, ed.), pp. 337–397, Pergamon Press, Oxford.

McCracken, J. A., Carlson, J. C., Glew, M. E., Goding, J. R., Baird, D. T., Green, K., and Samuelsson, B., 1972, Prostaglandin F$_2\alpha$ identified as a luteolytic hormone in sheep, *Nature (New Biol.)* **238**:129.

Menon, K. M. J., and Gunaga, K. P., 1976, Cytoplasmic and nuclear receptor–estradiol complex in the hypothalamus and pituitary: Relationship with pituitary sensitivity to gonadotropin releasing hormone and gonadotropin secretion in the rat, *Neuroendocrinology* **22**:8.

Meyerson, B. J., 1967, Relationship between the anesthetic and gestagenic action and estrous behavior-inducing activity of different progestins, *Endocrinology* **81**:369.

Meyerson, B. J., 1972, Latency between i.v. injection of progestins and the appearance of estrous behavior in estrogen-treated ovariectomized rats, *Horm. Behav.* **3**:1.

Michael, R. P., and Scott, P. P., 1957, Quantitative studies on mating behaviour of spayed female cats stimulated by treatment with oestrogens, *J. Physiol (Lond.)* **138**:46P.

Mills, J. M., and Schwartz, N. B., 1961, Ovarian ascorbic acid as an endogenous and exogenous assay for cyclic proestrous LH release, *Endocrinology* **69**:844.

Miyake, F., 1974, Blood concentration and interplay of pituitary and gonadal hormones governing the reproductive cycle in female mammals, in: *Reproductive Physiology*, Physiology Series One, Vol. 8 (R. O. Greep, ed.), pp. 155–178, MTP International Review of Science, University Park Press, Baltimore.

Monroe, S. E., Rebar, R. W., Gay, V. L., and Midgley, A. R., Jr., 1969, Radioimmunoassay determination of luteinizing hormone during the estrous cycle of the rat, *Endocrinology* **85**:720.

Moor, R. M., 1974, The ovarian follicle of the sheep: Inhibition of oestrogen secretion by luteinizing hormone, *J. Endocrinol.* **61**:455.

Moor, R. M., Hay, M. F., and Caldwell, B. V., 1971, The sheep follicle: Relation between sites of steroid dehydrogenase activity, gonadotrophic stimulation and steroid production, *J. Reprod. Fertil.* **27**:484.

Moor, R. M., Hay, M. F., and Seamark, R. F., 1975, The sheep ovary: Regulation of steroidogenic, haemodynamic and structural changes in the largest follicle and adjacent tissue before ovulation, *J. Reprod. Fertil.* **45**:595.

Moore, N. W., Barratt, S., Brown, J. B., Schindler, I., Smith, M. A., and Smyth, B., 1969, Oestrogen and progesterone content of ovarian vein blood of the ewe during the oestrous cycle, *J. Endocrinol.* **44**:55.

Morin, L. P., Fitzgerald, K. M., and Zucker, I., 1977a, Estradiol shortens the period of hamster circadian rhythms, *Science* **196**:305.

Morin, L. P., Fitzgerald, K. M., Rusak, B., and Zucker, I., 1977b, Circadian organization and neural mediation of hamster reproductive rhythms, *Psychoneuroendocrinology* **2**:73.

Moss, R. L., and McCann, S. M., 1973, Induction of mating behavior in rats by luteinizing hormone-releasing factor, *Science* **181**:177.

Moss, R. L., and McCann, S. M., 1975, Action of luteinizing hormone-releasing factor (LRF) in the initiation of lordosis behavior in the estrone-primed ovariectomized female rat, *Neuroendocrinology* **17**:309.

Mossman, H. W., and Duke, K. L., 1973, *Comparative Morphology of the Mammalian Ovary*, The University of Wisconsin Press, Madison.

Moudgal, N. R., MacDonald, G. J., and Greep, R. O., 1971, Effect of HCG antiserum on ovulation and corpus luteum formation in the monkey (*Macaca fascicularis*), *J. Clin. Endocrinol.* **32**:579.

Myers, H. I., Young, W. C., and Dempsey, E. W., 1937, Graafian follicle development throughout the reproductive cycle in the guinea pig, with especial reference to changes during oestrus (sexual receptivity), *Anat. Rec.* **65**:381.

Naftolin, F., Brown-Grant, K., and Corker, C. S., 1972, Plasma and pituitary luteinizing hormone and peripheral plasma oestradiol concentrations in the normal oestrous cycle of the rat and after experimental manipulation of the cycle, *J. Endocrinol.* **53**:17.

Nakai, Y., Plant, T. M., Hess, D. L., Keogh, E. J., and Knobil, E., 1978, On the sites of the negative and positive feedback action of estradiol in the control of gonadotropin secretion in the rhesus monkey, *Endocrinology* **102**:1008.

Nalbandov, A. V., 1958, *Reproductive Physiology*, W. H. Freeman and Company, San Francisco.

Nalbandov, A. V., and Cook, B., 1968, Reproduction, *Annu. Rev. Physiol.* **30**:245.

Neill, J. D., 1972, Effect of "stress" on serum prolactin and luteinizing hormone levels during the estrous cycle of the rat, *Endocrinology* **87**:1192.

Neill, J. D., and Smith, M. S., 1974, Pituitary–ovarian interrelationships in the rat, in: *Current Topics in Experimental Endocrinology*, Vol. II (V. H. T. James and L. Martini, eds.), pp. 73–106, Academic Press, New York.

Neill, J. D., Freeman, M. E., and Tillson, S. A., 1971, Control of the proestrus surge of prolactin and luteinizing hormone secretion by estrogens in the rat, *Endocrinology* **89**:1448.

Neill, J. D., Patton, J. M., Dailey, R. A., Tsou, R. C., and Tindall, G. T., 1977, Luteinizing hormone releasing hormone (LHRH) in pituitary stalk blood of rhesus monkeys: Relationship to level of LH release, *Endocrinology* **101**:430.

Nequin, L. G., and Schwartz, N. B., 1971, Adrenal participation in the timing of mating and LH release in the cyclic rat, *Endocrinology* **88**:325.

Nequin, L. G., Alvarez, J., and Schwartz, N. B., 1975, Steroid control of gonadotropin release, *J. Steroid Biochem.* **6**:1007.

Nett, T. M., Akbar, A. M., Phemister, R. D., Holst, P. A., Reichert, L. E., Jr., and Niswender, G. D., 1975, Levels of luteinizing hormone, estradiol and progesterone in serum during the estrous cycle and pregnancy in the beagle bitch, *Proc. Soc. Exp. Biol. Med.* **148**:134.

Niswender, G. D., 1974, Influence of 2-Br-α-ergocryptine on serum levels of prolactin and the estrous cycle in sheep, *Endocrinology* **94**:612.

Niswender, G. D., Roche, J. F., Foster, D. L., and Midgley, A. R., 1968, Radioimmunoassay of serum levels of luteinizing hormone during the cycle and early pregnancy in ewes, *Proc. Soc. Exp. Biol. Med.* **129**:901.

Niswender, G. D., Moore, R. T., Akbar, A. M., Nett, T. M., and Diekman, M. A., 1975, Flow of blood to the ovaries of ewes throughout the estrous cycle, *Biol. Reprod.* **13**:381.

Norman, R. L., 1975, Estrogen and progesterone effects on the neural control of the preovulatory LH release in the golden hamster, *Biol. Reprod.* **13**:218.

Norman, R. L., and Greenwald, G. S., 1971, Effect of phenobarbital, hypophysectomy and X-irradiation on preovulatory progesterone levels in the cyclic hamster, *Endocrinology* **89**:598.

Norman, R. L., and Spies, H. G., 1974, Neural control of the estrogen-dependent twenty-four-hour periodicity of LH release in the golden hamster, *Endocrinology* **95**:1367.

Norman, R. L., Blake, C. A., and Sawyer, C. H., 1973, Estrogen-dependent twenty-four-hour periodicity in pituitary LH release in the female hamster, *Endocrinology* **93**:965.

Ohta, Y., and Iguchi, T., 1976, Development of the vaginal epithelium showing estrogen-independent proliferation and cornification in neonatally androgenized mice, *Endocrinol. Jpn.* **23**:333.

Paape, S. R., Shille, V. M., Seto, H., and Stabenfeldt, G. H., 1975, Luteal activity in the pseudopregnant cat, *Biol. Reprod.* **13**:470.

Pant, H. C., 1977, Effect of oestradiol infusion on plasma gonadotrophins and ovarian activity in progesterone-primed and unprimed anoestrous ewes, *J. Endocrinol.* **75**:227.

Pant, H. C., Hopkinson, C. R. N., and Fitzpatrick, R. J., 1977, Concentration of oestradiol, progesterone, luteinizing hormone and follicle-stimulating hormone in the jugular venous plasma of ewes during the oestrous cycle, *J. Endocrinol.* **73**:247.

Parkes, A. S., and Deanesly, R., 1966, The ovarian hormones, in: *Marshall's Physiology of Reproduction*, Third Edition, Vol. 3 (A. S. Parkes, ed.), pp. 570–828, Longmans, Green, London.

Pelletier, J., Kann, G., Dolais, J., and Rosselin, G., 1968, Dosage radioimmunologique de l'hormone luteinisante plasmatique chez le mouton. Comparaison avec le dosage biologique de LH par la diminution de l'acide ascorbique ovarien, et exemple de l'application aux mesures de la LH sanguine chez la brebis, *C. R. Acad. Sci. [D] (Paris)* **266**:2352.

Peters, H., and Levy, E., 1966, Cell dynamics of the ovarian cycle, *J. Reprod. Fertil.* **11**:227.

Pfaff, D. W., 1973, Luteinizing hormone-releasing factor potentiates lordosis behavior in hypophysectomized ovariectomized female rats, *Science* **182**:1148.

Phemister, R. D., Holst, P. A., Spano, J. S., and Hopwood, M. L., 1973, Time of ovulation in the beagle bitch, *Biol. Reprod.* **8**:74.

Piacsek, B. E., Schneider, T. C., and Gay, V. L., 1971, Sequential study of luteinizing hormone (LH) and "progestin" secretion on the afternoon of proestrus in the rat, *Endocrinology* **89**:39.

Piva, F., Gagliano, P., Motta, M., and Martini, L., 1973, Adrenal progesterone: Factors controlling its secretion, *Endocrinology* **93**:1178.

Polkowska, J., Wolinska, E., and Domanski, E., 1976, Cyclic activity of the pituitary prolactin cells and plasma prolactin levels in the oestrous cycle of the ewe, *J. Reprod. Fertil.* **46**:295.

Powers, J. B., 1970, Hormonal control of sexual receptivity during the estrus cycle of the rat, *Physiol. Behav.* **5**:831.

Powers, J. B., 1972, Facilitation of lordosis in ovariectomized rats by intracerebral progesterone implants, *Brain Res.* **48**:311.

Poyser, N. L., Horton, E. W., Thompson, C. J., and Los, M., 1971, Identification of prostaglandin $F_2\alpha$ released by distension of the guinea-pig uterus *in vitro*, *Nature* **230**:526.

Pupkin, M., Bratt, H., Weisz, J., Lloyd, C. W., and Balogh, K., 1966, Dehydrogenases in the rat ovary. I. A histochemical study of Δ^5-3β- and 20α-hydroxysteroid dehydrogenases and enzymes of carbohydrate oxidation during the estrous cycle, *Endocrinology* **79**:316.

Purves, H. D., and Griesbach, W. E., 1954, The site of follicle stimulating and luteinizing hormone production in the rat pituitary, *Endocrinology* **55**:785.

Quadri, S. K., and Spies, H. G., 1976, Cyclic and diurnal patterns of serum prolactin in the rhesus monkey, *Biol. Reprod.* **14**:495.

Quinn, D. L., and Everett, J. W., 1967, Delayed pseudopregnancy induced by selective hypothalamic stimulation, *Endocrinology* **80**:155.

Radford, H. M., Wheatley, I. S., and Wallace, A. L. C., 1969, The effects of oestradiol benzoate and progesterone on secretion of luteinizing hormone in the ovariectomized ewe, *J. Endocrinol.* **44**:135.

Ramirez, V. D., and Sawyer, C. H., 1965, Fluctuations in hypothalamic LH-RF (Luteinizing hormone-releasing factor) during the rat estrous cycle, *Endocrinology* **76**:282.

Rani, C. S., and Moudgal, N. R., 1977, Role of the proestrous surge of gonadotropins in the initiation of follicular maturation in the cyclic hamster: A study using antisera to follicle stimulating hormone and luteinizing hormone, *Endocrinology* **101**:1484.

Rao, A. J., Moudgal, N. R., Raj, H. G., Lipner, H., and Greep, R. O., 1974, The role of FSH and LH in the initiation of ovulation in rats and hamsters: A study using rabbit antisera to ovine FSH and LH, *J. Reprod. Fertil.* **37**:323.

Reece, R. P., 1939, Lactogen content of female guinea pig pituitary, *Proc. Soc. Exp. Biol. Med.* **42**:54.

Resko, J. A., Norman, R. L., Niswender, G. D., and Spies, H. G., 1974, The relationship between progestins and gonadotropins during the late luteal phase of the menstrual cycle in rhesus monkeys, *Endocrinology* **94**:128.

Richards, J. S., and Midgley, A. R., Jr., 1976, Protein hormone action: A key to understanding ovarian follicular and luteal cell development, *Biol. Reprod.* **14**:82.

Ridley, K., and Greenwald, G. S., 1975, Progesterone levels measured every two hours in the cyclic hamster, *Proc. Soc. Exp. Biol. Med.* **149**:10.

Robertson, H. A., 1977, Reproduction in the ewe and goat, in: *Reproduction in Domestic Animals,* Third Edition (H. H. Cole and P. T. Cupps, eds.), pp. 477–498, Academic Press, New York.

Roche, J. F., Karsch, F. J., Foster, D. L., and Dziuk, P. J., 1974, Serum LH in ewes following sequential removal of ovarian follicles, corpora lutea and stroma, *J. Reprod. Fertil.* **40**:215.

Rodgers, C. H., and Law, O. T., 1968, Effects of chemical stimulation of the "limbic system" on lordosis in female rats, *Physiol. Behav.* **3**:241.

Roser, S., and Bloch, R. B., 1971, Etude comparative des variations de la progesterone plasmatique ovarienne au cours de cycles de respectinement 4 et 5 jours, chez la ratte, *C. R. Soc. Biol. (Paris)* **165**:1995.

Ross, J., Claybaugh, C., Clemens, L. G., and Gorski, R. A., 1971, Short latency induction of estrous behavior with intracerebral gonadal hormones in ovariectomized rats, *Endocrinology* **89**:32.

Rothchild, I., 1965, The corpus luteum–hypophysis relationship, *Acta Endocrinol. (Kbh.)* **49**:107.

Rowlands, I. W., 1956, The corpus luteum of the guinea pig, *Ciba Found. Colloq. Ageing* **2**:69.

Rowlands, I. W., 1962, The effect of oestrogens, prolactin and hypophysectomy on the corpora lutea and vagina of hysterectomized guinea-pigs, *J. Endocrinol.* **24**:105.

Rowlands, I. W., and Williams, P. C., 1943, Production of ovulation in hypophysectomized rats, *J. Endocrinol.* **3**:310.

Saba, N., Cunningham, N. F., Symons, A. M., and Millar, P. G., 1975, The effect of progesterone implants on ovulation and plasma levels of LH, FSH and progesterone in anoestrous ewes, *J. Reprod. Fertil.* **44**:59.

Saidapur, S- K., and Greenwald, G. S., 1978, Peripheral blood and ovarian levels of sex steroids in the cyclic hamster, *Biol. Reprod.* **18**:401.

Salamonsen, L. A., Jonas, H. A., Burger, H. A., Buckmaster, J. M., Chamley, W. A., Cumming, I. A., Findlay, J. K., and Goding, J. R., 1973, A heterologous radioimmunoassay for follicle stimulating hormone: Application to measurement of FSH in the ovine estrous cycle and in several other species including man, *Endocrinology* **93**:610.

Sar, M., and Meites, J., 1967, Changes in pituitary prolactin release and hypothalamic PIF content during the estrous cycle of rats, *Proc. Soc. Exp. Biol. Med.* **125**:1018.

Sarkar, D. K., Chiappa, S. A., and Fink, G., 1976, Gonadotropin-releasing hormone surge in pro-oestrous rats, *Nature* **264**:461.

Sasaki, Y., and Hanson, G. C., 1974, Correlation between the activities of enzymes involved in glucose oxidation in corpus luteum and the concentration of sex steroids in systemic plasma during the reproductive cycle of the guinea pig, *Endocrinology* **95**:1213.

Sawyer, C. H., 1959, Seasonal variation in the incidence of spontaneous ovulation in rabbits following estrogen treatment, *Endocrinology* **65**:523.

Sawyer, C. H., Markee, J. E., and Townsend, B. F., 1949, Cholinergic and adrenergic components in the neurohumoral control of the release of LH in the rabbit, *Endocrinology* **44**:18.

Scaramuzzi, R. J., 1975, Inhibition of oestrous behaviour in ewes by passive immunization against oestradiol-17β, *J. Reprod. Fertil.* **42**:145.

Scaramuzzi, R. J., and Baird, D. T., 1976, The oestrous cycle of the ewe after active immunization against prostaglandin F$_2$α, *J. Reprod. Fertil.* **46**:39.

Scaramuzzi, R. J., and Baird, D. T., 1977, Pulsatile release of luteinizing hormone and the secretion of ovarian steroids in sheep during anestrus, *Endocrinology* **101**:1801.

Scaramuzzi, R. J., Caldwell, B. V., and Moor, R. M., 1970, Radioimmunoassay of LH and estrogen during the estrous cycle of the ewe, *Biol. Reprod.* **3**:110.

Scaramuzzi, R. J., Blake, C. A., Papkoff, H., Hilliard, J., and Sawyer, C. H., 1972, Radioimmunoassay of rabbit luteinizing hormone: Serum levels during various reproductive states, *Endocrinology* **90**:1285.

Schally, A. V., Coy, D. H., and Meyers, C. A., 1978, Hypothalamic regulatory hormones, *Annu. Rev. Biochem.* **47**:89.

Schroff, C., Klindt, J. M., Kaltenbach, C. C., Graber, J. W., and Niswender, G. D., 1971, Maintenance of corpora lutea in hypophysectomized ewes, *J. Anim. Sci.* **33**:268.

Schwartz, N. B., 1964, Acute effects of ovariectomy on pituitary LH, uterine weight, and vaginal cornification, *Am. J. Physiol.* **207**:1251.

Schwartz, N. B., 1968, Newer concepts of gonadotrophin and steroid feedback control mechanisms, in: *Textbook of Gynecologic Endocrinology* (J. J. Gold, ed.), pp. 33–50, Hoeber Division of Harper & Row, New York.

Schwartz, N. B., 1969, A model for the regulation of ovulation in the rat, *Recent Prog. Horm. Res.* **25**:1.

Schwartz, N. B., 1970, Control of rhythmic secretion of gonadotrophins, in: *The Hypothalamus* (L. Martini, M. Motta, and F. Fraschini, eds.), pp. 515–528, Academic Press, New York.

Schwartz, N. B., 1974, The role of FSH and LH and of their antibodies on follicle growth and on ovulation, *Biol. Reprod.* **10**:236.

Schwartz, N. B., and Bartosik, D., 1962, Changes in pituitary LH content during the rat estrous cycle, *Endocrinology* **71**:756.

Schwartz, N. B., and Caldarelli, D., 1965, Plasma LH in cyclic female rats, *Proc. Soc. Exp. Biol. Med.* **119**:16.

Schwartz, N. B., and Gold, J. J., 1967, Effect of a single dose of anti-LH-serum at proestrus on the rat estrous cycle, *Anat. Rec.* **157**:137.

Schwartz, N. B., and Lawton, I. E., 1968, Effects of barbiturate injection on the day before proestrus in the rat, *Neuroendocrinology* **3**:9.

Schwartz, N. B., and Talley, W. L., 1965, Effect of acute ovariectomy on mating in the cyclic rat, *J. Reprod. Fertil.* **10**:463.

Schwartz, N. B., Cobbs, S. B., Talley, W. L., and Ely, C. A., 1975, Induction of ovulation by LH and FSH in the presence of antigonadotrophic sera, *Endocrinology* **96**:1171.

Scott, P. P., and Lloyd, M. A., 1959, Reduction in the anoestrus period of laboratory cats by increased illumination, *Nature* **184**:2022.

Self, L. W., and Lloyd, C. W., 1966, The pituitary during the oestrous and menstrual cycle, in: *The Pituitary Gland,* Vol. 2 (G. W. Harris and B. T. Donovan, eds.), pp. 346–363, University of California Press, Berkeley.

Sen, K. K., and Menon, M. J., 1978, Oestradiol receptors in the rat anterior pituitary gland during the oestrous cycle: Quantitation of receptor activity in relation to gonadotrophin releasing hormone-mediated luteinizing hormone release, *J. Endocrinol.* **76**:211.

Shaikh, A. A., 1971, Estrone and estradiol levels in the ovarian venous blood from rats during the estrous cycle and pregnancy, *Biol. Reprod.* **5**:297.

Shaikh, A. A., 1972, Estrone, estradiol, progesterone and 17α-hydroxyprogesterone in the ovarian venous plasma during the estrous cycle of the hamster, *Endocrinology* **91**:1136.

Shaikh, A. A., and Shaikh, S. A., 1975, Adrenal and ovarian steroid secretion in the rat estrous cycle temporally related to gonadotropins and steroid levels found in peripheral plasma, *Endocrinology* **96**:37.

Sherwood, N. M., Chiappa, S. A., and Fink, G., 1976, Immunoreactive luteinizing hormone releasing factor in pituitary stalk blood from female rats: Sex steroid modulation of response to electrical stimulation of preoptic area or median eminence, *J. Endocrinol.* **70**:501.

Shirley, B., Wolinsky, J., and Schwartz, N. B., 1968, Effects of a single injection of an estrogen antagonist on the estrous cycle of the rat, *Endocrinology* **82**:959.

Short, R. V., 1964, IV. Steroid hormones. Ovarian steroid synthesis and secretion *in vitro, Recent Prog. Horm. Res.* **20**:303.

Short, R. V., McDonald, M. E., and Rowson, L. E. A., 1963, Steroids in the ovarian venous blood of ewes before and after gonadotrophic stimulation, *J. Endocrinol.* **26**:155.

Siegel, H. I., Bast, J. D., and Greenwald, G. S., 1976, The effects of phenobarbital and gonadal steroids on periovulatory serum levels of luteinizing hormone and follicle-stimulating hormone in the hamster, *Endocrinology* **98**:48.

Smeaton, T. C., and Robertson, H. A., 1971, Studies on the growth and atresia of Graafian follicles in the ovary of the sheep, *J. Reprod. Fertil.* **25**:243.

Smith, E. R., Bowers, C. Y., and Davidson, J. M., 1973, Circulating levels of plasma gonadotropins in 4- and 5-day cycling rats, *Endocrinology* **93**:756.

Smith, M. S. and McDonald, L. E., 1974, Serum levels of luteinizing hormone and progesterone during the estrous cycle, pseudopregnancy and pregnancy in the dog, *Endocrinology* **94**:404.

Smith, M. S., Freeman, M. E., and Neill, J. D., 1975, The control of progesterone secretion during the estrous cycle and early pseudopregnancy in the rat: Prolactin, gonadotropin and steroid levels associated with rescue of the corpus luteum of pseudopregnancy, *Endocrinology* **96**:219.

Snabes, M. C., Kelch, R. P., and Karsch, F. J., 1977, A daily neural signal for luteinizing hormone release in the untreated ovariectomized rat: Changes in gonadotropin-releasing hormone content of the preoptic area and hypothalamus throughout the day, *Endocrinology* **100**:1521.

Stabenfeldt, G. H., and Shille, V. M., 1977, Reproduction in the dog and cat, in: *Reproduction in Domestic Animals,* Third Edition (H. H. Cole, and P. T. Cupps, eds.), pp. 499–528, Academic Press, New York.

Stabenfeldt, G. H., Holt, J. A., and Ewing, L. L., 1969, Peripheral plasma progesterone levels during the bovine estrous cycle, *Endocrinology* **85**:11.

Stetson, M. H., and Watson-Whitmyre, M., 1976, Nucleus suprachiasmaticus: The biological clock in the hamster? *Science* **191**:197.

Stetson, M. H., and Watson-Whitmyre, M., 1977, The neural clock regulating estrous cyclicity in hamsters: Gonadotropin release following barbiturate blockade, *Biol. Reprod.* **16**:536.

Stockard, C. R., and Papanicolaou, G. N., 1917, The existence of a typical oestrous cycle in the guinea-pig with a study of its histological and physiological changes, *Am. J. Anat.* **22**:225.

Stouffer, R. L., Nixon, W. E., and Hodgen, G. D., 1977, Estrogen inhibition of basal and gonadotropin-stimulated progesterone production by rhesus monkey luteal cells *in vitro, Endocrinology* **101**:1157.

Swerdloff, R. S., Jacobs, H. S., and Odell, W. D., 1972, Synergistic role of progestogens in estrogen induction of LH and FSH surge, *Endocrinology* **90**:1529.

Szego, C. M., and Roberts, S., 1953, Steroid action and interaction in uterine metabolism, *Recent Prog. Horm. Res.* **8**:419.

Takahashi, M., Ford, J. J., Yoshinaga, K., and Greep, R. O., 1974, Induction of ovulation in hypophysectomized rats by progesterone, *Endocrinology* **95**:1322.

Tapper, C. M., Greig, F., and Brown-Grant, K., 1974, Effects of steroid hormones on gonadotrophin secretion in female rats after ovariectomy during the oestrous cycle, *J. Endocrinol.* **62**:511.

Taya, K., and Igarashi, M., 1973, Changes in FSH, LH and prolactin secretion during estrous cycle in rats, *Endocrinol. Jpn.* **20**:199.

Telegdy, G., and Endröczi, E., 1963, The ovarian secretion of progesterone and 20α-hydroxy-pregn-4-en-3-one in rats during the estrous cycle, *Steroids* **2**:119.

Terranova, P. F., and Greenwald, G. S., 1978, Steroid and gonadotropin levels during the luteal–follicular shift of the cyclic hamster, *Biol. Reprod.* **18**:170.

Thorburn, G. D., Bassett, J. M., and Smith, I. D., 1969, Progesterone concentration in the peripheral plasma of sheep during the oestrous cycle, *J. Endocrinol.* **45**:459.

Tsou, R. C., Dailey, R. A., McLanahan, C. S., Parent, A. D., Tindall, G. T., and Neill, J. D., 1977, Luteinizing hormone releasing hormone (LHRH) levels in pituitary stalk plasma during the preovulatory gonadotropin surge of rabbits, *Endocrinology* **101**:534.

Turgeon, J. L., and Barraclough, C. A., 1977, Regulatory role of estradiol in pituitary responsiveness to luteinizing hormone-releasing hormone on proestrus in the rat, *Endocrinology* **101**:548.

Turner, C. D., 1966, *General Endocrinology*, W. B. Saunders, Philadelphia.

Uchida, K., Kadowaki, M., and Miyake, T., 1969a, Ovarian secretion of progesterone and 20α-hydroxypregn-4-en-3-one during rat estrous cycle in chronological relation to pituitary release of luteinizing hormone, *Endocrinol. Jpn.* **16**:227.

Uchida, K., Kadowaki, M., and Miyake, T., 1969b, Acute effects of various gonadotropins and other pituitary hormones on preovulatory ovarian progestin secretion in hypophysectomized rats, *Endocrinol. Jpn.* **16**:239.

Uchida, K., Kadowaki, M., and Miyake, T., 1969c, Effect of exogenous progesterone on the preovulatory progesterone secretion in the rat, *Endocrinol. Jpn.* **16**:485.

Velardo, J. T., 1960, Induction of ovulation in immature hypophysectomized rats, *Science* **131**:357.

Verhage, H. G., Beamer, N. B., and Brenner, R. M., 1976, Plasma levels of estradiol and progesterone in the cat during polyestrus, pregnancy and pseudopregnancy, *Biol. Reprod.* **14**:579.

Ward, I. L., Crowley, W. R., Zemlan, F. P., and Margules, D. L., 1975, Monoaminergic mediation of female sexual behavior, *J. Comp. Physiol. Psychol.* **88**:53.

Weick, R. F., Dierschke, D. J., Karsch, F. J., Butler, W. R., Hotchkiss, J., and Knobil, E., 1973, Periovulatory time courses of circulating gonadotropic and ovarian hormones in the rhesus monkey, *Endocrinology* **93**:1140.

Welschen, R., and Dullaart, J., 1976, Administration of antiserum against ovine follicle-stimulating hormone or ovine luteinizing hormone at pro-oestrus in the rat: Effects on follicular development during the oncoming cycle, *J. Endocrinol.* **70**:301.

Whalen, R. E., and Gorzalka, B. B., 1972, The effects of progesterone and its metabolites on the induction of sexual receptivity in rats, *Horm. Behav.* **3**:221.

Wheatley, I. S., and Radford, H. M., 1969, Luteinizing hormone secretion during the oestrous cycle of the ewe as determined by radioimmunoassay, *J. Reprod. Fertil.* **19**:211.

Wheeler, A. G., Baird, D. T., Land, R. B., and Scaramuzzi, 1975, Increased secretion of progesterone from the ovary of the ewe during the preovulatory period, *J. Reprod. Fertil.* **45**:519.

Wildt, D. E., Chakraborty, P. K., Panko, W. B., and Seager, S. W. J., 1978, Relationship of reproductive behavior, serum luteinizing hormone and time of ovulation in the bitch, *Biol. Reprod.* **18**:561.

Wise, P. M., Rance, N., Barr, G. D., and Barraclough, C. A., 1979, Further evidence that luteinizing hormone-releasing hormone also is follicle-stimulating hormone-releasing hormone, *Endocrinology* **104**:940.

Wolfe, J. M., 1935, The normal level of the various cell types in the anterior pituitaries of mature and immature female rats and further observations of cyclic changes, *Anat. Rec.* **61**:321.

Wolfe, J. M., and Cleveland, R., 1933, Cyclic histological variations in the anterior hypophysis of the albino rat, *Anat. Rec.* **55**:233.

Wu, C. H., Blasco, L., Flickinger, G. F., and Mikhail, G., 1977, Ovarian function in the preovulatory rabbit, *Biol. Reprod.* **17**:304.

Wuttke, W., and Meites, J., 1971, Luteolytic role of prolactin during the estrous cycle of the rat, *Proc. Soc. Exp. Biol. Med.* **137**:988.

Yamaji, T., Peckham, W. D., Atkinson, L. E., Dierschke, D. J., and Knobil, E., 1973, Radioimmunoassay of rhesus monkey follicle-stimulating hormone (RhFSH), *Endocrinology* **92**:1652.

Yanase, M., and Gorski, R. A., 1976, Sites of estrogen and progesterone facilitation of lordosis behavior in the spayed rat, *Biol. Reprod.* **15**:536.

Yokoyama, A., Tomogane, H., and Ota, K., 1971, Prolactin surge on the afternoon of pro-oestrus in the rat and its blockade by pentobarbitone, *Experientia* **27**:578.

Yoshinaga, K., Grieves, S. A., and Short, R. V., 1967, Steroidogenic effects of luteinizing hormone and prolactin on the rat ovary *in vivo, J. Endocrinol.* **38**:423.

Yoshinaga, K., Hawkins, R. A., and Stocker, J. F., 1969, Estrogen secretion by the rat ovary *in vivo* during the estrous cycle and pregnancy, *Endocrinology* **85**:103.

Young, W. C., 1961, The hormones and mating behavior, in: *Sex and Internal Secretions,* Third Edition, Vol. 2 (W. C. Young, ed.), pp. 1173–1239, Williams & Wilkins, Baltimore.

Young, W. C., 1969, Psychobiology of sexual behavior in the guinea pig, in: *Advances in the Study of Behavior,* Vol. 2 (D. S. Lehrman, R. A. Hinde, and E. Shaw, eds.), pp. 1–110, Academic Press, New York.

Younglai, E. V., 1975, Rapid interaction between luteinizing hormone and isolated rabbit follicles, *J. Endocrinol.* **67**:289.

Younglai, E. V., 1977, Effect of 20α-hydroxy-4-pregnen-3-one on luteinizing hormone secretion in the female rabbit, *Acta Endocrinol. (Kbh.)* **84**:45.

Yu, J. Y. L., Namiki, H., and Gorbman, A., 1978, Differential actions of GnRH and rat hypothalamic extracts in release of hypophysial FSH and LH *in vitro, Life Sci.* **22**:269.

Yuthasastrakosol, P., Palmer, W. M., and Howland, B. E., 1975, Luteinizing hormone, oestrogen and progesterone levels in peripheral serum of anoestrous and cyclic ewes as determined by radioimmunoassay, *J. Reprod. Fertil.* **43**:57.

Zarrow, M. X., and Clark, J. H., 1968, Ovulation following vaginal stimulation in a spontaneous ovulator and its implications, *J. Endocrinol.* **40**:343.

Zarrow, M. X., Yochim, J. M., and McCarthy, J. M., 1964, *Experimental Endocrinology,* Academic Press, New York.

Zeilmaker, G. H., 1966, The biphasic effect of progesterone on ovulation in the rat, *Acta Endocrinol. (Kbh.)* **41**:461.

Zucker, I., 1967, Actions of progesterone in the control of sexual receptivity of the spayed female rat, *J. Comp. Physiol. Psychol.* **63**:313.

11

How the Brain Mediates Ovarian Responses to Environmental Stimuli

Neuroanatomy and Neurophysiology

B. R. KOMISARUK, E. TERASAWA, AND
J. F. RODRIGUEZ-SIERRA

I. INTRODUCTION

In the preceding three chapters, we have examined the regulation of the gonads in general and the mammalian ovary in particular. In this analysis, we saw how interactions between the steroid-secreting organs, the brain, and the pituitary result in orderly reproductive events like the estrous cycle. In this chapter, we discuss many issues related to this basic theme of neuroendocrine integration, but with the emphasis on the specific role of the central nervous system.

Vertebrate neuroendocrinology is based on the recognition that pituitary-dependent hormonal secretion is mediated by the central nervous system. Since the response of the brain to an environmental stimulus can alter the secretory activity of the pituitary and consequently its target glands (e.g., the ovaries), the nervous system functions as the interpreter and mediator of the external environment on the endocrine system. Similarly, the nervous system can also mediate the internal environment's effects on endocrine function. For

B. R. KOMISARUK • Institute of Animal Behavior, Rutgers University, Newark, New Jersey 07102. E. TERASAWA • Wisconsin Regional Primate Research Center, University of Wisconsin, Madison, Wisconsin 53706. J. F. RODRIGUEZ-SIERRA • Department of Anatomy, School of Medicine, University of Nebraska, Omaha, Nebraska 68105.

example, the hormones that are secreted by the pituitary and the ovaries in turn act on the brain, thereby further modulating pituitary secretion and affecting behavior. This interplay between the internal and external milieus via the neuroendocrine system leads to the sequential changes in hormone secretion and behavior that characterize the reproductive cycle (e.g., courtship, mating, pregnancy or incubation of eggs, and caring for the young).

In this chapter we shall analyze some of the specific ways in which the nervous system mediates the internal and external influences on endocrine secretion.

II. ENVIRONMENTAL INFLUENCES ON HORMONE SECRETION

A. Visual and Auditory

Seasonal changes in gonadal activity provided some of the earliest examples of environmental influences on hormone secretion (see review by Lehrman, 1961). One of the first and clearest experimental cases of visual stimuli acting on reproductive function was that of Warren and Scott (1936) who showed that chickens laid eggs almost exclusively during the 12-hr period when the lights were on. When the light schedule was changed to constant illumination, the egg-laying pattern shifted gradually for 15 days until the chickens were laying approximately equal numbers of eggs during daytime and nighttime hours. When the light cycle was subsequently reversed, within 10 days the eggs were laid almost exclusively during the nighttime hours while the lights were on. Finally, when the light cycle was changed back to the original schedule, within 10 days the eggs were again laid exclusively during the daytime hours when the lights were on. Chapter 12 of this volume is devoted to the specific ways in which light affects estrous and seasonal cyclicity. In the context of the present chapter, light represents but one class of external stimulation that has potent effects on hormone function.

The timing of the lighting cycle has also been shown to regulate (entrain) the time of ovulation in rats. Under the controlled lighting condition of 14 hr lights on (5 a.m. to 7 p.m.) and 10 hr lights off, cycling rats spontaneously ovulate between 1–3 a.m. on the day of estrus (Everett and Sawyer, 1949). If a barbiturate (a central nervous system depressant) is administered to rats just prior to 2 p.m. on the day of proestrus, the time of spontaneous ovulation is postponed for 24 hr (Everett and Sawyer, 1950). If these animals receive another injection of barbiturate just prior to 2 p.m. on the day of estrus, the time of ovulation is again postponed for 24 hr. The time between 2–4 p.m. on the day of proestrus is called the "critical period" for the release of ovulatory hormone, i.e., luteinizing hormone, from the anterior pituitary gland (for review, see Everett, 1964). If the lighting schedule is reversed to lights on from

5 p.m. to 7 a.m., the critical period of female rats shifts 12 hr (Hoffman, 1969). Furthermore, exposure to constant illumination results in a cessation of ovulatory cycles and induces a state of "anovulatory persistent estrus" (Fiske, 1941) in female rats. Thus light stimulation modulates reproduction function in some species.

Removal of the eyes or the optic nerve blocks persistent estrus caused by constant illumination, whereas cutting of the optic tract does not interrupt light-induced persistent estrus (Critchlow, 1963). The difference between these two procedures can be accounted for by the findings of projections from the optic nerve directly into the hypothalamus (suprachiasmatic nucleus) (Moore and Lenn, 1972). Thus, there is no effect of nerve section when the visual pathway beyond the entry point is cut.

It would be an oversimplification to characterize light's effects on reproduction as the impinging of photic stimulation on a passive organism. For many species (e.g., hamster), light does not merely trigger a reflexive response, since there is an endogenous rhythm of sensitivity to light (see Chapter 12) as Elliot, *et al.* (1972) have shown in hamsters. That is, when light is presented in certain rhythms (i.e., for 6 hr every 36 or 60 hr), the testes and accessory organ sizes are maintained in the adult condition; but if light is presented in different rhythms (i.e., for 6 hr every 24 or 48 hr), they are not comparably maintained. The demonstration of differential gonadal activation is especially striking since organisms receiving more total light per unit time (e.g., 6 hr every 24 hr) do not respond reproductively, whereas organisms receiving less light (6 hr every 36 hr) do respond.

The previous examples deal with qualitative aspects of photic stimulation (amount and timing of illumination). The specific pattern of visual stimulation that the individual sees in the light also affects hormonal status. Isolated ring doves provided with a mirror are more likely to ovulate than individuals in a control group that were provided with a transparent glass plate (Lott and Brody, 1966). Furthermore, under appropriate conditions, when male ring doves are permitted to see a female dove incubating eggs, they show an increase in the prolactin-dependent secretion of "crop milk" which they use to feed their young (Friedman and Lehrman, 1968).

Loud noise (ringing of a bell) has been shown to stimulate adrenal corticoid secretion (Feldman *et al.,* 1968). In more naturalistic contexts, certain calls of budgerigars are much more effective than others (Brockway, 1965) in stimulating ovum development (measured as follicle diameter) and in inducing ovulation. Similarly, when sounds from a ring dove colony are played through a loudspeaker to isolated female doves, they show ovarian development greater than that of control females that do not receive the sound. Furthermore, the sounds augment the ovarian response of the doves to seeing their mirror image. A greater ovarian response is obtained when the females can obtain coordinated visual and auditory stimuli, that is, when they are paired with a male, but separated from the male by a glass partition (Lott and Brody, 1966; Lott *et al.,* 1967). A "dose–response" relationship was observed between the magnitude of the female's ovarian development and the amount of time she was exposed to a male across a glass partition, the male providing at least visual and auditory stimulation (Barfield, 1971). When female ring doves were exposed to castrated males that showed little or no courtship behavior, there was no oviduct development (Erickson and Lehrman, 1964) unless the female was in an advanced stage of ovarian development (Cheng, 1974). However, when the castrated males were injected with selected dosages of testosterone propionate, the oviduct weight of the females showed a dose–response relationship to the androgen dose which the males received. Thus, the visual and auditory stimuli provided by the hormonally stimulated behavior of the male induce ovarian hormonal changes in the female with which he is paired.

B. Tactile

Tactile stimulation elicits a diverse array of hormonal effects in vertebrates. Certain mammals, including cats, rabbits, ferrets, mink, and voles (Rowlands, 1966), normally ovulate reflexively in response to the tactile stimulation provided by copulation, whereas others (e.g., humans, rats, mice, cattle) normally ovulate spontaneously in response to cyclical changes in hormone levels (see Chapter 10). As pointed out by Zarrow and Clark (1968), the difference may be one of degree, for under appropriate circumstances, such as blocking the neural activity preceding spontaneous ovulation by anesthetics, rats ovulate reflexively in response to mating (Harrington *et al.,* 1967). Similarly, when rats are mated early in the estrous cycle, ovulation occurs earlier than usual (Aron *et al.,* 1966).

From early studies in rabbits, the time course of the events leading to reflex ovulation can be estimated as follows. If anesthesia is injected intravenously in rabbits within 30 sec of a brief mating stimulus (lasting several seconds), ovulation is blocked. However, if the anesthetic is injected more than 30 sec after mating, ovulation proceeds. Thus, the neural "trigger" for ovulation does not need to be active for more than 30 sec (Sawyer *et al.,* 1950a,b). If the blood of mated rabbits is removed and replaced with blood of unmated rabbits between 75 and 90 min after mating, ovulation is blocked. However, if the blood of mated rabbits is removed, and blood of unmated rabbits is substituted within 30 min after mating, ovulation does occur. This indicates that an amount of hormone sufficient for ovulation is released between 30 and 90 min after mating. Before 30 min, not enough has yet been released for ovulation, but an adequate amount will be released in the following 60 min (Westman and Jacobsohn, 1936).

Ovulation occurs 10–12 hr after mating, which is the latency period required for the ovulatory hormone, luteinizing hormone (LH), to cause the follicular membrane to rupture, releasing ova from the ovaries. In more recent studies using direct measurement of LH in pituitary and blood, significant depletion of pituitary LH has been shown to occur within 15 min of mating in rabbits (Desjardins *et al.*, 1967).

In rats exposed to constant light, ovulation occurs reflexively in response to mating, and LH increases in the blood within 10 min (Brown-Grant *et al.*, 1973). In anesthetized rats, the latency for the increase in LH in response to vaginal stimulation is somewhat longer (30 min); neural activity in the hypothalamus increases concurrently and persists for about 2 hr (Blake and Sawyer, 1972). Even in normal females, mating stimuli increase LH significantly (Moss and Cooper, 1973), but the function of this effect is not known, except that there is a small but significant increment in the number of ova released in mated versus nonmated rats (Rodgers, 1971; for review, see Komisaruk, 1974). Ovulation can also be induced in rabbits by vaginal stimulation, and estrogen facilitates the proportion of rabbits ovulating in response to this stimulus (Sawyer *et al.*, 1950a,b; Sawyer and Markee, 1959).

Mating also initiates the secretion of prolactin from the anterior pituitary in rats (Terkel *et al.*, 1978). A function of prolactin release in this context is to initiate the secretion of ovarian progesterone in amounts sufficient to stimulate the growth of the uterus and prepare it for implantation of the fertilized ova. The more intromissions the female receives, the more progesterone is secreted (Adler, 1969; Adler *et al.*, 1970), presumably as a consequence of prolactin release. This reflexive release of prolactin depends mainly on an intact sensory innervation of the vaginal canal (Spies and Niswender, 1971). If the female receives too few (fewer than three) intromissions before the male ejaculates, she does not become pregnant (Adler, 1969). Thus, the sensory input from the female's genital tract releases prolactin from the pituitary, prolactin stimulates progesterone secretion from the corpus luteum, and progesterone, in turn, stimulates the uterine growth necessary for implantation.

Vaginal stimulation alone can induce these progestational effects in the uterus without fertilization. This is a condition known as pseudopregnancy, during which the estrous cycle is suspended for 2 weeks (the normal gestation period in rats is 3 weeks). If the sensory nerve from the genital tract (vagina, cervix, and uterus) is cut, vaginal–cervical stimulation does not induce pseudopregnancy (Carlson and DeFeo, 1965).

Delayed pseudopregnancy (Everett, 1967) is an effect in which ovulation occurs after vaginal stimulation, and the following day pseudopregnancy begins. This is probably caused by the daily surges of prolactin occurring after vaginal stimulation (Freeman and Neill, 1972). After mating occurs, the circadian surges of prolactin probably stimulate progesterone secretion from the corpus luteum, thereby preparing the uterus for implantation and pregnancy.

Tactile stimulation can also inhibit reproductive function. In certain species of birds, for example, when the typical number of eggs are in the nest, ovulation is inhibited, thus limiting the clutch size. If the eggs are removed, ovulation (release of the ovum from the ovary) and oviposition (laying of the egg) resume until the normal number in the nest is reestablished, and then ovulation is inhibited. This process characterizes "indeterminate" egg-laying species (e.g., domestic hen, sparrows, pheasants). Species in which the number of eggs is limited, even if the eggs are removed from the nest, are called "determinate layers" (e.g., pigeons; see Lehrman, 1961, for review).

The mechanical stimulation provided by the egg in the oviduct also inhibits a pending ovulation. Huston and Nalbandov (1953) found that simply inserting a thread into the oviduct in chickens could inhibit ovulation for more than 25 days, demonstrating that the mechanical stimulation in some way inhibits ovulation.

Mechanical stimulation also plays a significant role in "milk letdown" and uterine contractions, processes which are mediated by oxytocin, a hormone released from the posterior (neural) lobe of the pituitary. Milk is secreted in the glandular alveoli of the mammary glands, which are surrounded by smooth muscle ("myoepithelium") (Zaks, 1962). Oxytocin induces the contraction of this smooth muscle, thereby forcibly ejecting the milk into the mouth of the suckling young. The oxytocin is released reflexively by the suckling stimulus (see Brooks et al., 1966). If the mother is anesthetized, the milk ejection is blocked (for an extensive review, see Beyer and Mena, 1969).

Oxytocin is also released reflexively by copulatory stimuli in cows and may facilitate sperm transport (Vandemark and Hays, 1952). The oxytocin thus released also stimulates milk letdown. This process has been utilized by the Hottentot tribe, who blow air through a tube inserted into the vagina in cows and thereby facilitate milking (Folley, 1969). Similarly, milk letdown has been reported in lactating women during sexual intercourse (Folley, 1969).

The release of oxytocin by genital tract stimulation also plays a role in parturition by stimulating the smooth muscle of the uterus. As outlined by Cross (1959), mechanical stimulation of the birth canal as the fetuses are expelled reflexively stimulates further oxytocin release which in turn promotes uterine contraction and expulsion of the fetuses. This is an example of a positive feedback system. As Cross pointed out, in rabbits, the first newborn pups start to suckle before their littermates are born. This may increase the release of oxytocin which could facilitate uterine contractions. Thus, by suckling, the newborn pups may facilitate the birth of their siblings.

The reflexive release of oxytocin by tactile stimulation can, like other reflexes, be conditioned to previously neutral stimuli. Thus, milk letdown in cows occurs in response to the rattling of milk pails prior to milking (Folley, 1969). Milk letdown in lactating women sometimes occurs in response to the sound of a crying baby, apparently another example of conditioned release of oxytocin. Increase of oxytocin secretion in mother rats exposed to ultrasonic calls of the young has been demonstrated (Terkel et al., 1978). The higher neural pathways involved in this process may include the cingulate gyrus of the cerebral cortex (Beyer et al., 1961). In addition, Mena and Beyer (1963) have suggested that the spinothalamic pathway mediates the suckling response, and Tindal et al. (1967) have delineated an ascending route from the lateral tegmentum and mesencephalic central gray to the hypothalamus in which electrical stimulation induces oxytocin release.

C. Olfactory

Olfactory stimuli have been shown to influence the latency of onset of puberty, estrous cyclicity, ovulation, and pregnancy in rodents. Female mice housed together show a delay in onset of puberty (Vandenbergh *et al.,* 1972; Drickamer, 1974; McIntosh and Drickamer, 1977), but when they are exposed to the odor of males (Vandenbergh, 1967), they show an accelerated onset of puberty. Adult female mice housed together show an inhibition of estrous cycles (Lee and Boot, 1955; Whitten, 1957), and when a male is placed in their cage, they resume estrous cyclicity in synchrony with each other (Whitten, 1956a). Bronson and Desjardins (1974) have shown that in the prepubertal female mouse, exposure to males induces an increase in plasma LH within 1 hr and an increase in plasma estradiol within 12 hr. An effect of the odor of female rats on the estrous cyclicity of other rats has been shown recently by McClintock (1974). When three groups of female rats were separated physically from each other but were connected by an "in-series" air supply, the group that was "downwind" from the center group showed a greater tendency to have synchronized estrous cycles than the group that was "upwind" from the center group. This suggests that the odor of one group synchronizes the estrous cycles of another group. Ablation of the olfactory bulbs has been shown to reduce ovarian and uterine weight in mice (Whitten, 1956b).

Ovulation has been induced in light-induced persistent estrous rats by placing them in contact with cage bedding soiled by male rats (Johns *et al.,* 1978). Direct contact with the bedding is necessary for this effect, for if the females are separated 1 inch above the bedding by a wire mesh floor, ovulation is not induced. The effect seems to be mediated by the vomeronasal organ which lies at the end of a pair of blind tubes in the base of the nasal canal, for if the openings to the tubes are occluded, ovulation does not occur. The ovulation-blocking effect of this occlusion is not caused by inability to secrete LH, since the occluded females ovulate when mated. Efferent neural activity from the vomeronasal organ projects to the accessory olfactory bulb; this in turn projects to the medial and cortical amygdaloid nuclei which project to the basal hypothalamus (Winans and Scalia, 1970), thus suggesting a possible neural pathway for this effect.

Olfactory stimulation provided by males has been shown to block pregnancy in mice. If female mice made pregnant by males of one strain are exposed to males of a different strain ("alien" males) within 5 days of copulation, they soon show estrous cycles again, indicating that their pregnancy was blocked. If different individual males of the same strain as the impregnating strain ("strange" males) are placed with the females, they show significantly less tendency to pregnancy blockage. The critical factor for the pregnancy block is the difference in strain between the male that impregnates and the male that is subsequently placed with the female. (It does not matter whether the impregnating male is of the same or different strain as the female.)

The pregnancy-blocking effect seems to be an olfactory phenomenon since it occurs even if the females are placed in the cages soiled and then vacated by the males (Bruce, 1960; Parkes and Bruce, 1961). Furthermore, the pregnancy-blocking effect is prevented by removing the olfactory bulbs of the females—that is, they remain pregnant even when exposed to alien males (Bruce and Parrott, 1962). The pregnancy-blocking effect is apparently brought about by an inhibition of prolactin secretion and consequent reduction in progesterone secretion in response to the alien male substance (Bruce, 1963); for administration of progesterone (Dominic, 1965, 1966) or prolactin (Dominic, 1967) prevents the pregnancy blockage. Lactating females, which presumably have increased prolactin secretion, are not susceptible to the pregnancy-blocking effect (Parkes, 1963).

Although there seems to be a wide variety of reproductive effects of olfactory stimulation on reproduction, Zarrow (1973) has suggested a unifying formulation. He postulates that a basic reciprocal relationship exists between the secretion of gonadotropins (FSH and LH) and prolactin. Olfactory stimulation may primarily increase gonadotropin secretion (leading to ovulation and early puberty) while it inhibits prolactin secretion (hence blocking pregnancy). The adaptive significance of these intriguing effects has yet to be elucidated.

III. HOW NEURAL STIMULI PRODUCE HORMONAL CHANGES

A. Role of the Anterior versus Posterior Divisions of the Pituitary Gland

The hormonal responses to environmental stimuli that were discussed in the preceding sections require the presence of the pituitary. Hypophysectomy (removal of the pituitary) results in atrophy of the target glands. In the following section, we shall present some of the underlying anatomical and physiological mechanisms. The anatomy of the pituitary gives the first indication of its relationship to the brain and thus hints at how its function may be controlled by environmental stimuli. The pituitary gland (hypophysis) consists of three main divisions—an anterior lobe ("adenohypophysis") a posterior lobe ("neurohypophysis"), and an intermediate lobe (Fig. 1). The posterior lobe is itself part of the nervous system: it contains axons and neuronal terminals whose cell bodies are situated in the supraoptic and paraventricular nuclei of the hypothalamus (Harris, 1955). These neurons secrete oxytocin and vasopressin, substances (called neurosecretions) that are drained from the posterior lobe via venous capillaries and from there enter the general body circulation. The effect of these hormones is to stimulate contraction of smooth muscle—vasopression

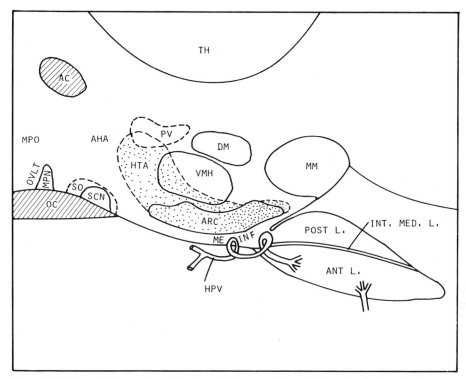

Figure 1. Schematic illustration of the hypothalamus and the pituitary gland. AC, anterior commissure; AHA, anterior hypothalamic area; ANT L., anterior lobe; ARC, arcuate nucleus; DM, dorsomedial nucleus; HPV, hypophyseal portal vessels; HTA, hypophysiotrophic area; INF, infundibular stalk; INT. MED. L., intermediate lobe; ME, median eminence; MM, mammillary nucleus; MPN, medial preoptic nucleus; MPO, medial preoptic area; OC, optic chiasm; OVLT, organum vasculosum of lamina terminalis; POST L., posterior lobe; PV, paraventricular nucleus; SCN, suprachiasmatic nucleus; SO, supraoptic nucleus; TH, thalamus; VMH, ventromedial hypothalamic nucleus.

stimulates blood vessel constriction, thereby increasing blood pressure, and oxytocin stimulates the smooth muscle of the uterus and mammary glands, thereby accelerating parturition and inducing milk ejection.

Vasopression also has an antidiuretic effect, i.e., it increases the reabsorption of water from the distal kidney tubules, thereby reducing the rate of urine production. It is of anatomical interest that antidiuresis may occur even after complete removal of the pituitary. A possible explanation is that these neurosecretions are synthesized in the brain and, in the absence of the posterior pituitary, "leak" out into the systemic circulation, thus exerting their effect (Harris, 1955).

The anterior lobe of the pituitary has a different connection to the hypothalamus. It does not contain axons or axon terminals. Instead, it is connected to the brain via the "hypophyseal portal system." A portal system consists of blood vessels that have capillaries at both ends. In the hypophyseal portal system, the lower capillary bed is in the adenohypophysis, whereas the upper capillary bed is in the region of the hypothalamic median eminence and upper ("proximal") end of the pituitary stalk (infundibulum). Axon terminals of neurosecretory cells terminate on the upper capillaries in the median eminence and infundibulum. The vascular arrangement makes it possible for secretory products of brain neurons to be transported to the adenohypophysis where they influence its secretory activity (Szentagothai *et al.*, 1968). These neurosecretory products are polypeptides that stimulate or inhibit the secretion of anterior pituitary hormones; they have, therefore, been termed "releasing hormones" and "inhibiting hormones" (Schally, 1978). The pituitary secretions then enter the systemic circulation and stimulate the target glands (e.g., ovaries).

Thus, the anterior and posterior lobes of the pituitary are both connected to the brain. But the nature of the connection is distinctly different for each lobe. The former is connected humorally via a local vascular system (hypothalamo–hypophyseal portal vessels) while the latter is a storage organ that is itself part of the nervous system. See Scharrer (1976, 1977) for an interesting discussion of the comparative evolution of these two kinds of neuroendocrine transduction mechanisms.

Although the anatomy of the hypothalamus–portal system–anterior pituitary suggests a potential mechanism for CNS control of hypophyseal function, it was the classic physiological experimentation of G. W. Harris and his coworkers that in fact demonstrated the existence and nature of this control. These investigators observed that direct application of electrical stimulation to the brain induced ovulation (see Harris, 1955, 1961, for review). In an ingenious series of experiments, Harris and Jacobsohn (1952) removed the pituitary and then transplanted pituitaries from other donors back to either the sella turcica, the bony cavity that encases the pituitary, or to a site several millimeters lateral to the sella turcica, under the temporal lobe of the brain. Animals receiving pituitary transplants under the temporal lobe did not resume ovarian cyclicity. In those animals bearing the pituitary transplants in the sella turcica, however, ovarian functions (estrous cycles) were restored, and normal pregnancy and lactation were maintained if the transplants were adequately revascularized.

This study suggested that reconnection to the hypophyseal portal vessels was essential for restoration of pituitary functioning. In a further test of this hypothesis, Harris transplanted the pituitaries back under the median eminence and inserted a cotton or waxed paper barrier between the pituitary and the median eminence. The cotton-barrier individuals resumed ovarian function, but the waxed paper-barrier individuals failed to do so unless the portal vessels regenerated around the edges of the barrier (see Harris, 1955). Subsequent studies showed that if the anterior lobe of the pituitary were transplanted elsewhere in the body, e.g., to the kidney capsule, ovarian function could not be restored unless extracts of hypothalamic tissue were infused into the pituitary (Nikitovitch-Winer and Everett, 1958). It was interesting to note that ovarian cycles could be maintained by pituitaries from either male or female rats, indicating that the specificity for maintaining the ovaries was not a function of the gender of the pituitary (Harris, 1955) but depended on differences in the CNS (see Chapters 5 and 9).

B. The Hypothalamus as the Final Common Pathway to the Pituitary Gland

The role of the hypothalamus as the final common pathway in the CNS to the pituitary was shown with lesions of the median eminence and tuberal region, resulting in the abolition of gonadal cyclicity and leading to gonadal atrophy (Dey, 1943; Taleisnik and McCann, 1961). Further evidence was provided by experiments in which local electrical stimulation of the basal hypothalamus resulted in ovulation (Markee *et al.*, 1946). Similarly, hypothalamic lesions prevented the increase in pituitary function that is typically induced by removal of one ovary. (When one ovary is surgically removed, the secretion of pituitary gonadotropins increases because of removal of the negative feedback effect of the ovarian hormones.) A compensatory increase in size and secretory activity of the remaining ovary then occurs. This effect, named compensatory hypertrophy, was blocked by basal hypothalamic lesions (Flerkó and Bardos, 1959).

Hormones from the target glands (e.g., ovaries, adrenals) in turn inhibit the secretion of pituitary hormones in part via hypothalamic neurons. Flerkó and Szentagothai (1957) pioneered this type of investigation by implanting pieces of ovary into the rat hypothalamus. They demonstrated uterine atrophy after implantation of ovarian fragments into the rostral hypothalamus but not after placements in the lateral hypothalamus. Implantation of small amounts of crystalline estrogen had similar effects (Lisk, 1960), and implantation of testosterone propionate into the basal hypothalamus was effective in decreasing testicular weight in male dogs (Davidson and Sawyer, 1961). A decrease in neuronal function by locally applied hormone was demonstrated by a decrease in nucleolar size at the site of implant of crystalline estrogen in the basal hypothalamus (Lisk and Newlon, 1963). In addition to the CNS-mediated actions of hormones implanted into the brain, there may also be a direct effect on the pituitary as a result of diffusion into the hypophysis (Bogdanove, 1963).

Reasoning that hypothalamic secretions stimulate the release of hormones from the anterior pituitary, Halász and co-workers (Halász and Pupp, 1965; Halász *et al.*, 1965) implanted a small piece of anterior pituitary into the hypothalamus of hypophysectomized rats and then observed both ovarian function and the histology of the pituitary transplants. They found that when pituitary fragments were transplanted into the hypothalamic region between the anterior hypothalamus and median eminence, the fragments retained their normal cytological characteristics, and ovarian cycles were maintained. When, however, pituitary fragments were transplanted outside this area, the tissue showed atrophic cells, and ovarian cycles were disrupted. Furthermore, when on occasion transplants were situated partly inside and partly outside the region, the portion of the transplant that was inside the region showed viable cells, whereas the portion outside the region was atrophic. They named this crescent-shaped hypothalamic region that could maintain the pituitary cells the "hypophysiotrophic area" (HTA). Subsequent studies using immunocytochemical methods have shown that the major part of the luteinizing hormone–releasing hormone (LHRH) distribution is in the HTA (Fig. 1) (McCann *et al.*, 1960; Harris, 1961; Palkovits *et al.*, 1974; Wheaton *et al.*, 1975; Kordon *et al.*, 1974; Naik, 1975; Hoffman *et al.*, 1978; also see Chapter 13). Immunoreactive perikarya of LHRH neurons are found in the arcuate nucleus of the mouse (Zimmerman *et al.*, 1974), guinea pig (Barry *et al.*, 1974; Silverman, 1976), and monkey (Barry *et al.*, 1975; Silverman *et al.*, 1977). These neurons project in the hypothalamo–infundibular tract to endings on the proximal capillary plexus of the portal vessels (Barry *et al.*, 1975) (Fig. 2). Luteinizing hormone-releasing hormone nerve fibers are extraordinarily rich in the external zone of the median eminence, especially in its lateral margin (Zimmerman, 1976). It appears that LHRH is also secreted into the ventricular cerebrospinal fluid and delivered to capillaries via the tanycyte ependymal cells at the base of the third ventricle (Knigge *et al.*, 1973). Thus, the medial basal hypothalamus (MBH) is involved in the basal secretion of LHRH.

In contrast to lesions in the median eminence and tuberal region which produced ovarian atrophy and led to the persistent diestrous anovulatory syndrome, lesions in the rostral hypothalamus–preoptic area blocked ovulation but did not induce ovarian atrophy. That is, the follicles grew, but ovulation did not occur. These animals remained in a state of persistent vaginal estrus (Dey, 1943; Hillarp, 1949; Greer, 1953; Flerkó, 1953, 1954; Flerkó and Bardos, 1960; see reviews by Flerkó, 1963; Barraclough, 1973). These and other studies (see Gorski, 1968, for review) led to the concept of a tonic mechanism maintaining basic ovarian function by the medial basal hypothalamus and a phasic mechanism controlling cyclic ovulation.

This concept of a dual mechanism was supported by studies of hypothalamic deafferentation. The medial basal portion of the hypothalamus, the HTA, was isolated from the rest of the brain by a knife cut but left in place with its connection to the pituitary intact, allowing the maintenance of vascularization via the portal system (Halász, 1969). After this operation, the rats maintained nonatrophic ovaries that did not, however, ovulate, suggesting that the HTA was competent to maintain tonic gonadotropin secretion but was not capable of stimulating the phasic release of gonadotropins. Some degree of compensatory hypertrophy of the ovaries could be induced in these animals bearing the HTA island (Halász, 1969).

Furthermore, an anterior cut of the hypothalamus (placed just caudal to the optic chiasm) that separated the HTA from its rostral inputs induced the anovulatory persistent estrous syndrome, suggesting that the stimulus for the phasic release of gonadotropin arises rostral to the hypothalamus (Halász and Pupp, 1965; Halász and Gorski, 1967). When the cuts were made rostral to the

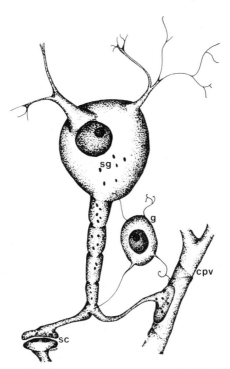

Figure 2. Schematic illustration of a neurosecretory neuron depicting its termination on a capillary blood vessel of the hypothalamo–hypophyseal portal system and on another neuron. Abbreviations: cpv, capillary of portal blood vessel; g, glial cell; sc, synaptic cleft; sg, secretory granules of neurosecretory neuron.

preoptic area, so that the continuity with the HTA was intact, cyclic ovulation could be maintained, although the cycles tended to be irregular (Kövecs and Halász, 1970; Taleisnik *et al.*, 1970). Since after the knife cuts were made, the maintenance of estrous cyclicity depended on the location in the rostro–caudal extent of the hypothalamus in which the cuts were made, the authors concluded that a neuronal system situated in the preoptic area is necessary for triggering the release of ovulatory hormones.

Electrical or electrochemical stimulation of the medial preoptic area induced ovulation in rats in which spontaneous ovulation had been blocked by barbiturate anesthesia (Everett and Radford, 1961; Gorski and Barraclough, 1963; Everett, 1964; Terasawa and Sawyer, 1969; Cramer and Barraclough, 1971), suggesting that activation of the medial preoptic area may normally trigger ovulation. This was further indicated by Tejasen and Everett (1967) who showed that ovulation induced by unilateral preoptic stimulation was blocked when knife cuts were made ipsilaterally, but not contralaterally, between the preoptic area and the basal hypothalamus. These studies imply that the neurons that trigger the release of an ovulatory surge of LH lie rostral to the basal hypothalamus, in the preoptic area or its afferents. This mechanism seems also to operate in hamsters, another species that has short estrous cycles (polyestrous) (Norman *et al.,* 1972).

Within the medial preoptic region, there may exist two distinct neural mechanisms for cyclic ovulation. Cyclic ovulation in rats occurs every 4–5 days following the LH surge during the "critical period" on the afternoon of proestrus. At least two factors are involved in this cyclicity: first, increments of estrogen titer, and second, a ciradian signal that is entrained to the light–dark cycle (Kawakami *et al.,* 1972b; Hoffman, 1973). Daily signals entrained to the lighting schedule may arise from the suprachiasmatic nucleus (SCN), since this nucleus receives a direct retinohypothalamic projection (Moore and Lenn, 1972). Lesion of the suprachiasmatic nucleus abolishes a number of circadian rhythms for which the environmental light–dark cycle is the Zeitgeber (Zucker *et al.,* 1976). The anovulatory persistent estrous syndrome can also be induced by small lesions in the posterior part of the preoptic area, specifically the suprachiasmatic nucleus (Barraclough *et al.,* 1964; Clemens *et al.,* 1976; Brown-Grant and Raisman, 1977; Raisman and Brown-Grant, 1977; Gray *et al.,* 1978), or by lesions in a small nucleus, termed the medial preoptic nucleus (MPN, Wiegand *et al.,* 1978), which is located just dorsal to the rostral end of the optic chiasma and caudal to the organum vasculosum of the lamina terminalis (OVLT). These two distinctive neural structures, the MPN–OVLT and the SCN, may be involved in two different mechanisms of cyclic release of LH described above. Although persistent estrus is induced by lesions of either the SCN or MPN–OVLT (Wiegand *et al.,* 1978), estrogen injection followed by progesterone induces the LH surge in the SCN-lesioned animals, whereas the same hormone treatments do not induce the LH surge in the MPN–OVLT-lesioned animals (Wiegand *et al.,* 1978; Kawakami *et al.,* 1978).

Thus, lesions of the SCN may destroy the mechanism for the circadian signal, whereas lesions of the MPN–OVLT abolish the estrogen–progesterone-sensitive positive feedback system. In the latter case, it is possible that (a) neural elements located in the vicinity of the MPN–OVLT produce and/or transport LHRH necessary for the ovulatory release of gonadotropins and (b) steroid-concentrating cells located in the vicinity of the MPN–OVLT mediate the action of ovarian hormones that trigger the release of LHRH. An abundance of estrogen- and progesterone-concentrating neurons have been found in the vicinity of the OVLT–MPN (Sar and Stumpf, 1973; Pfaff and Keiner, 1973; Stumpf *et al.,* 1974). In addition, perikarya of LHRH neurons as well as neural fibers have been found in the OVLT, preoptic area, septum, nucleus of the diagonal band of Broca, and the suprachiasmatic and periventricular region of the preoptic area in the rat (Sétaló *et al.,* 1976a,b; Kizer *et al.,* 1976; King *et al.,* 1978), guinea pig (Barry *et al.,* 1974; Silverman, 1976), dog (Barry and DuBois, 1975), and monkey (Barry *et al.,* 1975; Silverman *et al.,* 1977). The LHRH neurons were identified using an immunocytochemical technique in which a native hormone is made to react with a specific antibody, thereby giving a histologically visible precipitate. The OVLT, a circumventricular organ located at the anterior border of the optic recess of the third ventricle, resembles structurally the median eminence; in both brain regions neurosecretory neurons terminate upon the perivascular space of fenestrated capillaries (Weindl, 1973).

The role of the medial preoptic–anterior hypothalamus on reproductive function in animals other than polyestrous rodents is not well known. Blockade of ovulation, formation of polyfollicular ovaries, and absence of an LH surge in response to exogenous estrogen in animals bearing lesions in the medial preoptic–anterior hypothalamus or anterior deafferentation of the MBH has been reported for guinea pigs (Butler and Donovan, 1971; Terasawa and Wiegand, 1978), pigs (Döcke and Busch, 1974), and sheep (Jackson *et al.*, 1976). In contrast, anterior deafferentation of the MBH in the rhesus monkey appears not to interfere with gonadotropin secretion (Krey *et al.*, 1975). Furthermore, the MBH in the monkey is almost entirely autonomous (Knobil, 1974; Krey *et al.*, 1975; Hess *et al.*, 1977). Although some influence from the anterior part of the hypothalamus has been suggested in the monkey (Norman *et al.*, 1976), direct influence by external input such as visual, olfactory, and auditory in this primate may be minimal; the basal hypothalamus may be relatively independent of stimuli that affect other parts of the central nervous system. Thus, it is possible that species differences in the neuroendocrine control of gonadotropin function are related to the relative significance of environmental stimuli and the relative accessibility of these stimuli to the MBH.

IV. EXTRAHYPOTHALAMIC INFLUENCES ON HORMONE SECRETION

Thus far, we have discussed examples of environmental influences on hormone secretion and evidence that the MBH is the final common pathway for this effect. Except in the case of visual input to the SCN, however, sensory stimuli do not travel directly to the hypothalamus but are instead first integrated by extrahypothalamic structures. There are a number of brain structures outside the hypothalamus that project to the hypothalamus and have been shown to affect hormone secretion (Fig. 3). Although little is known about the nature of sensory influences on these extrahypothalamic structures, we can make some educated guesses as to possible pathways involved from sensory input to hormonal output. Thus, in the following section we shall describe a variety of effects on hormone secretion that result from stimulating or lesioning the olfactory bulbs, septum, amygdala, hippocampus, and midbrain reticular formation.

The status of this problem is exemplified in the study by Sawyer (1959) who showed that reflex ovulation in the rabbit persisted even after lesions or ablations of septum, amygdala, fornix, or olfactory bulbs. However, since electrical stimulation of the amygdala can induce ovulation in rabbits (Koikegami *et al.*, 1954; see more extensive review in Section IV. 2. C.) it is not

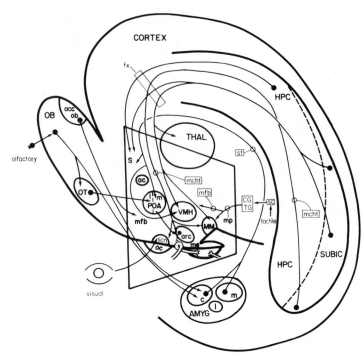

Figure 3. Schematic illustration of some afferent pathways to the hypothalamus. Abbreviations in addition to those in Fig. 1: acc ob, accessory olfactory bulb; amyg (c, m. l), amygdala (cortical, medial, lateral nucleus); cg, central gray; fx, fornix; hpc, hippocampus; mcht, medial cortico-hypothalamic tract; mfb, medial forebrain bundle; OB, olfactory bulb; OT, olfactory tubercle; POA (m, l), preoptic area (medial, lateral); S, septum; SC, spinal cord; st, stria terminalis; SUBIC, subiculum; TG, tegmentum; THAL, thalamus. For further details on these pathways, see Halász *et al.* (1975); Hamilton (1976); Heimer (1974); Lammers and Lohman (1974); Leonard and Scott (1971); Meibach and Siegel (1977); and Swanson and Cowan (1977).

yet clear whether the amygdala mediates ovulation during natural mating, and, if so, what its role is. In other words, the integrity of extrahypothalamic structures is apparently not necessary for a variety of hormonal responses, although the structures do modify hormonal responses. This then generates the intriguing question of their natural neuroendocrine function. With this disclaimer, let us now review some of the studies on extrahypothalamic influences on hormone secretion.

A. Olfactory Bulbs

In reviewing the clinical evidence of congenital absence of the olfactory bulbs in humans, Morsier and Gauthier (1963) found a high positive correlation between absence of the olfactory bulbs and the incidence of genital under-development (hypoplasia). Similarly, genital hypoplasia occurs in immature mice after bulbectomy (Whitten, 1956b; Lamond, 1958). In rats, olfactory bulbectomy delays the onset of puberty (Kling, 1964; Ohrbach and Kling, 1966), but once puberty is reached, ovarian cyclicity and ovulation do not differ from normal female rats.

Ovulation is blocked by olfactory bulbectomy in mice (Whitten, 1956b). However, Terasawa and Kawakami (1973a) found that olfactory bulbectomy in rats did not influence vaginal cyclicity. Curry (1974), using bulbectomized, pentobarbital-blocked rats, found a decline in the incidence of animals ovulating after copulation, and those bulbectomized animals that ovulated shed significantly fewer ova than sham-operated controls. On the other hand, Peppler *et al.*, (1973) have found no difference in the number of ova shed or in uterine weights of bulbectomized rats, although ovarian weight was reduced. Terasawa and Kawakami (1973a) found no changes in the serum and pituitary gonadotropins in rats after bulbectomy, but Signoret (1964) reported a decline in FSH in bulbectomized ewes. After electrical stimulation of olfactory bulbs, Donovan and Kopriva (1965) found no effect on the estrous cycles of guinea pigs.

B. Septum

Septal ablation in rats resulted in diestrous smears or irregular vaginal cycles with prolonged diestrus that persisted for more than a month; uterine weight was also reduced (Terasawa and Kawakami, 1973a). Rats with knife cuts above the septum, involving the fornix, showed reduced pituitary LH levels and increased FSH serum levels on the day of proestrus and increased serum prolactin on the day of estrus (Kawakami and Terasawa, 1972). Clemens *et al.* (1971) reported high levels of plasma LH and FSH 3 hr after electrical stimulation of the medial septum. L-shaped transections of the septum on the day prior to the gonadotropin surges resulted in an inhibition of the LH surge (Kawakami *et al.*, 1973). In addition, septal lesions delayed the onset of puberty in the female rat (Rodriguez-Sierra and Terasawa, 1978) and blocked the estrogen-induced LH surge in prepuberal rats (Clough and Rodriguez-Sierra, unpublished data).

C. Amygdala

A tentative generalization about the role of the amygdala in LH release and ovulation is that in general the intact corticomedial amygdala is facilitatory (Bunn and Everett, 1957; Velasco and Taleisnik, 1969a) and the lateral amygdala is inhibitory (Kawakami and Kimura, 1975; Velasco and Taleisnik, 1969a). Lesions of the corticomedial nucleus of the amygdala (Velasco and Taleisnik, 1971) or the bed nucleus of the stria terminalis (Brown-Grant and Raisman, 1972) block ovulation. Such lesions also prevent compensatory ovarian hypertrophy (Smith and Lawton, 1972), suggesting an inhibition of FSH secretion.

Electrical stimulation of the medial nuclei induced ovulation in rats (Bunn and Everett, 1957), rabbits (Koikegami *et al.,* 1954; Hayward *et al.,* 1964), and cats (Shealy and Peele, 1957). Electrical, electrochemical, or chemical stimulation of the corticomedial amygdala increased plasma levels of LH and FSH, whereas stimulation of the lateral amygdala decreased plasma levels of LH and FSH (Velasco and Taleisnik, 1969a; Kawakami and Kimura, 1975). Consistent with these findings, electrochemical stimulation of the basolateral amygdala in the awake, freely moving rat resulted in a delayed and diminished LH surge, whereas electrochemical stimulation of the corticomedial nucleus of the amygdala resulted in an early onset of the LH surge (Carrillo *et al.,* 1977). Estrogen implanted into the medial nuclear complex of the amygdala inhibited LH secretion (Lawton and Sawyer, 1970), and progesterone implants increased LH and decreased LHRH (Piva *et al.,* 1973). Although Velasco and Taleisnik (1969a) induced ovulation in rats by electrical stimulation or chemical (carbachol) implants in the basolateral as well as medial amygdaloid nuclei, Ellendorff *et al.* (1973) found that electrical stimulation of the medial nuclear complex of the amygdala inhibited LH release and ovulation. Moreover, Smith and Lawton (1972) found that lesions of the corticomedial nucleus of the amygdala did not change pituitary, ovarian, or uterine weights. Failure to block ovulation with amygdaloid lesions does not necessarily contradict induction of ovulation by stimulation of the amygdala. It is also of interest that lesions of the stria terminalis in prepubertal rats resulted in precocious puberty (Elwers and Critchlow, 1960, 1961; for further reviews of this literature, see Sawyer, 1972; Kawakami and Terasawa, 1974; and Ellendorff, 1978).

D. Hippocampus

Whereas most studies have shown the amygdala capable of stimulating LH secretion, the hippocampus has been shown to be predominantly inhibitory with respect to LH secretion. Early studies were contradictory and could not be interpreted readily in terms of gonadotropin secretion; hippocampal ablations were found to disrupt estrous cycles [prolongation of diestrus (Rodrigues, 1959); irregular appearance of cornified cells (Koikegami *et al.,* 1960)], but hippocampal ablation or transection of the fornix caudal to the anterior commissure or cuts of the medial corticohypothalamic tract (MCHT), which projects from the subiculum to the MBH (Gurdjian, 1927; Raisman *et al.,* 1966), did not prevent vaginal cyclicity in rats (Terasawa and Kawakami, 1973a). Brown-Grant and Raisman (1972) found that puberty was advanced in immature rats following hippocampal ablation.

However, later studies in which gonadotropins were measured directly were somewhat more consistent. Ablation of the hippocampus induced a rise in the serum levels of LH and FSH on the day of proestrus and of FSH on the day of estrus in rats (Terasawa and Kawakami, 1973a). Velasco and Taleisnik (1971) showed an increase of LH in the rat resulting from transection of the

MCHT (Raisman, 1970a,b). Electrochemical stimulation of the dorsal hippocampus in the freely moving rat resulted in blockade of the LH surge during proestrus (Carrillo *et al.*, 1977). Consistent with this, electrical stimulation of the hippocampus blocked spontaneous ovulation and ovulation induced by electrical stimulation of the preoptic area or the amygdala in rats (Kawakami *et al.*, 1972a, 1973; Velasco and Taleisnik, 1969b). This inhibitory effect of hippocampal stimulation was prevented by transection of the MCHT (Velasco and Taleisnik, 1971). Kawakami *et al.* (1973) have shown that when hippocampal stimulation blocks ovulation induced by preoptic stimulation, it also inhibits the elevation in LH and FSH that typically results from preoptic stimulation.

The effects of manipulations of the hippocampus on FSH secretion are contradictory (for review, see Kawakami and Terasawa, 1974).

E. Mesencephalic Reticular Formation

The midbrain reticular formation system is morphologically and functionally related to the diencephalon (Nauta, 1960). Critchlow (1958) described areas that include the basal mesodiencephalic junction that, when lesioned, blocked ovulation. Electrical stimulation of the ventral tegmental area (VTA) has been found to induce ovulation in light-induced persistent estrous rats, and electrical stimulation of VTA has been found to increase plasma LH in ovariectomized rats. Transections of the stria terminalis abolished this effect, suggesting that it is mediated via the amygdala (Carrer and Taleisnik, 1970).

A medial tegmental area appears to be involved in inhibiting ovulation. Stimulation along the path of the dorsal longitudinal fasciculus (FLD) inhibited spontaneous ovulation in the rats (Carrer and Taleisnik, 1972), and transections of the FLD, MCHT, or the medial forebrain bundle blocked the inhibiting effect of electrochemical stimulation. This suggests that at least part of this inhibitory effect is mediated by the hippocampus. The most effective inhibitory sites were found in an area along the ventromedial tegmentum extending from the caudal region of the mammillary bodies to the rostral part of the interpeduncular nucleus. Electrical stimulation of the medial raphe nucleus, which is further caudal, was also found to be inhibitory to ovulation. These inhibitory areas also decreased plasma LH levels when stimulated electrically (Carrer and Taleisnik, 1972).

Thus, extrahypothalamic brain systems modulate the action of the hypothalamus in controlling the pituitary. The role of these systems in analyzing and transducing species-specific complex patterns of environmental stimuli into hormonal changes has thus far received scant attention but raises interesting questions for future research.

In conclusion, besides the endogenous hormonal regulatory processes, sensory stimulation of internal or external origin can exert influences on hormone secretion. These may be considered as neuroendocrine reflexes in which the endocrine glands rather than muscles are the effectors. The mediobasal hypothalamus funneling into the median eminence is the final common neural pathway to the endocrine system via the pituitary gland. Certain sensory stimuli (i.e., light) have direct access to the hypothalamic pathway to the pituitary. Other modalities of sensory stimulation have access to the final common hypothalamic pathway via multisynaptic extrahypothalamic neural systems. These modulate the neuroendocrine reflexes via neural circuits that are arranged "in parallel" or "in series" with the sensory input.

REFERENCES

Adler, N. T., 1969, The effect of the male's copulatory behavior on successful pregnancy of the female rat, *J. Comp. Physiol. Psychol.* **69**:613.

Adler, N. T., Resko, J. A., and Goy, R. W, 1970, The effect of copulatory behavior on hormonal change in the female rat prior to implantation, *Physiol. Behav.* **5**:1003.

Aron, C., Asch, G., and Roos, J., 1966, Triggering of ovulation by coitus in the rat, *Int. Rev. Cytol.* **20**:139.

Barfield, R. J., 1971, Gonadotrophic hormone secretion in the female ring dove in response to visual and auditory stimulation by the male, *J. Endocrinol.* **49**:305.

Barraclough, C. A., 1973, Sex steroid regulation of reproductive neuroendocrine processes, in: *Handbook of Physiology*, Section 7, Vol. II (R. O. Greep, ed.), pp. 29–56, American Physiological Society, Washington.

Barraclough, C. A., Yrarrazaval, S., and Hatton, R., 1964, A possible hypothalamic site of action of progesterone in the facilitation of ovulation in the rat, *Endocrinology* **75**:838.

Barry, J., DuBois, M. P., 1975, Immunofluorescence study of LRF-producing neurons in the cat and dog, *Neuroendocrinology* **18**:290.

Barry, J., DuBois, M. P., and Carette, B., 1974, Immunofluorescence study of the preoptic–infundibular pathway in the normal, castrated or testosterone-treated male guinea pig, *Endocrinology* **95**:1416.

Barry, J., Girod, C., and DuBois, M. P., 1975, Topographie des neurones elaborateurs de LRF chez les primates, *Bull. Assoc. Anat. (Nancy)* **59**:102.

Beyer, C., and Mena, F., 1969, Neural factors in lactation, in: *Physiology and Pathology of Adaptation Mechanisms* (R. Bajusz, ed.), pp. 310–344, Pergamon Press, New York.

Beyer, C., Guillermo, A. L., and Mena, F., 1961, Ocytocin release in response to stimulation of cingulate gyrus, *Am. J. Physiol.* **200**:625.

Blake, C. A., and Sawyer, C. H., 1972, Effects of vaginal stimulation on hypothalamic multiple-unit activity and pituitary LH release in the rat, *Neuroendocrinology* **10**:358.

Bogdanove, E. M., 1963, Direct gonado–pituitary feedback: An analysis of effects of intracranial estrogenic depots on gonadotrophin secretion, *Endocrinology* **73**:696.

Brockway, B., 1965, Stimulation of ovarian development and egg-laying by male courtship vocalization in Budgerigars *(Melopsittacus undulatus)*, *Anim. Behav.* **13**:575.

Bronson, F. H., and Desjardins, C., 1974, Relationships between scent marking by male mice and the pheromone-induced secretion of the gonadotropic and ovarian hormones that accompany puberty in female mice, in: *Reproductive Behavior* (W. Montagna and W. A. Sadler, eds.), p. 157, Plenum Press, New York.

Brooks, C. McC., Ishikawa, T., Koizumi, K. and Lu, H.-H., 1966, Activity of neurones in the paraventricular nucleus of the hypothalamus and its control, *J. Physiol. (Lond.)* **182**:217.

Brown-Grant, K., and Raisman, G., 1972, Reproductive function in the rat following selective destruction of afferent fibres to the hypothalamus from the limbic system, *Brain Res.* **46**:23.

Brown-Grant, K., and Raisman, G., 1977, Abnormalities in reproductive function associated with the destruction of the suprachiasmatic nuclei in female rats, *Proc. R. Soc. Lond. [Biol.]* **198**:279.

Brown-Grant, K., Davidson, J. M., and Greig, F., 1973, Induced ovulation in albino rats exposed to constant light, *J. Endocrinol.* **57**:7.

Bruce, H. M., 1960, A block to pregnancy in the mouse caused by proximity of strange males, *J. Reprod. Fertil.* **1**:96.

Bruce, H. M., 1963, Secretion and release of prolactin: Discussion, in: *Advances in Neuroendocrinology* (A. V. Nalbandov, ed.), p. 282, University of Illinois Press, Urbana.

Bruce, H. M., and Parrott, D. M. V., 1962, Role of olfactory sense in pregnancy block by strange males, *Science* **131**:1526.

Bunn, J. P., and Everett, J. W., 1957, Ovulation in persistent estrous rats after electrical stimulation of the brain, *Proc. Soc. Exp. Biol. Med.* **96**:369.

Butler, J. E. M., and Donovan, B. T., 1971, The effect of surgical isolation of the hypothalamus upon reproductive function in the female guinea pig, *J. Endocrinol.* **50**:507.

Carrillo, A. J., Rabii, J., Carrer, H. F., and Sawyer, C. H., 1977, Modulation of the proestrous surge of luteinizing hormone by electrochemical stimulation of the amygdala and hippocampus in the unanesthetized rat, *Brain Res.* **128**:81.

Carlson, R. R., and DeFeo, V. J., 1965, Role of the pelvic nerve vs. the abdominal sympathetic nerves in the reproductive function of the female rat, *Endocrinology* **77**:1014.

Carrer, H. F., and Taleisnik, S., 1970, Effect of mesencephalic stimulation on the release of gonadotrophins, *J. Endocrinol.* **48**:527.

Carrer, H. F., and Taleisnik, S., 1972, Neural pathways associated with the mesencephalic inhibitory influence on gonadotropin secretion, *Brain Res.* **38**:299.

Cheng, M.-F., 1974, Ovarian development in the female ring dove in response to stimulation by intact and castrated male ring doves, *J. Endocrinol.* **63**:43.

Clemens, J. A., Shaar, C. J., Kleber, J. W., and Tandy, W. A., 1971, Reciprocal control by the preoptic area of LH and prolactin, *Exp. Brain Res.* **12**:250.

Clemens, J. A., Smalstig, E. B., and Sawyer, B. D., 1976, Studies on the role of the preoptic area in the control of reproductive function in the rat, *Endocrinology* **99**:728.

Cramer, O. M., and Barraclough, C. A., 1971, Effect of electrical stimulation of the preoptic area on plasma LH concentrations in proestrous rats, *Endocrinology* **88**:1175.

Critchlow, V., 1958, Blockade of ovulation in the rat by mesencephalic lesion, *Endocrinology* **63**:596.

Critchlow, V., 1963, Role of light on the neuroendocrine system, in: *Advances in Neuroendocrinology* (A. V. Nalbandov, ed.), p. 377, University of Illinois Press, Urbana.

Cross, B. A., 1959, Neurohypophyseal control of parturition, in: *Endocrinology of Reproduction* (C. L. Lloyd, ed.), p. 441, Academic Press, New York.

Curry, J. J., 1974, Alterations in incidence of mating and copulation-induced ovulation after olfactory bulb ablation in female rats, *J. Endocrinol.* **62**:245.

Davidson, J. M., 1977, Reproductive behavior in a neuroendocrine perspective, in: *Reproductive Behavior and Evolution* (J.S. Rosenblatt and B. R. Komisaruk, eds.), pp. 125, Plenum Press, New York.

Davidson, J. M., and Sawyer, C. H., 1961, Evidence for an hypothalamic focus of inhibition of gonadotropin by androgen in the male, *Proc. Soc. Exp. Biol. Med.* **107**:4.

Desjardins, C., Kirton, K. T., and Hafs, H. D., 1967, Anterior pituitary levels of FSH, LH, ACTH and Prolactin after mating in female rabbits, *Proc. Soc. Exp. Biol. Med.* **126**:23.

Dey, F. L., 1943, Evidence of hypothalamic control of hypophyseal gonadotrophic function in the female guinea pig, *Endocrinology* **33**:75.

Döcke, F., and Busch, W., 1974, Evidence for anterior hypothalamic control of cyclic gonadotrophin secretion in female pigs, *Endokrinologie* **63**:415.

Dominic, C. J., 1965, The origin of the pheromones causing pregnancy block in mice, *J. Reprod. Fertil.* **10**:469.

Dominic, C. J., 1966, Observations on the reproductive pheromones of mice. II. Neuroendocrine mechanisms involved in the olfactory block of pregnancy, *J. Reprod. Fertil.* **11**:415.

Dominic, C. J., 1967, Effect of exogenous prolactin on olfactory block of pregnancy in mice exposed to urine of alien males, *Indian J. Exp. Biol.* **5**:47.

Donovan, B. T., and Kopriva, P. C., 1965, Effect of removal or stimulation of the olfactory bulbs on the estrous cycle of the guinea pig, *Endocrinology* **77**:213.

Drickamer, L. C., 1974, Sexual maturation of female house mice: Social inhibition, *Dev. Psychobiol.* **7**:257.

Ellendorff, F., 1978, Extra-hypothalamic centres involved in the control of ovulation, in: *Control of Ovulation*, (D. B. Crighton, G. R. Foxcroft, N. B. Haynes, and G. E. Lamming, eds.), p. 1, Butterworths, London.

Ellendorff, F., Colombo, J. A., Blake, C. A., Whitmoyer, D. I., and Sawyer, C. H., 1973, Effects of electrical stimulation of the amygdala on gonadotrophin release and ovulation in rat, *Proc. Soc. Exp. Biol. Med.* **142**:417.

Elliott, J. A., Stetson, M. H., and Menaker, M., 1972, Regulation of testis function in golden hamsters: A circadian clock measures photoperiodic time, *Science* **178**:771.

Elwers, M., and Critchlow, V. B., 1960, Precocious ovarian stimulation following hypothalamic amygdaloid lesions in rats, *Am. J. Physiol.* **198**:381.

Elwers, M., and Critchlow, V. B., 1961, Precocious ovarian stimulation following interruption of the stria terminalis, *Am. J. Physiol.* **201**:281.

Erickson, C. J., and Lehrman, D. S., 1964, Effect of castration of male ring doves upon ovarian activity of females, *J. Comp. Physiol. Psychol.* **58**:164.

Everett, J. W., 1964, Central neural control of reproductive functions of the adenohypophysis, *Physiol. Rev.* **44**:374.

Everett, J. W., 1967, Provoked ovulation of long-delayed pseudopregnancy from coital stimuli in barbiturate-blocked rats, *Endocrinology* **80**:145.

Everett, J. W., and Radford, H. M., 1961, Irritative deposits from stainless steel electrodes in the preoptic rat brain causing release of pituitary gonadotropin, *Proc. Soc. Exp. Biol. Med.* **108**:604.

Everett, J. W., and Sawyer, C. H., 1949, A neural timing factor in the mechanism by which progesterone advances ovulation in the cyclic rat, *Endocrinology* **45**:581.

Everett, J. W., and Sawyer, C. H., 1950, A 24-hour periodicity in the "LH-release apparatus" of female rats, disclosed by barbiturate sedation, *Endocrinology* **47**:198.

Feldman, S., Conforti, N., Chowers, I., and Davidson, J. M., 1968, Differential effects of hypothalamic deafferentation on responses to different stresses, *Is. J. Med. Sci.* **4**:908.

Fiske, V. M., 1941, Effect of light on sexual maturation, estrous cycles, and anterior pituitary of the rat, *Endocrinology* **29**:187.

Flerkó, B., 1953, Einfluss experimenteller Hypothalamus-laesionen auf die Function des Sekretionsapparatus in weiblichen Genitaltrakt, *Acta Morphol. Acad. Sci. Hung.* **3**:67.

Flerkó, B., 1954, Zur hypothalamischen Steuerung der gonadotrophen Function der Hypophyse, *Acta Morphol. Acad. Sci. Hung.* **4**:475.

Flerkó, B., 1963, CNS and the secretion and release of LH and FSH, in: *Advances in Neuroendocrinology* (A. V. Nalbandov, ed.), p. 221, University of Illinois Press, Urbana.

Flerkó, B., and Bardos, V., 1959, Zwei verschiedene Effekte experimenteller Laision des Hypothalamus auf die Gonaden, *Acta Neuroveg.* **20**:248.

Flerkó, B., and Bardos, V., 1960, Pituitary hypertrophy after anterior hypothalamic lesion, *Acta Endocrinol. (Kbh.)* **35**:375.

Flerkó, B., and Szentagothai, J., 1957, Oestrogen sensitive nervous structures in the hypothalamus, *Acta Endocrinol.* **26**:121.

Folley, S. J., 1969, The milk-ejection reflex: A neuroendocrine theme in biology, myth and art, *J. Endocrinol.* **44**:x.

Freeman, M. E., and Neill, J. D., 1972, The pattern of prolactin secretion during pseudopregnancy in the rat: A daily nocturnal surge, *Endocrinology* **90**:1292.

Friedman, M., and Lehrman, D. S., 1968, Physiological conditions for the stimulation of prolactin secretion by external stimuli in the male ring dove, *Anim. Behav.* **16**:233.

Gorski, R. A., 1968, The neural control of ovulation, in: *Biology of Gestation*, Vol. I (N.S. Assali, ed.), pp. 1, Academic Press, New York.

Gorski, R. A., and Barraclough, C. A., 1963, Effects of low dosages of androgen on the differentiation of hypothalamic regulatory control of ovulation in the rat, *Endocrinology* **73**:210.

Gray, G. D., Sodersten, P., Tallentire, D., and Davidson, J. M., 1978, Effects of lesions in various structures of the suprachiasmatic–preoptic region on LH regulation and sexual behavior in female rats, *Neuroendocrinology* **25**:174.

Greer, M. A., 1953, Effects of progesterone on persistent estrus produced hypothalamic lesions in the rat, *Endocrinology* **53**:390.

Gurdjian, E. S., 1927, The diencephalon of the albino rat, *J. Comp. Neurol.* **43**:1.

Halász, B., 1969, The endocrine effects of isolation of the hypothalamus from the rest of the brain, in: *Frontiers in Neuroendocrinology* (W. F. Ganong and L. Martini, eds.), p. 307, Oxford University Press, New York.

Halász, B., and Gorski, R. A., 1967, Gonadotrophic hormone secretion in female rats after partial or total interruption of neural afferents to the medial basal hypothalamus, *Endocrinology* **80**:608.

Halász, B., and Pupp. L., 1965, Hormone secretion of the anterior pituitary gland after physical interruption of all neuron pathways to the hypophysiotrophic area, *Endocrinology* **77**:553.

Halász, B., Pupp, L., Uhlarik, S., and Tima, L., 1965, Further studies on the hormone secretion of the anterior pituitary transplanted into the hypophysiotrophic area of the rat hypothalamus, *Endocrinology* **77**:343.

Halász, B., Koves, K., Rethely, M., Bodoky, M., and Koritsanszky, S., 1975, Recent data on neuronal connections between nervous structures involved in the control of the adenohypophysis, in: *Anatomical Neuroendocrinology* (W. E. Stumpf and L. D. Grant, eds.), pp. 9–14, S. Karger, New York.

Hamilton, L. W., 1976, *Basic Limbic System Anatomy of the Rat,* Plenum Press, New York.

Harrington, R. E., Egger, R. G., and Wilbur, R. D., 1967, Induction of ovulation in chlorpromazine-blocked rats, *Endocrinology* **81**:877.

Harris, G. W., 1955, Neural control of the pituitary gland, *Monogr. Physiol. Soc.* **3**:1.

Harris, G. W., 1961, The pituitary stalk and ovulation, in: *Control of Ovulation* (C. A. Villie, ed.), p. 56, Pergamon Press, New York.

Harris, G. W., and Jacobsohn, D., 1952, Functional grafts of the anterior pituitary gland, *Proc. R. Soc. Lond. [Biol.]* **139**:263.

Hayward, J. N., Hilliard, J., and Sawyer, C. H., 1964, Time of release of pituitary gonadotropin induced by electrical stimulation of the rabbit brain, *Endocrinology* **74**:108.

Heimer, L., 1975, Olfactory projections to the diencephalon, in: *Anatomical Neuroendocrinology* (W. E. Stumpf and L. D. Grant, eds.), pp. 30–39, S. Karger, New York.

Hess, D. L., Wilkins, R. H., Moossy, J., Chang, J. L., Plant, T. M., McCormack, J. T., Nakai, Y., and Knobil, E., 1977, Estrogen-induced gonadotropin surges in decerebrated female rhesus monkeys with medial basal hypothalamic peninsulae, *Endocrinology* **101**:1264.

Hillarp, N. A., 1949, Studies on the localization of hypothalamic centers controlling the gonadotrophic function of the hypophysis, *Acta Endocrinol. (Kbh.)* **2**:11.

Hoffman, G. E., Melnyk, V., Hayes, T., Bennett-Clarke, C., and Fowler, C., 1978, Immunocytology of LHRH neurons, in: *Brain-Endocrine Interactions, III. Neural Hormones and Reproduction* (D. E. Scott, G. P. Kozlowski, and A. Weindl, eds.), p. 65, S. Karger, Basel.

Hoffman, J. C., 1969, Light and reproduction in the rat: Effect of lighting schedule on ovulation in blockade, *Biol. Reprod.* **1**:185.

Hoffman, V. C., 1973, The influence of photoperiods on reproductive functions in female mammals, in: *Handbook of Physiology,* Section 7, Vol. II, Part 1 (R. O. Greep, ed.), p. 57, American Physiological Society, Washington.

Huston, T. M., and Nalbandov, A. V., 1953, Neurohumoral control of the pituitary in the fowl, *Endocrinology* **52**:149.

Jackson, G. L., Kuehl, D., and Zuleski, A., 1976, Effects of anterior hypothalamic deafferentation of LH secretion in the ewe, in: *Ninth Annual Meeting of the Society for the Study of Reproduction.*

Johns, M. A., Feder, H. H., Komisaruk, B. R., and Mayer, A. D., 1978, Urine-induced reflex ovulation in anovulatory rats may be a vomeronasal effect, *Nature* **272**:446.

Kawakami, M., and Kimura, F., 1975, Inhibition of ovulation in the rat by electrical stimulation of the lateral amygdala, *Endocrinol. Jpn.* **22**:61.

Kawakami, M., and Terasawa, E., 1972, Acute effect of neural deafferentation on timing of gonadotropin secretion before proestrus in the female rat, *Endocrinol. Jpn.* **19**:449.

Kawakami, M., and Terasawa, E., 1974, Role of limbic forebrain structures on reproductive cycles, in: *Biological Rhythms in Neuroendocrine Activity* (M. Kawakami, ed.), pp. 197–219, Gaku Shoin Ltd., Tokyo.

Kawakami, M., Kimura, F., and Wakabayashi, K., 1972a, Electrical stimulation of the hippocampus under the chronic preparation and changes of LH, FSH and prolactin levels in serum and pituitary, *Endocrinol. Jpn.* **19**:85.

Kawakami, M., Terasawa, E., and Ibuki, T., 1972b, Changes in multiple unit activity of the brain during the estrous cycle, *Neuroendocrinology* **6**:30.

Kawakami, M., Terasawa, E., Kimura, F., and Wakabuyashi, K., 1973, Modulating effect of limbic structures on gonadotropin release, *Neuroendocrinology* **12**:1.

Kawakami, M., Yoshioka, E., Konda, N., Arita, J., and Visessuvan, S., 1978, Data on the sites of stimulatory feedback action of gonadal steroids indispensable for luteinizing hormone release in the rat, *Endocrinology* **102**:971.

King, J. C., Elkind, K. E., Gerall, A. A., and Miller, R. P., 1978, Investigations of the LH-RH system in the normal and neonatally steroid-treated male and female rats, in: *Brain–Endocrine Interaction, III. Neural Hormone and Reproduction* (D. E. Scott, G. P. Kozlowski, and A. Weindl, eds.), p. 57, Karger, Basel.

Kizer, J. S., Palkovits, M., and Brownstein, J. J., 1976, Releasing factors in the circumventricular organs of the rat brain, *Endocrinology* **98**:311.

Kling, A., 1964, Effects of rhinencephalic lesion on endocrine and somatic development in the rat, *Am. J. Physiol.* **206**:1395.

Knigge, K. M., Joseph, S. A., Silverman, A. J., and Vaala, S., 1973, Further observations on the structure and function of median eminence, with reference to the organization of RF-producing elements in the endocrine hypothalamus, *Prog. Brain Res.* **39**:7.

Knobil, E., 1974, On the control of gonadotropin secretion in the rhesus monkey, *Recent Prog. Horm. Res.* **30**:46.

Koikegami, H., Yamada, T., and Usui, K., 1954, Stimulation of amygdaloid nuclei and periamygdaloid cortex with special reference to its effect on uterine movements and ovulation, *Folia Psychiat. Neurol. Jpn.* **8**:7.

Koikegami, H. H., Fuse, H., and Kawakami, K., 1960, Bilateral destruction experiments of hippocampus or amygdaloid nuclear region. *Neurol. Med. Chir. (Tokyo)* **2**:49.

Komisaruk, B. R., 1974, Neural and hormonal interactions in the reproductive behavior of female rats, in: *Reproductive Behavior* (W. Montagna and W. A. Sadler, eds.), p. 97, Plenum Press, New York.

Kordon, C., Kerdelhue, B., Puttou, E., and Jutisz, M., 1974, Immunocytochemical localization of LHRH in axons and nerve terminals of the rat median eminence, *Proc. Soc. Exp. Biol. Med.* **147**:122.

Kövecs, K., and Halász, B., 1970, Location of the neural structures triggering ovulation in the rat, *Neuroendocrinology* **6**:180.

Krey, L. C., Butler, W. R., and Knobil, E., 1975, Surgical disconnection of the medial basal hypothalamus and pituitary function in the rhesus monkey. I. Gonadotropin secretion, *Endocrinology* **96**:1073.

Lammers, H. J., and Lohman, A. H. M., 1974, Structure and fiber connections of the hypothalamus in mammals, in: *Progress in Brain Research*, Vol. 41 (D. F. Swaab and J. P. Schade, eds.), *Integrative Hypothalamic Activity,* pp. 61–78, Elsevier, New York.

Lamond, D. R., 1958, Infertility associated with extirpation of the olfactory bulbs in female albino mice, *Aust. J. Exp. Biol. Med. Sci.* **36**:103.

Lawton, I. E., and Sawyer, C. H., 1970, Role of amygdala in regulating LH secretion in the adult female rat, *Am. J. Physiol.* **218**:622.

Lee, S. van der, and Boot, L. M., 1955, Spontaneous pseudopregnancy in mice, *Acta Physiol. Pharmacol. Neerl.* **4**:442.

Lehrman, D. S., 1961, Hormonal regulation of parental behavior in birds and infrahuman mammals, in: *Sex and Internal Secretions, Third Edition,* Vol. 2 (W. C. Young, ed.), p. 1268, Williams & Wilkins, Baltimore.

Leonard, C. M., and Scott, J. W., 1971, Origin and distribution of the amygdalofugal pathways in the rat: An experimental neuroanatomical study, *J. Comp. Neurol.* **141**:313.

Lisk, R. D., 1960, Estrogen-sensitive center in the hypothalamus of the rat, *J. Exp. Zool.* **145**:197.

Lisk, R. D., and Newlon, M., 1963, Estradiol: Evidence for its direct effect on hypothalamic neurons, *Science* **139**:223.

Lott, D., and Brody, P. N., 1966, Support of ovulation in the ring dove by auditory and visual stimuli, *J. Comp. Physiol. Psychol.* **62**:311.

Lott, D., Scholz, S. D., and Lehrman, D. S., 1967, Exteroceptive stimulation of the reproductive system of the female ring dove *(Streptopelia risoria)* by the mate and by the colony milieu, *Ani. Behav.* **15**:433.

Markee, J. E., Sawyer, C. H., and Hollinshead, W. H., 1946, Activation of the anterior hypophysis by electrical stimulation in the rabbit, *Endocrinology* **38**:345.

McCann, S. M., Taleisnik, S., and Friedman, H. M., 1960, LH-releasing activity in hypothalamic extract, *Proc. Soc. Exp. Biol. Med.* **104**:432.

McClintock, M. K., 1974, Sociobiology of reproduction in the Norway rat *(Rattus norvegicus)*, unpublished doctoral dissertation, University of Pennsylvania.

McClintock, T. K., and Drickamer, L. C., 1977, Excreted urine, bladder urine, and the delay of sexual maturation in female house mice, *Anim. Behav.* **25**:999.

McNeilly, A. S., 1979, Effects of lactation on fertility, *Br. Med. Bull.* **35**:151.

Meibach, R. C., and Siegel, A., 1977, Efferent connections of the hippocampal formation in the rat, *Brain Res.* **124**:197

Mena, F., and Beyer, C., 1963, Effect of high spinal section on established lactation in the rabbit, *Am. J. Physiol.* **205**:313.

Moore, R. Y., and Lenn, N. J., 1972, A retinohypothalamic projection in the rat, *J. Comp. Neurol.* **146**:1.

Morsier, C., and Gauthier, G., 1963, La Dysplasie olfactogenitale, *Pathol. Biol. (Paris)* **11**:1267.

Moss, R. L., and Cooper, K. J., 1973, Temporal relationship of spontaneous and coitus-induced release of luteinizing hormone in the normal cyclic rat, *Endocrinology* **92**:1748.

Naik, D. V., 1975, Immunoreactive LH-RH neurons in the hypothalamus identified by light and fluorescent microscopy, *Cell Tissue Res.* **157**:437.

Nauta, W. J. H., 1960, Some neural pathways related to the limbic system, in: *Electrical Studies on the Unanesthetized Brain* (E. R. Ramey, and D. S. O'Doherty, eds.), pp. 1–6, Hoeber, New York.

Nikitovitch-Winer, M., and Everett, J. W., 1958, Functional restitution of pituitary grafts retransplanted from kidney to median eminence, *Endocrinology* **63**:916.

Norman, R. L., Blake, C. A., and Sawyer, C. H., 1972, Effects of hypothalamic deafferentation on LH secretion and the estrous cycle in the hamster, *Endocrinology* **91**:95.

Norman, R. L., Resko, J. A., and Spies, H. G., 1976, The anterior hypothalamus: How it affects gonadotropin secretion in the rhesus monkey, *Endocrinology* **99**:59.

Ohrbach, J., and Kling, A., 1966, Effects of sensory deprivation on onset of puberty, mating, fertility and gonadal weight in rats, *Brain Res.* **3**:141.

Palkovits, M., Arimura, A., Brownstein, M., Schally, A. V., and Saavedra, J. M., 1974, Luteinizing hormone-releasing hormone (LH-RH) content of the hypothalamic nuclei in rat, *Endocrinology* **95**:554.

Parkes, A. S., 1963, Secretion and release of prolactin: Discussion, in: *Advances in Neuroendocrinology* (A. V. Nalbandov, ed.), p. 285, University of Illinois Press, Urbana.

Parkes, A. S., and Bruce, H. M., 1961, Olfactory stimuli in mammalian reproduction, *Science* **134**:1049.

Peppler, R. D., Bennett, M. H., and Dunn, J. D., 1973, Compensatory ovulation in blinded rats and/or those from which the olfactory bulb had been removed, *J. Reprod. Fertil.* **34**:501.

Pfaff, D., and Keiner, M., 1973, Atlas of estradiol-concentrating cells in the central nervous system of the female rat, *J. Comp. Neurol.* **151**:121.

Piva, F., Schieffini, O., Kalra, P. S., and Martini, L., 1973, The limbic system and the control of gonadotropin secretion, in: *Hormones, Metabolism, and Stress. Recent Progress and Perspectives* (S. Nemeth, ed.), p. 103, Publishing House Slovak Academy of Sciences, Bratislava.

Raisman, G., 1970a, An evaluation of the basis pattern of connections between the limkic system and the hypothalamus, *Am. J. Anat.* **129**:197.

Raisman, G., 1970b, Some aspects of the neural connections of the hypothalamus, in: *The Hypothalamus* (L. Martini, M. Motta, and F. Fraschini, eds.), p. 1, Academic Press, New York.

Raisman, G., and Brown-Grant, K., 1977, The suprachiasmatic syndrome, endocrine and behavioral abnormalities following lesions of the suprachiasmatic nuclei in the female rat, *Proc. R. Soc. Lond. [Biol.]* **198**:297.

Raisman, G., Cowan, W. H., and Powell, T. P. S., 1966, An experimental analysis of the efferent projection of the hippocampus, *Brain* **86**:83.

Rodgers, C. H., 1971, Influence of copulation on ovulation in the cycling rat, *Endocrinology* **88**:433.

Rodrigues, A., 1959, Influence de l'ecorce cérébrale sur le cycle sexual de rat blanc, *C. R. Soc. Biol. (Paris)* **153**:1271.

Rodriguez-Sierra, J. F., and Terasawa, E., 1978, Similar and differential roles for the septum and medial preoptic area on estrogen-dependent neuroendocrine processes, Abstract of the 8th Annual Meeting of the Society for Neuroscience no. 1127.

Roth, L. L., and Rosenblatt, J. S., 1968, Self-licking and mammary development during pregnancy in the rat, *J. Endocrinol.* **42**:363.

Rowlands, I. W., 1966, Comparative biology of reproduction in mammals, *Zool. Soc. Lond. Symposia*, No. 15, Academic Press, New York.

Sar, M., and Stumpf, W. E., 1975, Atlas of estrogen target cells in rat brain, in: *Anatomical Neuroendocrinology* (W. E. Stumpf and L. D. Grant, eds.), p. 104, Karger, Basel.

Sawyer, C. H., 1959, Effects of brain lesions on estrous behavior and reflexogenous ovulation in the rabbit, *J. Exp. Zool.* **142**:227.

Sawyer, C. H., 1972, Functions of the amygdala related to the feedback actions of gonadal steroid hormones, in: *Advances in Behavioral Biology*, Vol. 2, *The Neurobiology of the Amygdala* (B. E. Eleftheriou, ed.), pp. 745–762, Plenum Press, New York.

Sawyer, C. H., and Markee, J. E., 1959, Estrogen facilitation of release of pituitary ovulating hormone in the rabbit in response to vaginal stimulation, *Endocrinology* **65**:614.

Sawyer, C. H., Markee, J. E., and Everett, J. W., 1950a, "Spontaneous" ovulation in the rabbit following combined estrogen-progesterone treatment, *Proc. Soc. Exp. Biol. Med.* **74**:185.

Sawyer, C. H., Markee, and Everett, J. W., 1950b, Further experiments on blocking pituitary activation in the rabbit and the rat, *J. Exp. Zool.* **113**:659.

Schally, A. V., 1978, Aspects of hypothalamic regulation of the pituitary gland, *Science* **202**:18.

Scharrer, B., 1976, Neurosecretion—Comparative and evolutionary aspects, *Prog. Brain Res.* **45**:125.

Scharrer, B., 1977, Evolutionary aspects of neuroendocrine control processes, in: *Reproductive Behavior and Evolution* (J. S. Rosenblatt and B. R. Komisaruk, eds.), p. 111, Plenum Press, New York.

Sétáló, G., Vigh, S., Schally, A. V., Arimura, A., and Flerkó, B., 1976a, Immunohistological study of the origin of LH-RH containing nerve fibers of the rat hypothalamus, *Brain Res.* **103**:597.

Sétáló, G., Vigh, S., Schally, A. V., Arimura, A., and Flerkó, B., 1976b, Immunohistological investigations of the LH-RH-synthesizing neuron system of the rat, in: *Cellular and Molecular Bases of Neuroendocrinology* (O. Endrocz, ed.), pp. 77–78, Academiai Kiado, Budapest.

Shealy, C. N., and Peele, T. L., 1957, Studies on amygaloid nucleus of cat, *J. Neurophysiol.* **20**:125.

Signoret, J. P., 1964, Action de l'ablation des bulbes olfactifs sur les mechanismes de la reproduction, in: *Excerpta Medica International Congress Series* Vol. 83, *Proceedings of the Second International Congress of Endocrinology*, p. 198, Excerpta Medica, Amsterdam.

Silverman, A. J., 1976, Distribution of luteinizing hormone-releasing hormone (LHRH) in the guinea pig brain, *Endocrinology* **99**:30.

Silverman, A. J., Antumes, J. L., Ferin, M., and Zimmerman, E. A., 1977, The distribution of luteinizing hormone releasing hormone (LHRH) in the hypothalamus of the rhesus monkey. Light microscopic studies using immuno peroxidase technique, *Endocrinology* **101**:134.

Smith, S. W., and Lawton, J. E., 1972, Involvement of the amygdala in the ovarian compensatory hypertrophy response, *Neuroendocrinology* **9**:228.

Spies, H. G., and Niswender, G. D., 1971, Levels of prolactin, LH, and FSH in the serum of intact and pelvic-neurectomized rats, *Endocrinology* **88**:937.

Stumpf, W. E., Sar, M., and Keefer, S. A., 1974, Atlas of estrogen target cells in the rat brain, in: *Anatomical Neuroendocrinology* (W. E. Stumpf and L. D. Grant, eds.), pp. 104, Karger, Basel.

Swanson, L. W., and Cowan, W. M., 1977, An autoradiographic study of the organization of the efferent connections of the hippocampal formation in the rat, *J. Comp. Neurol.* **172**:49.

Szentágothai, J., Flerkó, B., Mess, B., and Halász, B., 1968, *Hypothalamic Control of the Anterior Pituitary*, Akademiai Kiado, Budapest.

Taleisnik, S., and McCann, S. M., 1961, Effects of hypothalamic lesions in the secretion and storage of hypophyseal luteinizing hormone, *Endocrinology* **68**:263.

Taleisnik, S., Velasco, M. E., and Astrada, J. J., 1970, Effect of hypothalamic deafferentation on the control of luteinizing hormone secretions, *J. Endocrinol.* **46**:1.

Tejasen, T., and Everett, J. W., 1967, Surgical analysis of the preoptic–tuberal pathway controlling ovulatory release of gonadotropins in the rat, *Endocrinology* **81**:1387.

Terasawa, E., and Kawakami, M., 1973a, Effects of limbic forebrain ablation on pituitary gonadal function in the female rat, *Endocrinol. Jpn.* **20**:277.

Terasawa, E., and Kawakami, M., 1973b, Sexual differentiation of the hippocampus; Effects of immobilization stress on gonadotropin secretion in the rat, in: *Psychoneuroendocrinology* (N. Hatotanai and M. Tsu, eds.), p. 144, Karger, Basel.

Terasawa, E., and Sawyer, C. H., 1969, Electrical and electrochemical stimulation of the hypothalamus–adenophypophyseal system with stainless steel electrodes, *Endocrinology* **84**:918.

Terasawa, E., and Wiegand, S. J., 1978, Effects of hypothalamic deafferentation on ovulation and estrous cyclicity in the female guinea pig, *Neuroendocrinology* **26**:229.

Terkel, J., Damassa, D. A., and Sawyer, C. H., 1978, Ultrasonic vocalizations of infant rats stimulate prolactin release in lactating females, *Endocrine Society Program and Abstracts, 60th Ann. Mtg.*, p. 190.

Tindal, J. S., Knaggs, G. S., and Turvey, A., 1967, The afferent path of the milk ejection reflex in the brain of the guinea pig, *J. Endocrinol.* **38**:337.

Vandemark, N. L., and Hays, R. L., 1952, Uterine motility responses to mating, *Am. J. Physiol.* **170**:518.

Vandenbergh, J. G., 1967, Effect of the presence of a male on the sexual maturation of female mice, *Endocrinology* **81**:345.

Vandenbergh, J. G., Drickamer, L. C., and Colby, D. R., 1972, Social and dietary factors in the sexual maturation of female mice, *J. Reprod. Fertil.* **28**:397.

Velasco, M. E., and Taleisnik, S., 1969a, Release of gonadotropins induced by amygdaloid stimulation in the rat, *Endocrinology* **84**:132.

Velasco, M. E., and Taleisnik, S., 1969b, Effect of hippocampal stimulation on the release of gonadotropins, *Endocrinology* **85**:1154.

Velasco, M. E., and Taleisnik, S., 1971, Effects of the interruption of amygdaloid and hippocampal afferents to the medial hypothalamus on gonadotrophin release, *J. Endocrinol.* **51**:41.

Warren, D. C., and Scott, H. M., 1936, Influence of light on ovulation in the fowl, *J. Exp. Zool.* **74**:137.

Weindl, A., 1973, Neuroendocrine aspects of circumventricular organs, in: *Frontiers in Neuroendocrinology* (W. Ganong and L. Martini, eds.), pp. 3–32, Oxford University Press, London.

Westman, A., and Jacobsohn, D., 1936, Uber Ovarialveranderungen beim Kaninchen nach Hypophysektomie, *Acta Obstet. Gynecol. Scand.* **16**:483.

Wheaton, J. E., Krulich, L., and McCann, S. M., 1975, Localization of luteinizing hormone-releasing hormone in the preoptic area and hypothalamus of the rat using radioimmunoassay, *Endocrinology* **97**:30.

Whitten, W. K., 1956a, Modification of the oestrous cycle of the mouse by external stimuli associated with the male, *J. Endocrinol.* **13**:399.

Whitten, W. K., 1956b, The effect of removal of the olfactory bulbs on the gonads of mice, *J. Endocrinol.* **14**:160.

Whitten, W. K., 1957, Effect of exteroceptive factors on the oestrous cycle of mice, *Nature* **180**:1436.

Wiegand, S., Terasawa, E., and Bridson, W. E., 1978, Persistent estrus and blockade of progesterone-induced LH release follows lesions which do not damage the suprachiasmatic nucleus, *Endocrinology* **102**:1645.

Winans, S., and Scalia, F., 1970, Amygdaloid nucleus: New afferent input from the vomeronasal organ, *Science* **170**:330.

Zaks, M. G., 1962, *The Motor Apparatus of the Mammary Gland,* Oliver and Boyd, London.

Zarrow, M. X., 1973, Pheromonal activation of the pituitary gland of mice and rats, unpublished manuscript.

Zarrow, M. X., and Clark, J. H., 1968, Ovulation following vaginal stimulation in spontaneous ovulator and its implications, *J. Endocrinol.* **40**:343.

Zimmerman, E. A., Hsu, K. G., Ferin, M., and Kuzlowski, G. P., 1974, Localization of gonadotropin releasing hormone (Gn-RH) in the hypothalamus of the mouse by immunoperoxidase technique, *Endocrinology* **95**:1.

Zimmerman, E. A., 1976, Localization of hypothalamic hormones by immunocytochemical techniques, in: *Frontier in Neuroendocrinology* (W. F. Ganong, and L. Martini, eds.), pp. 25–62, Raven Press, New York.

Zucker, I., Rusak, B., and King, R. G., Jr., 1976, Neural bases for circadian rhythms in rodent behavior, *Adv. Biosci.* **3**:35.

Seasonal Reproduction

Photoperiodism and Biological Clocks

JEFFREY A. ELLIOTT and BRUCE D. GOLDMAN

I. PHYSIOLOGICAL MEDIATORS

A. Photoperiod and Seasonality

Most organisms undergo seasonal changes in physiology and behavior. These changes enable the various species to adapt to annual cycles in a variety of environmental factors, such as temperature, rainfall, and food availability. It is not surprising that most species have developed adaptations so that most or all of their reproductive activity occurs during a particular portion of the annual cycle. In some organisms, reproduction is confined to a very restricted interval. For example, the short-tailed shearwater is a bird that arrives on islands north of Tasmania in late September and lays almost all of its eggs between November 24 and November 27. The sooty tern breeds on Ascension Island in the Atlantic on every tenth full moon, whereas the same species breeds every 6 months on islands in the central Pacific (Sadleir, 1973).

Before proceeding with a discussion of the mechanisms involved in the regulation of biological rhythms in general, it is important to define a few terms. A rhythm is a regularly recurring cyclic fluctuation. The period of a rhythm is the length of time required to pass through one complete cycle. Most

JEFFREY A. ELLIOTT • Hopkins Marine Station, Department of Biological Sciences, Stanford University, Pacific Grove, California 93950.   BRUCE D. GOLDMAN • Department of Bio-Behavioral Sciences, University of Connecticut, Storrs, Connecticut 06268.

organisms appear to be capable of exhibiting a variety of endogenous rhythms; that is, organisms are able to generate rhythms even when they are prevented from receiving rhythmic cues from their environment. In most cases, these endogenous rhythms can be "finetuned" by rhythmic environmental cues. The process of achieving synchrony between internal (endogenous) and external (environmental) rhythms is called entrainment. The environmental cue that is employed for entrainment is referrrd to by the term Zeitgeber (literally, "time-giver"). The most commonly used Zeitgeber is the alternating cycle of light and dark (day/light) which occurs with such precise regularity. A glossary providing definitions of terms, abbreviations, and symbols used in the discussion of biological rhythms is provided in Table 1.

B. Photosensitivity and Photorefractoriness

Seasonal rhythms are cycles with a periodicity of 1 year. Some animals, e.g., ground squirrels, exhibit endogenous rhythms with a periodicity of approximately 1 year (circannual rhythms) when deprived of any obvious environmental cues. Photoperiod (i.e., day length) is perhaps the single most widely used environmental cue in entraining seasonal rhythms. The widespread use of day length as a seasonal Zeitgeber is no doubt related to the reliability of the length of the photophase as an indicator of time of year. For example, in Connecticut, the amount of daylight reaches a maximum of 15 hr during the summer and reaches a minimum of 9 hr during the winter. Reliance on photoperiod as an environmental cue to indicate season does entail one serious problem. The same photoperiod occurs at two different times of year. For example, day-lengths of 12 hr occur at both the spring (March 21) and autumnal (September 21) equinoxes. For animals living in the northern hemisphere, the occurrence of 12 hr of daylight in the spring signifies the advent of summer—a season appropriate for the production and rearing of progeny. In the fall, on the other hand, the 12-hr photoperiod predicts winter. Obviously, it is of adaptive value for the organism to be able to distinguish between these two times of year. Many animals appear to have solved this ambiguity in the photoperiod by showing an annual cycle that incorporates alternating phases of photosensitivity and photorefractoriness. Let us take the Syrian hamster as an example. This rodent undergoes gonadal regression in the fall when the day lengths fall below 12.5 hr of illumination daily. The gonads undergo spontaneous recrudescence about 4 to 5 months later without photoperiod stimulation (Fig. 1). This regrowth of the gonads occurs even in hamsters kept in continuous darkness. The hamster is said to have become photorefractory during the recrudescent phase—i.e., at this phase of the annual cycle the gonads regrow independent of the length of the daily photoperiod. One consequence of photorefractoriness is that gonadal function begins in the spring before the environmental photoperiod reaches 12.5 hr, which would be required for continued gonadal maintenance in the fall (Gaston and Menaker, 1967; Reiter, 1973a).

Table 1. Glossary of Terms and Symbols Used to Describe Biological Rhythms

Activity time (α): The portion of an activity–rest or "sleep–wake" cycle during which the animal is active.

Circadian rhythm: An endogenous oscillation with free-running period (τ) that is close to the period (24 hr) of the solar day.

Circadian system: The sum of all of the circadian oscillations, including the pacemakers (driving oscillators), slave (driven) oscillators, and overt circadian rhythms of an organism.

Circadian time (ct): A time scale measured in circadian hours and covering one full circadian cycle normalized to 24 hr (ct 00 to ct 24).

Circannual rhythm: An endogenous oscillation that persists in seasonally constant conditions (e.g., continuous LD 12:12 and constant temperature) with a period of approximately 1 year.

Entrainment: The process by which an endogenous rhythm becomes coupled to and assumes the period of an environmental cycle (Zeitgeber).

Free-running period: The period of an endogenous rhythm (τ) when it is not entrained by an external cycle.

Period: The length of time between recurring phase reference points (ϕ_r) in a continuing oscillation, i.e., the time required for a rhythm to complete one full cycle.

Phase (ϕ): An instantaneous state in an oscillation or some larger fraction of its period.

Phase angle difference (ψ): The time (e.g., in hours or degrees) between phase reference points (ϕ_r) in a rhythm and a Zeitgeber or between ϕ_r of two rhythms.

Phase–response curve (PRC): Plot of the magnitude and direction (+/−) of the phase shift ($\Delta\phi$) caused by a standard perturbation (e.g., light pulse) applied at different phases (ϕ) or circadian times (ct) of a free-running rhythm.

Phase shift ($\Delta\phi$): A single displacement of an oscillation along its time axis involving a temporary change in the rhythm's period.

Photoinducible phase (ϕ_i): That phase or portion of the circadian cycle in which light can trigger a long-day photoperiodic response.

Photoperiod: Day length; the length (hours) of the light phase in a light–dark (LD) cycle.

Rest time (ρ): Time in a "sleep–wake" or activity–rest cycle during which the animal is inactive.

Skeleton photoperiod (PPs): A light regime using two shorter pulses of light to simulate dawn and dusk effects of a longer, continuous photoperiod (PPc). If the two pulses are of equal duration, the skeleton is symmetric; if they are unequal, it is asymmetric.

Subjective day (SD): The first half of the circadian cycle (ct 00 to ct 12) and that half that normally occurs in the light of an LD 12:12 cycle.

Subjective night (SN): The second half of the circadian cycle (ct 12 to ct 24). In the Syrian hamster, the onset of nocturnal wheel-running is designated as ct 12 and marks the beginning of the SN.

Zeitgeber: An environmental cycle or perturbation that is capable of entraining a biological rhythm.

Symbols

LD $X{:}Y$	Light–dark cycle with X hours of light (L) and Y hours of dark (D) per cycle
LL	Continuous light
DD	Continuous dark
τ	Period of an endogenous rhythm. Usually the free-running period expressed in DD (τ_{DD})
T	Period length of the Zeitgeber
ϕ_i	Photoinducible phase
$\Delta\phi$	Phase shift. $+\Delta\phi$ denotes an advance phase shift, and $-\Delta\phi$ denotes a phase delay.
ψ	Phase angle difference. ψ_{RL} denotes a ψ value measured between an endogenous rhythm and a light–dark cycle (the subscripts are often omitted).
PTM	Photoperiodic time measurement (day length measurement)

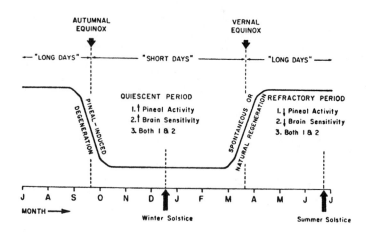

Figure 1. Theoretical role of the pineal gland in seasonal reproductive phenomena in the golden hamster. During the winter months ("short days"), reproductive organ growth is held in check by increased pineal activity and probably by an increased sensitivity of the brain to pineal substances. During the summer ("long days"), the neuroendocrine–gonadal axis may be refractory to the pineal influence. (Reproduced with permission from Reiter, 1973b.)

Exposure to the long days of summer terminates photorefractoriness. That is, after being exposed to long photoperiods again, the gonads once more become sensitive to day length as a reproductive cue. The hamster then responds to the short days of fall with gonadal regression (Reiter, 1972a). An analogous situation occurs in many birds. Gonadal growth is initiated by increasing day lengths in the spring, and the gonads remain functional for several weeks. Photorefractoriness in this case is accompanied by gonadal regression and occurs before the advent of short days in the fall. Exposure to short day lengths during fall and winter induces a return to the photosensitive state so that the entire cycle can be repeated in the next year (Follett and Davies, 1975; Follett, 1978). Note that the analogy between the hamster and the bird also provides an asymmetry. That is, in the hamster photosensitivity is reintroduced following long day lengths and is seen as a return of the response (gonadal regression) to short days, whereas in the bird, short day lengths restore photosensitivity which reappears as a return of the response (gonadal growth) to long days.

In considering the examples presented above, it is important to note that if the hamster (and the bird) were unable to develop the state of photorefractoriness it would be constrained to begin and end the breeding season at seasonal times that encompass the same day lengths. That is, the length of the breeding season would depend on the critical photoperiod and would include June 21 at its approximate midpoint with equal segments of time before and after that date included in the period of reproductive activity. The inclusion of the photorefractory mechanism along with its associated gonadal changes (recrudescence in the hamster and regression in the bird) allows considerably greater flexibility in the "choice" of an appropriate breeding season. For example, without the photorefractory mechanism, hamsters would produce fewer offspring because the breeding season would be shorter—photoperiodically induced gonadal recrudescence would not occur until after the spring equinox (i.e., not until day lengths reach 12.5 hr), and the first young would not be conceived until May. On the other hand, the bird would be forced to extend its breeding season until the occurrence of short days in the fall. The extra energy spent on reproduction late in the year would be a serious threat to the survival of both parents and offspring, neither of which would have the fat stores necessary to survive fall migration or the severities of winter.

It should be further noted that two time-measuring mechanisms are important in regulating the annual breeding cycle of the hamster. First, the ability to measure photoperiod during early fall is crucial in allowing for the termination of the breeding season at the "proper" time. Second, the spontaneous recrudescence of the gonads in anticipation of spring implies that during the fall and winter the hamster must measure a long time interval of approximately 4 to 5 months so that the gonads will develop at the "proper" time to initiate the next breeding season. Once the hamster has become photorefractory, the reproductive system will remain functional and cannot be suppressed by exposure to short days until a state of photosensitivity is regained through exposure to long days. In this species, the photosensitive state can be restored in the laboratory by exposure to long days for 10–12 weeks (Stetson *et al.*, 1977). In the wild, hamsters are exposed to long days (i.e., 12.5 hr of daylight) for several months during the summer. Thus, the animals presumably have ample opportunity to regain photosensitivity in time to respond to the decreasing day lengths during the ensuing fall season.

The mechansim by which the photosensitive hamster measures day length in the fall is discussed in detail in Section II of this chapter. It involves the use of the animal's circadian system. The method by which the animal measures the four to five months until the photorefractory condition and gonadal recrudescence ensue is completely unknown. However, it seems clear that changes in day length are not involved as cues in this process, since hamsters appear to require about the same period of time to complete a cycle of gonadal regression and eventual recrudescence in continuous darkness as in various short photoperiods (LD 10:14, LD 6:18). Indeed, even blinded hamsters exhibit one cycle of gonadal regression followed by recrudescence just as if intact animals had been transferred to short days at the time of blinding (Reiter, 1972a). Thus, it would seem that two different types of time measurement must be employed in this species for regulating the initiation and termination, respectively, of the gonadally inactive portion of the annual cycle. To summarize, initiation of gonadal inactivity is triggered by the occurrence of the short days of fall, and the termination of gonadal inactivity occurs spontaneously—or more precisely, occurs independently of the light cycle.

C. The Pineal Gland and Annual Reproductive Cycles in the Syrian Hamster

1. Effect of Pineal Removal

We must now ask how photoperiodic information is transmitted to the reproductive system. Removal of the pineal gland totally prevents gonadal involution in hamsters exposed to short photoperiods (Hoffman and Reiter, 1965). The pineal may therefore be involved in the flow of information from the circadian system to the reproductive system. Since the mammalian pineal does not appear to send out neural efferents, the influences of the gland on the hamster's annual reproductive cycle would be hormonally mediated (Reiter, 1972b).

Although the output of the pineal appears to be humoral, environmental stimulation of this gland is mediated by the nervous system. The pineal is richly innervated by a noradrenergic pathway originating in the superior cervical ganglion, and both ablation of this ganglion and section of its efferents to the pineal have been shown to prevent the "antigonadal" effects of short photoperiod in the hamster. Since these operations have an effect similar to pinealectomy, it seems clear that neural input to the pineal gland is essential for its function (Reiter, 1972b).

2. Role of Melatonin

The vertebrate pineal produces several indoleamines of which melatonin has received the most attention (see Chapters 1 and 4). The pineal gland is capable of converting serotonin to melatonin via the action of two enzymes, N-acetyltransferase and hydroxy-inole-O-methyltransferase, and melatonin seems to be critical in regulating the hamster's annual reproductive cycle. The specific effect of melatonin treatments depends on both the dose of melatonin as well as the photoperiod to which the hamsters are exposed (Turek and Campbell, 1979). For example, implants that release melatonin at a constant rate can cause testicular regression when the hamsters are exposed to long days and can cause gonadal recrudescence when the animals are exposed to short days. Daily injections of melatonin can also induce gonadal involution (Tamarkin et al., 1976b; 1977).

Although other substances present in pineal tissue may possess antigonadal activity, the case for melatonin as a key compound is strengthened by the striking parallels between the action of this substance and the effects produced by exposure to a short photoperiod. Daily injection of melatonin in male hamsters leads to decreases in circulating LH, FSH, and prolactin concentrations, but these changes occur only after several weeks of treatment. Similar changes have been observed to occur following exposure to short photoperiods (Fig. 2), and in this case as well, several weeks of exposure is required before decreases in the blood levels of these hormones take place

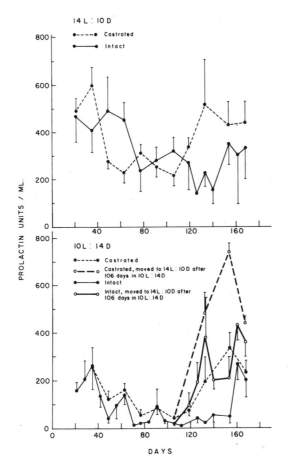

Figure 2. Serum prolactin concentrations in intact and castrated male hamsters exposed to long-day and short-day photoperiods, respectively. Animals represented in the lower panel were transferred to the short-day photoperiod on day 0; all castrations were also performed at this time. One group of castrated males and one group of intacts were returned to long days after 106 days' exposure to the short photoperiod. Most of the points represent the mean value for 4–7 animals, and the bars indicate standard error of the mean (SE). Five of the points for the intact, long-photo-period group represent only 2–3 animals.

(Tamarkin, 1977; Goldman *et al.*, 1979). The changes in gonadotropin secretion patterns that result from exposure of female hamsters to short photoperiod include the appearance of daily afternoon peaks in LH and FSH release. These same changes also appear during chronic daily treatment with melatonin (Tamarkin *et al.*, 1976b). When daily injections of melatonin are continued for a very long time in male hamsters kept on a long photoperiod, the testes first undergo regression, and this is followed by complete recrudescence after about 20 weeks of treatment. This phenomenon appears to parallel the spontaneous recrudescence that occurs following long-term exposure to short days. Finally, photorefractory hamsters do not respond to daily injections of melatonin (Table 2); suggesting an interesting parallel between the ability to respond to melatonin and the ability to respond to changes in photoperiod (Bittman, 1978; Goldman, unpublished data).

3. Pattern of Melatonin Production

It appears that melatonin production and release follow a fairly rigid diurnal pattern in a wide variety of vertebrate species, with peak secretion always occuring at night (Rollag and Niswender, 1976; Klein and Weller, 1970; Binkley, 1976). There is some evidence that the rhythmic production of melatonin in mammals is at least partially governed by an endogenous circadian clock, perhaps associated with the suprachiasmatic nuclei of the brain. Superimposed on this "clock" control is a brake mechanism by which melatonin is promptly and markedly decreased following acute exposure to light in most species (Rollag and Niswender, 1976; Reppert et al., 1979).

Because of the close relationship between environmental lighting and the production of melatonin, it has been widely believed that the pattern of secretion of this compound might serve as an indicator of the photoperiod. However, this hypothesis has never been put to a critical test; and it is not obvious from recent data in the Syrian hamster that the pattern of melatonin secretion accurately reflects changes in the photoperiod to which this species is exposed (Tamarkin et al., 1979; Panke et al., 1979). When pineal melatonin content was monitored, a pronounced daily rhythm was observed; but the duration of the melatonin "peak" was not clearly different as a function of photoperiod (Fig. 3). Even hamsters kept in continuous darkness failed to show any obvious increase in the duration of the "daily" melatonin peak (Fig. 4) as compared to animals in LD 14:10 or LD 10:14 (Tamarkin, Pratt, and Goldman, unpublished data). Indeed, it might be argued that the apparent conservation of a similar nocturnal rhythm of melatonin production throughout most of vertebrate evolution suggests some sort of time-measuring role for this compound. It should be remembered, however, that photoperiodic time measurement is not the only determinant of the hamster's annual reproductive cycle. Is it possible that melatonin might be involved in the ability of this species to measure the period of time intervening between gonadal involution and subsequent "spontaneous" recrudescence? Could it be that the 24-hr cycle of melatonin release is used in conjunction with some sort of digital counting, "calendar" mechanism?

It should be noted that the hamster has been discussed at length here only

Table 2. Failure of Photorefractory Hamsters to Respond to Melatonin

Condition at time of pinealectomy	N	Treatment	Testis wt. (mg)
Photorefractory	5	Oil	3919 ± 163
Photorefractory	11	Melatonin	3951 ± 189
Photosensitive	11	Melatonin	1163 ± 252

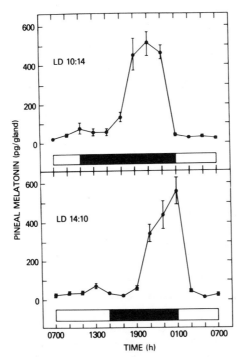

Figure 3. The amount of melatonin in the pineal glands of Syrian hamsters maintained in LD 10:14 or LD 14:10. The lighting schedules are represented by the open (L) and shaded (D) portions of the bar below. Data are presented as the mean ± SE of seven determinations. (Reproduced with permission from Tamarkin *et al.*, 1979.)

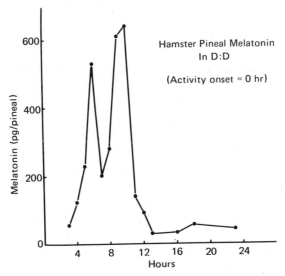

Figure 4. Pineal melatonin contents in hamsters housed in continuous darkness (DD). The animals were in DD for 3–4 weeks. Values are plotted in relation to the time of activity onset (wheel-running activity) on the day preceding sacrifice. Each point is the average value for two animals. (Reproduced with permission from Tamarkin *et al.*, 1980.)

because this species has been investigated so extensively. It is already clear that the hamster system differs from that of some seasonally breeding mammals, for example the ferret. The female ferret normally comes into estrus in early spring (March/April). Exposure to an artificially lengthened photoperiod during the winter months can advance the onset of estrus by many weeks. However, if the ferret is pinealectomized during the winter, subsequent exposure to long photoperiods cannot advance the onset of estrus, and gonadal development occurs at the usual time (Herbert, 1972). When ferrets are kept on natural photoperiods, they remain in estrus from March/April until July/August. In August a state of photorefractoriness ensues, in this case accompanied by the cessation of reproductive activity. Pinealectomized ferrets show a loss of normal synchrony and a loss of "proper" timing with respect to season. They tend to come into estrus much later than the expected time and show considerably greater interindividual variability as compared to intact ferrets (Herbert, 1972). Indeed, in the ferret and also in the Djungarian hamster, pinealectomy can promote or inhibit reproductive activity depending on the photoperiod and the phase of the gonadal cycle at which the surgery is done. By comparison, although pinealectomy has not been observed to inhibit gonadal function in the Syrian hamster, melatonin can either promote or inhibit reproductive activity depending on the photoperiod (Turek and Campbell, 1979). Thus, although the precise effects of pinealectomy (and melatonin) are different in hamsters and ferrets, it can be said that the pineal is involved in synchronizing reproductive events to seasonal time in both species.

4. Site of Action of Melatonin

The site of action of melatonin in mammals is not known. Since lesions in the suprachiasmatic nuclei (SCN) prevented hamsters from responding to changes in photoperiod (Stetson and Watson-Whitmyre, 1976; Morin et al., 1977), it seemed possible that melatonin might act on the SCN. However, since destruction of the suprachiasmatic nuclei failed to prevent the gonadal response to exogenous melatonin, it does not appear that the SCN are essential targets (Bittman et al., 1979). When melatonin is administered to hamsters by daily injections, changes in the blood levels of LH, FSH, and prolactin occur. As described, these hormonal changes are remarkably similar to those induced by exposure to a short photoperiod. These observations do not, however, suggest that melatonin acts directly on the pituitary gland. Indeed, both male and female hamsters respond about equally well to injections of LRF regardless of photoperiod (Turek et al., 1977). Also, ectopic pituitary grafts continue to secrete large amounts of prolactin during exposure to short days, although prolactin secretion from the in situ gland is greatly diminished (Bartke et al., 1978).

Thus, it seems that the changes in pituitary hormone release following exposure to short days or to melatonin treatment may be secondary to alterations in the production and release of hypothalamic hormones. Despite these observations, it remains possible that melatonin may have multiple sites of action and that the pituitary gland and the gonads might be additional targets. In the rat, melatonin inhibits the response of the neonatal pituitary to LRF *in vitro* (Martin and Klein, 1976). However, it is not clear what the physiological significance of this response might be, since pinealectomy has little effect on reproduction in the rat.

D. The Pituitary–Gonadal Axis and Annual Reproductive Cycles

1. Significance of Changes in Blood Levels of Pituitary Hormones

The decreased secretions of LH, FSH, and prolactin in short-day-exposed male hamsters may all be involved in causing the regression of the testes. Dramatic seasonal fluctuations in prolactin have also been observed in rams (Ravault, 1976), and photoperiod influences prolactin secretion in bulls (Leining *et al.,* 1979; Bourne and Tucker, 1975). Both LH and FSH appear to be required for the maintenance of testicular function. Prolactin may not have a direct stimulatory effect, but this hormone does appear to be required for maintaining an adequate level of LH receptor activity in the hamster (Bex *et al.,* 1978). Thus, the marked decrease in serum prolactin level, accompanied by a more modest decline in the LH concentration in short days, may produce a "cascade" effect.

When male hamsters bearing an ectopic pituitary transplant (in addition to their own *in situ* gland) were exposed to a short photoperiod, their testes required longer to regress and did not regress as completely as did those of animals without ectopic pituitary tissue. The pituitary grafts maintained high serum prolactin concentrations, apparently because of their removal from the inhibitory influence (prolactin-inhibiting factor) of the hypothalamus; this influence appears to be increased in short days. Serum FSH was increased to a much lesser extent, and serum LH was unaffected by the grafts. These observations seem to confirm a role of prolactin in testicular function (Bartke *et al.,* 1978). The causal relation between changes in gonadotropin secretion and the onset of the anovulatory state during exposure to short days is less well understood.

2. Regulation of Pituitary Hormones by Photoperiod

The decreases in serum prolactin levels in short-day-exposed male hamsters occur even in castrated animals, and prolactin levels are not affected by exogenous androgen. Castration also does not alter serum prolactin concentrations in males kept on a long photoperiod. Thus, the photoperiod-induced changes in serum prolactin do not result from alterations in the levels of testicular hormones in this species (Bex *et al.,* 1978; Stetson, Matt, Roychoudhury and Goldman, unpublished data). The decrease in serum gonadotropins in male hamsters kept in short photoperiod appears to be at least partly caused by a greatly increased sensitivity of the hypothalamic–pituitary axis to the negative feedback effects of androgen (Tamarkin *et al.*, 1976a; Turek, 1977). However, there is some evidence for an androgen-independent suppression of gonadotropins in short photoperiods in the male (Ellis and Turek, 1979), and the pattern of LH secretion in the short-photoperiod-exposed female shows little or no change even after combined ovariectomy and adrenalectomy (Bittman and Goldman, 1979).

In the ewe, it appears that seasonal changes in LH secretion are mediated by alterations in sensitivity to the negative feedback effect of estrogen. Ovariectomized ewes maintain high serum LH levels throughout the year, but when ovariectomized animals were administered a constant dose of estradiol, they showed pronounced seasonal fluctuations in serum LH concentrations, with the highest levels occurring during the normal breeding season (Fig. 5). These seasonal changes in sensitivity to estrogen feedback are apparently mediated by photoperiod. In sheep, the reproductive system becomes activated by exposure to short days (Legan *et al.*, 1977). The seasonal regulation of reproduction in rams seems to be analogous to the system described for the ewes, since rams show an increased sensitivity to the negative feedback action of testosterone on LH secretion when exposed to a long photoperiod (Pelletier and Ortavant, 1975).

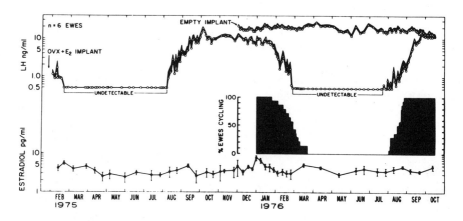

Figure 5. Seasonal variation in serum LH concentrations in estradiol-treated ovariectomized ewes. The upper portion of the figure depicts mean (± SE) serum LH levels (open circles and shaded area) in two groups of six ewes each. One group was treated so with Silastic capsules containing estradiol-17β (subcutaneous implants) immediately after ovariectomy (OVX + E₂ IMPLANT). The lower portion of the figure depicts mean (± SE) serum estradiol concentrations (closed circles) in the ewes receiving estradiol implants. The histogram illustrates the time course of the onset and end of the anestrous season in 1976 as determined from observations of estrus in a group of 14 intact ewes. Ewes were considered to be "cycling" until the day of the last estrus in the spring and from the day of the first ovulation in the fall (17 days before the first estrus). (Reproduced with permission from Legan *et al.*, 1977.)

E. Annual Rhythms in Other Physiological Functions

Seasonal changes in several physiological and behavioral phenomena have been observed, and some of these phenomena do not bear any obvious direct relationship to reproduction per se. Indeed, the first scientific report of a photoperiodically regulated function in vertebrates was that of Rowan (1925) who noted that migratory restlessness, or *Zugunruhe*, appeared to be regulated by day length in the junco. However, in this bird, the change in behavior was accompanied by changes in body fat stores and by a dramatic change in gonadal function. Most mammalian species that undergo seasonal rhythms in gonadal function show corresponding changes in sexual behavior. In some cases, it seems that the behavioral changes are not solely the result of seasonal fluctuations of the sex hormones. For example, male deer and male hamsters show decreased sexual behavior during the nonbreeding season even when androgens are administered in an attempt to stimulate the behavior (Lincoln *et al.*, 1972; Morin and Zucker, 1978; Campbell *et al.*, 1978).

1. Hibernation

Several species of mammalian hibernators undergo impressive annual fluctuations in body weight, primarily resulting from the successive periods of accumulation and then loss of body fat (Mrosovsky, 1971). Maximum body weight is generally achieved just before entrance into hibernation so that the accumulation of fat in late summer/early fall can be viewed as an adaptation to achieve a store of energy to be utilized during the winter months.

In some cases, this cyclicity can occur independently from changes in photoperiod since ground squirrels show circannual rhythms in accumulation of body fat and in hibernation when kept in the laboratory under constant conditions of temperature and photoperiod (Pengelley and Asmundson, 1974). The period lengths of these rhythms may be considerably shorter than one year, although some individuals show rhythms with periods of longer than 365 days. Virtually nothing is known regarding the physiological mechanisms that regulate these circannual cycles; nor do we know what environmental cues are used to entrain these rhythms in the wild so that the squirrels are able to remain "in synchrony" with the seasons.

In another species of hibernator, the Turkish hamster *(Mesocricetus brandti)*, it appears that photoperiod may have an indirect role in determining the time of hibernation. When exposed to cold (10 °C) in the laboratory, male Turkish hamsters will enter hibernation much more readily if they have small, nonfunctional testes than if they are reproductively active. Also, when hibernating males are administered constant release capsules of testosterone or dihydrotestosterone, they almost invariably terminate hibernation. In order to achieve this effect, the testosterone capsule need only be large enough to maintain a serum hormone level intermediate between those observed in males with functional testes and those observed in males with regressed testes. In addition to the observations cited above, it is known that exposure to short days results in testicular regression in the Turkish hamster. Therefore, it seems that exposure to the decreasing day lengths of autumn may indirectly prepare this species for entry into hibernation by causing testicular regression and the accompanying decrease in androgen production (Hall and Goldman, 1980).

A further link between annual reproductive cycles and hibernation was suggested by the following observations. Male Turkish hamsters with regressed testes were placed in a cold room along with a group of castrated males. The testes of the intact animals were measured at various intervals during bouts of spontaneous arousal from torpor. In most of these animals, testicular size began to increase after about 5 months of hiberation. When the testes reached about 60–80% of their maximum size, the males stopped hibernating. In contrast, the castrated males and three males that showed no sign of testicular growth continued to hibernate (Fig. 6). Four castrated males have hibernated for more than 15 months. Thus, it appears that a spontaneous recrudescence of the testes may occur after several months of hibernation, and this growth of the testes may result in increased androgen secretion which then terminates hibernation. This mechanism could serve to insure that the animals become active and are prepared to begin breeding early in the spring. The spontaneous testicular recrudescence in this species may be regulated by a mechanism similar to that which determines the time of testicular recrudescence and the development of the photorefractory state in the short-day exposed Syrian hamster, a closely related species. Note that in the scheme proposed here, the Turkish hamster may respond differently to the same environmental temperatures in the fall than in the spring as a result of its internal state (difference in circulating androgen concentrations), just as responses to day length are different depending on whether the animal is in the photosensitive or photorefractory state.

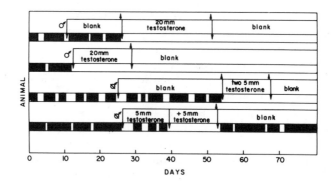

Figure 6. Effect of testosterone implants on the pattern of hibernation in intact (♂) and castrated (♂̶) Turkish hamsters. Blackened areas represent days in torpor; uncolored areas represent days of arousal. Arrows indicate times of implantation and removal of implants. (Reproduced with permission from Hall and Goldman, 1980.)

We have recently obtained even more striking evidence of the way in which an internal time-measuring device linked to the reproductive system may be involved in synchronizing seasonal cycles of reproduction and hibernation in the Turkish hamster. One group of male hamsters was exposed to short days (LD 10:14) beginning at T = 0. These animals were maintained at an ambient temperature of 22°C. A second group of males was placed in a cold room (10°C) on long days (LD 16:8) at the same time. After 8 weeks, both groups had undergone testicular regression, and the cold-exposed animals had begun to hibernate. At this time some of the short-day animals were moved into a second cold room which was kept on a short-day schedule. These males soon entered hibernation. All three groups of Turkish hamsters (i.e., long-day and cold-exposed, short-day, short-day and cold-exposed) began to undergo testicular recrudescence at the same time. This process began approximately 5–6 months after T = 0. All the cold-exposed males terminated hibernation shortly following the initiation of testicular growth. These results suggest that the Turkish hamster begins to measure time to gonadal recrudescence dating from the time of exposure to either short photoperiod or cold, both of which may serve as potential cues to initiate regression of the gonads (Hall and Goldman, unpublished data).

In migratory birds, the phase of the circadian locomotor activity rhythm relative to the light–dark cycle may shift dramatically during the migratory season. This corresponds to the fact that many avian species that are normally day-active carry out a large proportion of their migratory flying at night. The appearance of nocturnal locomotor activity results in an increase in the total duration of activity (α) in each 24-hr cycle. In the male starling, seasonal changes in the duration of the active phase appear to be at least partly dependent on circulating androgen levels (Gwinner, 1975). This species shows a circannual periodicity in testicular function when kept in the laboratory under a constant LD 12:12 photoperiod but not under constant photoperiods (e.g., 11 hr, 13 hr) either shorter or longer than 12 hr (Schwab, 1971). While the basis for the circannual periodicity under LD 12:12 is unknown, it appears that the annual rhythm is normally synchronized to the seasons via photoperiodic cues.

2. Photoperiodism in Birds and Reptiles

Many birds use day length as the major environmental cue to regulate annual reproductive rhythms. As with the mammalian species described in Section I.E.1, an alternation between photosensitive and photorefractory states appears to be characteristic of a number of avian species. However, thus far there is little evidence for a role of the pineal in bird reproduction. Rather, in at least the house sparrow *(Passer domesticus)* and the starling, recent evidence suggests that the pineal gland acts as an oscillator that "drives" daily rhythms in activity and body temperature (Zimmerman and Menaker, 1975; Gwinner, 1978). When sparrows are maintained in continuous darkness (DD), they manifest a circadian rhythm in locomotor activity that can be assessed by recording perch-hopping behavior via an event-recorder. Following pinealectomy, the activity rhythm begins to damp, and within a few days, episodes of perch-hopping become randomly spread across time (i.e., locomotor activity becomes arrhythmic). Recent evidence suggests that the pineal may indeed be a pacemaking oscillator in this system. Thus, when a pineal is transplanted into a previously pinealectomized arrhythmic sparrow housed in DD, the recipient becomes rhythmic again, and the phase of its activity (Ψ) with respect to local time is closely correlated with the phase of the donor bird (Zimmerman and Menaker, 1979). Furthermore, melatonin synthesis in the avian pineal shows an endogenous circadian periodicity in DD, and in a light–dark cycle this rhythm becomes entrained (Binkley, 1979). Finally, there is evidence to suggest that the melatonin rhythm may be involved in the regulation of the circadian rhythm in locomotor activity (Turek et al., 1976; Gwinner and Benzinger, 1978).

The reception of light cues that influence reproduction in birds is not exclusively via the retina, as appears to be true for mammals. Blinded birds are still capable of displaying characteristic reproductive responses to changes in photoperiod (McMillan et al., 1975). These responses can be prevented by shielding the head, suggesting that the extraretinal photoreceptors reside in the brain (Menaker and Underwood, 1976). Recently it has been discovered that birds can respond to light that is delivered directly into the hypothalamus by means of optic fibers (Yokoyama and Farner, 1978).

Unlike the Syrian hamster, which does not show changes in gonadotropin secretion for several weeks following exposure to short days, several avian species show very rapid responses to altered photoperiod. A single pulse of light given during the photoinductive phase can lead to an increase in LH release within a few hours (Follett et al., 1975). One might speculate that the delayed response to a photoperiodic change in the hamster could be an adaptation to its nocturnal and fossorial habits. Thus, despite the accuracy of the hamster's physiological mechanism for photoperiodic time measurement, the behavior of this rodent may place restraints on its ability to closely monitor day length in nature. Since the hamster probably receives light cues only when it emerges from its burrow, and since emergences occur only infrequently during the light phase (Pratt and Goldman, unpublished data), it may be that the hamster would be less accurate than the bird in daily monitoring of photoperiod. If this is so, it would seem that it might be of adaptive value for the hamster to have a system that reacts more slowly to changes in day length, thereby decreasing the likelihood of alterations in gonadal function being induced by occasional misreadings of day length. Two other fossorial mammals, the Djungarian hamster and the ferret, also show delayed responses to changes in day length.

The lizard, Anolis carolinesis, is photoperiodic and has been widely studied because of its ready availability. Exposure to short days in the summer results in premature regression of the testes in this species, whereas exposure to long days can induce testicular recrudescence. These responses to photoperiod are similar in blinded *Anolis* (Underwood, 1975). The biological clock that controls circadian locomotor activity in *Anolis* can also be entrained to light–dark cycles after blinding (Underwood, 1973). Unlike the birds and mammals discussed above, *Anolis* does not appear to utilize its circadian system for photoperiodic time measurement. Rather, this lizard seems to use a nonoscillatory or "hourglass" type of mechanism to measure day length and regulate reproductive status (Underwood, 1979).

II. CIRCADIAN RHYTHMS AND DAY LENGTH MEASUREMENT

A. Biological Time Measurement

The major topic in this chapter is time—that is, the way that an animal's reproductive life is synchronized with the external seasons. In Section I, we examined some of the neuroendocrine variables that mediate temporal synchronization of the organism with its environment. We pointed out that there were several ways in which time had to be measured for this to be accomplished. The major time measurement is, of course, the annual cycle. Indeed, some species display cycles with a period of approximately one year (circannual) even when placed in constant environmental conditions. For these organisms, environmental cycles (e.g., photoperiod) presumably entrain the circannual rhythm to a period of one year under natural conditions, but in the laboratory, the persistance of the rhythm under constant conditions argues that the rhythm itself is generated endogenously. So far little is known about the physiological processes responsible for the generation and entrainment of circannual rhythms. On the other hand, the species that have received the most attention here are those, like the Syrian hamster, that fail to show a circannual rhythm under constant conditions but do display endogenously timed changes in their response to photoperiod. For these species, an alternation of long and short day lengths is required for expression of the gonadal cycle.

It should be obvious by now that the way in which day length is used as a cue for seasonal biological rhythms is a complex one. It was pointed out already that at least two time-measuring mechanisms are important in regulating the annual breeding cycle of the hamster. First, the ability to measure photoperiod during early fall is crucial in terminating the breeding season at the proper time. Second, the spontaneous recrudescence of the gonads in the spring implies that during the fall and winter the hamster must measure a long time interval (approximately four to five months) so that the gonads will develop at their proper time to initiate the next breeding season during the following spring.

In the remainder of the chapter, we shall consider the ways in which organisms can accurately assess the length of light per day, this assessment in turn permitting the temporal control of reproduction by the environment. The mechanism of response to photoperiodic cues must involve a timing device or photoperiod clock that measures day length and triggers the appropriate response. In theory, this time measurement could involve a passive process (like an hourglass timer) that is forced to oscillate by the light–dark cycle. Or it might depend on an endogenous oscillation (circadian clock) that interacts with the light cycle but does not depend on it to sustain an oscillation. Over the years, the question of hourglass versus oscillator has largely given way to a broader field of investigation which is the comparative study of the photoperiodic clock in a number of plant and animal species. In this formal analysis, the internal clock is treated as a "black box" whose properties are inferred from overt responses to environmental light cycles and pulses. As we shall see, this analysis has shown us that circadian rhythms participate in the photoperiodic control of the annual reproductive rhythms of a variety of birds and mammals. The formal analysis has also given us information about the light requirements for photoperiodic responses and has taught us something of the ways in which circadian rhythms are involved in photoperiodic phenomena. Our concern with the relationship between circadian and annual rhythms will begin in the next two sections with a discussion of the conceptual framework behind the formal analysis. We shall then turn our attention to the study of the mechanism of the day length measurement in the Syrian hamster.

B. Models for the Photoperiodic Clock

Although there exists an extensive literature on the photoperiodic responses of birds and mammals, the major theories concerning the mechanism of photoperiodic time measurement (PTM) come largely from earlier work with plants and insects. Two fundamentally different mechanisms have been proposed on theoretical grounds, and both have been found to occur in some organisms. The first hypothesis assumes that the time measurement is based on a passive "hourglass" or "interval timer." A common feature of this model is the involvement of some photochemical process occurring during the light (or the dark) period that is reversed in the other portion of the light–dark cycle. If enough of a hypothetical reaction product accumulates as a result of the organism's being exposed to a long day (or night), then a threshold is exceeded, and a photoperiodic response is observed (e.g., stimulation of gonadal growth). The distinguishing feature of an hourglass timer is its predicted requirement for a critical duration of light or dark, or a critical ratio of light : dark in each cycle. The hourglass timer is thought to lack inherent rhythmicity. The underlying metabolic process is forced by the environmental cycle of light and dark. A convincing case for an hourglass timer has been established in at least two insect species (Lees, 1966; Skopik and Bowen, 1976). In both cases, the time-measuring system requires daily resetting by light but measures the duration of uninterrupted darkness. As discussed in Section I, a converse mechanism has been found in the lizard *Anolis carolinenis* (Underwood, 1979). In this vertebrate, testicular function is regulated by an hourglass timer that measures the absolute length of the light period. Although the occurrence of "hourglass timers" has not been convincingly demonstrated in a wide variety of species, there is some evidence that they may be widespread phenomena in insects (Beck, 1968).

A modified hourglass mechanism was invoked to explain the results of many early photoperiod experiments with birds (e.g., Jenner and Engels, 1952; Kirkpatrick and Leopold, 1952) and one recent study with hamsters (Hoffman and Melvin, 1974), but the results of these experiments are most adequately interpreted on the basis of a fundamentally different mechanism, one in which PTM is based on an endogenous oscillation with a circadian periodicity.

This alternative to the hourglass hypothesis was first suggested in 1936 by Bünning who proposed that circadian rhythms were involved in the measurement of day length by plants. In its modern version, Bünning's hypothesis assumes that PTM is based on a circadian rhythm of responsiveness to light with two qualitatively distinct halves: during the first half cycle (subjective day), the organism is nonresponsive to light; during the second half cycle (subjective night), the organism becomes responsive to light. The essence of the Bünning model is that the photoperiodic effect of a particular LD cycle depends on the temporal position of light relative to what we shall call the circadian rhythm of photoperiodic photoresponsivity or photoinducibility (CRPP). According to the model, photoperiodic stimulation by long days occurs when light extends into the responsive portion of the CRPP, whereas short days fail to stimulate because light is restricted to the nonresponsive portion of the rhythm (Bünning, 1960; Elliott, 1976).

In Bünning's model, the light sensitive "scotophil" phase of the oscillation was assumed to occur at a fixed time after dawn regardless of the duration of the photoperiod (Bünning, 1960). In more recent discussions, this feature of the model has been changed to incorporate advances in our knowledge of the mechanism of entrainment of circadian rhythms by light cycles (Pittendrigh and Minis, 1964, 1971; Pittendrigh, 1965, 1966). Thus, in describing their "external coincidence" model, Pittendrigh and Minis postulate a "photo-inducible phase" (ϕ_i) whose position with respect to the phase of the light cycle is expected to vary as a function of entrainment. In the external coincidence model, light has two conceptually distinct roles. Its primary action is to entrain the organism's CRPP, but it also entrains all the other circadian rhythms of the organism. Secondly, light acts as inducer of the photoperiodic response when ϕ_i is illuminated, but the temporal coincidence of light and ϕ_i depends on precisely how the CRPP is entrained to the LD cycle and not simply on the duration of the photoperiod. It is for this reason that Pittendrigh and Minis stressed the importance of studying the entraining action of light in addition to its photoperiodic effects in any attempt to test predictions arising from Bünning's general hypothesis.

Another possible mechanism for the role of circadian rhythms in PTM derives from the now widely established concept that multicellular organisms possess a circadian system comprised of many oscillations whose mutual phase relationships may have a significant impact on a variety of physiological functions (Pittendrigh, 1960, 1974; Menaker, 1974; Aschoff and Wever, 1976; Moore-Ede *et al.,* 1976). In this model, if an organism is taken from one photoperiod and reentrained to another, the phase relationships among the multiple biological oscillators change. When the phase relationships of these internal rhythms are in the appropriate configuration (i.e., under some photoperiods but not others), the photoperiodically controlled process is initiated. In recent discussions, Pittendrigh (1972, 1974) has introduced the term "internal coincidence" to refer to this class of model. In internal coincidence, light serves only as an entraining agent that differentially controls the phase of internal rhythms, and, therefore, it does not play a direct role in inducing the photoperiodic response (Turek and Campbell, 1979).

C. Entrainment of Circadian Rhythms

Before considering experimental evidence for the participation of circadian rhythms in the photoperiodic control of annual cycles, it is important to briefly discuss a few of the basic properties of circadian rhythms and especially their responses to changes in external lighting. Circadian rhythms are a universal characteristic of eukaryotic life, and in complex multicellular organisms they exist at all levels of organization. In nature, most of any animal's activity—biochemical and behavioral—is undertaken at some appropriate, restricted time in the daily cycle of changing conditions (e.g., light, temperature, availability of food, susceptibility to predation). In general, this daily cycle of biological activity is dictated by an innate temporal program or "biological clock": under laboratory conditions of continuous darkness (DD) and constant temperature, most daily rhythms persist as free-running circadian rhythms. The period (τ) of the free-running rhythm is often remarkably stable and is usually close to, but rarely exactly 24 hr. This fact implies that the rhythms we observe are driven by, and hence are overt manifestations of, some metabolic process or system pacemaker capable of continued, self-generated oscillation. This circadian pacemaker is conceptually and physiologically discrete from the components of the system (e.g., slave oscillations, overt rhythms) that it drives. In birds and mammals and a number of invertebrates the pacemaker for circadian rhythms has been localized to some small fraction of the central nervous system (reviewed in Menaker *et al.,* 1978; Rusak and Zucker, 1979).

The major action of the environment is not to generate the rhythmicity but rather to entrain the internal pacemaker to a period of precisely 24 hr and to control its phase so that the pacemaker and the many rhythms it drives will maintain an adaptive temporal relationship to the periodicities of the natural environment. In general, only a few environmental variables are capable of entraining circadian pacemakers. In mammals and birds (homeotherms), light is by far the dominant entraining agent. In many other organisms, including reptiles, temperature cycles are also effective in entraining circadian rhythms, but the light–dark cycle is the principle Zeitgeber.

Let us consider a specific case. The Syrian hamster is a burrowing, nocturnally active rodent. In nature, these animals presumably spend much of the day sleeping in their underground burrows. At dusk, they emerge from their burrows to forage for food and to mate. In the laboratory, the clock system that times nocturnal activity is usually studied by monitoring wheel-running behavior. Hamsters are placed in individual cages each equipped with a running wheel and a supply of food and water. Each cage is placed in a ventilated light-proof cabinet equipped with a clock-controlled light source. A microswitch is mounted on the side of each cage and wired so that each wheel revolution is recorded as a pen deflection on one channel of a multichannel operations recorder.

On a 14-hr photoperiod (LD 14:10), activity is strictly nocturnal—most hamsters begin vigorous wheel-running approximately 20 min after dark, day after day (Fig. 7). The activity pattern may be unimodal with one nightly bout of nearly continuous running, or it may be bimodal with two peaks of activity each night. In the bimodal pattern, an intense 3- to 6-hr bout of activity in the

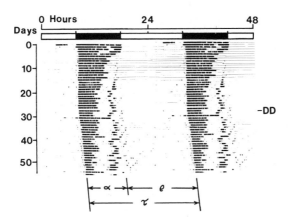

Figure 7. Record of the circadian rhythm of wheel-running activity of an individual Syrian hamster entrained to a 14-hr photoperiod (LD 14:10) and free-running in continuous darkness (DD). Revolutions of the exercise wheel produced deflections of the recording pen on one channel of an event recorder. Each line on the left is one day's record (0 to 24 hr) cut from noon to noon and pasted beneath the reccord of the preceding day. For illustration, the entire record is shown again on the right (24 to 48 hr). The heavy bands indicate nearly continuous running. Days 0–27 show 4 weeks of entrainment to the LD 14:10 cycle diagrammed above (lights on 0600 to 2000). In entrainment, activity begins about 0.3 hr after lights-out each day, so that the average period of the rhythm (τ_{LD}) matches the 24-hr period (T) of the LD cycle. Days 28–56 show the rhythm free-running in DD. The activity cycle is divided into activity time (α) and rest time (ρ). In this example, the period of the free-run (τ_{DD}) is 24.07 hr and α is 8.5 hr. Note that the heavy band of activity from 1525 to 1800 on day 0 represents the animal's initial response to the activity monitor. Thereafter, wheel-running activity is almost entirely nocturnal but switches from a predominately unimodal to a bimodal pattern as the "novelty" of the wheel is reduced (Elliott, unpublished data).

early night (evening component) is followed several hours later by a shorter, less precisely timed bout (morning component) marking the end of the animal's night. In either pattern (unimodal or bimodal), activity onset is the most regular and precisely timed feature of the rhythm, and the active phase (activity time, α) usually lasts 6 to 10 hr. In entrainment, the period (τ_{DD}) of the activity rhythm comes to match the period (T) of the light cycle ($\tau_{DD} \rightarrow \tau_{LD} = T$), and a stable phase relationship is established between the rhythm and the light cycle. On LD 14:10, τ is 24.0 hr and the phase angle difference (ψ_{RL}) measured between activity onset and the onset of the photoperiod is stable at about 9.7 hr. In DD, the activity rhythm persists with a remarkably stable free-running period (τ_{DD}). The period of the free-running rhythm is circadian. It is close to, but rarely exactly 24 hr. As a consequence, in DD, the rhythm gradually drifts out of phase with local time. In most hamsters, τ_{DD} is about 24.1 hr—activity onset occurs about 6 min later each day that the animal remains in constant darkness.

The phase of a circadian rhythm free-running* in DD can be shifted (reset) to an earlier or later time by a single brief light pulse. In records of hamster wheel-running, the phase shift ($\Delta\phi$) is seen as a displacement of the rhythm along the horizontal (24 hr) time scale (Fig. 8). Both the magnitude and direction (advance or delay) of the $\Delta\phi$ response to a standard pulse are characteristic of the particular phase (ϕ), or circadian time (ct) at which the pulse is given. The dependence of $\Delta\phi$ on ct is summarized graphically in a phase–response curve (PRC). In the PRC graph (Fig. 8), one full circadian cycle (360°) with period τ is divided into 24 circadian hours, each lasting $\tau/24$ hr of real time. In the hamster, activity onset is designated ct 12 and marks the beginning of the subjective night (ct 12 to ct 24). The half-cycle immediately before onset is defined as subjective day (ct 0 to ct 12). Phase delays ($-\Delta\phi$) are caused by light falling in the very late subjective day and early subjective night (ct 11 to ct 15). Phase advances ($+\Delta\phi$) peak in the middle of the subjective night (around ct 18) and continue with diminishing magnitude into the early subjective day. Most of the subjective day (e.g., ct 1 to ct 11), the hamster is very unresponsive to light. These features of the hamster PRC are characteristic of the PRCs of all circadian pacemakers (Pittendrigh, 1965; Daan and Pittendrigh, 1976).

The PRC describes the resetting response to light that mediates the entrainment of a circadian pacemaker to a light cycle. In each cycle of entrainment, the phase of the pacemaker is shifted or reset by an amount ($\Delta\phi$) equal to the difference between the freerunning period (τ) of the pacemaker and the period (T) of the LD cycle ($\tau - T = \Delta\phi$). For given values of τ and T, there is a unique pacemaker phase (ct) at which light must fall to produce stable entrainment (Pittendrigh, 1965; Pittendrigh and Daan, 1976b). Thus, if τ is known, and one has measured a PRC for a standard light pulse, then it is possible to predict the circadian time at which the light pulse must fall in entrainment to different Ts. For example, if a hamster whose τ is 24.3 hr is to entrain to a light

*See Table 1 and comment on bottom of page 406.

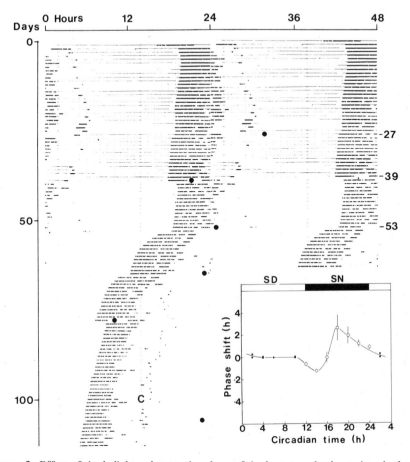

Figure 8. Effect of single light pulses on the phase of the hamster wheel-running rhythm free-running in DD. The main body of the figure is a continuous record of the activity of one animal in which the upper portion is shown twice (double plotted) to aid in visual scanning of the data. The rhythm free-ran unperturbed for the first 26 days of the experiment with a period of slightly less than 24 hr. The solid circles (•) indicate the time (midpoint) of single light pulses given on days 27, 39, 53, 65, 78, and 106 of DD. The pulse on day 78 was 2 hr long; all other pulses were 1 hr. Phase advances (+Δφ) were elicited by pulses 1, 3, and 4; phase delays (−Δφ) were elicited by pulses 2 and 5. The last pulse and a control disturbance (C) on day 100 (cage moved with the aid of a dim red light) failed to cause detectable phase shifts. The inset summarizes the data from 18 animals and many (n = 47) estimates of the Δφ responses to 1 hr light pulses (50–100 lux) given at different phases of the cycle. Open circles plot the mean ± SE for Δφ responses averaged over 2-hr bins of circadian time. Solid circles plot individual responses. An eye-fit line drawn through the points gives a phase response curve (data from Elliott, 1974).

cycle with a period of 24.0 hr, the light pulse must cause a phase advance of +0.3 hr. To do this, the pulse must fall near the end of the subjective night (e.g., around ct 23.5). We shall consider other examples of entrainment as we discuss the various kinds of experiments that have been used to study the formal properties of the photoperiodic clock.

1. The Resonance Experiment

Is PTM based on an hourglass or an oscillator? To determine which of the different models for photoperiodic time measurement is correct, it is necessary to expose photosensitive animals to light cycle treatments specifically designed to reveal which feature of the LD cycle is measured. For reasons that will soon become clear, this usually requires the use of exotic light cycles with periods (T) differing from 24 hr; hence, several of the most widely used paradigms are collectively known as T experiments. Of these tests, the so called resonance experiment introduced by Nanda and Hamner (1958) is one of the most powerful. In this paradigm, a short photoperiod (e.g., 6 hr) is coupled to different durations of darkness to generate LD cycles of increasing period length. In a typical experiment, D is lengthened in 12-hr increments to give Ts of 24, 36, 48, 60, and 72 hr. Thus, in a typical resonance experiment, an animal exposed to a T36 cycle would receive 6 hr of light alternating with 30 hr of dark in a repeating 36-hr cycle (LD 6:30).

Although the choice of LD cycles may appear strange, the rationale is a simple one. If the photoperiodic clock is based on the hourglass principle, none of the LD cycles described above is expected to induce a long-day response. On the other hand, if photoperiodic induction rises and falls as a periodic function of T, this demonstrates that neither the duration of light, nor the duration of dark, nor the light/dark ratio is the determining factor and at the same time provides strong evidence in favor of a circadian mechanism. This is best illustrated by considering a specific example.

Figure 9 gives data from two experiments with male hamsters. In the first experiment (Fig. 9a), animals reared on a photostimulatory light cycle (LD 14:10) were divided into four treatment groups, and each group was exposed to a different resonance light cycle. After 13 weeks, only the animals exposed to the T36 (LD 6:30) and T60 (LD 6:54) cycles had large testes. In the T 24 (LD 6:18) and T48 (LD 6:42) cycles, the testes regressed. In the second experiment, (Fig. 9b) hamsters whose testes were regressed after a 10-week exposure to LD 6:18 were subjected to the same lighting schedules to test their effectiveness for the photoperiodic induction of gonadal growth.

The results of these two experiments clearly defy explanation on the basis of an hourglass mechanism for PTM. Hamsters do not measure the absolute duration of light or darkness per cycle or the light-to-dark ratio. If they did, none of the experimental light cycles would have simulated the action of a long photoperiod, since in a T24 cycle, a 12.5-hr photoperiod (LD 12.5:11.5) is the minimum day length necessary for photoperiodic induction of gonadal activity

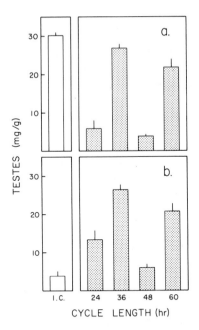

Figure 9. Testicular responses of hamsters to resonance light cycles. A. Testis weight (mg/g body weight) of LD 14:10 initial controls (I.C.) and groups of hamsters sacrificed after 89 days of exposure to light cycles in which a 6-hr photoperiod was repeated either once every 24 (LD 6:18), 36 (LD 6:30), 48 (LD 6:42), or 60 (LD 6:54) hr. B. Testis weights of initial controls (10 weeks prior exposure to LD 6:18) and of hamsters exposed to resonance light cycles and sacrificed after 63 days. Photostimulation of testicular maintenance and testicular recrudescence is obtained only in the 36- and 60-hr cycles, indicating the participation of a circadian rhythm of photosensitivity in the hamster's photoperiodic testicular response. Each histogram represents the mean and standard error (vertical line) of 7 to 11 animals (Reproduced with permission from Elliott, 1976, *Fed. Proc.* **35**:2334.)

(Gaston and Menaker, 1967; Elliott, 1976). Instead, both the LD 6:30 and LD 6:54 cycles are clearly photostimulatory, and gonadal weight rises and falls as a periodic function of T, indicating that PTM is based on a circadian rhythm. This implies that the 24- and 48-hr cycles are nonstimulatory because light falls only in the subjective day, whereas the 36- and 60-hr cycles are photo-stimulatory because light also coincides with the subjective night where it illuminates ϕ_i. Similar results have been reported for the vole, *Microtus agrestis* (Grococh and Clarke, 1974) and also for several species of birds (Hamner, 1963; Follett and Sharp, 1969; Turek, 1972, 1974). The resonance paradigm has also produced similar results in a number of plants and insects, and in yet another study on the Syrian hamster, Stetson and co-workers showed that the day length measurement required for the termination of photorefractoriness is also based on a circadian mechanism (Stetson *et al.*, 1976).

    In an attempt to learn more about the properties of the time-measuring system, several investigators have recorded the locomotor activity rhythms of animals subjected to resonance light cycles. The idea is to use the locomotor rhythm as an indicator of the rhythm of photoinducibility (the postulated CRPP), because in principle it is not possible to use a single assay to study both photoperiodic induction and circadian entrainment (see Pittendrigh and Minis, 1964, 1971). This technique was employed by Hamner and Enright (1967) in their studies with house finches, *Carpodoxus mexicanus*, and it was also used in the hamster experiments discussed above. In both species, the data demonstrate an excellent correlation between the photoperiodic response and the pattern of locomotor activity. Although house finches are day-active, and hamsters are night-active, both species are most sensitive to photoperiodic stimuli when they occur in the subjective night.

Representative activity records from hamsters entrained to resonance light cycles are reproduced in Fig. 10. Even under the non-24-hr cycles, the activity rhythms show an average period of almost precisely 24 hr, although the circadian phase of light differs markedly between the photostimulatory and nonphotostimulatory regimes. The entrainment of the rhythm to the 24-hr and 48-hr cycles is not surprising; a light stimulus occurring at the same time every day or every other day is sufficient to entrain the rhythm to a 24-hr

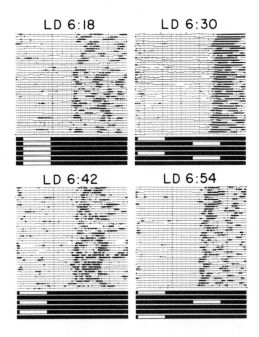

Figure 10. Temporal relationship between the light cycle and the circadian rhythm of locomotor (wheel-running) activity in hamsters, one from each of the four resonance treatments. The light cycle is diagrammed at the bottom of each record on a 24-hr scale (solid black, darkness; white, fluorescent light). Only days 47 through 89 of the experiment (Fig. 9A) are shown. On the LD 6:18 and LD 6:42 cycles, the activity rhythm entrains such that light is present only during the hamster's subjective day and fails to stimulate the gonads. On the LD 6:30 and LD 6:54 cycles, light is present both early and late in the subjective night and is photostimulatory to the reproductive system. (Reproduced with permission from Elliott, 1976.)

period. Entrainment to a 24-hr period by the 36-hr and 60-hr cycles is also easily explained by plotting these cycles on a 24-hr time scale (see bottom of each panel in Fig. 10). In both regimes there is an alternation of light in the morning with light in the evening the following day (LD 6:30) or 2 days later (LD 6:54). Since the duration of darkness in the two regimes differs by exactly 24 hr, the phases of the 6-hr light periods relative to real time are the same, and if the morning and evening pulses occurred together on the same day, they would form a "skeleton" (6L; 6D; 6L; 6D) of an 18-hr photoperiod (LD 18:6). The extra day or two of darkness between light pulses has little effect on the pattern of entrainment because the free-running period of the hamster's clock is very close to 24 hr. For this reason, entrainment to LD 6:42 closely resembles entrainment to LD 6:18, and entrainment to both LD 6:30 and LD 6:54 closely resembles entrainment to LD 18:6.

This pattern of entrainment is consistent with Bünning's hypothesis. On the nonstimulatory cycles (LD 6:18; LD 6:42), the light is on only during the subjective day, whereas in the photoinductive cycles (LD 6:30; LD 6:54), each light pulse runs into either the beginning or the end of the subjective night. Although these observations definitely indicate that a circadian light response rhythm participates in the photoperiodic response, neither the waveform of this rhythm nor its phase relationship to wheel running can be accurately determined because the light pulses are 6 hr long ($\frac{1}{4}\tau$), and it is not known whether light falling early and/or late in the subjective night is critical to the photostimulatory effects of the 36-hr and 60-hr cycles (Elliott, *et al.*, 1972).

Although it has been possible to infer the existence of a circadian rhythm of responsiveness to photoperiodic stimuli from successful resonance experiments by studying the correlation between entrainment and photoperiodic induction, it would be more satisfying if we could observe the rhythm more directly and show it running free for several cycles in constant darkness. In work with vertebrates, the possibility of such an experiment is usually precluded by the requirement for exposing animals to lighting schedules for weeks or even months before a photoperiodic response can be observed. However, the availability of a radioimmunoassay for avian LH led to the discovery in quail and white-crowned sparrows that exposure to a single long day can lead to a significant increase in LH titers (Nicholls and Follett, 1974; Follett *et al.*, 1974). This made possible the experiment shown in Fig. 11. White-crowned sparrows were transferred from a short photoperiod to darkness, and at different times thereafter, each bird was subjected to a single 8-hr pulse of light. Plasma LH was measured before and after the treatment, and the photoperiodic response assessed by the change in LH. In this system, a significant increase in LH indicates a long-day response, and the effectiveness of the light pulses in promoting such increases clearly varies with a circadian rhythm. The rhythm persists in constant darkness without damping for four complete cycles, providing unusually direct evidence that the photoperiodic response involves a self-sustained circadian oscillation (Follett, 1978). The analogous experiment has not been possible in hamsters where stable changes in LH and FSH titers

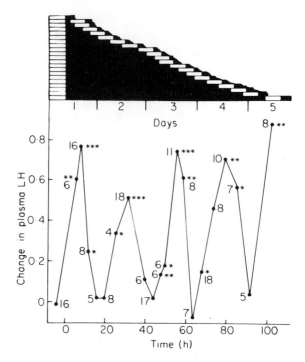

Figure 11. Results from an experiment testing for the presence of free-running circadian rhythm of photoperiodic photosensitivity in white-crowned sparrows, *Zonatrichia leucophrys*. The birds were held on a short photoperiod (LD 8:16) until the beginning of the experiment when they were placed in continuous darkness. At prescribed times thereafter, each bird was subjected to a single 8-hr light exposure. Twenty of the treatments are represented in the schematic above the graph. Blood samples taken before transfer to darkness and again a few hours after the light pulse were assayed for LH. The change in LH concentration (ng/ml) is plotted on the ordinate against the time of the pulse. The number of birds exposed to a treatment is shown by each point together with an assessment of whether the change was significant (no stars $p > 0.05$*; $p < 0.05$**; $p < 0.01$***; $p < 0.001$). The data demonstrate a rhythm in the response to light that runs free in darkness with a circadian period. (Reproduced with permission from Follett *et al.*, 1974.)

develop only gradually over several days or weeks after a change in photoperiod (Berndtson and Desjardins, 1974; Turek *et al.*, 1976; Turek and Elliottt, unpublished data).

D. Entrainment and Photoperiodic Induction by Skeleton Photoperiods

In the study of photoperiodic time measurement, it has often proven difficult to devise experimental tests that adequately discriminate among competing theories. The history of so called "night-interruption" or asymmetric "skeleton photoperiod" experiments presents an interesting example.* It appears that this type of experiment was originally designed to test whether the length of the light period or the length of the dark period was critical for photoperiodic induction. To answer this question, the long night of a short photoperiod was interrupted at various points with a brief light exposure to determine whether the two light pulses acting together could promote a long-day response. When it was found that light pulses placed in the middle of the long night were inductive, it was concluded that the response depended on an hourglass that measured the duration of uninterrupted darkness; that is, a brief light exposure could apparently override the effect of many hours of darkness by resetting the hourglass. However, other researchers soon pointed out that the inductive effect of a night interruption is also consistent with a circadian mechanism, since photoperiodic induction would be expected when the night interruption illuminates ϕ_i. Obviously, night-interruption experiments alone do not allow one to discriminate between hourglass and circadian oscillator mechanisms. For this reason, it is more informative to begin the investigation with the Nanda–Hamner experiment.

When other experiments (e.g., Nanda–Hamner resonance) indicate a circadian basis for PTM, night-interruption experiments can help to locate the position of ϕ_i in the night; however, there are a number of difficulties. The first is that the temporal position of the maximally effective night interruption (and, hence, the presumed location of ϕ_i) shifts when either the duration of the main photoperiod or the length of the night interruption is changed (Follett, 1973). This shifting of the peak response appears to be linked to the entrainment of circadian rhythms to asymmetric skeletons, since in the several cases where this has been studied, both the duration of the main photoperiod and the timing of the night interruption affect the phase of the entrained rhythm (Pittendrigh and Minis, 1964, 1971; Saunders, 1976). Since an inductive night interruption is expected to alter the pattern of entrainment of the circadian system with respect to the main photoperiod, the photoperiodic response is open to either of two interpretations: (a) the night interruption may itself coincide with ϕ_i in steady-state entrainment, or (b) it may shift the phase of ϕ_i causing it to be illuminated by the main photoperiod. It should be obvious that these considerations (phase shift of ϕ_i, two light pulses per cycle) pose serious difficulties for any attempt to pinpoint the exact location of ϕ_i within the circadian cycle even for the case where one has studied the entrainment of an overt rhythm.

Although skeleton photoperiod experiments are not well suited to identifying the location of ϕ_i, under appropriate conditions they can provide exceptionally strong evidence that day length is measured by a circadian

*A "skeleton photoperiod" is an LD cycle in which two pulses in combination effectively simulate the action of a single pulse (complete photoperiod) with duration equal to the interval from the beginning of the first pulse to the end of the second pulse of the two-pulse regime. Asymmetric refers to the unequal length of the two pulses in classical night-interruption experiments.

mechanism (Pittendrigh, 1966; Saunders, 1976). This is illustrated by an experiment in which a single skeleton photoperiod is shown to be photoinductive or noninductive depending on which of two stable entrainment patterns is assumed by the circadian system. A group of 20 male hamsters was transferred from LD 14:10 to DD, permitting their activity rhythms to free-run* independently in continuous darkness for 34 days (see Fig. 12). From day 35 to day 100 of the experiment, all of the animals were exposed to a skeleton photoperiod regime consisting of two 15-min light pulses separated by intervals of darkness lasting 13.5 hr and 10 hr (0.25L : 13.5D : 0.25L : 10D). All of the hamsters entrained to the skeleton regime, but the approach to entrainment and the phase angle (Ψ) characteristic of the steady state depended on the phase of the circadian activity cycle illuminated by the first pulse. Although the first 15-min light pulse occurred at the same time with respect to the solar day (2:40 a.m.) in all cases, the pulse occurred at different times with reference to the circadian activity cycle in each animal because the hamsters had been free-running* with slightly different circadian periods. In all, their free-running periods (τ) ranged from 23.95 hr to 24.19 hr, and after 34 days of running free in darkness, the time of the solar day at which individual hamsters began their activity ranged from 6:40 p.m. to 2:10 a.m.

Depending on the circadian time of the first pulse, individual hamsters either phase-advanced (e.g., animal #C15) or phase-delayed (e.g., #C16) into entrainment, and this determined the subsequent gonadal response. In every case (n = 10), the testes were maintained when activity occurred in the shorter 10-hr dark interval but regressed (n = 8) when activity occurred in the longer 13.5-hr dark interval. (Two animals died before the testes were measured by surgical laporotomy on day 97.)† Thus, for both the entrainment of the activity rhythm and the response of the testes, it is as if the animal on the left (#C15) interpreted the skeleton regime as a 14-hr photoperiod (LD 14:10), whereas the one on the right (#C16) interpreted it as a 10.5-hr photoperiod (LD 10.5:13.5). Since the two animals experienced exactly the same conditions and, in fact, were subjected simultaneously to exactly the same light cycle, the pattern of entrainment to the skeleton regime is the only variable that can account for the difference in their gonadal response. When one compares the records of all 18 hamsters, there are two consistent differences between the

---

*The terms "free-run" and "free-running" are used extensively in the literature—see Table 1 (page 379) for definition of "free-running" period.

†To control for differences in free-running period, the animals were divided into two treatment groups. The animals in the first group (I) were exposed to a skeleton in which the first interval between light pulses was 13.5 hr (as for the two animals in Fig. 12). The animals in the second group (II) were exposed to a skeleton in which the first interval seen was 10 hr. In Group I only, the animals that phase-advanced into entrainment (shorter τs) showed activity in the 10-hr dark period (interpreted the skeleton as LD 14:10). In Group II, only the animals that phase-delayed into entrainment (longer τs) interpreted the skeleton as a long day. Thus, when both groups are considered together, the only reliable predictor of the gonadal response is the pattern of entrainment to the skeleton: τ_{DD} whether measured before or after the skeleton, does not correlate with the gonadal response.

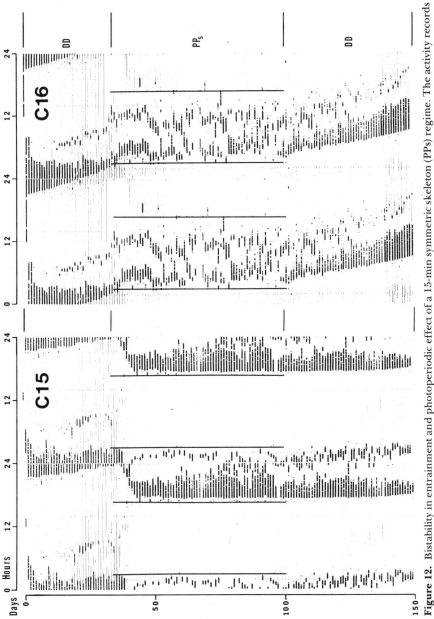

Figure 12. Bistability in entrainment and photoperiodic effect of a 15-min symmetric skeleton (PPs) regime. The activity records have been double-plotted to aid in interpretation of the results. The animals were transferred from LD 14:10 to DD on day 0. On days 35–100, they were exposed to the symmetric skeleton light cycle consisting of two 15-min light pulses (ink lines) alternating with dark periods of 13.5 hr and 10 hr (0.25 LD : 13.50D : 0.25L : 10D) (Elliott, unpublished).

activity patterns of those animals whose testes were maintained (TM) and those whose testes regressed (TR). The major difference, already described, is in the phase of entrainment to the skeleton: only the TM animals chose the shorter, 10-hr dark period as night. As a consequence of the decreased length of their night, these animals also experienced a reduction in activity time (α). That is, during entrainment to the skeleton, the fraction of the circadian cycle given to activity was smaller in the TM than in the TR animals. The activity rhythms of several of the TR animals also became noticeably less regular and precise during exposure to the skeleton regime. The physiological basis of this loss of precision in the overt rhythm is not known, but the phenomenon is frequently correlated with testicular regression (Elliott, 1974; Eskes and Zucker, 1978).

The occurrence of two alternative patterns of stable entrainment to skeleton photoperiods intended to simulate complete photoperiods in the neighborhood of 10–14 hr is a well-known property of circadian rhythms. This "bistability phenomenon" was first encountered in computer simulations of entrainment and subsequently verified in experiments with the *Drosophila* eclosion rhythm (Pittendrigh and Minis, 1964). In cases where the circadian system is involved in PTM, bistability obviously leads to rather complex expectations with regard to the photoperiodic effects of skeleton photoperiods. When those expectations are upheld (as in the above experiment), the conclusion that day length is measured by the circadian system is beyond question. How the circadian system performs the measurement is not known, and this is a much more difficult question to answer. In the next two sections we shall examine the formal properties of the hamster's photoperiodic clock in greater depth in an effort to provide some answers to this question.

E. Entrainment and Photoperiodic Induction When T Is Close to τ

If a circadian rhythm of photoinducibility (CRPP) mediates hamster PTM, then it should be possible to describe the rhythm in some detail by examining the photoperiodic effect of brief light pulses applied at numerous discrete phase points in the circadian cycle. For example, in theory, a single 1-hr pulse of light each day should prevent testicular regression or support testicular recrudescence provided it can be timed to illuminate ϕ_i. An equivalent light pulse should fail to promote testicular activity when it occurs elsewhere in the circadian cycle. In practice, the best way to make this temporal relationship explicit is to measure the location of ϕ_i with reference to the rhythm of locomotor activity which can be continuously recorded. However, one problem remains. How can one vary the phase point in the circadian cycle to be tested with light and at the same time insure that the light pulse will fall at the same circadian time each day? One obvious approach would be to observe the time of activity onset each day and then set the time of the light pulse accordingly, so that one animal would receive, for example, an hour of light every day 5 hr after activity onset, whereas another would receive light 12 hr after activity onset. This could be done manually or with the aide of an electronic activity counter and a "computer" circuit designed to switch the light on at the pre-scribed interval after activity onset. However, there is a simpler way, and that is to deliberately exploit the action of light as entraining agent for the circadian system. Since entrainment involves control over both the phase and the period of a rhythm, it is easy to vary the circadian time of a light pulse (e.g., steady-state Ψ of activity onset to light) by simply varying T, the period length of the LD cycle. The special advantage of this paradigm (hereafter called a T experiment) is that a brief light pulse seen only once per circadian cycle serves both as Zeitgeber for the circadian system and as photoperiodic stimulus, so for each value of T selected, the photoperiodic effect of the stimulus is tested at a single unique phase point in the circadian cycle (Pittendrigh and Minis, 1964; Elliott, 1976).

T experiments have been employed in insects (Pittendrigh and Minis, 1964, 1971; Saunders, 1979), lizards (Underwood, 1979), birds (Hamner and Enright, 1967; Farner et al., 1977), and mammals (Elliott, 1974, 1976) with varying degrees of success. For example, T experiments failed to demonstrate circadian involvement in PTM in two cases (lizard: Underwood, 1979; pink bollworm: Pittendrigh and Minis, 1964, 1971) where the majority of the other evidence (e.g., resonance data) also points to an hourglass mechanism. On the other hand, experiments with house sparrows (Farner et al., 1977) dem-onstrated a positive correlation between the rate of testicular growth and Ψ for a 3-hr photoperiod given in cycles of T = 20 to T = 28 hr. A similar but very weak correlation was also observed in house finches (Hamner and En-right, 1967). In the flesh fly (Saunders, 1979) and the hamster (Elliott, 1976), the goal of describing the position of ϕ_i within the circadian cycle has been largely realized in experiments utilizing a 1-hr standard light pulse and many different T values.

Examples of the activity rhythms of individual hamsters entrained to light cycles with periods of T = 23.34 hr, T = 24.00 hr, and T = 24.67 hr are shown in Fig. 13. In each case the rhythm free-ran in DD with a circadian period (τ) of close to 24 hr and then rapidly entrained following the initiation of the light cycle on day 13. The expected circadian time of the light pulse in entrainment can be predicted from the equation $\tau - T = \Delta\phi$ and the PRC. Where T = 23.34 hr, and T is therefore less than τ, the light pulse falls in the late subjective night (approximately ct 21) where it elicits the advance phase shift required to produce stable entrainment (see Fig. 8 and Pittendrigh, 1965; Pittendrigh and Daan, 1976b). Where T = 24.67 hr (T $>\tau$), the light pulse falls at the beginning of the subjective night near activity onset (ct 12) where in this case it elicits the phase delay required for stable entrainment. Where T = 24.00 hr (T $\cong \tau$), the position of the light pulse required for stable entrainment varies widely from animal to animal and depends markedly on whether τ is greater or less than T. Where (in the majority of cases) τ is greater than 24 hr, the light pulse falls at the beginning of the subjective day (ct 0) and produces the small phase advance required for entrainment (e.g., Fig. 13). In the case where τ is less than 24 hr (not shown), entrainment must involve a small phase delay in each cycle, and

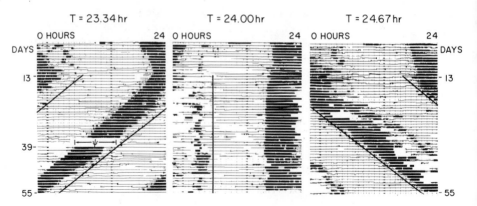

Figure 13. Circadian activity rhythm of hamsters in DD and during entrainment to light cycles with periods of T = 23.34, 24.00, and 24.67 hr. Activity recording began on the hamster's last day in LD 6:18 (lights-on 0800 to 1400). Days 2–12 of each record show the rhythm free-running in DD. The experimental light cycles were initiated on day 13. In each record, the light cycle is represented by a heavy line that connects the midpoints of 1-hr light pulses. Note the immediate effect of the light cycle on the period and phase of the activity rhythm and the dependence of ψ on T. (Reproduced with permission from Elliott, 1976.)

this can occur only if the light pulse falls in the late subjective day (e.g., ct 11). In each case described above, the entrained activity rhythm adopts the period length of the light cycle (τ_{LD} = T), and a unique and stable phase angle (Ψ) is established between the activity rhythm and the light pulse. Thus, the circadian time of the light pulse can be varied almost at will simply by varying T. In practice, the approximate limits of T to which the hamster's activity rhythm can entrain (i.e., T = 23 to 25 hr) and the value of Ψ for any given T within this range can be predicted from the relationship $\tau - T = \Delta\phi$ and the phase–response curve (Pittendrigh, 1965; Pittendrigh and Daan, 1976b). Now that we have seen how the dependence of Ψ on T can be exploited to vary the phase of the circadian cycle illuminated by a standard light pulse, we are ready to examine the photoperiodic response.

As expected, the hamster's photoperiodic response to a 1-hr light stimulus also depends markedly on T (Fig. 14). The response is, therefore, also strongly correlated with the phase of the entrained activity rhythm which is exposed to light (Fig. 15), and this correlation yields information on the precise location of ϕ_i (Elliott, 1976). In these studies ϕ_i was found to begin about 0.5 hr before activity onset and to last for 10 to 12 hr. During the remainder of the circadian cycle, including most of the subjective day, the reproductive system of hamsters is relatively insensitive to stimulation by light. Figure 14 illustrates the dependence of testicular maintenance on T observed when males raised on a 14-hr photoperiod were subjected to different T cycles or to DD for either 6, 9, or 12.5 weeks. When T is exactly 24 hr (LD 1:23), the testes regress at the normal rate (same as DD), indicating that hamsters "read" this as a short day. In contrast, testicular regression is partially (e.g., T = 23.89 hr, T = 24.27 hr) or

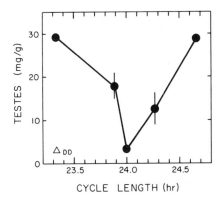

Figure 14. Photoperiodic testicular response to a 1-hr light pulse plotted as a function of the period length of the light cycle. Each point represents the mean testis weight of a group of 10 to 12 hamsters exposed to one of five experimental light cycles and sacrificed after 64 days. The experiment employed light cycles with Ts of 23.34, 23.89, 24.00, 24.27, and 24.66 hr. The testes regressed fully in DD (Δ) and in LD 1:23 (T24) control groups, but regression was partially or completely blocked in all non-24-hr T cycles. The results are most adequately interpreted with reference to the way in which the various light cycles entrain the circadian system. See text and Fig. 13. (Reproduced with permission from Elliott, 1976.)

completely (e.g., T = 23.34 hr, T = 24.66 hr) blocked in hamsters exposed to non-24 hr T cycles. In general, the closer T is to 24.1 hr (i.e., the average value of τ in DD), the greater is the extent of testicular regression observed within a given duration of treatment. When T differs from τ by ≥ 0.5 hr, the testes are maintained, indicating that hamsters interpret these T cycles as a long day (Elliott, 1974). These data clearly establish that a 1-hr light pulse can be an effective photoperiodic stimulus when T $\neq$ 24 hr, but what about the location of ϕ_i?

Figure 15 summarizes the results of a series of experiments used to examine the effectiveness of various Ts for the photoperiodic induction of testicular recrudescence. In this case, the photoperiodic response has been plotted with reference to the average circadian time of the light pulse, with activity onset designated as ct 12. The resulting graph is a circadian photoperiodic response curve. It provides specific information on the phase and duration of ϕ_i with respect to wheel-running activity and may be viewed as an empirical representation of the rhythm of photoinducibility (CRPP) thought to be responsible for the measurement of day length. Whether the assay is testicular maintenance (not shown) or testicular recrudescence (Fig. 15), the waveform of the rhythm is essentially the same. The photoinducible portion of the circadian cycle includes phase points in both the early and late subjective night, and if ϕ_i can be assumed to be continuous, it must encompass a large (10–12 hr) portion of the circadian cycle (Fig. 15). There are two portions of the circadian cycle not examined in T experiments. The "dead zone" of the hamster's phase–response curve lies between ct 1 and ct 9 (see Fig. 8)—a 1-hr light pulse falling in this region fails to shift the phase of the free-running rhythm, cannot

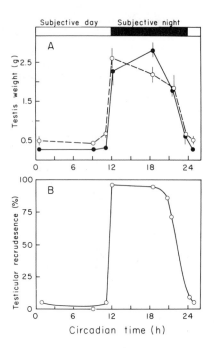

Figure 15. Circadian photoperiodic response curve for testicular recrudescence. A. Hamsters with regressed testes were transferred to one of seven different T cycles and sacrificed after 40 days of exposure. The experiment employed light cycles with periods of between T = 23.27 hr and T = 24.67 hr. Each point represents the mean testis weight of a group of 9–10 hamsters subjected to a particular light cycle, and points are plotted as a function of the mean circadian time of the light pulse for the group. Open circles, hamsters housed in individual activity cages; closed circles, hamsters housed in groups in cages without wheels. B. Circadian photoperiodic response curve for the induction of testicular recrudescence. Each point represents a percentage value based on the testicular responses of a group of 17 to 40 hamsters subjected to a particular T cycle and plotted as a function of the mean circadian time of light (1-hr pulse) as assayed from the entrainment of the activity rhythm. (Reproduced with permission from Elliott and Menaker, 1981.)

entrain the rhythm, and therefore cannot be tested for photoperiodic effect using the T cycle paradigm. However, this portion of the circadian cycle is known to be nonresponsive to photoperiodic stimuli because it is illuminated when the circadian system is entrained by standard nonstimulatory photoperiods such as LD 6:18 or LD 10:14 (see Figs. 16–18). Figure 15 also lacks points in the early subjective night between ct 12 and ct 18. This "gap" in the curve corresponds to the transition between delays and advances in the PRC. Stable entrainment is not possible with 1-hr light pulses falling in this portion of the PRC, and its photoperiodic photosensitivity could not be tested in T experiments.

To test this portion of the cycle for photoinducibility, groups of hamsters were transferred from LD 14:10 to DD and then pulsed with light (15 min) at different phases (ct) of the activity cycle approximately once every 10 days during the first month of DD. For the rest of the experiment, the animals remained in uninterrupted darkness. Ten weeks after transfer to DD, hamsters pulsed with light at cts 13, 14, 15, 16, or 18 had significantly larger testes than controls receiving no pulses. Pulses at ct 10, 12, 21, or 24 failed to alter the time course of gonadal regression in DD (Elliott, 1981). These data emphasize the overriding importance of the circadian time of the light stimulus as opposed to its duration or frequency: a 15-min pulse once every 10 circadian cycles is sufficient for induction provided it coincides with ϕ_i. The data also establish a close correlation between the magnitude of the phase shifts induced in the free-running rhythm and the size of the testes at week 10 of DD, and they indicate that ϕ_i does include the portion of the subjective night (ct 13–18) that could not be tested in T experiments. In the hamster, ϕ_i clearly encompasses a major fraction of the subjective night. This contrasts markedly with the T experiment data of Saunders (1979) that indicated that in the fleshfly, *Sarcophaga*, ϕ_i is restricted to a brief interval in the late subjective night (*ca*. ct 20).

F. Entrainment and Induction by 24-Hour LD Cycles with Different Photoperiods

In the preceding sections, we examined the formal properties of the photoperiodic clock by studying the responses of hamsters to exotic non-24-hr cycles (resonance and T experiments) and to two-pulse symmetric skeleton photoperiods. First, these experiments constitute tests of the circadian hypothesis for photoperiodic time measurement, and, as we have seen, the results provide compelling evidence in support of its general validity. Second, the information on the specific location of ϕ_i developed in T cycle experiments provides the data base for an unusually specific version of the circadian (Bünning–Pittendrigh) model for the physiological mechanism of photoperiodic time measurement. This model for the hamster's photoperiodic clock assumes (a) that the phase and duration of ϕ_i are precisely defined by the circadian photoperiodic response curve (Fig. 15B, 50% induction) and (b) that the phase angle (Ψ_{Ai}) between activity onset (ϕ_A) and the photoinducible phase (ϕ_i) remains relatively constant under a variety of conditions including entrainment of the circadian system to light cycles with different Ts and varied durations of light and dark. From these two assumptions, it follows that the model predicts photoperiodic induction to occur whenever entrainment of the circadian system exposes some fraction of ϕ_i to light. One obvious and important further test of the model is to ask how well it accommodates the system's response to the range of photoperiods (T = 24 hr) observed in nature. Does the model explain how hamsters discriminate long from short daily photoperiods? And does it accurately predict the critical day length? To obtain answers to these questions, one has simply to study rhythm of hamsters subjected to different photoperiods.

It may be helpful to begin with a comparison between photoperiods of 14 and 6 hr (Fig. 16), since these two photoperiods are employed in the laboratory to simulate summer and winter conditions. On a 14-hr photoperiod, hamsters begin wheel running shortly after dark (i.e., 9.7 hr before "dawn"), whereas on a 6-hr photoperiod, activity onset typically occurs 5–6 hr after dark (i.e., 12–13 hr before "dawn"). Since ϕ_i was found to begin 0.5 hr before activity onset and to last for a minimum of about 10 hr thereafter (Fig. 15B), it follows that a 14-hr photoperiod must illuminate ϕ_i. Indeed, it appears that the photostimulatory effect of LD 14:10 involves two separate events: light at dusk falls at the beginning, and light at dawn at the end of ϕ_i. On a 6-hr photoperiod, all of ϕ_i occurs in the dark, and this is consistent with the observation that a 6-hr photoperiod promotes regression of the testes. Thus, the model clearly accommodates the gonadal responses to long and short photoperiods (T = 24 hr) that are representative of those typically employed in laboratory studies of hamster photoperiodism. However, a more exacting test is to examine how well the model "predicts" the gonadal response to photoperiods in the neighborhood of 12 hr.

In studies of photoperiodic time measurement, it is customary to begin by obtaining a standard photoperiodic response curve that plots the photoperiodic response as a function of photoperiod (hours of light/24 hr). The critical day length is then defined as the point where the switchover from "short-" to "long-day" responses occurs or as the minimum (or maximum) photoperiod that will induce a particular response. Figure 17 shows the results

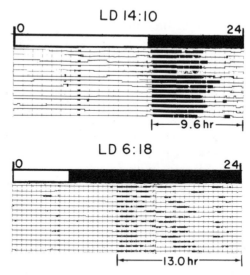

Figure 16. Entrainment to photoperiods of 6 and 14 light per day. The circadian activity rhythms of two hamsters, one entrained to LD 14:10, and one to LD 6:18, are shown. The light cycle is diagrammed at the top of a 14-day portion of data from each hamster. The arrow beneath the last day of each record indicates the ψ value (14-day average) for the individual whose record is shown. The difference in the value of ψ on a 14-hr as compared to a 6-hr photoperiod correlates well with the photoperiodic response. See text for discussion. (Reproduced with permission from Elliott, 1976.)

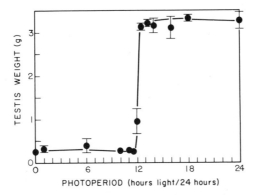

Figure 17. Testicular response to photoperiods ranging in short steps from 0 to 24 hr light per day. Each point represents the mean paired testis weight of a group of hamsters subjected to the indicated photoperiod for the previous 95–96 days (except for 6-hr photoperiod, 85 days). Note that only photoperiods of at least 12.5 hr light/day result in maintenance of the testes. The "critical" day length lies between 12 and 12.5 hr. (Reproduced with permission from Elliott, 1976.)

obtained with male hamsters subjected to photoperiods ranging in short steps from 0 to 24 hr light per day. The data shows that day length measurement by hamsters is remarkably precise, with a clear "break" occurring between photoperiods of 12.0 and 12.5 hr. The data in Fig. 17 are for the photoperiodic maintenance of the testes, but essentially the same result is obtained when the assay is photostimulated testicular growth; at least 12.5 hr of light per day is required for photoperiodic stimulation of testicular function (Elliott, 1974).

Figure 18 shows how the phase angle (Ψ) of entrained wheel-running activity measured with reference to dawn varies with the duration of the photoperiod for photoperiods of 1 to 8 hr. The first point of interest is that Ψ remains essentially constant for all photoperiods of less than 11.5 hr. On very short photoperiods, the phase of the activity rhythm is usually determined solely by the time of the lights-on transition because τ is (nearly always) longer than 24 hr. In such cases, entrainment is achieved entirely via a small phase advance elicited each morning when the lights come on, and this typically occurs 12–13 hr after the onset of activity the previous night. As the length of the photoperiod is increased (up to 11 or 11.5 hr), the only significant change is that more and more of the subjective day is exposed to light, while ϕ_i remains in the dark. When the photoperiod is increased beyond 11 hr, entrainment begins to involve a balance between phase delays elicited by light in the evening near activity onset and phase advances elicited by light in the morning. As a result of this interaction, the phase of the activity rhythm changes with reference to both the lights-on and the lights-off transitions. Thus, as the photoperiod is increased from 11.5 hr to 18 hr, there is a stepwise decrease in Ψ with increased duration of the photoperiod, and this is consistent with the switch from a "short-day" to a "long-day" photoperiodic response. On a 12-hr photoperiod, the longest photoperiod inducing a short-day response, activity onset precedes

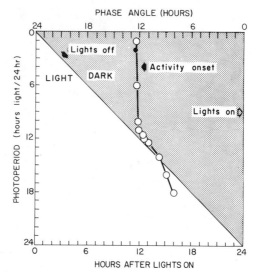

Figure 18. Temporal relationships between activity onset and the light and dark portions of the LD cycle during entrainment to photoperiods of 1 to 18 hr light/day. The vertical sides of the square represent the time of lights-on, and the diagonal line the time of lights-off for each photoperiod indicated on the vertical axis. Each point (open circle) represents the mean phase at which a group of hamsters began their daily activity while entrained to the indicated photoperiod (the small filled circle represents the phase of one hamster entrained to LD 2:22). The phase angle scale reads "backwards" because ψ is measured from activity onsets to lights-on. Note that the phase of activity is not much affected by the time of lights-off until a photoperiod of 11.5 hr is reached; as the photoperiod becomes longer, there is a progressive reduction in ψ as light penetrates into the subjective night. The switch from a "short-day" to a "long-day" reproductive response between photoperiods of 12 and 12.5 hr is correlated with a very slight (0. 6 hr) but critical change in ψ. (Reproduced with permission from Elliott, 1976.)

lights-on by approximately 11.5 hr ($\bar{\Psi} = 11.5 \pm 0.1$ hr), whereas on a 12.5-hr photoperiod, which is the shortest long day, onset occurs about 11 hr before lights-on ($\bar{\Psi} = 10.9 \pm 0.1$ hr). On both photoperiods, activity onset occurs approximately 0.5 hr after the lights go out.

The potential significance of this small change in Ψ (between photoperiods of 12 and 12.5 hr) should be clear from earlier discussions. A photoperiod of 12.5 hr is just long enough to bring ϕ_i into the light. One way to see how well the model accommodates these results is to use the present data to derive an independent estimate of the phase and duration of ϕ_i with reference to the activity rhythm. To do this, one must assume that the limits of ϕ_i are defined by those points in the circadian cycle that escape illumination on a 12-hr photoperiod but that are illuminated on a 12.5-hr photoperiod and that ϕ_i is continuous between these two phase points. According to this, one estimates that ϕ_i should begin about 0.5 hr before activity onset and end approximately 11 or 11.5 hr thereafter. The agreement between this estimate based on 24-hr LD cycles with different photoperiods and the data on the location of ϕ_i obtained in T experiments (Fig. 15) is very good. One is forced to conclude that the impressive difference in the response of the reproductive system to photo-periods of 12 and 12.5 hr can be traced to what would otherwise appear to be a very subtle change in the characteristics of entrainment of the circadian system.

G. Photoperiodic Time Measurement and the Regulation of the Annual Cycle

The study of photoperiodic time measurement and the formal properties of circadian rhythms can sometimes appear complicated to a student first approaching the subject. Its power lies in the fact that a quantitative formal model with relatively few parameters can account for so many aspects of biological rhythmicity. A basic understanding of circadian physiology includ-ing the entrainment of circadian rhythms by light can provide a framework for understanding other aspects of physiology including the photoperiodic control of reproduction. On this note, we return to the subject posed at the beginning of this chapter, how photoperiod regulates the timing of the annual cycle.

The critical event initiating the annual gonadal cycle is the autumnal decrease in photoperiod below 12.5 hr (see Figs. 1, 17). When this occurs, light fails to illuminate ϕ_i, and gonadal regression is initiated. After they regress, the gonads remain quiescent for an additional 8–10 weeks before gradual changes in the activity of the neuroendocrine–gonadal axis (Turek et al., 1975) eventu-ally culminate in spontaneous gonadal recrudescence and a complete recovery of the testes before the spring equinox (Vandreley et al., 1972). On the basis of this account, it can be seen that the critical role of photoperiodic time mea-surement is to insure that the breeding season is terminated in the fall in advance of the less favorable conditions of winter. Moreover, since the re-growth of the testes in the "late winter phase" of the gonadal cycle occurs spontaneously before day length reaches 12.5 hr, the timing of testicular regression in the fall must be regarded as the primary event that sets the phase of the entire annual cycle.

Although the long photoperiods of spring and summer are clearly not important for the initiation of gonadal recrudescence, they do play a significant role in the regulation of the annual cycle, since the exposure to long photo-periods is necessary to terminate refractoriness and to reinstate photo-sensitivity (Reiter, 1972a). This sets the stage so that the short days of fall can once again initiate the gonadal cycle. Thus, PTM mediated by the circadian system plays an essential role both in reinstating photosensitivity in the summer and in initiating gonadal regression at the proper time in the fall. The value of entrusting this function to the circadian system may lie in the history depen-dence and plasticity of circadian oscillators as well as in their remarkable stability and precision under constant conditions (Pittendrigh and Daan, 1976a–c). In the hamster, for example, it is clear that a 2% change in either T (Elliott, 1974, 1976) or τ (Eskes and Zucker, 1978) is sufficient to disrupt PTM so that a short photoperiod becomes inductive. A corollary of this is that, at least in this species, natural selection could achieve a substantial change in the length and timing of the breeding season or abolish seasonality entirely simply by producing a 2% (0.5-hr) change in the species τ or in the phase relation between ϕ_i and the PRC of the circadian pacemaker. Natural selection could also adjust the critical day length by changing the duration of ϕ_i. Its duration in the hamster is long compared with that in *Sarcophaga* (Saunders, 1979), and it will be of interest to see whether this feature is peculiar to the hamster or will prove to be generally characteristic of species with nocturnal and fossorial habits (see related discussion in Section I.E.2).

III. SUMMARY AND OUTLOOK

Seasonal reproduction regulated by daylength is widespread among organisms. In this chapter, we have focused our attention on a few species of mammals and birds and, in particular, the Syrian hamster to illustrate concepts and methodology that we hope will apply more generally to research on other species. In Section I, we discussed some aspects of neuroendocrinology related to vertebrate photoperiodism. In mammals, the pineal gland and its hormone melatonin appear essential for the photoperiodic response of the reproductive system. The pronounced circadian rhythmicity in pineal melatonin synthesis combined with a rapid suppression of the nocturnal peak by light suggested that this hormone might be involved in transmitting information about day length from the circadian system to the reproductive system. However, in the Syrian hamster, the nocturnal peak in pineal melatonin appears to be about the same duration and to occur at the same phase in relation to the activity cycle whether hamsters are entrained to long or short photoperiods or are free-running in continuous darkness. Another possibility is that the melatonin rhythm is involved as part of the machinery for timing the long interval between photoperiodic induction of gonadal regression and the occurrence of spontaneous gonadal recrudescence and the associated period of photorefractoriness. However, this "calendar" hypothesis has not been tested, and further research is also needed on the photoperiodic control of pineal melatonin synthesis. It may be that a very small change in the pattern of melatonin synthesis or its phase relationship to some other rhythm is critical in triggering the photoperiodic response. If so, careful and more frequent measurements and/or the identification of other component(s) of the photoperiodic control mechanism may be required before we can hope to understand the role of the pineal gland. Successful experiments based on precisely controlled temporal patterning of exogenous melatonin administered by infusion to pinealectomized animals could resolve many of these questions about pineal function. Similar investigations should also be undertaken in other species.

In mammals and birds, the photoperiodic timing of the annual cycle is mediated by the circadian system. In Section II, we discussed the formal properties of the photoperiodic clock. The clock is based on a circadian rhythm of response to light that is entrained to the daily photoperiod. The photoinducible phase (ϕ_i) of the rhythm has been described by assaying the response of the reproductive system to light occurring at different phases of the circadian cycle. In the case of the Syrian hamster, this analysis has been used to define the phase and duration of ϕ_i with respect to the circadian activity rhythm. This provides the basis of a model that accounts for photoperiodic control of the annual cycle in terms of entrainment of the circadian rhythm. In entrainment to a long photoperiod, ϕ_i is illuminated, and the gonads are maintained; on a short photoperiod, ϕ_i lies in the dark, and the gonads regress. Although this model accounts for the circadian basis and precision of day length measurement in the hamster, in its present form, it is solely descriptive. The major challenge ahead is to unveil the cellular and neuroendocrine machinery responsible for the time measurement and for the transfer of photoperiodic information from the circadian system to the reproductive system.

As discussed in Section I, some progress has already been made in this direction. The pineal gland and its circadian rhythm of melatonin synthesis are surely involved, but precisely how remains to be determined. The suprachiasmatic nuclei (SCN) of the anterior hypothalamus are also essential for the photoperiodic response as well as for the normal entrainment of a variety of rodent circadian rhythms. In addition, the SCN appear to function as a pacemaker or as part of the pacemaking system for many rodent circadian rhythms including the rhythm of pineal melatonin synthesis (see reviews by Menaker *et al.,* 1978; Rusak and Zucker, 1979). Thus, it seems likely that the SCN are directly involved in photoperiodic time measurement, perhaps via circadian regulation of pineal melatonin synthesis. However, this remains an open question, and further experiments are required to clarify the role of the pineal and the SCN in photoperiodic time measurement. At present, it appears that one goal of this research should be to understand the circadian rhythm of photoinducibility in terms of the physiological action of light on SCN and pineal function.

REFERENCES

Aschoff, J., and Wever, R., 1976, Human circadian rhythms: A multioscillatory system, *Fed. Proc.* **35**:2326.

Bartke, A., Goldman, B. D., Bex, F. J., and Dalterio, S., 1978, Mechanism of reversible loss of reproductive capacity in a seasonally-breeding mammal, *Int. J. Androl.* (Suppl. 2), pp. 345–353.

Beck, S. D., 1968, *Insect Photoperiodism,* Academic Press, New York.

Berndtson, W., and Desjardins, C., 1974, Circulating LH and FSH levels and testicular function in hamsters during light deprivation and subsequent photoperiodic stimulation, *Endocrinology* **95**:195.

Bex, F., Bartke, A., Goldman, B. D., and Dalterio, S., 1978, Prolactin, growth hormone, luteinizing hormone receptors, and seasonal changes in testicular activity in the golden hamster, *Endocrinology* **103**:2069.

Binkley, S., 1976, Pineal gland biorhythms: N-Acetyltransferase in chickens and rats, *Fed. Proc.* **35**:2347.

Binkley, S., 1979, A timekeeping enzyme in the pineal gland, *Sci. Am.* **240**:66.

Bittman, E. L., 1978, Hamster refractoriness: The role of insensitivity of pineal target tissues, *Science* **202**:648.

Bittman, E. L., and Goldman, B. D., 1979, Serum gonadotropin levels in hamsters exposed to short photoperiods: Effects of adrenalectomy and ovarectomy, *Endocrinology* **83**:113.

Bittman, E. L., Goldman, B. D., and Zucker, I., 1979, Testicular responses to melatonin are altered by lesions of the suprachiasmatic nuclei in golden hamsters, *Biol. Reprod.* **21**:647.

Bourne, R. A., and Tucker, H. A., 1975, Serum prolactin and LH responses to photoperiod in bull calves, *Endocrinology* **97**:473.

Bünning, E., 1936, Die endogene Togesrhythmik als Grundlage der photoperiodischen Reaktion, *Ber. Dtsch. Bot. Ges.* **54**:590.

Bünning, E., 1960, Circadian rhythms and time measurement in photoperiodism, *Cold Spring Harbor Symp. Quant. Biol.* **25**:249.

Campbell, C. S., Finkelstein, J. S., and Turek, F. W., 1978, The interaction of photoperiod and testosterone on the development of copulatory behavior in castrated male hamsters, *Physiol. Behav.* **21**:409.

Daan, S., and Pittendrigh, C. S., 1976, A functional analysis of circadian pacemakers in nocturnal rodents II. The variability of phase response curves. *J. Comp. Physiol.* **106**:253.

Elliott, J. A., 1974, Photoperiodic regulation of testis function in the golden hamster: Relation to the circadian system, Ph.D. Thesis, University of Texas, Austin.

Elliott, J. A., 1976, Circadian rhythms and photoperiodic time measurement in mammals, *Fed. Proc.* **35**:2339.

Elliott, J. A., 1981, Circadian rhythms, entrainment and photoperiodism in the Syrian hamster, in: *Biological Clocks in Seasonal Reproductive Cycles* (B. K. Follett, ed.), J. Wright, Bristol, England (in press).

Elliott, J. A., and Menaker, M., 1981, Circadian basis of photoperiodic time measurement in male golden hamsters I. Entrainment and induction by T cycles, *Biol. Reprod.* (submitted).

Elliott, J. A., Stetson, M. J., and Menaker, M., 1972, Regulation of testis function in golden hamsters: A circadian clock measures photoperiodic time, *Science* **178**:771.

Ellis, G. B., and Turek, F. W., 1979, Time course of the photoperiod-induced change in sensitivity of the hypothalamic–pituitary axis to testosterone feedback in castrated male hamsters, *Endocrinology* **104**:625.

Eskes, G. A., and Zucker, I., 1978, Photoperiodic regulation of the hamster testis: Dependence on circadian rhythms, *Proc. Natl. Acad. Sci. USA* **75**:1034.

Farner, D. S., Donham, R. S., Lewis, R. A., Mattocks, P. W., Jr., Darden, T. R., and Smith, J. P., 1977, The circadian component in the photoperiodic mechanism of the house sparrow, *Passer domesticus, Physiol. Zool.* **50**:247.

Follett, B. K., 1973, Circadian rhythms and photoperiodic time measurement in birds. *J. Reprod. Fertil. (Suppl.)* **19**:5.

Follett, B. K., 1978, Photoperiodism and seasonal breeding in birds and mammals, in: *Control of Ovulation* (G. E. Lamming and D. B. Crighton, eds.), pp. 267–293, Butterworth Press, London.

Follett, B. K., and Davies, D. T., 1975, Photoperiodicity and the neuroendocrine control of reproduction in birds, *Symp. Zool. Soc. Lond.* **35**:199.

Follett, B. K., and Sharp, P. J., 1969, Circadian rhythmicity in photoperiodically induced gonadotropin release and gonadol growth in the quail, *Nature* **223**:968.

Follett, B. K., Mattocks, P. W., Jr., and Farner, D. S., 1974, Circadian function in the photoperiodic induction of gonadotropin secretion in the white-crowned sparrow, *Zonotrichia leucophrys gambellii, Proc. Natl. Acad. Sci. USA* **71**:1666.

Follett, B. K., Farner, D. S., and Mattocks, P. W., Jr., 1975, Luteinizing hormone in the plasma of white-crowned sparrows *(Zontorichia Leucophrys gambelii)* during artificial photostimulation, *Gen. Comp. Endocrinol.* **26**:126.

Gaston, S., and Menaker, M., 1967, Photoperiodic control of hamster testis, *Science* **167**:925.

Goldman, B., Hall, V., Hollister, C., Roychoudhury, P., Tamarkin, L., and Westrom, W., 1979,

Effects of melatonin on the reproductive system in Syrian hamsters maintained under various photoperiods, *Endocrinology* **104**:82.

Grococh, C. A., and Clarke, J. R., 1974, Photoperiodic control of testis activity in the vole, *Microtus agrestis, J. Reprod. Fertil.* **43**:461.

Gwinner, E., 1975, Effects of season and external testosterone on the free-running circadian activity rhythm of European starlings *(Sturnus vulgaris), J. Comp. Physiol.* **103**:315.

Gwinner, E., 1978, Effects of pinealectomy on circadian locomotor activity rhythms in European starlings, *Sturnus vulgaris, J. Comp. Physiol.* **126**:123.

Gwinner, E., and Benzinger, J., 1978, Synchronization of circadian rhythm in pinealectomized European starlings by daily injection of melatonin, *J. Comp. Physiol.* **127**:209.

Hall, V., and Goldman, B., 1980. Effects of gonadal steroid hormones on hibernation in the Turkish hamster *(Mesocricetus brandti), J. Comp. Physiol.* **135**:107.

Hamner, W. M., 1963, Diurnal rhythm and photoperiodism in testicular recrudescence in the house finch, *Science* **142**:1294.

Hamner, W. M., and Enright, J. T., 1967, Relationships between photoperiodism and circadian rhythms of activity in the house finch, *J. Exp. Biol.* **46**:43.

Herbert, J., 1972, Initial observations on pinealectomized ferrets kept for long periods in either daylight or artificial illumination, *J. Endocrinol.* **55**:591.

Hoffman, R. A., and Melvin, H., 1974, Gonadal responses of hamsters to interrupted dark periods, *Biol. Reprod.* **10**:19.

Hoffman, R. A., and Reiter, R. J., 1965, Pineal gland: Influence on gonads of male hamsters, *Science* **148**:1609.

Jenner, C. E., and Engels, W. L., 1952, The significance of the dark period in the photoperiod response of male juncos and white throated sparrows, *Biol. Bull.* **103**:345.

Kirkpatrick, C. M., and Leopold, A. C., 1952, The role of darkness in the sexual activity of the quail, *Science* **116**:280.

Klein, D. C., and Weller, J., 1970. Indole metabolism in the pineal gland: A circadian rhythm in *N*-acetyltransferase, *Science* **169**:1093.

Lees, A. D., 1966, Photoperiodic timing mechanisms in insects, *Nature* **210**:986.

Legan, S. J., Karsch, F. J., and Foster, D. L., 1977, The endocrine control of seasonal reproductive function in the ewe: A marked change in response to the negative feedback action of estradiol on luteinizing hormone secretion, *Endocrinology* **101**:818.

Leining, K. B., Bourne, R. A., and Tucker, H. A., 1979, Prolactin response to duration and wavelength of light in prepubertal bulls, *Endocrinology* **104**:289.

Lincoln, G. A., Guinness, F., and Short, R. V., 1972, The way in which testosterone controls the social and sexual behavior of the red deer stag *(Cervus elaphus), Horm. Behav.* **3**:375.

Martin, J., and Klein, D., 1976, Melatonin inhibition of the neonatal pituitary response to luteinizing-hormone-releasing factor, *Science* **191**:301.

McMillan, J. P., Underwood, H. A., Elliott, J. A., Stetson, M. H., and Menaker, M., 1975, Extraretinal light perception in the sparrow. IV. Further evidence that the eyes do not participate in photoperiodic photoreception, *J. Comp. Physiol.* **97**:205.

Menaker, M., 1974, Aspects of the physiology of circadian rhythmicity in the vertebrate nervous system, in: *The Neurosciences: Third Study Program* (F. O. Schmitt and F. G. Worden, eds.), pp. 479–489, MIT Press, Cambridge, Massachusetts.

Menaker, M., and Underwood, H., 1976, Extraretinal photoreception in birds, *Photochem. Photobiol.* **23**:299.

Menaker, M., Takahashi, J. S., and Eskin, A., 1978, The physiology of circadian pacemakers, *Annu. Rev. Physiol.* **40**:501.

Moore-Ede, M. C., Schmelzer, W. S., Koss, D. A., and Herd, A. J., 1976, Internal organization of the circadian timing system in multicellular animals, *Fed. Proc.* **35**:2333.

Morin, L. P., and Zucker, I., 1978, Photoperiodic regulation of copulatory behavior in the male hamster, *J. Endocrinol.* **77**:249.

Morin, L. P., Fitzgerald, K. M., Rusak, B., and Zucker, I., 1977, Circadian organization and neural mediation of hamster reproductive rhythms, *Psychoneuroendocrinology* **2**:73.

Mrosovsky, N., 1971, *Hibernation and the Hypothalamus*, Appleton-Century-Crofts, New York.

Nanda, K. K., and Hamner, K. C., 1958, Studies on the nature of the endogenous rhythm affecting photoperiodic response of Biloxi soybean, *Bot. Gaz.* **120**:14.

Nicholls, T. J., and Follett, B. K., 1974, The photoperiodic control of reproduction in *Coturnix* quail: The temporal pattern of LH secretion, *J. Comp. Physiol.* **93**:301.

Panke, E. S., Rollag, M. D., and Reiter, R. J., 1979, Pineal melatonin concentrations in the Syrian hamster, *Endocrinology* **104**:194.

Pelletier, J., and Ortavant, R., 1975, Photoperiodic control of LH release in the ram. II Light–androgens interaction, *Acta Endocrinol. (Kbh.)* **78**:442.

Pengelley, E. T., and Asmundson, S. J., 1974, Circannual rhythmicity in hibernating mammals, in: *Circannual Clocks* (E. T. Pengelley, ed.), pp. 95–160, Academic Press, New York.

Pittendrigh, C. S., 1960, Circadian rhythms and the circadian organization of living systems, *Cold Spring Harbor Symp. Quant. Biol.* **25**:159.

Pittendrigh, C. S., 1965, On the mechanism of entrainment of a circadian rhythm by light cycles, in: *Circadian Clocks* (J. Aschoff, ed.), pp. 277–297, North-Holland, Amsterdam.

Pittendrigh, C. S., 1966, The circadian oscillation in *Drosophila pseudoobscura pupae:* A model for the photoperiodic clock, *Z. Pflanzenphysiol.* **54**:275.

Pittendrigh, C. S., 1972, Circadian surfaces and the diversity of possible roles of circadian organization in photoperiodic induction, *Proc. Natl. Acad. Sci. USA* **69**:2734.

Pittendrigh, C. S., 1974, Circadian oscillations in cells and the circadian organization of multicellular systems, in: *The Neurosciences: Third Study Program* (F. O. Schmitt and F. G. Worden, eds.), pp. 437–458, MIT Press, Cambridge, Massachusetts.

Pittendrigh, C. S., and Daan, S., 1976a, A functional analysis of circadian pacemakers in noctural rodents, I. The stability and lability of spontaneous frequency, *J. Comp. Physiol.* **106**:223.

Pittendrigh, C. S., and Daan, S., 1976b, A functional analysis of circadian pacemakers in nocturnal rodents IV. Entrainment: Pacemaker as clock, *J. Comp. Physiol.* **106**:291.

Pittendrigh, C. S., and Daan, S., 1976c, A functional analysis of circadian pacemakers in nocturnal rodents, V. Pacemaker structure: A clock for all seasons, *J. Comp. Physiol.* **106**:333.

Pittendrigh, C. S., and Minis, D. H., 1964, The entrainment of circadian oscillations by light and their role as photoperiodic clocks, *Am. Natur.* **98**:261.

Pittendrigh, C. S., and Minis, D. H., 1971, The photoperiodic time measurement in *Pectinophora gossypiella* and its relation to the circadian system in that species, in: *Biochronometry* (M. Menaker, ed.), p. 212–247, National Academy of Sciences, Washington.

Ravault, J. P., 1976, Prolactin in the ram: Seasonal variations in the concentration of blood plasma from birth until three years old, *Acta Endocrinol. (Kbh.)* **83**:720.

Reiter, R. J., 1972a, Evidence for refractoriness of the pituitary gonadal axis to the pineal gland in golden hamsters and its possible implications in annual reproductive rhythms, *Anat. Rec.* **173**:365.

Reiter, R. J., 1972b, Surgical procedures involving the pineal gland which prevent gonadal degeneration in adult male hamsters, *Ann. Endocrinol. (Paris)* **33**:571.

Reiter, R. J., 1973a, Pineal control of a seasonal reproductive rhythm in male golden hamsters exposed to natural daylight and temperature, *Endocrinology* **92**:423.

Reiter, R. J., 1973b, *Annu. Rev. Physiol.* **35**:305.

Reppert, S. M., Perlow, M. J., Tamarkin, L., and Klein, D. C., 1979, A diurnal melatonin rhythm in primate cerebrospineal fluid, *Endocrinology* **104**:295.

Rollag, M. D., and Niswender, G. D., 1976, Radioimmunoassay of serum concentrations of melatonin in sheep exposed to different lighting regimes, *Endocrinology* **98**:482.

Rowan, W., 1925, Relation of light to bird migration and development changes, *Nature* **115**:494.

Rusak, B., and Zucker, I., 1979, Neural regulation of circadian rhythms, *Physiol. Rev.* **59**:449.

Sadleir, M. F. S., 1973, *The Reproduction of Vertebrates*, Academic Press, New York.

Saunders, D. S., 1976, The circadian eclosion rhythm in *Sarcophaga argyrostoma:* Some comparisons with the photoperiodic clock, *J. Comp. Physiol.* **110**:111.

Saunders, D. S., 1979, External coincidence and the photoinducible phase on the *Sarcophaga* photoperiodic clock, *J. Comp. Physiol.* **132**:179.

Schwab, R. S., 1971, Circannian testicular periodicity in the European starling in the absence of the photoperiodic change, in: *Biochronometry* (M. Menaker, ed.), pp. 428–447, National Academy of Sciences, Washington.

Skopik, S. D., and Bowen, M. F., 1976, Insect photoperiodism: An hourglass measures photoperiodic time in *Ostrinia nubilalis, J. Comp. Physiol.* **111**:249.

Stetson, M. H., and Watson-Whitmyre, M., 1976, Nucleus suprachiasmaticus: The biological clock in Hamsters? *Science* **191**:197.

Stetson, M. H., Matt, K. S., and Watson-Whitmyre, M., 1976, Photoperiodism and reproduction in golden hamsters: Circadian organization and the termination of photorefractoriness, *Biol. Reprod.* **14**:531.

Stetson, M. H., Watson-Whitmyre, M., and Matt, K. S., 1977, Termination of photorefractoriness in golden hamsters: Photoperiodic requirements, *J. Exp. Zool.* **202**:81.

Tamarkin, L., 1977, Photoperiod and melatonin: Effects on the reproductive system of the Syrian hamster, Ph.D. Thesis, University of Connecticut.

Tamarkin, L., Hutchison, J. S., and Goldman, B. D., 1976a, Regulation of serum gonadotropins by photoperiod and testicular hormone in the Syrian hamster, *Endocrinology* **99**:1528.

Tamarkin, L., Westrom, W. K., Hamill, A. I., and Goldman, B. D., 1976b, Effect of melatonin on the reproductive systems of male and female Syrian hamsters: A diurnal rhythm in sensitivity to melatonin, *Endocrinology* **99**:1534.

Tamarkin, L., Hollister, C. W., Lefebvre, N. G., and Goldman, B. D., 1977, Melatonin induction of gonadal quiescence in pinealectomized Syrian hamsters, *Science* **198**:953.

Tamarkin, L. S., Reppert, S. M., and Klein, D. C., 1979, Regulation of pineal melatonin in the Syrian hamster, *Endocrinology* **104**:395.

Tamarkin, L., Reppert, S. M., Klein, D. C., Pratt, B., and Goldman, B. D., 1980, Studies on the daily pattern of pineal melatonin in the Syrian hamster, *Endocrinology* **107**:1525.

Turek, F. W., 1972, Circadian involvement in termination of the refractory period in two sparrows, *Science* **178**:1112.

Turek, F. W., 1974, Circadian rhythmicity and the initiation of gonadal growth in sparrows, *J. Comp. Physiol.* **96**:27.

Turek, F. W., 1977, The interaction of the photoperiod and testosterone in regulating serum gonadotropin levels in castrated male hamsters, *Endocrinology* **101**:1210.

Turek, F. W., and Campbell, C. S., 1979, Photoperiodic regulation of neuroendocrine–gonadal activity, *Biol. Reprod.* **20**:32.

Turek, F. W., Elliott, J. A., Alvis, J. D., and Menaker, M., 1975, Effect of prolonged exposure to non-stimulatory photoperiods in the activity of the neuroendocrine–testicular axis of the golden hamster, *Biol. Reprod.* **13**:475.

Turek, F. W., McMillan, J. P., and Menaker, M., 1976, Melatonin: Effects on the circadian locomotor rhythms of sparrows, *Science* **194**:1441.

Turek, F. W., Alvis, J. P., and Menaker, M., 1977, Pituitary responsiveness to LRF in castrated male hamsters exposed to different photoperiodic conditions, *Neuroendocrinology* **24**:140.

Underwood, H., 1973, Retinal and extraretinal photoreceptors mediate entrainment of the circadian locomotor rhythm in lizards, *J. Comp. Physiol.* **83**:187.

Underwood, H., 1975, Extraretinal light receptors can mediate photoperiodic photoreception in the male lizard *Anolis carolinensis, J. Comp. Physiol.* **99**:71.

Underwood, H., 1979, Photoperiodic time measurement in the male lizard *Anolis carolinensis, J. Comp. Physiol.* **125**:143.

Vendreley, E., Guerrilot, C., and Da Lage, C., 1972, Variations saissonaires de l'activite des cellules de Sertoli et de Leydig dans le testicule du Hamster dore: Etude caryometrique, *C. R. Acad. Sci. [D] (Paris)* **275**:1143.

Yokoyama, K., and Farner, D. S., 1978, Induction of Zugunruhe by photostimulation of encephalic receptors in white-crowned sparrows, *Science* **201**:76.

Zimmerman, N. H., and Menaker, M., 1975, Neural connections of sparrow pineal: Role in circadian control of activity, *Science* **190**:477.

Zimmerman, N. H., and Menaker, M., 1979, The pineal gland: A pacemaker within the circadian system of the house sparrow, *Proc. Natl. Acad. Sci. USA* **76**:999.

IV

Control of Reproduction on the Cellular and Chemical Level

CNS Control of the Pituitary

Neurochemistry of Hypothalamic Releasing and Inhibitory Hormones

SAMUEL McCANN

I. INTRODUCTION

In this chapter I should like to describe the saga of the discovery of the hypothalamic neurohormones that regulate the secretion of anterior pituitary hormones, discuss the current status of their chemistry and the factors that influence their release, and allude briefly to some possible clinical applications of these neurohormones. I shall try to present the current status of this rapidly advancing field but shall not document all statements with references. Instead, I shall provide key references, mostly to reviews, that should enable the interested student to delve further into the literature.

II. EVIDENCE FOR HYPOTHALAMIC CONTROL OF ANTERIOR PITUITARY HORMONE RELEASE

Evidence for hypothalamic control of the anterior pituitary has come primarily from studies employing hypothalamic lesions or stimulation. As early as the 1920s, Bailey and Bremer reported that lesions in the hypothalamus could induce gonadal atrophy in the dog, even in the presence of what ap-

SAMUEL McCANN • Department of Physiology, University of Texas Southwestern Medical School at Dallas, Dallas, Texas 75235.

peared to be a histologically normal pituitary gland. Shortly after he developed the technique for hypophysectomy in the rat, P.E. Smith described what he called the "tuberal syndrome," a term that encompassed the reproductive disorders induced by lesions in the basal tuberal region. Subsequent work by Dey in Ranson's laboratory clarified two syndromes. One, which followed lesions in the region of the median eminence, was associated with gonadal atrophy in both sexes and cessation of reproductive cycles in the female, whereas the other syndrome, induced by large lesions over the optic chiasm, was associated with large ovarian follicles and evidence of constant stimulation of the accessory sex organs by estrogen in females. These animals fail to ovulate because of suppression of LH release. Dey's work was done in the guinea pig, but subsequent studies clearly showed that the same two syndromes could be obtained in the rat. Some time later, it was shown that lesions in the region of the median eminence also interfered with ACTH secretion, and, thereafter, anterior hypothalamic and median eminence lesions were shown to block at least partially the secretion of TSH. Massive basal hypothalamic lesions were shown to interfere with the secretion of growth hormone as well.

In contrast to the deficiences obtained in the secretion of the hormones just listed, the secretion of two hormones appeared to be enhanced by hypothalamic lesions. These two hormones were prolactin and MSH.

Even as early as the mid-1930s, it was shown that hypothalamic stimulation could induce ovulation in the rabbit. Later, Sawyer, Everett, and Markee were able to show that similar stimulation delivered to the anterior lobe itself was ineffective, indicating that the anterior lobe itself was not electrically excitable. Subsequent work by many investigators has shown that hypothalamic stimulation can induce a release of FSH, LH, ACTH, growth hormone, and TSH. Thus, on the basis of these lesion and stimulation studies, it would appear that the hypothalamus exerts a net stimulatory influence on the secretion of all anterior pituitary hormones with the exception of prolactin, which is inhibited. The predominant influence on the secretion of MSH by the intermediate lobe also appears to be inhibitory.

These lesion and stimulation studies have also delimited, to some extent at least, the regions of the hypothalamus that are concerned with the secretion of particular anterior pituitary hormones. This has been most clearly worked out in the case of the gonadotropins. In this case, lesions in the median eminence of the tuber cinereum interfere drastically with the secretion of both FSH and LH and result in cessation of estrous cycles and suppression of follicular growth in females and the atrophy of the testis and male accessory organs in the male. In the female, because of the fact that these lesions also augment prolactin secretion, corpora lutea are maintained.

Lesions over the optic chiasm, so-called suprachiasmatic lesions, lead to another syndrome in which the ovaries are filled with large follicles that appear poised on the brink of ovulation, but ovulation does not occur. These animals secrete estrogen, which produces vaginal cornification. They exhibit more or less constant vaginal cornification, which is frequently called "constant estrus."

It is noteworthy, however, that these animals are not in estrus in a behavioral sense, although they are not totally unreceptive.

Examination of the endocrine deficiences in these animals, utilizing radioimmunoassay of gonadotropins, has revealed that the defect appears to be in the stimulatory action of the gonadal steroids that normally evoke the preovulatory discharge of FSH and LH in the intact female. In these animals with suprachiasmatic lesions, it has been shown by radioimmunoassay of plasma FSH and LH that the stimulatory action of progesterone on LH secretion is absent, but that on FSH secretion is retained, suggesting a selective deficiency in LH release. This, of course, could account for the failure of these animals to ovulate. In contrast to the normal animal which ovulates as the result of an estrogen-induced preovulatory gonadotropin surge, in the lesioned animals, the preovulatory estrogen fails to stimulate LH release, and, consequently, the animals do not ovulate. Thus, these lesions appear to destroy a region that mediates the stimulatory action of estrogen and progesterone on LH release while leaving the stimulatory action on FSH intact. Basal release of FSH and LH is not abolished, and this results in the follicular development and estrogen secretion.

Conversely, electrochemical stimulation of the same suprachiasmatic region evokes only LH and not FSH release (Fig. 1). Stimulation more caudally in an area extending caudally and ventrally from the chiasm into the median eminence–arcuate region evokes release of both gonadotropins. Thus, it would appear that there are overlapping regions that control gonadotropin secretion in the female rat. The LH-controlling region extends from the suprachiasmatic–medial preoptic area caudally to the arcuate–median eminence region,

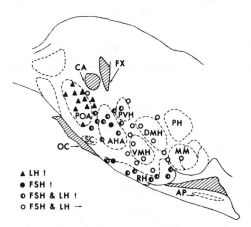

Figure 1. Location of stimulating electrodes projected on a parasagittal section through the rat brain. Symbols on figure refer to alterations in plasma FSH and LH (↑, increase; →, no change). OC, optic chiasm; CA, anterior commissure; SC, suprachiasmatic nucleus; FX, fornix; PVH, paraventricular nucleus; AHA, anterior hypothalamic area; DMH, dorsomedial nucleus; RH, arcuate nucleus; PH, posterior hypothalamic nucleus; MM, medial mamillary nucleus; AP, anterior pituitary, POA, preoptic area. (Reproduced with permission from Kalra *et al.*, 1971.)

whereas the FSH-controlling region appears to begin in the anterior hypothalamic area and extend caudally to the arcuate–median eminence region.

Stimulation and lesion studies suggest that a region extending from the anterior hypothalamus caudally to the median eminence–arcuate region is concerned with the secretion of TSH. ACTH secretion is clearly interfered with by median eminence lesions. Lesions elsewhere have not uniformly interfered with secretion of this trophic hormone which suggests that the region concerned may be closely limited to the basal tuberal region. The regions involved in growth hormone and prolactin secretion have not been so clearly delimited, but I shall discuss this further in Section VIII. Thus, the lesion and stimulation studies that we have briefly alluded to here have clearly established that the hypothalamus controls the release of pituitary hormones but does not provide evidence as to the mechanism by which this control is exerted (McCann, 1974; McCann *et al.*, 1974).

III. THE NEUROHUMORAL HYPOTHESIS OF CONTROL OF ANTERIOR PITUITARY HORMONE SECRETION

There were two possibilities to explain the mechanism by which the hypothalamus controls the anterior pituitary. One was by a direct secretomotor innervation, but this potential mechanism was eliminated by the absence of a clear innervation to the anterior lobe except by vascular autonomic fibers and also by the evidence cited in Section II that the gland is not electrically excitable. The presence of the hypophyseal portal system of veins that drain blood from capillary loops in the median eminence down the hypophyseal stalk to the adenohypophyseal sinusoids suggested the possibility of the brain's exerting neurohumoral control on the pituitary (Fig. 2).

Early evidence for the neurohumoral hypothesis was confusing, since experiments in which the pituitary stalk was sectioned gave variable results. This question was settled by Harris (1961) who showed that if an impervious plate were placed between the cut ends of the stalk, a permanent derangement of pituitary function resulted. The earlier discrepancies had resulted from variable regeneration of hypophyseal portal vessels across the cut edges of the stalk. Further strong circumstantial evidence for the neurohumoral hypothesis was provided by ingenious grafting experiments in which the gland was removed from the hypophyseal capsule and then reimplanted under the median eminence of the tuber cinereum so that it could be revascularized by hypophyseal portal vessels. These experiments carried out by Harris and Jacobsohn indicated that such grafts were associated with the return of normal anterior pituitary function, whereas grafts placed in other loci at a distance from the portal vessels so that they had to be revascularized by other arterial twigs led to a permanent dysfunction of the gland. In a further ramification of this type of experiment. Nikitovitch-Winer and Everett placed grafts under the kidney

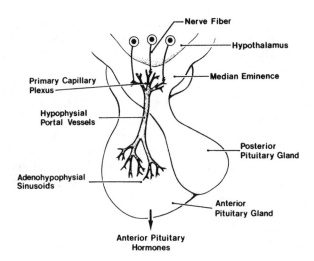

Figure 2. Diagram of the hypothalamo–pituitary region. (Reproduced with permission from McCann, 1977.)

capsule and then, after the pituitary deficiency had developed, removed the grafts and replaced them under the median eminence. This was followed by the return of normal anterior pituitary function.

IV. HYPOTHALAMIC RELEASING AND INHIBITING HORMONES

The next logical step was to make extracts of the median eminence region, the area that is drained by the portal vessels, and to inject these into animals to determine if they could alter anterior pituitary function. Because of the availability of a relatively simple sensitive assay for adrenocortical function, the adrenal ascorbic acid depletion assay of Sayers, interest initially focused on a possible factor to control the secretion of ACTH. It was early shown that extracts of the posterior pituitary could release ACTH. This occurred in animals in which the ACTH release induced by nonspecific stress had been blocked either by hypothalamic lesions or by administration of drugs, such as pentobarbital–morphine, that were capable of blocking the stress response.

At about this time, it was also shown that neurohypophyseal extracts could increase the release of ACTH from anterior pituitaries incubated *in vitro*. A controversy soon ensued. Although synthetic vasopressin could release ACTH, some workers were able to separate a substance in the neurohypophyseal extracts, apparently different from vasopressin, that would also release ACTH. Unfortunately, this substance was present in trace amounts or not uniformly present in neurohypophyseal extracts. The controversy cleared when it was shown that extracts of median eminence tissue contained more corticotropin-releasing activity than could be accounted for by the amount of vasopressin present. Consequently, it was clear that a corticotropin-releasing factor (CRF) existed in addition to vasopressin (Table 1) (McCann and Dhariwal, 1966; McCann and Porter, 1969).

Vasopressin may still have a physiological role in the control of ACTH release since a slight but definite deficiency in ACTH release is present in animals with hereditary diabetes insipidus; such animals lack endogenously produced vasopressin. Another bit of evidence supporting vasopressin as a CRF is that it has a direct action to stimulate ACTH release in a dose-related fashion from the pituitary incubated *in vitro*. Finally, vasopressin has been shown to be present in high concentrations in portal blood collected from the stalk of monkeys; these concentrations are in the range that should stimulate ACTH release, at least under stressful conditions, at a time when vasopressin is released in large amounts.

The discovery of a CRF distinct from vasopressin stimulated a search for other similar factors to stimulate release of other anterior pituitary hormones; and, in rapid succession an LH-releasing factor, FSH-releasing factor, growth hormone-releasing factor, TSH-releasing factor, and prolactin-inhibiting factor were discovered. Evidence for both an MSH-releasing and -inhibiting factor was obtained, and a growth hormone-inhibiting factor was also described. There is now some evidence for a prolactin-releasing factor (Table 1).

There followed an intensive effort to purify these new substances, to separate them from other activities in hypothalamic extracts, and to determine their structure so that this could be confirmed by synthesis.

Since only very small amounts of these substances are present in hypothalamic tissue, this proved to be a herculean task. Apparently because of their ready access to the anterior lobe via the hypophyseal portal vessels, there is no need to flood the general circulation with these releasing hormones and, therefore, no need to store large amounts in the hypothalamus. Consequently, isolation and determination of structure of these factors required the processing of hundreds of thousands and even millions of hypothalamic fragments. There were two keys in the elucidation of these structures. The first was the realization that neurohypophyseal extracts that were commercially available were not suitable as starting material because of the small amounts of the releasing factors present. Therefore, it was necessary to process hypothalamic tissue. The second key was the realization that truly massive numbers of fragments had to be processed because of the small quantities of the active substances present even in hypothalamic tissue.

The first releasing factor to be characterized was thyrotropin-releasing factor (TRF), also known as thyrotropin-releasing hormone (TRH) or thyroliberin. The structure is that of a tripeptide, pyroglutamyl-histidyl-prolineamide (Table 2). The cyclic nature of the peptide caused problems in the elucidation of the structure, but this was eventually resolved by two groups (those of Schally and Guillemin) almost simultaneously in 1969 (Vale *et al.*, 1973). The synthetic hormone proved active, and this eliminated some of the doubt among a few diehards that releasing factors did in fact exist.

Table 1. History of the Releasing Factors

Releasing factor	Discovery	Purified	Structure determined by	Synthesized	Stimulates	Inhibits	Discoverers
Vasopressin	1954	Yes	DuVigneaud	Octapeptide	ACTH	0	McCann and Brobeck; Martini
Corticotropin-releasing factor (CRF)	1955–59	Yes	No	No	ACTH	0	Saffran and Schally; Guillemin; Sayers and Royce
LH-releasing hormone (LHRH)	1960	Yes	Matsuo and Schally; Burgus and Guillemin	Decapeptide	LH, FSH	0	McCann, Taleisnik and Friedman; Harris and Nikitovitch-Winer
FSH-releasing factor (FSH-RF)	1964	Yes	No	No	FSH	0	Igarashi and McCann
Thyrotropin-releasing hormone (TRH)	1958–62	Yes	Enzman, Folkers, and Schally; Burgus and Guillemin	Tripeptide	TSH, prolactin	0	Schreiber and Guillemin
Growth hormone-releasing factor (GRF)	1958–64	Yes	No	No	GH	0	Franz; Dueben and Meites
Growth hormone-inhibiting factor (GIF) (somatostatin)	1967	Yes	Brazeau, Vale, Burgus, and Guillemin	Tetradeca-peptide	0	GH, prolactin, TSH, gastrin, glucagon, insulin	Krulich, Dhariwal, and McCann
Prolactin-inhibiting factor (PIF)	1963	Yes	No	No	0	Prolactin	Pasteels; Talwalker, Ratner, and Meites
Prolactin-releasing factor (PRF)	1972	Yes	No	No	Prolactin	0	Valverde, Chiaffo, and Reichlin; Krulich, Quijada and McCann
MSH-releasing factor (MRF)	1965	Yes	?	?	MSH	0	Taleisnik and Orias
MSH-inhibiting factor (MIF)	1966	Yes	?	?	0	MSH	Kastin and Schally

Table 2. Structure of LHRH, TRH, and Somatostatin

TRH	(P-Glu-His-Pro-NH$_2$) 　1　　2　　3
LHRH	(P-Glu-His-Trp-Ser-Tyr-Gly-Leu-Arg-Pro-Gly-NH$_2$) 　1　2　3　4　5　6　7　8　9　10
GIF (Somatostatin)	NH$_2$-Ala-Gly-Cys-Lys-Asn-Phe-Phe-Trp-Lys-Thr-Phe-Thr-Ser-Cys-COOH 　1　2　3　4　5　6　7　8　9　10　11　12　13　14

In 1971, LH-releasing factor or hormone (LHRH) was shown to be a decapeptide (Table 2), and, once again, the synthetic hormone was active. The synthetic peptide released not only LH but to a lesser extent also FSH, which has led some to postulate that an LH-releasing hormone is sufficient to account for the hypothalamic stimulation if both FSH and LH release (Schally *et al.*, 1973). Since dissociation in FSH and LH release can occur following hypothalamic lesions and stimulations and also in a variety of physiological states, I still believe that an FSH-releasing factor will ultimately be isolated; however, this point is now controversial. Several groups have reported partial purifications of the FSH-releasing factor; however, others have not been able to find any evidence for a factor other than LHRH.

The third hypothalamic factor to be isolated was the growth hormone-inhibiting factor (GIF), a factor discovered by Krulich and associates (1972) in 1967 while attempting to purify the growth hormone-releasing factor by gel filtration on Sephadex. In essence, fractions from hypothalamic extract were eluted from the column that had an inhibitory action on growth hormone release from pituitaries incubated *in vitro*. This was particularly apparent using monolayer cultures of pituitary cells, and the sensitivity of this particular system to the inhibitory action led to its rapid purification, isolation, and determination of structure by Guillemin's group utilizing only 500,000 hypothalamic fragments. The structure of GIF (somatostatin) is that of a tetradecapeptide (Table 2), and, in contrast to TRH and LRF, there is no amino terminal pyroglutamyl group (Brazeau *et al.*, 1973). In the case of MSH, structures of both a postulated MSH-releasing and MSH-inhibiting factor have been proposed; however, more work is necessary to determine if these are in reality the proper structures (McCann *et al.*, 1974).

With the elucidation of the structures of at least three of these releasing and inhibiting hormones, it has been possible to prepare many analogues of each of the three factors. Some of these have inhibitory activity, and others are more active than the natural compound. In the case of LHRH, analogues may be particularly important clinically since the so-called super-LHRH analogues may be valuable in the induction of ovulation in infertile women, whereas the inhibitors are potential antifertility drugs that might be capable of blocking conception via an inhibition of ovulation. Some of these analogues are shown in Table 2.

V. MECHANISM OF ACTION OF RELEASING AND INHIBITING HORMONES ON THE PITUITARY

It is becoming increasingly clear that peptide and protein hormones act by combining with a receptor on the cell membrane. This contrasts with steroid hormones which are lipid soluble and penetrate the cell membrane only to combine with a receptor in the cytosol. Most peptide and protein hormones appear to act at least in part via the adenylate cyclase system (Fig. 3). This appears to be true at least in part for the releasing factors also. After their

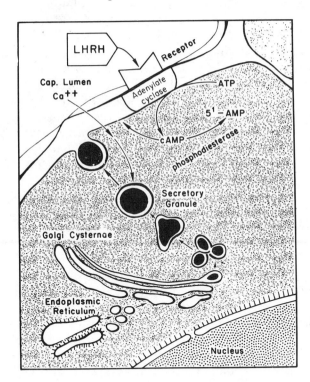

Figure 3. A schematic diagram of the possible mechanism of action of LHRH on the gonado-trophs. Hormone is stored in secretory granules. LHRH combines with a cell surface receptor, and this results in activation of adenylate cyclase and the generation of increased cyclic AMP. This is visualized as altering the membrane characteristics of the cell, possibly via a protein kinase which would dephosphorylate membrane constituents, thereby promoting reverse pinocytosis (exocytosis) as indicated. Calcium ions are required for the releasing action. (Reproduced with permission from McCann, 1971.)

combination with the membrane-bound receptor, they appear to activate adenylate cyclase, a membrane-bound enzyme, which then converts ATP into cyclic AMP. In most tissues, cyclic AMP then activates a protein kinase that can mediate most of the effects of the cyclic nucleotide. In the case of the pituitary, it has been suggested that a protein kinase is activated and that this then dephosphorylates certain membrane constituents, promoting exocytosis. In this process, hormone-containing secretory granules located in the cytoplasm migrate to and fuse with the cell membrane, and the granular core is extruded to the extracellular space, particularly at the vascular pole of the cell. Calcium is clearly required for the releasing process, since removal of this cation from the medium blocks the release of hormones from pituitaries *in vitro*.

The means by which the secretory granules migrate to the cell surface remains an enigma. It has been postulated that this might involve microtubules or microfilaments; however, colchicine, which disrupts microtubules, not only fails to block release of several pituitary hormones but actually augments it, suggesting the possibility that the tubules might hold the granules in the interior of the cell and, after dissolution of the tubules, the granules then migrate spontaneously to the surface, possibly because of electrostatic forces between the granules and the inside of the cell membrane.

If the cell membrane is depolarized by placing pituitaries in a high-potassium medium, release is also induced, and this finding has led some to suggest that the mechanism of release occurred according to the so-called secretion-coupling hypothesis of Douglas and Poisner which was put forward to explain the release of neurohypophyseal and medullary hormones. It is not clear as yet whether depolarization of the cell membrane actually accompanies the releasing process in normally secreting pituitary cells.

It is clear that the releasing factors act on the cell very rapidly, (within less than a minute) to either promote or inhibit release of particular pituitary hormones; however, their precise effect on the biosynthesis of these hormones has not been elucidated. It is apparent that with sufficient stimulation of release, synthesis is promoted, but it is not certain whether this is secondary to the release process or represents another primary action of the releasing factors on the biosynthetic process itself (McCann, 1971; Labrie *et al.*, 1976). (For a related discussion, see Chapter 4.)

Specificity of action of each releasing factor is probably provided by the presence of highly specific receptors on the target cell as well as by some degree of specificity in the chemical structure of the releasing factor. However, an absolute specificity of action of releasing factors, originally thought to obtain, now has a number of exceptions. As already indicated, LHRH stimulates FSH as well as LH release. Thyrotropin-releasing hormone can stimulate prolactin as well as TSH release, and somatostatin inhibits prolactin and TSH as well as GH release. In fact, somatostatin can inhibit a variety of secretory processes, e.g., secretion of saliva, gastrin, glucagon, and insulin. An important area of research is devoted to working out the "code" by which releasing factors mediate specific pituitary responses to environmental and endocrine input.

VI. LOCALIZATION OF RELEASING AND INHIBITING HORMONES WITHIN THE BRAIN

In order to understand the mechanisms controlling the release of the releasing factors, it is critical to know which CNS cell types synthesize and release these factors and also to know the anatomical distribution of these cells within the brain. Several techniques have been applied to this problem. The first has been to cut thick frozen sections serially through the hypothalamus in three planes at right angles to each other, to take thin sections before and after each thick section for histological control, and to extract the thick sections and assay them for releasing factors. The assays can be effected by bioassay, using the output of pituitary hormones from pituitaries incubated *in vitro,* or by immunoassay using immunoassays developed against the synthetic releasing factors (Fig. 4) (McCann *et al.,* 1975; Wheaton *et al.,* 1975).

Another approach to cell localization has been to punch out nuclei from frozen sections utilizing stereomicroscopic control, to extract these, and to assay them by radioimmunoassay (Brownstein *et al.,* 1976). Finally, the techniques of immunohistochemistry have permitted investigators to localize some of the releasing factors within cellular elements in the brain (Zimmerman, 1976). As a result of all of these approaches, it is now known that most of these neurohormones are stored particularly in the median eminence region and

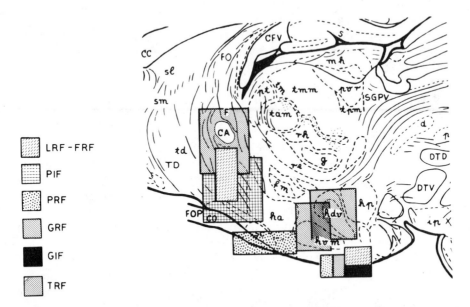

Figure 4. Schematic localization of various releasing and inhibiting factors in the preoptic–hypothalamic region. The areas indicated correspond to regions of relatively high activity. (Reproduced with permission from McCann *et al.,* 1975.) For abbreviations of hypothalamic structures, see legend to Fig. 5.

pituitary stalk. Smaller amounts may actually be found in the neural lobe itself. It appears that the factors are stored in granules in axon terminals, the cell bodies of which are located at some distance from these terminals.

In the case of the CRF, little is known, but here the cell bodies may be relatively close to the median eminence, perhaps in the arcuate nucleus immediately overlying it. In the case of LHRH, the activity is found in the very regions that when stimulated release LH and when destroyed lead to deficiencies in its secretion (Fig. 5). Most of the evidence favors the viewpoint that there are two populations of LHRH neurons. The first of these has cell bodies located in the medial preoptic area (labeled POM in Fig. 5) immediately overlying the optic chiasm and axons that project caudally to terminate in the median eminence. Another population of LHRH neurons may have cell bodies located in the vicinity of the arcuate nucleus (ar) and relatively short axons that project to the median eminence. The axon terminals in the median eminence have been found to end in juxtaposition to hypophyseal portal capillaries. Not only can LHRH be extracted from these regions, but also lesions in the suprachiasmatic region are followed by a decline in the content of LHRH stored in the median eminence as measured in assays subsequently; this loss would be consistent with the degeneration of the preoptico–tuberal LHRH neurons and loss of the stored LHRH in their axon terminals.

It is now clear also that LHRH is found in the organum vasculosum lamina terminalis, one of the circumventricular organs, which is at the rostral extent of the third ventricle. It is conceivable that LHRH may be secreted from axon terminals in this organ into the ventricular system and be transported to the base of the third ventricle where it could be taken up by specialized ependymal cells, the tanycytes, and transported to the median eminence.

In the case of TRH (Fig. 4), activity is also found in the preoptic region, this time in the region of the interstitial nucleus of the stria terminalis. The activity is present in a region extending caudally from this structure to the dorsomedial nucleus where a higher activity is present; activity then extends ventrally into the median eminence–arcuate region where the bulk of the activity is stored. In this case, the neurons have not yet been visualized by immunohistochemical techniques, but one could postulate that neurons with cell bodies in the interstitial nucleus of the stria terminalis have long axons that project caudally to the dorsomedial nucleus and ventrally to terminate in the median eminence. Alternatively, some neurons could have cell bodies there, another collection could have cell bodies in the dorsomedial nucleus, and the axons of both of these groups of TRH neurons could project to the median eminence. Thyrotropin-releasing hormone has been found outside the hypothalamus as well and even in the spinal cord, which has raised the possibility that it may be involved in other CNS functions as well as its well-known role of increasing TSH release by the adenohypophysis.

Growth hormone-releasing factor is found predominantly in the ventromedial nucleus. The growth hormone-inhibiting factor (somatostatin) is present in the suprachiasmatic nucleus, the ventromedial nucleus, and the

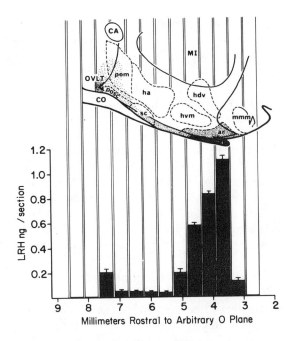

Figure 5. A parasagittal section through the hypothalamic region of the rat. The relative concentration of LHRH in a region is indicated by the intensity of the stippling. Note in particular the location of the organum vasculosum lamina terminalis (OVLT), the arcuate nucleus (AR) with overlying median eminence and pituitary stalk (I). Abbreviations for the remaining hypothalamic structures are as follows: ha, nucleus anterior (hypothalamus); hdv, nucleus dorsomedialis (hypothalamus); hvm, nucleus ventromedialis (hypothalamus); pom, nucleus preopticus medialis; posc, nucleus preopticus, pars suprachiasmatic; mmm, nucleus mamillaris medialis, pars medialis; sc, nucleus suprachiasmaticus; CA, commissura anterior; CO, chiasma opticum; MI, massa intermedia (Reproduced with permission from McCann, 1977.)

median eminence (Brownstein *et al.*, 1976; Krulich *et al.*, 1972). These localizations of releasing factors are consistent with the findings from electrical stimulation and lesion studies and give the best evidence for the precise regions of the hypothalamus that are involved in the control of particular hormone secretions.

VII. FACTORS AFFECTING RESPONSIVENESS OF THE ADENOHYPOPHYSIS TO RELEASING AND INHIBITING FACTORS

The hormonal state of the animal is very important in determining the responsiveness of the adenohypophysis to the various releasing factors. In the case of TRH, pituitary responsiveness is enhanced by removal of the thyroid and consequent loss of negative feedback by thyroxine and triodothyronine.

Conversely, responsiveness is supressed by administration of thyroid hormone. In fact, the negative feedback of thyroid hormone seems to be mediated predominantly on the pituitary gland to modulate its responsiveness to TRH.

It is also possible that TRH release is under inhibitory control via circulating thyroid hormones, but the evidence for this is less compelling. The mechanism by which the thyroid hormones suppress pituitary responsiveness to TRH may involve the uptake of the thyroid hormone by the thyrotroph. Under the influence of thyroid hormone, the pituitary cells' messenger RNA synthesis is modified with resultant stimulation of synthesis of an inhibitory peptide or protein that, in turn, then blocks the response of the cell to TRH. The evidence for this sequence is that inhibitors of DNA-directed RNA synthesis, such as actinomycin, and inhibitors of protein synthesis, such as cyclohexamide, can prevent the establishment of the thyroid hormone blockade and can even reverse it after a period of time. The "lag period" is presumably the time required for the inhibitory peptide or protein to be catabolized (Vale *et al.*, 1967).

In the case of corticotropin-releasing factor, there is also good evidence that adrenal steroids feed back directly at the pituitary to inhibit the response to CRF; however, this feedback may also take place at the hypothalamic level to alter release of CRF (McCann and Porter, 1969).

The interplay between gonadal steroids and the hypothalamic–pituitary axis is particularly complex. Following removal of the gonads and the elimination of feedback by the gonadal steroids, predominantly estrogen in the female and testosterone in the male, levels of both FSH and LH are elevated. The release of these pituitary hormones is pulsatile and occurs rhythmically. The timing of the discharge varies among species and even among individual animals within a species and is the so-called ultradian rhythm of LH release (Fig. 6). This rhythm is probably brought about by pulsatile release of LHRH and possibly FSH-RH as well (if a discrete FSH-RH actually exists). Following removal of negative feedback, the enhanced LHRH release not only increases the discharge of gonadotropins but also their synthesis, so the quantities stored in the gland increase. This augmented storage is associated with an increase in responsiveness to the neurohormone. Small doses of estrogen or androgen can suppress the responsiveness to LHRH, and this occurs quickly. At least in the case of estrogen administration, it can take place within 1 hr. With long-term therapy, there is not only suppression of release, but also of synthesis of LH, and pituitary content of gonadotropin consequently falls. This is associated with a further decline in responsiveness to the neurohormone.

In the intact female, complex relationships occur during the estrous or menstrual cycle. Responsiveness to LHRH is minimal on the day after ovulation in the rat (diestrus day 1), begins to increase on the afternoon of the second day of diestrus, and is clearly augmented by the morning of the next day (proestrus). Responsiveness increases through the day of proestrus and reaches its height at the time of the preovulatory discharge of LH on the afternoon of proestrus (Fig. 7). Treatment of ovariectomized animals with

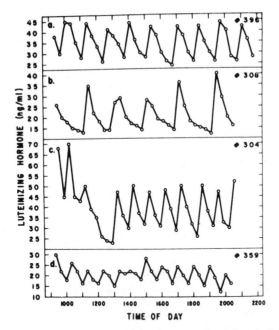

Figure 6. Circhoral changes in plasma luteinizing hormone from four individual castrate monkeys. (Reproduced with permission from Dierschke *et al.*, 1970.)

estrogen has a biphasic effect on pituitary responsiveness to LHRH (Fig. 8): the initial suppression reported above followed by an augmented responsiveness. Consequently, estrogen secreted by the preovulatory follicles is probably responsible for the enhanced responsiveness to LHRH that occurs in early proestrus.

In addition, during the preovulatory discharge of LH, the characteristics of the LH discharge in response to LHRH change, and the response becomes much more rapid and pulselike (Fig. 7). This further change in responsiveness is probably brought about by LHRH itself, since it can be induced by a priming injection of LHRH early in proestrus. Responsiveness then declines after the ovulatory discharge and is considerably lessened by the morning of estrus (Cooper and McCann, 1974; Zeballos and McCann, 1975).

Similar changes in responsiveness occur in the human menstrual cycle, with responsiveness increasing in the late proliferative phase, reaching a maximum during the preovulatory discharge, and becoming pulselike and then declining during the progestational phase of the cycle (Yen *et al.*, 1975).

The mechanism by which estrogen augments responsiveness to LHRH is not known. It might induce additional receptors for the neurohormone, or, alternatively, it might alter the synthesis of LH and provide a larger pool of releaseable LH. Similarly, the mechanism for the self-priming action (positive feedback) of LHRH remains to be elucidated, but this could be explained by an effect on synthesis of a releaseable pool of LH.

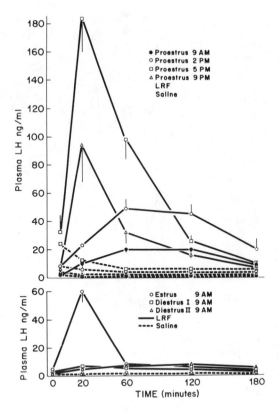

Figure 7. Plasma LH in response to sLRF (LHRH) or saline diluent injected s.c. at various stages of the estrous cycle. Vertical lines represent 1 standard error of the mean. (Reproduced with permission from Zeballos and McCann, 1975.) The preovulatory discharge of LH was in progress at 5 p.m. on proestrus as evidenced by the high initial plasma LH.

This remarkable increase in responsiveness to LHRH as a function of the steroid milieu undoubtedly accounts in part for the proestrous discharge of LH, but it is believed that an enhanced release of LHRH is also involved. This is probably induced once again by estrogen from the preovulatory follicle. In addition, there is a daily timing mechanism in the rat such that the increased release of LHRH occcurs on the afternoon of proestrus (McCann, 1974). This increased release of LHRH is probably responsible for bringing on the self-priming action of LHRH that characterizes the late proestrous phase. Evidence for the increased release of LHRH on the afternoon of proestrus includes the detection of increased titers of the hormone in peripheral blood in some animals (Wheaton and McCann, 1976) and the observation of very high titers in portal blood collected from the cut pituitary stalk of the monkey at this stage of the cycle.

It would appear, then, that the preovulatory discharge of LH is brought about by enhanced release of LHRH coupled with a marked increase in

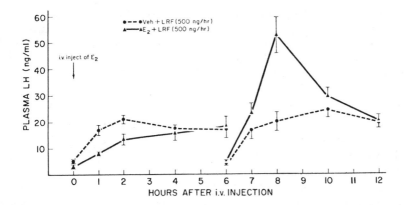

Figure 8. The effect of intravenous estradiol on the responsiveness of ovariectomized rats to LHRH (LRF). In the left hand portion of the figure, the animals were injected i.v. with estradiol (E₂) or the vehicle, and an infusion of LHRH at 500 ng/hr was started and continued for 6 hr. For the animals in the right hand portion of the figure, the injection of estradiol or diluent took place at time 0, and the infusion of LHRH was begun at 6 hr. Values shown are mean ± SEM.

responsiveness to the neurohormone. The result is a discharge of LH far greater than that necessary to induce ovulation. Perhaps this is part of a fail-safe mechanism to insure full ovulation even when follicular development is not optimal; it might serve to prolong the reproductive life of the individual.

VIII. PUTATIVE SYNAPTIC TRANSMITTERS INVOLVED IN CONTROLLING THE RELEASE OF RELEASING HORMONES

The releasing factor-producing neurons appear to be in synaptic contact with a host of putative synaptic transmitters. The hypothalamus is richly supplied with monoaminergic nerve fibers (see Chapters 4 and 14). There is a heavy input of noradrenergic fibers from neurons whose cell bodies lie in the brain stem. The distribution of these neurons has been mapped by fluorescent histochemistry, and the presence of norepinephrine in the region of the terminals has been confirmed by direct assay of norepinephrine either by classical fluorometric techniques or, more recently, by using the nuclear punch technique and assaying for the catecholamine by the ultrasensitive enzymatic radiometric technique. In this technique, ^{14}C-labeled S-adenosyl methionine reacts with the catecholamine in the extract in the presence of catechol-O-methyl transferase to produce a labeled product that can be isolated and counted. There are also terminals from epinephrine-containing neurons that end in the hypothalamus. These also appear to originate from neurons whose cell bodies are located in the brain stem.

Axons of serotonin-containing neurons whose cell bodies lie in the medial raphe nuclei project to the suprachiasmatic, anterior hypothalamic, and median eminence regions. Assays for choline acetyltransferase indicate the wide-spread distribution of cholinergic fibers within the hypothalamus as well. There is also an abundance of histamine that appears to be located in synaptosomelike structures, and this amine is particularly concentrated in the median eminence region where it may also serve as a synaptic transmitter (Brownstein *et al.*, 1976).

Consequently, a great deal of effort has been exerted in an attempt to determine the role of these possible transmitters in controlling the release of the various releasing hormones. The most extensive studies have been carried out in the case of the gonadotropins, where it appears that there is an excitatory noradrenergic synapse that may mediate not only the preovulatory release of LHRH but also the increased LHRH release that follows castration. In the case of the preovulatory release of LHRH, the synapse may be in the preoptic–anterior hypothalamic region, whereas in the case of the increased release in the castrate, the synapse may be on the other population of LHRH neurons, located in the arcuate nucleus. The evidence for these statements is the ability of α-adrenergic receptor-blocking drugs to prevent both the preovulatory type and the postcastration type of LH release. Furthermore, inhibitors of catecholamine synthesis interfere with gonadotropin release in these cir-cumstances, and if agents are given that bypass the block and reinitiate norepinephrine synthesis, the blockade of gonadotropin release is frequently reversed.

A site for the noradrenergic synapse in the preoptic–anterior hy-pothalamic area was suggested by studies in which inhibitors of norepineph-rine synthesis blocked the release of LH following preoptic stimulation. The blockade could be reversed by giving drugs that bypass the block in synthesis of the catecholamine. By contrast, inhibition of norepinephrine synthesis did not interfere with LH release induced by stimulation in the median eminence region. Presumably in this latter instance, the axons of the LHRH neurons themselves were being stimulated (Fig. 9).

Dopamine has been postulated to both stimulate and inhibit LH release. The evidence is confusing, but the view held at the present time is that this catecholamine may have only a minor role. Intraventricular administration of dopamine, norepinephrine, or epinephrine will clearly stimulate LH release. In this connection, it is conceivable that the effects that are now attributable to norepinephrine may in fact be caused by epinephrine, since we have no means for selectively blocking the synthesis of epinephrine.

Serotonin, when injected into the third ventricle, can inhibit LH release; this suggests that it is an inhibitory transmitter, but the evidence is not conclu-sive. Similarly, histamine can, in large doses, stimulate LH release following its intraventricular injection.

There is considerable evidence for a cholinergic link in gonadotropin release, since atropine can block gonadotropin release when it is administered systemically, microinjected into the third ventricle, or implanted within the hypothalamus. However, injections of cholinergic drugs have not been as

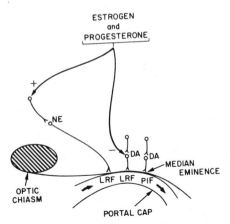

Figure 9. A schematic diagram indicating proposed sites of the stimulatory (+) and inhibitory (−) action of estrogen and progesterone on LH release and the postulated noradrenergic synapse (NE) involved in mediating the stimulatory action. Dopamine (DA) may be involved in mediating the inhibitory action of gonadal steroids. (Reproduced with permission from McCann *et al.*, 1971.)

successful in stimulating LH release, so the precise role of cholinergic synapses remains to be established.

In the case of ACTH, there is considerable evidence to suggest an inhibitory noradrenergic control over the release of this tropin, and there is some evidence to suggest cholinergic and serotoninergic stimulatory components as well. Thyrotropin has been little investigated but may be under adrenergic control. Growth hormone also appears to be under adrenergic control, but the relative importance of dopamine and norepinephrine has yet to be clearly established.

Prolactin is definitely under inhibitory control via dopamine. There is a tuberoinfundibular dopaminergic tract, the neurons of which have cell bodies lying in the arcuate nucleus and axons projecting to the external layer of the median eminence. Here, they terminate in juxtaposition to hypophyseal portal capillaries.

Dopamine has recently been demonstrated in portal blood, and it can inhibit the release of prolactin by a direct action on the pituitary following its injection into cannulated portal vessels or its incubation with pituitaries *in vitro*. Consequently, dopamine itself may be a prolactin-inhibiting factor. Considerable evidence also indicates that a peptidic prolactin-inhibiting factor probably exists, and dopamine may cause its release from terminals in the median eminence.

Norepinephrine may possibly have an excitatory role on prolactin release as evidenced by the results of pharmacological studies similar to those carried out for gonadotropins. It is conceivable that norepinephrine causes the release of prolactin-releasing factor from neurons whose cell bodies lie in the region of the suprachiasmatic nucleus (McCann and Moss, 1975; McCann and Ojeda, 1979).

IX. THE ROLE OF PROSTAGLANDINS IN CONTROLLING THE RELEASE OF RELEASING FACTORS AND IN STIMULATING THE RELEASE OF PITUITARY HORMONES BY DIRECT ACTION ON THE PITUITARY GLAND

It is now clear from a variety of studies that prostaglandins can stimulate the release of pituitary hormones by a direct action on the gland. The addition of prostaglandins to pituitaries incubated *in vitro* causes a marked increase in adenylate cyclase and cyclic AMP within the gland. There is a stimulation of growth hormone release; stimulation of release of other hormones is more variable. Whether prostaglandins play any role within the cell in the normal releasing process remains to be established.

Similarly, it is established that the prostaglandins can also act on the hypothalamus to stimulate release of a variety of pituitary hormones: ACTH, FSH, LH, and prolactin. It is possible to interfere with gonadotropin release using inhibitors of prostaglandin synthetase (the enzyme that catalyzes synthesis of prostaglandins) such as indomethacin; however, since there is a lag period before systemic administration of the drug is effective and since the dose required is rather large, it is still not certain that the prostaglandins are an essential link in the release of the releasing factors (McCann and Ojeda, 1979).

X. EXTRAPITUITARY ACTIONS OF RELEASING FACTORS

The distribution of releasing factors in brain regions outside the hypothalamus (e.g., brainstem, cortex) has stimulated a search for extrapituitary actions of the releasing factors. As indicated earlier, TRH is found in other brain regions and even in the spinal cord; somatostatin is similarly distributed widely throughout the nervous system and also has been found in thd delta cells of the islets of Langerhans (Goldsmith *et al.,* 1975). Since somatostatin can inhibit the release of both insulin and glucagon, it is possible that it may act as a local hormone to control the release of these hormones from the islets.

The clearest behavioral effect of releasing factors is the induction of mating behavior by relatively low doses of LHRH in the ovariectomized, estrogen-primed rat. The occurrence of LHRH in the preoptic area, the same region of the brain that is known to be involved in mating behavior, plus the onset of this behavior shortly after the preovulatory discharge of LHRH suggested to us that LHRH might be involved in induction of mating behavior. When the synthetic hormone became available to us, we tested this hypothesis, and, indeed, LHRH would permit induction of the lordosis reflex in ovariectomized, estrogen-primed rats (Moss and McCann, 1973; Moss *et al.,* 1975) (Fig. 10). This effect was not caused by the gonadotropins released, since these hormones had no effect on mating behavior and since, as Pfaff showed, the effect of LHRH could be obtained in the hypophysectomized rat. Neither are the adrenal steroids important, since the effect could be obtained in

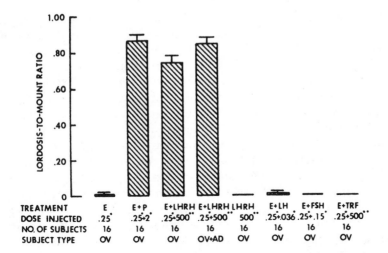

Figure 10. Effect of gonadotropins, ovarian hormones, and releasing factors on lordosis behavior in the female rat. * mg; **, ng; E, estrone; P, progesterone; OV, ovariectomy; AD, adrenalectomy. (Reproduced with permission from Moss *et al.,* 1975.)

ovariectomized–adrenalectomized rats. Further studies have shown that the effect can be obtained by microinjecting the LHRH into the preoptic–anterior hypothalamic and arcuate–median eminence regions, whereas similar injections into lateral hypothalamus or cortex proved ineffective. There is a latency between the injection of LHRH either into the brain or systemically and the onset of mating behavior, suggesting that the effect may not be a simple one but may involve some intervening steps. It is still not clear whether LHRH has any normal role in mating since the hormone did not advance or prolong mating in normal female rats.

Thyrotropin-releasing hormone has been shown to have effects that indicate an arousal action of the hormone, i.e., it shortens the duration of pentobarbital anesthesia. The doses required are very large; however, if the material is present at synaptic sites in other regions of the brain, it is conceivable that these responses to high doses could be physiological (Kastin *et al.,* 1972). Somatostatin, on the other hand, has been shown to depress animals (Brown and Vale, 1975). Thus, the concept is emerging that the releasing factors may have important extrapituitary actions. One could even visualize the possibility that they may serve as peptidic neurotransmitters and that this could be an even more important role than that of governing the release of anterior pituitary hormones.

XI. SUMMARY

Hypothalamic control over anterior pituitary hormone secretion is exerted by the release of a family of peptidic neurohormones termed releasing and inhibiting hormones that are synthesized in specialized neurosecretory neurons whose terminals end in the median eminence. In the axon terminals in the median eminence, the bulk of the releasing and inhibiting hormones are stored for release in response to the appropriate stimulus. Three of the neurohormones have been characterized and synthesized: TRH, LHRH, and growth hormone-inhibiting hormone (somatostatin). Responsiveness of the pituitary gland to these hormones is modulated by target gland hormones. The releasing and inhibiting hormones interact with membrane-bound receptors, and their action may be brought about largely through alterations in the adenylate cyclase–cyclic AMP system. The releasing factor neurons are in synaptic contact with a variety of other neurons, and there is strong evidence for adrenergic control of the release of most of these hormones. Considerable evidence also exists to suggest important cholinergic, serotoninergic, and even histaminergic inputs to the system. In addition to controlling the release of the various anterior pituitary hormones, some, at least, of the releasing factors are distributed outside of the hypothalamus and may exert important actions on the central nervous system. Among these may be the induction of mating behavior. Somatostatin is even found in the islets of Langerhans and may serve as a local hormone to inhibit release of insulin and glucagon.

REFERENCES

Brazeau, P., Vale, W., Burgus, R., Ling, N., Butcher, M., Rivier, J., and Guillemin, R., 1973, Hypothalamic polypeptide that inhibits the secretion of immunoreactive pituitary growth hormone, *Science* **179**:177.

Brown, M., and Vale, W., 1975, Central nervous system effects of hypothalamic peptides, *Endocrinology* **96**:1333.

Brownstein, M. J., Palkovits, M., Saavedra, J. M., and Kizer, J. S., 1976, Distribution of hypothalamic hormones and neurotransmitters within the diencephalon, in: *Frontiers in Neuroendocrinology* (L. Martini and W. F. Ganong, eds.), pp. 1–23, Raven Press, New York.

Cooper, K. J., and McCann, S. M., 1974, Influence of ovarian steroids on pituitary responsiveness to LH-releasing hormone (LH-RH) in the rat, in: *Hypothalamic Hormones: Chemistry, Physiology, Pharmacology and Clinical Uses* (M. Motta *et al.*, eds.), pp. 161–169, Academic Press, New York.

Dierschke, D. J., Bhattacharya, A. N., Atkinson, L. E., and Knobil, E., 1970, Circhoral oscillations of plasma LH levels in the ovariectomized Rhesus monkey, *Endocrinology* **87**:850–853.

Goldsmith, P. C., Rose, J. C., Arimura, A., and Ganong, W. F., 1975, Ultrastructural localization of somatostatin in pancreatic islets of the rat, *Endocrinology* **97**:1061.

Harris, G. W., 1961, The pituitary stalk and ovulation, in: *Control of Ovulation* (C. A. Villee, ed.), pp. 56–74, Pergamon Press, London.

Kalra, S. P., Ajika, K., Krulich, L., Fawcett, C. P., Quijada, M., and McCann, S. M., 1971, Effects of hypothalamic and preoptic electrochemical stimulation on gonadotropin and prolactin release in proestrus rats, *Endocrinology.* **88**:1150.

Kastin, A. J., Schalch, D. S., Ehrensing, R. H., and Anderson, M. S., 1972, Improvement in mental depression with decreased thyrotropin response after administration of thyrotropin-releasing hormone, *Lancet* **2**:740.

Krulich, L., Illner, P., Fawcett, C. P., Quijada, M., and McCann, S. M., 1972, Dual hypothalamic regulation of growth hormone secretion, in: *Growth and Growth Hormone* (A. Pecile and E. E. Muller, eds.), pp. 306–316, Excerpta Medica, Amsterdam.

Labrie, F., Pelletier, G., Borgeat, P., Drouin, J., Ferland, L., and Belanger, A., 1976, Mode of action of hypothalamic regulatory hormones in the adenohypophysis, in: *Frontiers in Neuroendocrinology* (L. Martini, and W. F. Ganong, eds.), pp. 63–93, Raven Press, New York.

McCann, S. M., 1971, Mechanism of action of hypothalamic hypophyseal stimulating and inhibiting hormones, in: *Frontiers in Neuroendocrinology* (L. Martini, and W. F. Ganong, eds.), pp. 209–235, Oxford University Press, New York.

McCann, S. M., 1974, Regulation of secretion of follicle-stimulating hormone and luteinizing hormone, in: *Handbook of Physiology* (R. O. Greep and E. B. Astwood, eds.), pp. 489–517, American Physiological Society, Washington.

McCann, S. M., 1977, Luteinizing-hormone-releasing hormone, *N. Engl. J. Med.* **296**:797–802.

McCann, S. M., and Dhariwal, A. P. S., 1966, Hypothalamic releasing factors and the neurovascular link between brain and anterior pituitary, in: *Neuroendocrinology* (L. Martini and W. F. Ganong, eds.), pp. 261–296, Academic Press, New York.

McCann, S. M., and Moss, R. L., 1975, Putative neurotransmitters involved in discharging gonadotropin-releasing neurohormones and the action of LH-releasing hormone on the CNS, *Life Sci.* **16**:833.

McCann, S. M., and Ojeda, S. R., 1979, The role of brain monoamines, acetylcholine, and prostaglandins in the control of anterior pituitary function, in: *Endocrinology*, Vol. 1 (L. J. DeGroot, G. F. Cahill, Jr., L. Martini, D. H. Nelson, W. D. Odell, J. T. Potts, Jr., E. Steinberger, and A. I. Winegrad, eds.), pp. 55–63, Grune and Stratton, New York.

McCann, S. M., and Porter, J. C., 1969, Hypothalamic pituitary stimulating and inhibiting hormones, *Physiol. Rev.* **49**:240.

McCann, S. M., Klana, P. S., Donoso, A. O., Bishop, W. Schneider, H. P. G., Fawcett, C. P., and Krulich, L., 1971, Role of monoamines in control of gonadotropin and prolactin secretions, in: *Brain–Endocrine Interaction. Median, Eminence: Structure and Function* (K. Knigge, D. E. Scott, and A. Weindl, eds.), pp. 224–235, Karger, Basel.

McCann, S. M., Fawcett, C. P., and Krulich, L., 1974, Hypothalamic hypophysial releasing and inhibiting hormones, in: *Endocrine Physiology* (S. M. McCann, ed.), pp. 31–65, MTP, Press, Lancaster, England.

McCann, S. M., Krulich, L., Quijada, M., Wheaton, J. E., and Moss, R. L., 1975, Gonadotropin-releasing factors. Sites of production, secretion and action in the brain, in: *Anatomical Neuroendocrinology* (W. Stumpf and G. Grant, eds.), pp. 192–199, S. Karger, Basel.

Moss, R. L., and McCann, S. M., 1973, Induction of mating behavior in rats by luteinizing hormone releasing factor, *Science* **181**:177.

Moss, R. L., McCann, S. M., and Dudley, C. A., 1975, Releasing hormones and sexual behavior, in: *Progress in Brain Research* (W. H. Gispen, T. B. van Dimersma Greidanus, B. Bohus, and D. de Wied, eds.), pp. 37–46, Elsevier, Amsterdam.

Schally, A. V., Kastin, A. J., Arimura, A., Coy, D., Coy, E., Debeljuk, L., and Redding, T. W., 1973, Basic and clinical studies with LHRH and its analogs, *J. Reprod. Fertil. (Suppl.)* **20**:119.

Vale, W., Burgus, R., and Guillemin, R., 1967, On the mechanism of action of TRF, *Neuroendocrinology* **3**:34.

Vale, W., Grant, G., and Guillemin, R., 1973, Chemistry of the hypothalamic releasing factors—Studies on structure-function relationships, in: *Frontiers in Neuroendocrinology* (W. F. Ganong and L. Martini, eds.), pp. 375–413, Oxford University Press, New York.

Wheaton, J. E., Krulich, L., and McCann, S. M., 1975, Localization of luteinizing hormone-releasing hormone in the preoptic area and hypothalamus of rat using radioimmunoassay, *Endocrinology* **97**:30.

Wheaton, J. E., and McCann, S. M., 1976, Luteinizing hormone-releasing hormone in peripheral plasma and hypothalamus of normal and ovariectomized rats, *Neuroendocrinology*, **20**:296–210.

Yen, S. S. C., Lasley, B. L., Wang, C. F., Leblanc, H., and Siler, T. M., 1975, The operating characteristics of the hypothalamic pituitary system during the menstrual cycle and observations of biological action of somatostatin, *Recent Prog. Horm. Res.* **31**:321.

Zeballos, G., and McCann, S. M., 1975, Alterations during the estrous cycle in the responsiveness of the pituitary to subcutaneous administration of synthetic LH-releasing hormone (LHRH), *Endocrinology* **96**:1377.

Zimmerman, E. A., 1976, Localization of hypothalamic hormones by immunocytochemical techniques, in: *Frontiers in Neuroendocrinology* (W. F. Ganong and L. Martini, eds.), pp. 25–62, Raven Press, New York.

14

The Neurochemical Control
of Mating Behavior

WILLIAM R. CROWLEY and FRANK P. ZEMLAN

I. INTRODUCTION

This chapter provides a survey of psychopharmacological studies of male and female sexual behavior, primarily conducted on rodent species. Because the expression of these behaviors normally requires the presence of gonadal hormones, this chapter attempts to integrate behavioral studies with studies on the effects of these hormones on neurotransmitter metabolism. The bulk of the literature in these fields focuses on norepinephrine (NE), dopamine (DA), serotonin (5-HT) and acetylcholine (ACh), all of which are involved in neuroendocrine regulation and in a variety of behaviors other than mating. For this reason, we also have attempted to place the neuropharmacology of reproductive behavior within a broader context. The other chapters in Part IV of this volume present closely related material.

II. NEUROPHARMACOLOGY OF FEMALE SEXUAL BEHAVIOR

A. Introduction

It is important to discuss briefly the behaviors shown by an estrous female and the ways in which they are measured (see also Gorski, 1974). As detailed in

WILLIAM R. CROWLEY • Department of Pharmacology, University of Tennessee Center for the Health Sciences, Memphis, Tennessee 38163.   FRANK P. ZEMLAN • Department of Pharmacology, University of Pennsylvania School of Medicine, Philadelphia, Pennsylvania 19104.

preceding chapters, female mammals display sexual behavior just prior to the time of ovulation to insure fertilization of the ova. Sexual receptivity in the female rat consists of the lordosis reflex and various soliciting behaviors. Lordosis is a posture characterized by immobilization, arching of the back such that the head and rump are elevated and the vaginal area is presented, and deflection of the tail to allow intromission (Komisaruk, 1974). Female rats also perform soliciting behaviors such as darting when in behavioral estrus. The behaviors of the mating male and female are coordinated so that the male's mount, which is actively solicited by the female through her behaviors, provides somatic stimulation that in turn elicits the full lordosis reflex by the female (Pfaff *et al.*, 1973, 1977). Each bout of mounting and lordosis is brief and is repeated a number of times until ejaculation occurs. The female guinea pig does not show similar solicitations but assumes and holds a lordosis posture with the back flattened while the male mounts and intromits (Young, 1969). Female hamsters also assume and hold a lordosis posture for long periods of time, even if not mounted by a male (Carter and Schein, 1971).

Many investigators use lordosis as the principal measure of female sexual behavior. Some simply note presence or absence of lordosis during a behavioral test, whereas others report the percentage of mounts that elicit lordosis (lordosis quotient, LQ). The intensity of lordosis also has been used as an index of receptivity (Hardy and DeBold, 1971). Gerall and Kenney (1970) and Ward (1972) have employed quality scoring systems for female rodent sexual behavior that take into account lordosis intensity, duration, and the presence of soliciting behaviors. Lordosis quotient scores are not employed in studies of lordosis in hamsters and guinea pigs which tend to hold the posture for long periods of time. Rather, in these species the duration of lordosis is usually recorded. These differences in assessing female sexual behavior should be remembered because drug treatments may selectively alter one component of estrous behavior without affecting another, leading to the possibility that such alterations may be more apparent with one scoring system than with another. For example, a drug may not increase the percentage of females that show lordosis during a test but may change the proportion of lordosis to mounts or the intensity of the responses in each female.

The regulation of the female rat's sexual activity by the ovarian hormones estradiol and progesterone is well established (Beach, 1942; Zemlan and Adler, 1977). The neurochemical mechanisms by which these steroids induce mating are currently under investigation, and we should like to examine the possibility that hormones change neural activity by altering neurotransmitter metabolism. The experiments reviewed in this section provide behavioral evidence for a hormone–neurotransmitter interaction. In Section IV, anatomical and biochemical evidence for such an interaction will be reviewed.

Two basic experimental protocols have been employed to assess the effects of drugs on female mating behavior. Strategy I involves treatment of an ovariectomized rat with estrogen alone or with estrogen and progesterone in doses sufficient to activate the full pattern of copulatory behavior. Drugs are then administered in an attempt to inhibit lordosis and/or soliciting behaviors. Strategy II consists of treating the ovariectomized animal with estrogen in doses that are too low to induce full receptivity. In this case, subsequent drug treatments attempt to produce the full mating pattern.

B. Monoamines and Female Sexual Behavior

1. Strategy I: Estrogen- and Progesterone-Treated Animals

Initial reports by Meyerson and co-workers (Meyerson, 1964a,c; Meyerson *et al.*, 1973) used drugs that affected the monoamines (NE, DA, 5-HT) non-selectively. For example, elevation of brain monoamine levels produced by the administration of monoamine oxidase (MAO) inhibitors such as pargyline markedly reduced the number of female rats, mice, hamsters, or rabbits displaying lordosis. Lordosis was also inhibited by treating receptive rats with imipramine or desmethylimipramine, drugs that prolong the action of monoamines at receptors by inhibiting the membrane pump reuptake process (Meyerson, 1966a).

2. Strategy II: Estrogen-Primed Animals

Because the above experiments show that increases in monoamines inhibit female sexual behavior, it follows that disruption of monoaminergic neuro-transmission should facilitate receptivity. Administration of reserpine or tetrabenazine increased the percentage of female rats showing lordosis (Meyerson, 1964b; Ahlenius *et al.*, 1972). These drugs, which deplete monoamines by displacing them from storage vesicles, could substitute for progesterone but not for estrogen. The facilitatory effects of reserpine and tetrabenazine were not obtained in hamsters, however (Meyerson, 1970).

3. The Adrenal Controversy

The use of drugs such as reserpine and tetrabenazine has been criticized because, in addition to their nonselective depleting action on monoamines, they cause the release of ACTH from the pituitary (cf. Van Loon, 1973). ACTH, in turn, promotes the release of adrenal steroids, including proges-terone, that can synergize with the exogenously administered estrogen to induce lordosis behavior (Meyerson, 1964b; Feder and Ruf, 1969). Thus, enhancement of receptivity by such drugs might be mediated by an indirect endocrine mechanism rather than by a direct effect on central monoaminergic neurons mediating lordosis. Indeed, reserpine induces a measurable increase in plasma progesterone soon after its administration (Paris *et al.*, 1971), and both reserpine and tetrabenazine failed to facilitate lordosis in rats or mice that had been adrenalectomized or pretreated with dexamethasone, a synthetic glucocorticoid that suppresses ACTH release (Uphouse *et al.*, 1970; Paris *et al.*, 1971; Larsson *et al.*, 1974). The possibility of indirect adrenal involvement in pharmacological induction of lordosis has become an important methodological consideration in designing and interpreting experiments in this area (see Whalen *et al.*, 1975).

C. Serotonin and Female Sexual Behavior

1. Strategy I: Estrogen- and Progesterone-Treated Animals

Drugs such as MAO inhibitors and reserpine do not allow identification of the specific transmitter or transmitters responsible for producing a behavioral effect because they act on all monoamines. Further experimentation (Meyerson, 1964a, c; Meyerson *et al.*, 1973) was necessary to clarify the role of 5-HT in suppressing lordosis. Selective increases in brain DA or NE (produced by administration of the precursor DOPA plus MAO inhibitor) did not inhibit lordosis, but an increase in 5-HT levels produced by treatment with 5-hydroxytryptophan (5-HTP) plus MAO inhibitor reduced the number of females mating. The inhibitory effect of the MAO inhibitor pargyline on female sexual behavior was prevented by first depleting the brain of 5-HT with a synthesis inhibitor. If the catecholamines but not 5-HT were first depleted, pargyline still inhibited lordosis. Increased brain 5-HT levels also decreased lordosis in mice, hamsters, and rabbits (Meyerson *et al.*, 1973).

A variety of 5-HT agonists also suppress lordosis behavior (as measured by number of animals showing lordosis or by *LQ*). These include α-methyltryptamine (Espino *et al.*, 1975), fenfluramine (Everitt *et al.*, 1974, 1975a), *p*-chloroamphetamine (Michanek and Meyerson, 1977), and hallucinogens such as LSD (Eliasson and Meyerson, 1977; Eliasson, 1976; Everitt *et al.*, 1974, 1975a), psilocybin, and dimethyltryptamine (Everitt and Fuxe, 1977a). LSD also produced a brief cessation of lordosis responding in guinea pigs (Crowley *et al.*, 1976).

2. Strategy II: Estrogen-Treated Animals

Treatment of nonreceptive, estrogen-primed rats with 5-HT antagonists can induce lordosis. Estrogen-treated female rats showed increased lordosis behavior after administration of the 5-HT synthesis inhibitor pCPA (Meyerson and Lewander, 1970; Lindström, 1971; Zemlan *et al.*, 1973; Everitt *et al.*, 1974, 1975a) or the 5-HT receptor blocker methysergide (Zemlan *et al.*, 1973; Henrik and Gerall, 1976). The effects of methysergide and pCPA were not abolished by adrenalectomy (Everitt *et al.*, 1975a; Zemlan *et al.*, 1973). *p*-Chorophenylalanine also increased the display of receptive behaviors in the ovariectomized rhesus monkey, and this was abolished by subsequent administration of 5-hydroxytryptophan, a treatment that restores 5-HT levels

(Gradwell *et al.*, 1975). Methysergide or pCPA induced lordosis behavior in estrogen-primed hamsters (Carter, 1977), but apparently neither drug can do so in estrogen-primed guinea pigs (Crowley *et al.*, 1976; Davis and English, 1977).

3. Biphasic Drug Effects

There are several interesting examples of biphasic effects of serotonergic drugs on female sexual behavior. As discussed in Chapter 4, low doses of monoamine agonists may stimulate presynaptic autoreceptors preferentially, thereby decreasing transmitter release and reducing functional activity in the system. Low doses of LSD and other hallucinogens facilitate lordosis behavior in estrogen-primed female rats, whereas higher doses of the same compounds suppress lordosis in estrogen- plus progesterone-primed rats (Everitt *et al.*, 1975a; Everitt and Fuxe, 1977a). These investigators have suggested that in lower dosages, the drugs induce lordosis by stimulating presynaptic autoreceptors that decrease activity in 5-HT neurons, whereas in higher doses, postsynaptic 5-HT receptor stimulation predominates and lordosis is inhibited.

A second example illustrates time-dependent biphasic effects. Zemlan (1978) and Zemlan *et al.* (1977) found that the 5-HT neurotoxin, *p*-chloroamphetamine, initially (within 15 min) reduced the display of lordosis in receptive rats but enhanced lordosis responding if animals were tested 3, 5, or 7 days afterward. These results are most likely caused by an initial release of 5-HT from damaged nerve terminals that is followed by a long-term depletion of 5-HT.

To summarize briefly, serotonergic systems have been shown to inhibit lordosis behavior in several species on the basis of the following evidence. Inhibition of receptivity has been observed after (a) activation of 5-HT receptors, (b) potentiation of 5-HT release, (c) blockade of 5-HT reuptake, and (d) increase in 5-HT levels. Conversely, the display of lordosis in estrogen-primed animals has been induced by (a) stimulation of inhibitory 5-HT autoreceptors, (b) blockade of postsynaptic 5-HT receptors, and (c) inhibition of 5-HT synthesis. It is not clear at present whether 5-HT affects both lordosis and soliciting behaviors or lordosis only. Everitt *et al.* (1975a) induced soliciting as well as lordosis with 5-HT antagonists, but Zemlan *et al.* (1973) and Ward *et al.* (1975) failed to activate soliciting behaviors with either systemic or central administration of 5-HT antagonists.

4. Neural Localization of Serotonin Lordosis Inhibitory Synapses

Several experiments have been carried out in an attempt to localize the neural sites at which 5-HT neurons inhibit lordosis. Ward *et al.* (1975) administered crystalline 5-HT receptor blockers (methysergide, cinanserin) via cannulae into areas known to contain estrogen receptors and 5-HT nerve terminals. Increases in *LQ* were observed when these drugs were placed into the preoptic–anterior hypothalamus, posterior hypothalamus, or basal telencephalon in estrogen-primed rats. Implants into the thalamus or dorsal neostriatum were ineffective. Methysergide also induced receptivity when placed into the amygdala (Franck and Ward, 1975) or microinjected into the arcuate nucleus (Foreman and Moss, 1978b). Foreman and Moss also found decreased lordosis responding in receptive rats after administration of 5-HT to the arcuate or medial preoptic areas.

  Display of lordosis behavior also was enhanced in estrogen-primed female rats following lesions of an ascending 5-HT pathway with the neurotoxin 5,7-dihydroxytryptamine (Everitt et al., 1975b). This fiber system supplies 5-HT terminals to the regions where Ward et al. (1975) and Foreman and Moss (1978b) induced lordosis with implants of 5-HT antagonists. More extensive mapping of sites where 5-HT agonists and antagonists affect female sexual behavior will be valuable in further characterizing the role of 5-HT in the mediation of female mating behavior.

D. Dopamine and Female Sexual Behavior

1. Strategy I: Estrogen- and Progesterone-Treated Animals

  Recent experiments have suggested that DA neurons, as well as serotonergic neurons, contribute to the overall monoaminergic inhibition of lordosis. Meyerson et al. (1974) and Everitt et al. (1974, 1975a) found that administration of DA receptor stimulants such as apomorphine or ET495 suppressed lordosis behavior in receptive rats. Apomorphine also produced a transient inhibition of receptivity in the guinea pig (Crowley et al., 1976). These findings may also explain the inhibition of lordosis behavior in rats that is observed after treatment with amphetamine, which promotes DA release (Meyerson, 1968a; Eliasson et al., 1972; Michanek and Meyerson, 1977).

2. Strategy II: Estrogen-Primed Animals

  Consistent with the above findings, administration of DA receptor blockers, such as pimozide or spiroperidol, activated lordosis behavior in female rats (Everitt et al., 1974, 1975a). These effects were not prevented by adrenalectomy. Dopamine antagonists do not facilitate lordosis behavior in guinea pigs, however (Crowley et al., 1976; Davis and English, 1977).

  Everitt and Fuxe (1977b) have demonstrated dose-dependent biphasic effects of DA agonists on female sexual behavior similar to their findings on 5-HT agonists (see Section II.C.3). That is, low doses of several DA receptor stimulants increased lordosis responding in estrogen-primed rats. In higher doses, this facilitatory effect disappeared, and the drugs abolished lordosis responding in estrogen- and progesterone-treated rats. As for 5-HT, this effect can be explained by postulating that low doses of these agonists primarily stimulate inhibitory presynaptic DA autoreceptors, whereas the higher doses primarily affect postsynaptic DA receptors. This suggestion is supported by their findings that the low-dose, lordosis-inducing effects were blocked by sulpiride, a putative presynaptic DA receptor blocker. This drug had no effect on the lordosis inhibition produced by the higher doses of DA agonists, presumably mediated by postsynaptic receptors.

3. Localization of Dopamine Lordosis-Inhibitory Synapses

Intraventricular injections of the catecholamine neurotoxin 6-hydroxydopamine (6-OHDA) produced depletion of forebrain NE and DA and markedly increased lordosis frequency and intensity in estrogen-pretreated rats (Herndon *et al.*, 1976; Caggiula *et al.*, 1977). Because soliciting behaviors were not increased and because lordosis responses were frequently of long duration, Herndon *et al.* (1976) suggested that the 6-OHDA lesion primarily enhanced the immobilization component of sexual receptivity. This finding suggests that the relevant catecholamine system is the nigrostriatal DA system. Lesions of this system produce akinesia and rigidity of the limbs (Andén *et al.*, 1971), and the lordosis posture is also characterized by such immobility and rigidity (Komisaruk, 1974). Further evidence on the locus for DA inhibition of female sexual behavior comes from studies with the guinea pig. Progesterone has two clear-cut effects on lordosis in this species, an initial facilitation followed by a period during which the female is refractory to stimulation by ovarian hormones (Zucker, 1966). Morin and Feder (1974a,b) localized the lordosis-inducing effects of progesterone to the medial basal hypothalamus, whereas the hormone inhibited lordosis when implanted into the substantia nigra, the origin of nigrostriatal DA neurons. These considerations, plus the findings that the DA agonist apomorphine inhibited lordosis, suggest the possibility that in guinea pigs, the progesterone-induced refractory period involves activation of nigrostriatal DA neurons.

4. Dopamine and Soliciting Behaviors

Because soliciting behaviors such as darting and hopping are active, stereotyped movements, it is likely that their neural control differs from that underlying the immobile lordosis posture, even though their appearance is coordinated. Caggiula *et al.* (1976) found that DA receptor blockade with haloperidol abolished soliciting behaviors but not lordosis in receptive female rats. This stands in contrast to the studies already cited that demonstrated increased lordosis after DA receptor blockade. Thus, central DA neurons appear to influence the two components of female receptivity differentially. Perhaps the nigrostriatal system, which is involved in many behaviors, must be activated during soliciting but must be turned off while the animal is in the lordosis posture. Dopamine receptor blockers may facilitate lordosis and suppress soliciting by enhancing a "stop" component, whereas the increased motor activity produced by DA agonists antagonizes the immobilization required for lordosis.

E. Norepinephrine and Female Sexual Behavior

1. Strategy I: Estrogen- and Progesterone-Treated Animals

Although 5-HT and DA systems clearly seem to inhibit lordosis, a role for NE in control of this behavior is much less certain at present. In receptive rats, inhibition of NE synthesis with the dopamine-β-hydroxylase inhibitor FLA63 produced a slight inhibition of lordosis responding (Everitt *et al.*, 1975a). Severe decrements in lordosis behavior have resulted from damage to the dorsal and ventral ascending NE bundles (Herndon, 1976). However, in receptive female guinea pigs, either the dopamine-β-hydroxylase inhibitor, U-14,624, or the NE receptor blocker, phenoxybenzamine, suppressed lordosis behavior (Crowley *et al.*, 1976; Nock and Feder, 1979). The inhibitory effect of U-14,624 was reversed by the noradrenergic agonist, clonidine (Nock and Feder, 1979).

2. Strategy II: Estrogen-Treated Animals

The NE agonist clonidine activated lordosis responding in nonreceptive, estrogen-primed guinea pigs (Crowley *et al.*, 1978a; Nock and Feder, 1979), but this drug suppressed lordosis responding in receptive rats (Davis and Kohl, 1977). The latter effect may have resulted from an action of the drug on inhibitory presynaptic NE autoreceptors analogous to the effects of DA and 5-HT agonists. This view is plausible because the inhibitory effect of clonidine was prevented by yohimbine, a presynaptic NE blocker, but not by phenoxybenzamine, a postsynaptic NE antagonist.

3. Localization of Noradrenergic Influences on Lordosis

Infusions of norepinephrine or epinephrine into the medial preoptic or arcuate nuclei activated lordosis behavior in nonreceptive, estrogen-primed female rats (Foreman and Moss, 1978a). However, these investigators showed further that the facilitation of lordosis behavior was mediated by β-receptors, whereas α-receptor stimulation appeared to exert inhibitory effects in animals already receptive.

Thus, some evidence suggests that NE systems are excitatory to the display of lordosis in rats and guinea pigs, an effect possibibly mediated by β-adrenergic receptors in the medial preoptic and arcuate nuclei.

F. Acetylcholine and Female Sexual Behavior

1. Strategy I: Estrogen- and Progesterone-Treated Animals

A series of experiments by Lindström and Meyerson (1967; Lindström, 1970, 1971) indicates that cholinergic neurons may interact with serotonergic neurons to inhibit lordosis. Muscarinic cholinergic agonists, such as pilocarpine, decreased the number of receptive females displaying lordosis. This effect was blocked by centrally acting muscarinic antagonists but not by antimuscarinics that do not cross the blood–brain barrier. The cholinergic inhibition of lordosis was potentiated by elevation of monoamine levels with MAO inhibitors. Furthermore, the cholinergic inhibition was not observed if lordosis was activated by estrogen and 5-HT antagonists.

From these data, Lindström concluded that 5-HT mechanisms must be intact for cholinergic stimulants to exert their inhibitory effects. The neuroanatomical basis for such an interaction is unknown at present. Analogous experiments with hamsters (Lindström, 1972) demonstrated cholinergic inhibition of lordosis, but no evidence of 5-HT–ACh interaction was obtained.

2. Strategy II: Estrogen-Treated Rats

Consistent with the hypothesis of an interaction with 5-HT mechanisms, muscarinic antagonists by themselves did not activate lordosis responding in estrogen-primed rats (Lindström, 1973). However, recent evidence indicates that nicotine can induce lordosis responding in estrogen-primed female rats (Fuxe *et al.*, 1977a). This raises the possibility of a nicotinic–muscarinic antagonism in female sexual behavior.

G. Monoamines and Lordosis in Male Rats

As discussed in Chapter 6, adult male rats rarely display lordosis when mounted and are less sensitive than females to treatment with ovarian hormones. This behavioral insensitivity is likely to be the result of perinatal androgen exposure. However, lordosis behavior has been induced in estrogen-primed male rats treated systemically with monoamine-depleting drugs (Meyerson, 1968b; Larsson and Södersten, 1971; Södersten and Ahlenius, 1972). Thus, monoaminergic inhibition of lordosis is characteristic of males as well as females. This conclusion is supported by the findings that estrogen-primed male rats showed increased lordosis behavior after placement of 5-HT or β-adrenergic antagonists into anterior and posterior hypothalamic sites similar to those effective in females (Crowley *et al.*, 1975). These investigators hypothesized that one action of ovarian hormones may be to remove monoaminergic inhibition of lordosis. Males seem less sensitive to this effect, leaving open the possibility, however, that experimental manipulation of monoaminergic transmission can reveal the existence of "lordosis circuitry" in males.

H. Peptides and Lordosis

Several studies have demonstrated a facilitatory role for LH-releasing hormone (LRH) in female sexual behavior. This peptide induced lordosis in estrogen-primed female rats after systemic administration, and the effects were not dependent on adrenal or pituitary hormone release (Moss and McCann, 1973, 1975; Pfaff, 1973). Infusion of LRH into preoptic or arcuate sites in estrogen-pretreated females also induced mating behavior and potentiated lordosis after repeated matings (Moss and Foreman, 1976; Foreman and Moss, 1977).

Thyrotropin releasing hormone (TRH) did not facilitate lordosis after systemic or central administration (Moss and McCann, 1973; Foreman and Moss, 1977). Rather, this peptide attenuated the increase in LQ produced by repeated matings, an effect localized to the arcuate region (Foreman and Moss, 1977). These intriguing findings raise the possibility that hypothalamic peptide hormones, perhaps functioning as "peptidergic" neurotransmitters, coordinate mating behavior and pituitary hormone secretion as part of a general neuroendocrine control mechanism.

I. Monoamines and Sexual Motivation

According to Meyerson and Lindström (1973), sexual motivation can be operationally defined as a state in which an animal seeks sexual contact with a conspecific. This may be analogous to those behaviors Beach (1976) has termed "proceptive." In a detailed parametric study, Meyerson and Lindström (1973) showed that estrogen treatment stimulated female rats to cross an electrified grid to reach male rats. Meyerson *et al.* (1974) have shown further that some drugs that affect female sexual behavior at the reflexive level (i.e., lordosis) also affect performance in sexual motivation tasks. For example, LSD and apomorphine, both of which diminish lordosis responding, also decreased the number of grid crossings for a male. The 5-HT synthesis inhibitor pCPA, which enhances lordosis in estrogen-pretreated females, also potentiated the effect of estrogen on grid crossings. These preliminary findings suggest that monoamines may have parallel roles in central motivational and copulatory reflex systems.

J. Monoamines and Maternal Behavior

Recent studies implicate NE systems in the expression of maternal behavior. Moltz *et al.* (1976) reported that an increase in hypothalamic noradrenergic activity occurred soon after parturition. A similar change was also observed in virgin rats that were induced to behave maternally towards foster pups (Rosenberg *et al.*, 1976). This group has suggested that NE neurons may control the initiation of maternal behavior because intraventricular administration of 6-OHDA during gestation interfered with the postpartum onset of maternal behavior (Rosenberg *et al.*, 1977). The neurotoxin had no effect if given during lactation, when maternal responsiveness had already been established.

K. Summary

Table 1 summarizes what is known at present concerning central neurotransmitter systems and female sexual behavior. It appears that 5-HT, DA, and ACh systems inhibit lordosis behavior, although there is some evidence for noradrenergic stimulation of lordosis. An active DA system appears to be required for the display of soliciting behaviors. Serotonin may also inhibit soliciting, but more anatomical and pharmacological studies on this behavior need to be performed. As indicated in the table, the neuroanatomical loci for monoaminergic and cholinergic control over female mating patterns are largely unknown. Serotonergic antagonists activate lordosis when implanted into various preoptic, hypothalamic, and amygdaloid sites. Circumstantial evidence implicates the neostriatum as a site for dopaminergic modulation of receptive behaviors. LH-releasing hormone and TRH have excitatory and inhibitory roles, respectively, in female mating behavior on the basis of systemic and central administration studies. These effects appear to involve the preoptic and arcuate regions.

Table 1. Effects of Neurotransmitters on Female Sexual Behavior

Transmitter	Effect on lordosis	Effect on soliciting	Neuroanatomical sites of effect
Serotonin	Inhibition	Inhibition	Anterior and posterior hypothalamus, preoptic area, arcuate, amygdala
Dopamine	Inhibition	Facilitation	Neostriatum (?)
Norepinephrine	Facilitation	?	?
β-Adrenergic (Epinephrine ?)	Facilitation	?	Anterior, posterior hypothalamus
Acetylcholine	Inhibition	?	?
Luteinizing hormone-releasing hormone	Facilitation	Facilitation	Preoptic, arcuate
Thyrotropin-releasing hormone	Inhibition	?	Arcuate

III. NEUROPHARMACOLOGY OF MALE SEXUAL BEHAVIOR

A. Introduction

This section reviews the involvement of neurotransmitter systems in masculine copulatory behavior. Nearly all of the studies cited have been performed on rats, whose copulatory pattern is characterized by series of mounts, some of which result in vaginal penetration (intromission). Ejaculation occurs after a number of intromissions and is followed by a period of behavioral inactivity (postejaculatory interval or PEI). The male rat will then resume mating and typically can achieve five or more ejaculatory series on a satiety test (see Dewsbury, 1972; Sachs and Barfield, 1976 for review). Besides noting such routine measures as percent of animals copulating and the number of mounts, intromissions, and ejaculations per test, studies of male rat sexual behavior frequently report latencies to first mount, intromission, or ejaculation, the interintromission interval, and the duration of the PEI. Drug effects may be limited to only one or several of these components, making interpretation of results sometimes complicated. The reader is referred to Dewsbury (1975) for an excellent discussion of methodological considerations in designing and interpreting pharmacological experiments on male copulatory behavior.

In contrast to the female, pharmacological studies of masculine behavior do not divide themselves into two clear-cut experimental strategies. Various studies have employed sexually vigorous males, sexually naive males, "sexually sluggish" males, or castrated males with or without testosterone replacement. With a few exceptions, pharmacologically consistent results generally have been obtained despite the variety of experimental designs. Therefore, in our discussions of the role of various transmitters, we shall present the results of increasing or decreasing functional activity in a particular transmitter system and, where possible, indicate the type of male studied and specific measures affected by drug treatment.

B. Monoamines and Male Sexual Behavior

1. Increased Monoamine Activity

As was true in the study of the female, earlier studies used drugs that elevated or depleted all monoamines nonselectively. For example, administration of MAO inhibitors such as pargyline and nialamide inhibited copulatory behavior by lengthening intromission and ejaculation latencies and prolonging the PEI in gonadally intact, experienced maters (Dewsbury *et al.*, 1972). These drugs also decreased the percentage of castrated, testosterone-maintained animals that mounted (Malmnäs, 1973).

2. Decreased Monoamine Activity

Conversely, several groups have reported that depletion of monoamines with reserpine or tetrabenazine produced a relatively specific facilitatory effect on male copulatory performance, i.e., a reduction in the number of intromissions prior to ejaculation and a consequent shortening of the ejaculatory latency (Dewsbury, 1971, 1972; Dewsbury and Davis, 1970; Soulairac and Soulairac, 1961, 1962). These effects, however, appeared to be dose dependent inasmuch as higher acute doses or chronic treatment with these agents inhibited copulation, as well as other behavioral activities (Dewsbury, 1972; Soulairac, 1963). Malmnäs (1973) also found that these drugs tended to reduce the display of copulatory behavior in castrated, testosterone-treated animals in doses that also depressed other behaviors.

Thus, the results of these studies, which parallel the initial findings in females, indicate that male sexual behavior is inhibited by a monoamine system or systems. The use of more selective drugs has revealed that 5-HT inhibits and DA enhances male copulatory performance.

C. Serotonin and Male Sexual Behavior

1. Increased Serotonin Activity

Malmnäs (1973) reported that administration of the 5-HT precursor 5-HTP in combination with MAO and peripheral decarboxylase inhibitors to prevent premature degradation or of the 5-HT agonist LSD decreased mating behavior in castrated, testosterone-maintained males. Neither treatment decreased general motor activity, but both did reduce the amount of activity by the male directed toward the receptive female.

2. Decreased Serotonin Activity

Consistent with the above studies, there are numerous reports of enhanced male copulatory performance after disruption of serotonergic neurotransmission. The most widely used 5-HT antagonist has been the tryptophan hydroxylase inhibitor pCPA. In several earlier studies (Tagliamonte et al., 1969; Gessa et al., 1970; Shillito, 1970; Gawienowski and Hodgen, 1971; Gawienowski et al., 1973; Hoyland et al., 1970; Ferguson et al., 1970), pCPA enhanced the display of "homosexual" mounting, i.e., male rats or cats housed in groups began mounting each other after treatment. It is difficult to evaluate the results of these unconventional experiments, but subsequent work demonstrated a marked stimulatory effect of pCPA on male copulatory performance in heterosexual testing situations. For example, pCPA increased the number of intact male rats that copulated and ejaculated (Gessa and Tagliamonte, 1973; Gessa et al., 1970). Similar effects have been reported to occur in castrated males maintained on a suboptimal testosterone regime (Malmnäs and Meyerson, 1971; Malmnäs, 1973) and in chronic noncopulators (Ginton, 1976). Increases in ejaculation frequency and decreases in ejaculatory latencies and postejaculatory intervals have been the most frequently noted changes in male sexual behavior after pCPA treatment (Mitler *et al.*, 1972; Malmnäs, 1973; Salis and Dewsbury, 1971; Ahlenius *et al.*, 1971). In contrast to rats, no stimulation of heterosexual copulation by pCPA has been observed in cats or monkeys (Zitrin *et al.*, 1970; Redmond *et al.*, 1971).

The stimulatory effect of pCPA on male–male mounting apparently requires both androgen and the presence of an intact pituitary gland (Gessa *et al.*, 1970; Gawienowski and Hodgen, 1971). That the effect is actually caused by depletion of 5-HT rather than some other nonspecific action is strongly suggested by the findings that 5-HTP treatment reverses the effect of pPCA (Tagliamonte *et al.*, 1969; Gessa *et al.*, 1970; Gessa and Tagliamonte, 1973; Malmnäs and Meyerson, 1971).

Interestingly, decreased ejaculatory latencies and shortening of the PEI also have been reported to occur in adult rats that were treated neonatally with pCPA (Hyyppä *et al.*, 1972). These behavioral effects are apparent long after the neurochemical effects of the drug have worn off and suggest a role for 5-HT in the processes of sexual differentiation.

Other serotonin antagonists such as methysergide also have been reported to facilitate male–male mounting behavior (Benkert and Eversmann, 1971; Soulairac and Soulairac, 1971). In addition, homosexual mounting in rats and rabbits has been increased after maintaining the animals on a tryptophan-free diet that markedly decreases central 5-HT content (Gessa and Tagliamonte, 1975).

3. Localization of Serotonin Inhibition of Male Sexual Behavior

There are no published reports on male sexual behavior after administration of serotonergic drugs to brain areas containing 5-HT nerve terminals. Intraventricular injections of the 5-HT neurotoxin 5,6-dihydroxytryptamine increased homosexual mounting in male rats (Da Prada *et al.*, 1972); the toxin also increased the number of sexually naive males copulating and ejaculating with a female after injection into the midbrain raphe, a site of 5-HT cell bodies that innervate forebrain areas (Gessa and Tagliamonte, 1975). Another neurotoxic indoleamine, 5,7-dihydroxytryptamine, increased the number of castrated, low-dose testosterone-treated males showing ejaculation after administration into the ascending 5-HT bundles (Södersten *et al.*, 1978).

D. Dopamine and Male Sexual Behavior

1. Increased Dopamine Activity

The inhibition of masculine copulatory behavior by 5-HT appears to be opposed by an excitatory DA system. Several studies have shown that male copulatory performance is enhanced after treatment with the catecholamine precursor L-DOPA. For example, in castrated male rats given a suboptimal testosterone replacement regimen, a combination of L-DOPA plus MAO and peripheral decarboxylase inhibitors increased the number of males mounting, intromitting, and ejaculating and reduced mount, intromission, and ejaculation latencies (Malmnäs, 1973, 1976). The facilitatory effect of DOPA was prevented by pretreatment with the DA receptor blocker pimozide (Malmnäs, 1976). Similarly, L-DOPA plus the peripheral decarboxylase inhibitor benserazide increased the display of mounts, intromissions, and ejaculations in intact but "sexually sluggish" male rats and shortened the ejaculatory latency and PEI in sexually experienced male rats. These effects were antagonized by a DA receptor blocker (Tagliamonte *et al.*, 1974). However, Hyyppä *et al.* (1971) and Gray *et al.* (1974) failed to enhance male copulatory behavior with L-DOPA and benserazide. It has been suggested that this failure may have resulted from the use of higher doses of DOPA in highly active males and the consequent appearance of competing responses such as stereotypies and sluggish motor activity (Malmnäs, 1976; Gray *et al.*, 1974).

Male copulatory behavior has also been increased by the DA receptor stimulant apomorphine. This drug increased the display of mounts, intromissions, and ejaculations in gonadally intact males (Tagliamonte *et al.*, 1974) and in castrated, testosterone-treated males (Malmnäs, 1973). As for DOPA, these effects were blocked by pretreatment with DA receptor antagonists. In contrast to the stimulatory effects of pCPA, which seem to require the presence of androgen, apomorphine treatment has been reported to induce copulatory behavior in castrated or castrated–adrenalectomized animals not receiving any exogenous androgen treatment (Malmnäs, 1977).

2. Decreased Dopamine Activity

Consistent with the above findings, male copulatory behavior has been disrupted by treatment with DA receptor blockers in doses that did not impair other motor behaviors both in castrated, testosterone-treated males and in intact males (Malmnäs, 1973; Tagliamonte *et al.*, 1974).

3. Localization of Dopamine Facilitation of Male Sexual Behavior

To date, there have been no published reports that specifically investigate the neural sites at which DA influences male sexual behavior. However, it appears likely that the nigrostriatal DA system is involved in control of many behaviors, including copulation. This will be discussed in more detail in Section V.

E. Norepinephrine and Male Sexual Behavior

In contrast to the reciprocal DA facilitatory/5-HT inhibitory control of masculine copulatory behavior, it seems that noradrenergic systems play a relatively minor role in control of this behavior. Malmnäs (1973) found that neither noradrenergic agonists nor antagonists influenced the number of males copulating. Administration of the NE receptor stimulant clonidine or the NE precursor dihydroxyphenylserine did reduce the number of mounts/min during a short test. Conversely, this parameter was increased by NE antagonists. This suggests a possible inhibitory role for NE, at least over some aspects of the male copulatory pattern. Consistent with this view, lesions in the region of the dorsal ascending NE bundle markedly reduced the PEI in sexually experienced male rats (Clark *et al.*, 1975). However, the same group (Caggiula *et al.*, 1977) subsequently failed to reproduce this effect with selective lesions of the dorsal NE bundle with 6-OHDA, thus casting some doubt on the role of NE in these effects.

F. Acetylcholine and Male Sexual Behavior

The role of cholinergic systems in male copulatory behavior is not well-defined at present. A possible modulating role is suggested by the following findings. The muscarinic blocker atropine antagonized the pCPA-induced homo- and heterosexual mounting (Gessa and Tagliamonte, 1973). This suggests a 5-HT/ACh interaction in control of male mating behavior and is reminiscent of a similar interaction postulated for female sexual behavior (Section II.F). Suppression of copulatory behavior was reported after treatment with either eserine, an acetylcholinesterase inhibitor that prolongs synaptic action of ACh, or the blocker atropine (Soulairac, 1963), leading to the proposal that any disruption of cholinergic function can impair sexual behavior. More recently, Soulairac and Soulairac (1975) reported an enhancement of male copulatory performance (increased ejaculation frequency and decreased ejaculatory latencies and postejaculatory intervals) following administration of nicotine.

G. Peptides and Male Sexual Behavior

1. ACTH-like Peptides

Intracerebroventricular injection of $ACTH_{1-24}$ (a fragment containing the first 24 amino acid residues of ACTH), α-or β-melanocyte-stimulating hormone (MSH), or β-lipotropin produces several behavioral syndromes in a variety of species (see Bertolini *et al.*, 1975, for review). One consists of repetitive erections, copulatory movements, and ejaculations, not necessarily directed towards another animal. As colorfully described by Bertolini (1971b), the ejaculations occur ". . . almost as in a dream, the animal having no interaction with its partners (male or female) and apparently being surprised at what is happening in its body" (p. LXXIV). Other pituitary hormones such as growth hormone, oxytocin, and vasopressin do not produce these effects (Bertolini, 1971b). In addition, intraventricular $ACTH_{1-24}$ shortened ejaculation latency in sexually experienced male rats, suggesting some role in control of the naturally occurring behavior pattern (Bertolini *et al.*, 1975).

Bertolini and co-workers (Bertolini, 1971a; Bertolini *et al.*, 1971, 1975) have determined the behaviorally active amino acid sequence to be $ACTH_{4-10}$. This sequence, present in all the above hormones, has been implicated in learning and memory (see Chapter 4) but is devoid of adrenocortical activating properties. Bertolini *et al.* (1971) have suggested that this or a similar peptide is synthesized in the hypothalamus and may be a corticotropin-releasing factor (CRF). If the active principle is a CRF, this would be analogous to the lordosis-inducing action of LRF in females.

2. Luteinizing Hormone-Releasing Hormone

Luteinizing hormone-releasing hormone may also be involved in regulation of masculine behavior. This peptide reduced the latencies to intromission and ejaculation in intact males and in castrated, testosterone-treated males (Moss, 1978) after systemic administration.

3. Endogenous Opiate Peptides

Another portion of the β-lipotropin molecule is the sequence encompassing amino acids 61–91 (β-endorphin), now thought to be an endogenous ligand for opiate receptors (see Chapter 4). In a recent study (Meyerson and Terenius, 1977), this peptide disrupted normal male copulatory behavior inasmuch as the treated males failed to mount or mounted after a long delay, even though they actively pursued and investigated the female. This effect was blocked by the opiate antagonist naltrexone, indicating involvement of opiate receptors. Furthermore, naltrexone increased the number of male rats ejaculating (Hetta, 1977). Similarly, intracerebroventricular injection of an enkephalin analogue decreased copulatory behavior in male rats without disrupting motor behavior (Pellegini Quarantotti *et al.*, 1978).

H. Monoamines and Mounting in Female Rats

Masculine copulatory behavior is not uncommon in female rodents, especially during sexual receptivity (Young, 1961, 1969). Several studies have shown that treatment of ovariectomized female rats with testosterone plus pCPA enhances mounting over that shown after each compound alone (Rodriguez-Sierra *et al.* 1976; Van de Poll *et al.*, 1977), suggesting that serotonergic inhibition of mounting is present in females as well as males. In contrast to the male, however, the DA agonist apomorphine has no stimulatory effect on mounting in testosterone-treated females (Rodriguez-Sierra *et al.*,

1976). Thus, the importance of DA in mounting behavior may be different for males and females.

I. Monoamines and Sexual Behavior in Humans

A number of drugs used in our culture today such as amphetamine, cocaine, marijuana, methaqualone, and LSD have been ballyhooed as aphrodisiacs. Even if such claims are true, it is difficult to ascertain whether such drugs enhance sexual performance and pleasure in humans by a specific action on neural pathways mediating sexual behavior or do so by altering perception, increasing arousal, or removing inhibitions. Several recent, interesting reviews treat this topic in more detail (Carter and Davis, 1976; Hollister, 1975a,b). However, there are some instances in which drug effects on sexual behavior in humans appear to parallel the animal work. In some cases, the animal literature has provided the rationale for attempts to use neuropharmacological agents to ameliorate sexual dysfunction. This section reviews briefly some of the studies implicating monoamine systems in human (mostly male) sexual behavior. The reader should be aware that some of this information appears to be based on somewhat casual observation, and even the more controlled studies are plagued with the various problems attendant on the study of sexual behavior in humans.

1. Catecholamines

Sexual stimulation has been reported after the use of amphetamine and cocaine (Hollister, 1975a). These drugs may exert this effect by enhancing overall arousal through an action on the autonomic system or by potentiation of central catecholaminergic neurotransmission. Conversely, impotence has been observed during treatment with tranquilizers, such as chlorpromazine, that block central catecholamine receptors (Belt, 1973).

Perhaps the best known parallel drug effect between animals and humans involves L-DOPA. Section III.D.1 discussed experiments in which this catecholamine precursor potentiated copulatory behavior in male rats. DOPA has been used clinically to treat the tremor and akinesia of Parkinson's disease, which is characterized by a loss of striatal DA because of lesions in the brainstem. Soon after the introduction of L-DOPA therapy, there were occasional reports of increased sexual activity in Parkinson's disease pateints (Barbeau, 1969). For example, one study reported that 7 of 19 male and female parkinsonian patients showed increased sexual behavior during treatment with L-DOPA (Bowers *et al.*, 1971). These investigators noted three patterns of sexual change associated with DOPA therapy. In one group, increased sexual behavior accompanied a more generalized improvement in health and mobility. A second group showed a specific stimulation of sexual activity that was relatively independent of overall improvement in health. The sexual behavior of the third group was thought to have resulted from a loss of inhibition. It is interesting to note that the scattered reports of a stimulatory effect of L-DOPA on sexual behavior in humans actually antedated experiments with this drug on animals.

Despite its occasional stimulation of sexual behavior in Parkinson's disease patients, L-DOPA has not proved useful in the treatment of impotence. Benkert and co-workers (Benkert *et al.,* 1972; Benkert, 1973) reported that although L-DOPA treatment did increase the degree of penile erection, this improvement was still insufficient to permit coitus.

2. Serotonin

Following the reports of the stimulatory effects of 5-HT antagonists, such as pCPA, on mating in male and female rats, several tests were made on humans. In one study (Sicuteri, 1974) performed on male headache sufferers who also complained of impotence, a combination of testosterone plus pCPA increased the number of daily erections. One detailed case history described a man who had been impotent for 2 years but was able to have sexual relations with his wife during pCPA plus testosterone therapy. Sicuteri also reported that treatment with the 5-HT precursor tryptophan, which elevates 5-HT levels, had a depressant effect on sexual behavior in some males. Treatment with androgen plus the 5-HT antagonists *p*-chloroamphetamine or methysergide also produced some increase in erectile strength and libido in impotent men (Benkert, 1973). Thus, in spite of the limited samples and other methodological problems, there are some intriguing hints that monoamine systems in humans play a role in sexual behavior and that neuropharmacological agents may one day be used to treat human sexual disorders.

J. Summary

There is strong evidence to support an excitatory role for DA and an inhibitory role for 5-HT in male copulatory behavior (see Table 2). Thus, 5-HT systems apparently inhibit both masculine and feminine sexual behavior pat-

Table 2. Effects of Neurotransmitters on Male Copulatory Behavior

Transmitter	Effect on male sexual behavior	Neuroanatomical site of action
Serotonin	Inhibition	?
Dopamine	Facilitation	Striatum (?)
Norepinephrine	Inhibition	?
Acetylcholine	Facilitation, inhibition	?
ACTH-like peptides	Facilitation	?
β-Endorphin	Inhibition	?

terns. These two transmitter systems may serve analogous functions in humans. Relatively little is known about the function of noradrenergic or cholinergic neurons in male behavior, although these systems may modulate the dopaminergic or serotonergic circuits. ACTH-like peptides produce a striking sexual arousal syndrome that is independent of the adrenal cortex and actually may be mediated by an ACTH-releasing factor synthesized by hypothalamic neurons. As indicated in Table 2, information concerning specific brain areas mediating these effects is virtually nonexistent.

IV. EFFECTS OF GONADAL HORMONES ON CENTRAL NEUROTRANSMITTERS

There is a good deal of research currently devoted to analysis of the neurochemical mechanisms by which gonadal hormones affect sexual behavior and other reproductive processes (cf. Chapters 13 and 15). Because the previous two sections presented evidence that sexual behavior can be influenced by monoaminergic and cholinergic drugs, it is reasonable to hypothesize that gonadal hormones affect copulatory behavior by interacting in some way with monoaminergic and cholinergic systems. This section examines evidence for this hypothesis by surveying the actions of estradiol, progesterone, and testosterone on monoaminergic neurotransmission. First, the effects of gonadal hormones on monamine turnover will be reviewed, followed by a discussion of possible mechanisms underlying these changes. The reader should recall from Chapter 4 that turnover provides an index of the state of activity in a system, i.e., a faster turnover indicates an active system. Our task is made difficult by the failure of many studies to relate their hormone treatment to known effects on gonadotropin secretion or mating behavior. Therefore, it is not always possible to determine whether a given endocrine manipulation mimics a physiological condition. We have emphasized those studies in which such a correlation is possible.

A. Effects of Estrogen and Progesterone

Estrogen and progesterone have several important actions during the estrous cycle, including inhibitory and stimulatory feedback effects on gonadotropin release and induction of female sexual behavior (cf. Chapter 10). A heuristic model for studying these effects has been developed in ovariectomized rats by McCann and co-workers (see Kalra and McCann, 1973) and used for studying drug effects. In this protocol, a single administration of estrogen to ovariectomized females reduces plasma LH levels, whereas subsequent treatment with either estrogen again or with progesterone stimulates LH secretion. These dual effects may mimic the inhibitory and stimulatory feedback actions of ovarian hormones during the estrous cycle. The combined estrogen plus progesterone treatment also induces sexual receptivity. There is evidence that some of the inhibitory and stimulatory feedback effects of ovarian hormones are associated with changes in monoaminergic neural activity.

1. Influence on Norepinephrine Turnover

In several studies, ovariectomy increased hypothalamic NE levels and turnover, an effect reversible by subsequent estrogen treatment (Donoso and Stefano, 1967; Coppola, 1969). Single injections of estrogen reduced NE turnover in the cortex, brainstem, and anterior hypothalamus after ovariectomy (Everitt *et al.,* 1974; Munaro, 1977). Recently, more discrete anatomical analyses have shown that estrogen treatment that reduced plasma levels of LH and FSH also reduced NE turnover in the medial preoptic nucleus, bed nucleus of stria terminalis, and central gray (Crowley *et al.,* 1978b; Fuxe *et al.,* 1977b; Löfström *et al.,* 1977). Progesterone administration to estrogen-primed rats (which elevates gonadotropins and induces sexual receptivity) increased NE turnover in the cerebral cortex, anterior hypothalamus (Everitt *et al.,* 1975a,b; Munaro, 1977), bed nucleus of stria terminalis, arcuate nucleus, and central gray (Crowley *et al.,* 1978b). Furthermore, hypothalamic NE turnover is increased during proestrus (Donoso and de Gutierrez Moyano, 1970; Löfström, 1977). Thus, during conditions of high gonadotropin secretion such as after ovariectomy, after estrogen plus progesterone treatment, or on the day of proestrus, NE activity tends to be high. Under conditions where gonadotropins are low, i.e., diestrus or ovariectomized and estrogen-primed, NE activity tends to be reduced.

2. Influence on Dopamine Turnover

Fuxe and co-workers (Fuxe *et al.,* 1967, 1969, 1977) have shown by several different techniques that an inhibitory feedback action of estrogen on LH secretion is associated with an increase in turnover of the tuberoinfundibular DA system. This system also showed reduced activity during the proestrus critical period (Ahren *et al.,* 1971). Ovarian hormones have not been reported to affect turnover in other major DA terminal areas such as the caudate nucleus, nucleus accumbens, or olfactory tubercle (Fuxe *et al.,* 1977; Crowley *et al.,* 1978b). However, ovarian hormones do influence the behavioral effects of DA agonists and antagonists (Bedard *et al.,* 1979; Nausieda *et al.,* 1979).

3. Influence on Serotonin Turnover

There is a prominent circadian rhythmicity in brain 5-HT levels in the rat, the highest levels being attained during the light and lowest during the dark (Hery *et al.,* 1972). According to Everitt *et al.* (1975a), ovarian hormones can exert opposite effects on 5-HT turnover depending on what time of day they are administered. For example, if injected at the beginning of the dark phase, estrogen increased and subsequent progesterone reduced 5-HT turnover. This is consistent with an inhibitory role of 5-HT in hormone-induced sexual receptivity (Section II.C). However, if the hormones were given at the beginning of the light phase, estrogen decreased and progesterone increased 5-HT turnover. The mechanisms underlying these opposite effects are unknown at present. Similarly, Munaro (1978) reported that estradiol decreased, and subsequent progesterone treatment elevated 5-HT turnover. These effects were observed in the morning, but not afternoon, hours.

B. Effects of Testosterone

Although the behavioral studies reviewed in Section III point to an interaction between testosterone and monoaminergic neurons in the regulation of male sexual behavior, little is known regarding the effects of androgens on neurotransmitter dynamics. According to fluorescence histochemical estimates of monoaminergic neural activity (Fuxe *et al.*, 1969; Fuxe and Hökfelt, 1970), castration of male rats produced a decrease in NE turnover in various brain regions but had no effect on the activity of the tuberoinfundibular DA system. Testosterone replacement, however, accelerated the activity of both NE and tuberoinfundibular DA. On the other hand, Donoso *et al.* (1969) reported a castration-induced increase in hypothalamic NE synthesis and release. More recently, Simpkins *et al.* (1980) found that administration of testosterone subcutaneously or directly into the medial basal hypothalamus reduced the turnover of NE in this area.

These various effects may be relevant to gonadotropin secretion, but their significance for male sexual behavior is unlikely. Because the psychopharmacological studies reviewed in Section III point to a DA excitatory/5-HT inhibitory modulation of masculine copulatory behavior, the effects of androgens on these systems should be studied.

C. Possible Mechanisms of Hormone-Induced Alterations in Neurotransmitter Function

To summarize briefly, the evidence generally indicates that a state of increased gonadotropin release, sometimes also corresponding with sexual receptivity, is associated with increased NE turnover and decreased DA and 5-HT turnover. Conversely, low gonadotropin levels are associated with low NE turnover and increased DA and 5-HT turnover. It is tempting but perhaps premature to relate these findings to female sexual behavior, especially as the evidence in Section II points to an excitatory role for NE and inhibitory roles for DA and 5-HT in lordosis behavior. No firm conclusions can be drawn at present concerning the effects of testosterone on monoaminergic systems. This section reviews briefly some possible mechanisms by which hormones may affect neurotransmitter turnover.

1. Neuroanatomical Considerations

Comparisons of atlases of estradiol- and testosterone-concentrating neurons (e.g., Stumpf et al., 1975; Sar and Stumpf, 1975; Pfaff and Keiner, 1973) with those of catecholamine-containing neurons (e.g., Fuxe, 1965; Jacobowitz and Palkovits, 1974; Palkovits and Jacobowitz, 1974; see also Grant and Stumpf, 1975) reveal that many areas in which estrogen and androgen accumulate receive a rich catecholaminergic innervation. These areas include the bed nucleus of stria terminalis, preoptic area, anterior, periventricular, paraventricular, and arcuate nuclei of the hypothalamus, midbrain central gray, and spinal dorsal horn. Many of these areas also receive substantial 5-HT innervation. These considerations suggest an anatomical basis for gonadal hormone–monoamine interaction in areas known to be involved in reproductive processes. More direct evidence (Grant and Stumpf 1975) using combined autoradiography and fluorescence histochemistry indicates that some estrogen-containing cells in the arcuate and paraventricular nuclei receive NE innervation. Furthermore, these investigators (Grant and Stumpf, 1973; Heritage et al., 1977) found that some arcuate DA cell bodies and some NE cell bodies in groups A1, A2, A5, A6, and A7 accumulate estrogen. Thus, gonadal hormones could exert their effects on monoaminergic cell bodies, nerve terminal areas, or both.

2. Effects on Enzymes

There is abundant evidence that in various peripheral tissues steroids produce their biological effects by altering genomic activity in target cell nuclei (Jensen and DeSombre, 1973; O'Malley and Means, 1974; Buller and O'Malley, 1976.) McEwen (1976) and McEwen et al. (1979) have reviewed evidence that this model may be applicable to steroid hormone interactions with neural tissue as well. Thus, in the brain, steroid hormones may stimulate synthesis of specific messenger RNAs (transcription) that code for specific proteins (translation).

Among the proteins that could be regulated by this mechanism are enzymes in the metabolic pathways of various neurotransmitters. There are several examples of steroid-induced changes in neurotransmitter enzyme activity in the brain. For example, Beattie et al. (1972) found that the activity of hypothalamic tyrosine hydroxylase, the rate-limiting enzyme in catecholamine biosynthesis, increased after ovariectomy. Daily estrogen treatment further increased enzyme activity, and subsequent progesterone treatment antagonized this effect. However, others have reported that daily estradiol reduced tyrosine hydroxylase activity (Luine *et al.*, 1977). These studies did not distinguish whether these changes occurred in NE or DA neurons.

In the median eminence of male rats, tyrosine hydroxylase activity was also elevated after gonadectomy, and testosterone replacement partially returned enzyme activity to baseline (Kizer *et al.*, 1974). Testosterone administration to males increased activity of the monoamine degradative enzyme MAO and of the ACh-synthesizing enzyme choline acetyltransferase (ChAT) in the medial preoptic area. Estradiol also elevated ChAT activity in the medial basal hypothalamus (Luine *et al.*, 1975).

3. Effects on Postsynaptic Receptors

Hormone-induced changes in monoamine turnover may be caused by some signal sent to afferent monoamine neurons from the postsynaptic steroid-target cell. Other proteins whose synthesis may be regulated by steroids include monoaminergic receptors. In a variety of species, steroids modify the sensitivity of uterine adrenergic receptors and the response of the uterus to adrenergic agonists (cf. Marshall, 1970). For example, estrogen treatment potentiates the uterine cyclic AMP rise produced by epinephrine (Chew and Rinaud, 1974; Rinaud and Chew, 1975). Recent evidence demonstrates that estrogen treatment actually increases the number of uterine α-adrenergic receptors (Roberts *et al.*, 1977). It is possible that a similar regulation occurs in brain (Fuxe *et al.*, 1979).

4. Effects on Nerve Terminals

Some other effects of hormones on processes occurring in monoaminergic nerve terminal regions include increased release of NE from brain slices by estradiol and progesterone (Janowsky and Davis, 1970). This is consistent with an increase in NE turnover produced by these hormones. Estrogen and progesterone also decrease uptake of NE and increase uptake of 5-HT into brain slices or synaptosome (nerve ending) preparations (Nixon *et al.*, 1974; Wirz-Justice *et al.*, 1974; Everitt *et al.*, 1975a). However, it is difficult to relate these effects with certainty to monoamine function, although it has been suggested that a decreased uptake of transmitter results in more transmitter available to occupy the receptor (Everitt *et al.*, 1975a). Moreover, it has not been demonstrated conclusively that steroids can be taken up by nerve terminals.

V. SUMMARY AND REVIEW

In summary, the following statements on the psychopharmacology of mating behavior in rodents seem to be well documented. (a) Male and female mating behaviors are inhibited by serotonergic systems. Furthermore, the display of female behavior by males or male behavior by females also is inhibited by 5-HT. The inhibition of lordosis behavior by 5-HT occurs in telencephalic and diencephalic sites, according to the limited mapping available. (b) Activation of a DA system is necessary for the expression of male copulatory behavior and female soliciting behaviors. However, DA inhibits the lordosis component of female sexual receptivity. (c) The role of NE in the mediation of masculine behaviors seems minor, but some evidence suggests that NE is facilitatory for lordosis and for the appearance of maternal behavior in the female. (d) Cholinergic systems participate in the inhibition of lordosis behavior in females, (e) Gonadal steroid hormones may induce sexual behavior by acting on monoaminergic systems. There is evidence that estrogen and progesterone affect NE, DA, and 5-HT turnover in complex ways and by mechanisms not understood. (f) Peptides, perhaps functioning as neurotransmitters or modulators, play a role in mating behavior. LRH induces lordosis behavior in estrogen-primed animals in an action independent of the pituitary. $ACTH_{4-10}$ and endorphins appear to be involved in the control of male ejaculatory patterns.

The study of the role of neurotransmitters in various behaviors primarily has been concerned with monoaminergic and cholinergic mechanisms because the anatomy, biochemistry, and pharmacology of these systems are relatively well-known. However, these systems comprise a relatively minor fraction of the total neuronal population of the CNS. Thus, one should not attempt to account for all facets of male and female sexual behavior in terms of NE, DA, 5-HT, and ACh. Yet, it is clear that these four systems exert a major influence on sexual and other behaviors, and it is on this point that we wish to speculate. It is likely that these neurochemical systems are not involved in the exclusive control of male or female sexual behavior, or any other behavior, in a "chemical code." Rather it is more profitable to view these systems as part of a more general modulation of behavior.

For example, several groups have proposed that nigrostriatal DA neurons are involved in arousal, sensorimotor regulation, and homeostatic regulation (Bolme et al., 1972; Marshall et al., 1974; Antelman et al., 1975; Antelman and Caggiula 1977; Zigmond and Stricker, 1974). Activation of DA neurons may be required for the appearance of many adaptive behaviors because they regulate sensory processing and motor output from the basal ganglia. Stein and co-workers (Stein et al., 1973; Wise et al., 1973) have described the ascending 5-HT pathways as behavior suppressant systems on the basis of operant and self-stimulation experiments. In addition to its effect on male and female sexual behavior, 5-HT has been reported to inhibit predatory aggression (Eichelman and Thoa, 1973; Grant et al., 1973), feeding (Breisch et al., 1976; Saller and Stricker, 1976), and responsiveness to noxious stimuli (Harvey et al., 1975). It has been suggested that ACh neurons also mediate behavioral inhibition, perhaps in an interaction with DA systems in the striatum (Carlton, 1963; Grossman 1972; Bolme et al., 1972). Noradrenergic systems also appear to be involved in arousal and reward mechanisms, neuroendocrine regulation, and modulation of DA and 5-HT systems (Bolme *et al.,* 1972; Antelman and Caggiula, 1977).

Thus, the results of psychopharmacological studies of mating behavior may be interpreted within this general framework. The inhibition of masculine and feminine sexual behavior by 5-HT systems would, therefore, be consistent with the role of this neurotransmitter in behavioral suppression. Similarly, male copulatory behavior and female soliciting provide additional examples of behaviors requiring activation of DA systems. Activity in this system may have to be suppressed in order for the immobile lordosis posture to be elicited.

An alternative, and not necessarily contradictory, interpretation is also possible. Some monoaminergic and cholinergic systems participate in neuroendocrine regulation (cf. Weiner and Ganong, 1978). It may be the case that these systems influence mating behavior as part of their control over other neuroendocrine processes. This could serve to coordinate sexual behavior with pituitary hormone secretion. For example, NE may stimulate, and DA and 5-HT may inhibit the release of LRH, which itself induces both LH release and female sexual behavior. Thus, the proposed excitatory role of NE and inhibitory role of DA and 5-HT in female sexual behavior primarily may involve control of these transmitters over LRH release.

REFERENCES

Ahlenius, S., Eriksson, H., Larsson, K., Modigh, K., and Södersten, P., 1971, Mating behavior in the male rat treated with *p*-chlorophenylalanine methyl ester alone and in combination with pargyline, *Psychopharmacologia* **20**:383.

Ahlenius, S., Eriksson, H., and Södersten, P., 1972, Effects of tetrabenazine on lordosis behavior and on brain monoamines in the female rat, *J. Neural Trans.* **33**:155.

Ahren, K., Fuxe, K. Hamberger, L., and Hökfelt, T., 1971, Turnover changes in the tuberoinfundibular dopamine neurons during the ovarian cycle of the rat, *Endocrinology* **88**:1415.

Andén, N.-E., Larsson, K., and Steg, G., 1971, The influence of the nigroneostriatal dopamine pathway on spinal motorneuron activity, *Acta Physiol. Scand.* **82**:268.

Antelman, S. M., and Caggiula, A. R., 1977, Norepinephrine–dopamine interactions and behavior, *Science* **195**:646.

Antelman, S. M., Szechtman, H., Chin, P., and Fisher, A. E., 1975. Tail pinch induced eating, gnawing, and licking behavior in rats: Dependence on the nigrostriatal dopamine system, *Brain Res.* **99**:319.

Barbeau, A., 1969, L-DOPA therapy in Parkinson's disease, a critical review of nine years' experience, *Can. Med. Assoc. J.* **101**:791.

Beach, F. A., 1942, Importance of progesterone to induction of sexual receptivity in spayed female rats, *Proc. Soc. Exp. Biol. Med.* **51**:369.

Beach, F. A., 1976, Sexual attractivity, proceptivity, and receptivity in female mammals, *Horm. Behav.* **7**:105.

Beattie, C. W., Rodgers, C. H., and Soyka, L. F., 1972, Influence of ovariectomy and ovarian steroids on hypothalamic tyrosine hydroxylase activity in the rat, *Endocrinology* **91**:276.

Bedard, P., Sanokova, J., Boucher, R., and Langelier, P., 1979, Effect of estrogens on apomorphine-induced circling behavior in the rat, *Can. J. Physiol. Pharmacol.* **56**:538.

Belt, B. G., 1973, Some organic causes of impotence, *Med. Asp. Hum. Sex.* **7**:152.

Benkert, O., 1973, Pharmacological experiments to stimulate human sexual behavior, in: *Psychopharmacology, Sexual Disorders, and Drug Abuse* (T. A. Ban, J. R. Boissier, G. J. Gessa, H. Heimann, L. Hollister, H. E. Lehmann, I. Munkvad, H. Steinberg, F. Sulser, A. Sundwall, and O. Vinar, eds.), pp. 489–495, North-Holland, Amsterdam.

Benkert, O., and Eversmann, T., 1971, Importance of the anti-serotonin effect for mounting behavior in rats, *Experientia* **28**:532.

Benkert, O., Crombach, G., and Kockott, G., 1972, Effect of L-DOPA on sexually impotent patients, *Psychopharmacologia* **23**:91.

Bertolini, A., 1971a, Behavioural effects of ovine β-LPH intraliquorally injected in the male rabbit, *Riv. Farm. Terap.* **2**:XLIII.

Bertolini, A., 1971b, Different type of sexual excitement produced in rats by intraliquoral ACTH and by intraperitoneal p-chlorophenylalanine, *Riv. Farm. Terap.* **2**:LXXIII.

Bertolini, A., Gentile, G., Greggia, A., Sternieri, F., and Ferrari, W., 1971, Possible role of hypothalamic corticotropin releasing factor in the induction of sexual excitation in adult male rats, *Riv. Farm. Terap.* **2**:243.

Bertolini, A., Gessa, G. L., and Ferrari, W., 1975, Penile erection and ejaculation: A central effect of ACTH-like peptides in mammals, in: *Sexual Behavior—Pharmacology and Biochemistry* (M. Sandler and G. L. Gessa, eds.), pp. 247–257, Raven Press, New York.

Bolme, P., Fuxe, K., and Lidbrink, P., 1972, On the function of central catecholamine neurons— Their role in cardiovascular and arousal mechanisms, *Res. Commun. Chem. Pathol. Pharmacol.* **4**:657.

Bowers, M. B., van Woert, M., and Davis, L., 1971, Sexual behavior during L-DOPA treatment for parkinsonism, *Am. J. Psychiatry* **127**:1691.

Breisch, S. T., Zemlan, F. P., and Hoebel, B. G., 1976, Hyperphagia and obesity following serotonin depletion by intraventricular p-chlorophenylalanine, *Science* **192**:382.

Buller, R. E., and O'Malley, B. W., 1976, The biology and mechanism of steroid hormone receptor interaction with the eukaryotic nucleus, *Biochem. Pharmacol.* **25**:1.

Caggiula, A. R., Shaw, D. H., Antelman, S. M., and Edwards, D. J., 1976, Interactive effects of brain catecholamines and variations in sexual and nonsexual arousal on copulatory behavior of male rats, *Brain Res.* **111**:321.

Caggiula, A., Herndon, J., Antelman, S., Sharp, D., Scanlon, R., Greenstone, D., and Bradshaw, W., 1977, Brain catecholamines and copulatory behavior of male and female rats, *Abstracts, East. Reg. Conf. Reprod. Behav.*, p. 29.

Carlton, P. L., 1963, Cholinergic mechanisms in the control of behavior by the brain, *Psychol. Rev.* **70**:19.

Carter, C. S., 1977, Pharmacological manipulations and sexual behavior in the hamster, *Abstracts: East. Reg. Conf. Reprod. Behav.* p. 3.

Carter, C. S., and Davis, J. M., 1976, Effects of drugs on sexual arousal and performance, in: *Clinical Management of Sexual Disorders* (J. Myer, ed.), pp. 195–205, Williams & Wilkins, Baltimore.

Carter, C. S., and Schein, M. W., 1971, Sexual receptivity and exhaustion in the female golden hamster, *Horm. Behav.* **2**:191.

Chew, L. S., and Rinaud, G. A., 1974, Estrogenic regulation of uterine cyclic AMP metabolism, *Biochem. Biophys. Acta* **362**:493.

Clark, T. K., Caggiula, A. R., McConnell, R. A., and Antelman, S. M., 1975, Sexual inhibition is reduced by rostral midbrain lesions in the male rat, *Science* **190**:169.

Coppola, J. A., 1969, Turnover of hypothalamic catecholamines during various states of gonadotrophin secretion, *Neuroendocrinology* **5**:75.

Crowley, W. R., Ward, I. L., and Margules, D. L., 1975, Female lordotic behavior mediated by monoamines in male rats, *J. Comp. Physiol. Psychol.* **88**:62.

Crowley, W. R., Feder. H. H., and Morin, L. P., 1976, Role of monoamines in sexual behavior of the female guinea pig, *Pharmacol. Biochem. Behav.* **4**:67.

Crowley, W. R., Nock, B. L., and Feder, H. H., 1978a, Facilitation of lordosis behavior by clonidine in female guinea pigs, *Pharmacol. Biochem. Behav.* **8**:207.

Crowley, W. R., O'Donohue, T. L., Wachslicht, H., and Jacobowitz, D. M., 1978b, Effects of estrogen and progesterone on plasma gonadotropins and on catecholamine levels and turnover in discrete brain regions of ovariectomized rats, *Brain Res.* **154**:345.

Da Prada, M., Carruba, M., O'Brien, R. A., Saner, A., and Pletscher, A., 1972, The effect of 5,6-dihydroxytryptamine on sexual behavior of male rats, *Eur. J. Pharmacol.* **19**:288.

Davis, G. A., and English, E., 1977, Monoamines and lordosis in the female guinea pig, *Horm. Behav.* **8**:88.

Davis, G. A., and Kohl, R., 1977, The influence of α-receptors on lordosis in the female rat, *Pharmacol. Biochem. Behav.* **6**:47.

Dewsbury, D. A., 1971, Copulatory behavior of male rats following reserpine administration, *Psychon. Sci.* **22**:177.

Dewsbury, D. A., 1972, Effects of tetrabenazine on the copulatory behavior of male rats, *Eur. J. Pharmacol.* **17**:221.

Dewsbury, D. A., 1975, The normal heterosexual pattern of copulatory behavior in the male rats: Effects of drugs that alter brain monoamine levels, in: *Sexual Behavior—Pharmacology and Biochemistry* (M. Sandler and G. L. Gessa, eds.), pp. 169–179, Raven Press, New York.

Dewsbury, D. A., and Davis, H. N., 1970, Effects of reserpine on the copulatory behavior of male rats, *Physiol. Behav.* **5**:1331.

Dewsbury, D. A., Davis, H. N., and Jansen, P. E., 1972, Effects of monoamine oxidase inhibitors on the copulatory behavior of male rats, *Psychopharmacologia* **24**:209.

Donoso, A. O., and de Gutierrez Moyano, M. B., 1970, Adrenergic activity in the hypothalamus and ovulation, *Proc. Soc. Exp. Biol. Med.* **135**:633.

Donoso, A. O., and Stefano, F. J. E., 1967, Sex hormones and concentration of noradrenaline and dopamine in the anterior hypothalamus, *Am. J. Physiol.* **212**:737.

Donoso, A. O., de Gutierrez Moyano, M. B., and Santolaya, R. C., 1969, Metabolism of noradrenaline in the hypothalamus of castrated rats, *Neuroendocrinology* **4**:12.

Eichelman, B. S., and Thoa, N. B., 1973, The aggressive monoamines, *Biol. Psychiatry* **6**:143.

Eliasson, M., 1976, Actions of repeated injections of LSD and apomorphine on the copulatory response of female rats, *Pharmacol. Biochem. Behav.* **5**:621.

Eliasson, M., and Meyerson, B. J., 1977, The effects of lysergic acid diethylamide on copulatory behaviour in the female rat, *Neuropharmacology* **16**:37.

Eliasson, M., Michanek, A., and Meyerson, B. J., 1972, A differential inhibitory action of LSD and amphetamine on copulatory behavior in the female rat, *Acta Pharmacol. Toxicol.* **31** (Suppl. 1):22.

Espino, C., Sano, M., and Wade, G. M., 1975, Alpha-methyltryptamine blocks facilitation of lordosis by progesterone in spayed, estrogen-primed rats, *Pharmacol. Biochem. Behav.* **3**:557.

Everitt, B. J., and Fuxe, K., 1977a, Dopamine and sexual behaviour in female rats. Effects of dopamine receptor agonists and sulpiride, *Neurosci. Lett.* **4**:209.

Everitt, B. J., and Fuxe, K., 1977b, Serotonin and sexual behaviour in female rats. Effects of hallucinogenic indolealkylamines and phenylethylamines, *Neurosci. Lett.* **4**:215.

Everitt, B. J., Fuxe, K., and Hökfelt, T., 1974, Inhibitory role of dopamine and 5-hydroxytryptamine in the sexual behavior of female rats, *Eur. J. Pharmacol.* **29**:187.

Everitt, B. J., Fuxe, K., Hökfelt, T., and Jonsson, G., 1975a, Role of monoamines in the control by hormones of sexual receptivity in the female rat, *J. Comp. Physiol. Psychol.* **89**:556.

Everitt, B. J., Fuxe, K., and Jonsson, G., 1975b, The effects of 5,7-dihydroxytryptamine lesions of ascending 5-hydroxytryptamine pathways on the sexual and aggressive behavior of female rats, *J. Pharmacol. (Paris)* **6**:25.

Feder, H. H., and Ruf, K. B., 1969, Stimulation of progesterone release and estrous behavior by ACTH in ovariectomized rodents, *Endocrinology* **84**:171.

Ferguson, J., Henriksen, S., Cohen, H., Mitchell, G., Barchas, J., and Dement, W., 1970, Hypersexuality and behavioral changes in cats caused by the administration of *p*-chlorophenylalanine, *Science* **168**:499.

Foreman, M. M., and Moss. R. L., 1977, Effects of subcutaneous injection and intrahypothalamic infusion of releasing hormones upon lordotic response to repetitive coital stimulation, *Horm. Behav.* **8**:219.

Foreman, M. M., and Moss, R. L., 1978a. Role of hypothalamic alpha and beta adrenergic receptors in the control of lordotic behavior in the ovariectomized–estrogen-primed rat, *Pharmacol. Biochem. Behav.* **9**:235.

Foreman, M. M., and Moss, R. L., 1978b, Role of hypothalamic serotonergic receptors in the control of lordosis behavior in the female rat. *Horm. Behav.* **10**:97.

Franck, J. A., and Ward, I. L., 1975, Amygdaloid mediation of female sexual behavior, Paper presented at the 46th Meeting of the Eastern Psychological Association, New York, April, 1975.

Fuxe, K., 1965, Evidence for the existence of monoamine-containing neurons in the central nervous system. IV. The distribution of monoamine nerve terminals in the central nervous system, *Acta Physiol. Scand. (Suppl.)* **247**:36.

Fuxe, K., and Hökfelt, T., 1970, Central monoaminergic systems and hypothalamic function, in: *The Hypothalamus* (L. Martini, M. Motta, and F. Fraschini, eds.), pp. 123–138, Academic Press, New York.

Fuxe, K., Hökfelt, T., and Nilsson, O., 1967, Activity changes in the tuberoinfundibular dopamine neurons of the rat during various states of the reproductive cycle, *Life Sci.* **6**:2057.

Fuxe, K., Hökfelt, T., and Nilsson, O., 1969, Castration, sex hormones and tuberoinfundibular dopamine neurons, *Neuroendocrinology* **5**:107.

Fuxe, K., Everitt, B. J., and Hökfelt, T., 1977a, Enhancement of sexual behavior in the female rat by nicotine, *Pharmacol. Biochem. Behav.* **7**:147.

Fuxe, K., Löfström, A., Eneroth, P., Gustaffson, J.-A., Skett, P., Hökfelt, T., Wiesel, F.-A., and Agnati, L., 1977b, Involvement of central catecholamines in the feedback actions of 17β-estradiolbenzoate on luteinizing hormone secretion in the ovariectomized female rat, *Psychoneuroendocrinology* **2**:203.

Fuxe, K., Andersson, K., Agnati, L. F., Ferland, L., Hökfelt, T., Eneroth, P., Gustaffson, J.-A., and Skett, P., 1979, Central catecholamine systems and neuroendocrine regulation. Controllers of anterior pituitary secretion, in: *Catecholamines: Basic and Clinical Frontiers* (E. Usdin, I. J. Kopin, and J. Barchas, eds.), pp. 1187–1203, Pergamon Press, New York.

Gawienowski, A. M., and Hodgen, D. M., 1971, Homosexual activity in male rats after p-chlorophenylalanine: Effects of hypophysectomy and testosterone, *Physiol. Behav.* **7**:551.

Gawienowski, A. M., Merker, J. W., and Damon, R. A., 1973, Alteration of sex accessory glands by p-chlorophenylalanine and testosterone, *Life Sci.* **12**:307.

Gerall, A. A., and Kenney, A., 1970, Neonatally androgenized female's responsiveness to estrogen and progesterone, *Endocrinology* **87**:560.

Gessa, G. L., and Tagliamonte, A., 1973, Role of brain monoamines in controlling sexual behavior in male animals, in: *Psychopharmacology, Sexual Disorders and Drug Abuse* (T. A. Ban, J. R. Boissier, G. J. Gessa, H. Heimann, L. Hollister, H. E. Lehmann, I. Munkvad, H. Steinberg. F. Sulser, A. Sundwall, and O. Vinar, eds.), pp. 451–462, North-Holland, Amsterdam.

Gessa, G. L., and Tagliamonte, A., 1975, Role of brain serotonin and dopamine in male sexual behavior, in: *Sexual Behavior—Pharmacology and Biochemistry* (M. Sandler and G. L. Gessa, eds.), pp. 117–128, Raven Press, New York.

Gessa, G. L., Tagliamonte, A., Tagliamonte, P., and Brodie, B. B., 1970, Essential role of testosterone in the sexual stimulation induced by p-chlorophenylalanine in male animals, *Nature* **227**:616.

Ginton, A., 1976, Copulation in noncopulators: Effect of pCPA in male rats, *Pharmacol. Biochem. Behav.* **4**:357.

Gorski, R. A., 1974, The neuroendocrine regulation of sexual behavior, in: *Advances in Psychobiology*, Vol. 2 (G. Newton, and H. H. Riesen, eds), pp. 1–58, John Wiley and Sons, New York.

Gradwell, P. B., Everitt, B. J., and Herbert, J., 1975, 5-Hydroxytryptamine in the central nervous system and sexual receptivity of female rhesus monkeys *Brain Res* **88**:281.

Grant, L. D., and Stumpf, W. E., 1973, Localization of ^{3}H-estradiol and catecholamines in identical neurons in the hypothalamus, *J. Histochem. Cytochem.* **21**:404.

Grant, L. D., and Stumpf, W. E., 1975, Hormone uptake sites in relation to CNS biogenic amine systems, in: *Anatomical Neuroendocrinology* (W. E. Stumpf and L. D. Grant, eds.), pp. 445–463, Karger, Basel.

Grant, L. D., Coscina, D. V., Grossman, S. P., and Freedman, D. X., 1973, Muricide after serotonin depleting lesions of midbrain raphe nuclei, *Pharmacol. Biochem. Behav.* **1**:77.

Gray, G. D., Davis, H. N., and Dewsbury, D. A., 1974, Effects of *l*-DOPA on the heterosexual copulatory behavior of male rats, *Br. J. Pharmacol.* **27**:367.

Grossman, S. P., 1972, Cholinergic synapses in the limbic system and behavioral inhibition, *Res. Publ. Assoc. Res. Nerv. Ment. Dis.* **50**:315.

Hardy, D. F., and DeBold, J. F., 1971, The relationship between levels of exogenous hormones and the display of lordosis by the female rat, *Horm. Behav.* **2**:287.

Harvey, J. A., Schlossberg, A. J., and Yunger, L. M., 1975, Behavioral correlates of serotonin depletion, *Fed. Proc.* **34**:1796.

Henrik, E., and Gerall, A. A., 1976, Facilitation of receptivity in estrogen-primed rats during successive mating tests with progestins and methysergide, *J. Comp. Physiol. Psychol.* **90**:590.

Heritage, A. S., Grant, L. D., and Stumpf, W. E., 1977, ³H-estradiol in catecholamine neurons of rat brain stem: Combined localization by autoradiography and formaldehyde-induced fluorescence, *J. Comp. Neurol.* **176**:607.

Herndon, J. G., Jr., 1976, Effects of midbrain lesions on female sexual behavior in the rat, *Physiol. Behav.* **17**:143.

Herndon, J. G., Jr., Caggiula, A. R., Sharp, D., Ellis, D., Zigmond, M. J., and Redgate, E. S., 1976, Alterations in reproductive behavior patterns of female rats following administration of catecholamine-depleting drugs, *Neurosci. Abstr.* **2**:851.

Hery, F., Rouer, E., and Glowinski, J., 1972, Daily variations of serotonin metabolism in the rat brain, *Brain Res.* **43**:445.

Hetta, J., 1977, Effects of morphine and naltrexone on sexual behaviour of the male rat, *Acta Pharmacol. Toxicol.* **41**(*Suppl.* IV):53.

Hollister, L. E., 1975a, Drugs and sexual behavior in man, *Life Sci.* **17**:661.

Hollister, L. E., 1975b, The mystique of social drugs and sex, in: *Sexual Behavior—Pharmacology and Biochemistry* (M. Sandler and G. L. Gessa, eds.), pp. 85–92, Raven Press, New York.

Hoyland, V. J., Shillito, E. E., and Vogt, M., 1970, The effect of parachlorophenylalanine on the behavior of cats, *Br. J. Pharmacol.* **40**:659.

Hyyppä, M., Lehtinen, P., and Rinne, U.K., 1971, Effect of *l*-DOPA on the hypothalamic, pineal and striatal monoamines and on the sexual behavior of the rat, *Brain Res.* **30**:265.

Hyyppä, M., Lampinen, P., and Lehtinen, P., 1972, Alteration in the sexual behavior of male and female rats after neonatal administration of *p*-chlorophenylalanine, *Psychopharmacologia* **25**:152.

Jacobowitz, D. M., and Palkovits, M., 1974, Topographic atlas of catecholamine and acetylcholinesterase-containing neurons in the rat brain. I. Forebrain (telencephalon, diencephalon), *J. Comp. Neurol.* **157**:13.

Janowsky, D. S., and Davis, J. M., 1970, Progesterone–estrogen effects on uptake and release of norepinephrine by synaptosomes, *Life Sci.* **9**:525.

Jensen, E. V., and DeSombre, E. R., 1973, Estrogen–receptor interaction, *Science* **182**:126.

Kalra, P. S., and McCann, S. M., 1973, Involvement of catecholoamines in feedback mechanisms, *Prog. Brain Res.* **39**:185.

Kizer, J. S., Palkovits, M., Zivin, J., Brownstein, M., Saavedra, J. M., and Kopin, I. J., 1974, The effect of endocrinological manipulations on tyrosine hydroxylase activity in individual hypothalamic nuclei of the adult male rat, *Endocrinology* **95**:799.

Komisaruk, B. R., 1974, Neural and hormonal interactions in the reproductive behavior of female rats, in: *Reproductive Behavior* (M. Montagna and W. A. Sadler, eds.), pp. 97–129, Plenum Press, New York.

Larsson, K., and Södersten, P., 1971, Lordosis behavior in male rats treated with estrogen in combination with tetrabenazine and nialamide, *Psychopharmacologia* **21**:13.

Larsson, K., Feder, H. H., and Komisaruk, B. R., 1974, Role of the adrenal glands, repeated matings, and monoamines in lordosis behavior of rats, *Pharmacol. Biochem. Behav.* **2**:685.

Lindström, L. H., 1970, The effect of pilocarpine in combination with monoamine oxidase inhibitors, imipramine or desmethylimipramine on oestrous behavior in female rats, *Psychopharmacologia* **17**:160.

Lindström, L. H., 1971, The effect of pilocarpine and oxotremorine on oestrous behavior in female rats after treatment with monoamine depletors or monoamine synthesis inhibitors, *Eur. J. Pharmacol.* **15**:60.

Lindström, L. H., 1972, The effect of pilocarpine and oxotremorine on hormone activated copulatory behavior in the ovariectomized hamster, *Naunyn-Schmiedebergs Arch. Pharmacol.* **275**:233.

Lindström, L. H., 1973, Further studies on cholinergic mechanisms and hormone-activated copulatory behavior in the female rat, *J. Endocrinol.* **56**:275.

Lindström, L. H., and Meyerson, B. J., 1967, The effect of pilocarpine, oxotremorine, and arecoline in combination with methyl-atropine or atropine on hormone-activated oestrous behavior in ovariectomized rats, *Psychopharmacologia* **11**:405.

Löfström, A., 1977, Catecholamine turnover alterations in discrete areas of the median eminence of the 4- and 5-day cyclic rat, *Brain Res.* **120**:113.

Löfström, A., Eneroth, P., Gustaffson, J.-A., and Skett, P., 1977, Effects of estradiol benzoate on catecholamine levels and turnover in discrete areas of the median eminence and the limbic forebrain, and on serum luteinizing hormone, follicle stimulating hormone and prolactin concentrations in the ovariectomized female rat, *Endocrinology* **101**:1559.

Luine, V. N., Khylchevskaya, R. I., and McEwen, B. S., 1975, Effect of gonadal steroids on activities of monoamine oxidase and choline acetylase in rat brain, *Brain Res.* **86**:293.

Luine, V. N., McEwen, B. S., and Black, I. B., 1977, Effect of 17β estradiol on hypothalamic tyrosine hydroxylase activity, *Brain Res.* **120**:188.

Malmnäs, C. O., 1973, Monoaminergic influence on testosterone-activated copulatory behavior in the castrated male rat. *Acta Physiol, Scand. (Suppl.)* **395**:1

Malmnäs, C. O., 1976, The significance of dopamine, versus other catecholamines, for *l*-DOPA induced facilitation of sexual behavior in the castrated male rat, *Pharmacol. Biochem. Behav.* **4**:521.

Malmnäs, C. O., 1977, Dopaminergic reversal of the decline after castration of rat copulatory behavior, *J. Endocrinol.* **73**:187.

Malmnäs, C. O., and Meyerson, B. J., 1971, *p*-Chlorophenylalanine and copulatory behavior in the male rat, *Nature* **232**:398.

Marshall, J. F., Richardson, J. S., and Teitelbaum, P., 1974, Nigrostriatal bundle damage and the lateral hypothalamic syndrome, *J. Comp. Physiol. Psychol.* **87**:808.

Marshall, J. M., 1970, Adrenergic innervation of the female reproductive tract: Anatomy, physiology and pharmacology, *Ergeb. Physiol.* **62**:6.

McEwen, B. S., 1976, Steroid receptors in neuroendocrine tissues: Topography, subcellular distribution, and functional implications, in: *Subcellular Mechanisms in Reproductive Neuroendocrinology* (F. Naftolin, K. J. Ryan, and J. Davies, eds.), pp. 277—304, Elsevier, Amsterdam.

McEwen, B. S., Davis, P. G., Parsons, B., and Pfaff, D. W., 1979, The brain as a target for steroid hormone action, *Annu. Rev. Neurosci.* **2**:65.

Meyerson, B. J., 1964a, Central nervous monoamines and hormone induced estrus behavior in the spayed rat, *Acta Physiol. Scand. (Suppl.)* **248**:5.

Meyerson, B. J., 1964b, Estrus behavior in spayed rats after estrogen or progesterone treatment in combination with reserpine or tetrabenazine, *Psychopharmacologia* **6**:210.

Meyerson, B. J., 1964c, The effect of neuropharmacological agents on hormone-activated estrus behavior in ovariectomized rats, *Arch. Int. Pharmacodyn. Ther.* **150**:4.

Meyerson, B. J., 1966, The effect of imipramine and related antidepressive drugs on estrus behavior in ovariectomized rats activated by progesterone, reserpine, or tetrabenazine in combination with estrogen, *Acta Physiol. Scand.* **67**:411.

Meyerson, B. J., 1968a, Amphetamine and 5-hydroxytryptamine inhibition of copulatory behavior in the female rat, *Ann. Med. Exp. Fenn.* **46**:394.

Meyerson, B. J., 1968b, Female copulatory behavior in male and androgenized female rats after oestrogen/amine depletor treatment, *Nature* **217**:683.

Meyerson, B. J., 1970, Monoamines and hormone activated oestrous behavior in the ovariectomized hamster, *Psychopharmacologia* **18**:50.

Meyerson, B. J., and Lewander, T., 1970, Serotonin synthesis inhibition and estrous behavior in female rats, *Life Sci.* **9**:661.

Meyerson, B. J., and Lindstrom, L. H., 1973, Sexual motivation in the female rat, *Acta Physiol. Scand. (Suppl.)* **389**:1.

Meyerson, B. J., and Terenius, L., 1977, β-Endorphin and male sexual behavior, *Eur. J. Pharmacol.* **42**:191.

Meyerson, B. J., Eliasson, M., Lindström, L., Michanek, A., and Söderlund, A., 1973, Monoamines and female sexual behavior, in: *Psychopharmacology, Sexual Disorders, and Drug Abuse* (T. A. Ban, J. R. Boissier, G. J. Gessa, H. Heimann, L. Hollister, H. E. Lehmann, I. Munkvad, H. Steinberg, F. Sulser, A. Sundwall, and O. Vinar, eds.), pp. 463–472, North-Holland Publishing Co., Amsterdam.

Meyerson, B. J., Carrer, H., and Eliasson, M., 1974, 5-hydroxytryptamine and sexual behavior in the female rat, *Adv. Biochem. Psychopharmacol.* **11**:229.

Michanek, A., and Meyerson, B. J., 1977, A comparative study of different amphetamines on copulatory behavior and stereotype activity in the female rat, *Psychopharmacology* **53**:175.

Mitler, M. M., Morden, B., Levine, S., and Dement, W., 1972, The effects of parachlorophenylalanine on the mating behavior of male rats, *Physiol. Behav.* **8**:1147.

Moltz, H., Rowland, D., Steele, M., and Halaris, A., 1976, Hypothalamic norepinephrine: Concentration and metabolism during pregnancy and lactation in the rat, *Neuroendocrinology* **19**:252.

Morin, L., and Feder, H. H., 1974a, Hypothalamic progesterone implants and facilitation of lordosis behavior in estrogen-primed ovariectomized guinea pigs, *Brain Res.* **70**:84.

Morin, L. P., and Feder, H. H., 1974b, Inhibition of lordosis behavior in ovariectomized guinea pigs by mesencephalic implants of progesterone, *Brain Res.* **70**:71.

Moss, R. L., 1978, Effects of hypothalamic peptides on sex behavior in animal and man, in: *Psychopharmacology: A Generation of Progesss* (M. A. Lipton, A. DiMascio, and K. F. Killam, eds.), pp. 431–440, Raven Press, New York.

Moss, R. L., and Foreman, M. M., 1976, Potentiation of lordosis behavior by intrahypothalamic infusion of synthetic luteinizing hormone-releasing hormone, *Neuroendocrinology* **20**:176.

Moss, R. L., and McCann, S. M., 1973, Induction of mating behavior in rats by luteinizing hormone releasing factor, *Science* **181**:177.

Moss, R. L., and McCann, S. M., 1975, Action of luteinizing hormone-releasing factor (LRF) in the initiation of lordosis behavior in the estrone-primed ovariectomized female rat, *Neuroendocrinology* **17**:309.

Munaro, N. I., 1977, The effect of ovarian steroids on hypothalamic norepinephrine neuronal activity, *Acta Endocrinol. (Kbh.)* **86**:235.

Munaro, N. I., 1978, The effect of ovarian steroids on hypothalamic 5-hydroxytryptamine neuronal activity, *Neuroendocrinology* **26**:270.

Nausieda, P. A., Kaller, W. C., Weiner, W. J., and Klawans, H. L., 1979, Modification of postsynaptic dopaminergic sensitivity by female sex hormones, *Life Sci.* **25**:521.

Nixon, R. L., Janowsky, D. S., and Davis, J. M., 1974, Effects of progesterone, beta-estradiol and testosterone on the uptake and metabolism of ^{3}H-norepinephrine, ^{3}H-dopamine and ^{3}H-serotonin in rat brain synaptosomes, *Res. Commun. Chem. Pathol. Pharmacol.* **7**:233.

Nock, B., and Feder, H. H., 1979, Noradrenergic transmission and female sexual behavior of guinea pigs, *Brain Res.* **66**:369.

O'Malley, B. W., and Means, A. R., 1974, Female steroid hormones and target cell nuclei, *Science* **183**:610.

Palkovits, M., and Jacobowitz, D. M., 1974, Topographic atlas of catecholamine and acetylcholinesterase-containing neurons in the rat brain II. Hindbrain (mesencephalon, rhombencephalon), *J. Comp. Neurol.* **157**:29.

Paris, C. A., Resko, J. A., and Goy, R. W., 1971, A possible mechanism for the induction of lordosis by reserpine in spayed rats, *Biol. Reprod.* **4**:23.

Pellegrini Quarantotti, B., Corda, M. G., Paglietti, E., Biggio, G., and Gessa, G. L., 1978, Inhibition of copulatory behavior in male rats by D-ala^2-met-enkephalinamide, *Life Sci.* **23**:673.

Pfaff, D. W., 1973, Luteinizing hormone-releasing factor potentiates lordosis behavior in hypophysectomized, ovariectomized female rats, *Science* **182**:1148.

Pfaff, D. W., and Keiner, M., 1973, Atlas of estradiol-concentrating cells in the central nervous system of the female rat, *J. Comp. Neurol.* **151**:121.

Pfaff, D., Lewis, C., Diakow, C., and Keiner, M., 1973, Neurophysiological analysis of mating behavior responses as hormone-sensitive reflexes, in: *Progress in Physiological Psychology*, Vol. 5 (E. Stellar and J. M. Sprague, eds.), pp. 253–297, Academic Press, New York.

Pfaff, D., Montgomery, M., and Lewis, C., 1977, Somatosensory determinants of lordosis in female rats: Behavioral definition of the estrogen effect, *J. Comp. Physiol. Psychol.* **91**:134.

Redmond, D. E., Mass, J. W., Kling, A., Graham, C. W., and Dekirmenjian, H., 1971, Social behavior of monkeys selectively depleted of monoamines, *Science* **174**:428.

Rinaud, G. A., and Chew, C. S., 1975, Interacting effects of estrogen, progesterone, and catecholamines on rat uterine cyclic AMP and glycogen phosphorylase, *Life Sci.* **16**:1507.

Roberts, J. M., Insel, P. A., Goldfien, R. D., and Goldfein, A., 1977, α-Adrenoreceptors but not β-adrenoreceptors increase in rabbit uterus with oestrogen, *Nature* **270**:624.

Rodriguez-Sierra, J. F., Naggar, A. N., and Komisaruk, B. R., 1976, Monoaminergic mediation of masculine and feminine copulatory behavior in female rats, *Pharmacol. Biochem. Behav.* **5**:457.

Rosenberg, P., Leidahl, L., Halaris, A., and Moltz, H., 1976, Changes in the metabolism of hypothalamic norepinephrine associated with the onset of maternal behavior in the nulliparous rat, *Pharmacol. Biochem. Behav.* **4**:647.

Rosenberg, P., Halaris, A., and Moltz, A., 1977, Effects of norepinephrine depletion on the initiation and maintainance of maternal behavior in the rat, *Pharmacol. Biochem. Behav.* **6**:21.

Sachs, B. D., and Barfield, R. J., 1976, Functional analysis of masculine copulatory behavior in the rat, in: *Advances in the Study of Behavior* (J. S. Rosenblatt, R. A. Hinde, E. Shaw, and C. Beer, eds.), pp. 91–154, Academic Press, New York.

Salis, P. J., and Dewsbury, D. A., 1971, *p*-Chlorophenylalanine facilitates copulatory behavior in male rats, *Nature* **232**:400.

Saller, C. F., and Stricker, E. M., 1976, Hyperphagia and increased growth in rats after intraventricular injection of 5, 7-dihydroxytryptamine, *Science* **192**:385.

Sar, M., and Stumpf, W. E., 1975, Distribution of androgen-concentrating neurons in rat brain, in: *Anatomical Neuroendocrinology* (W. E. Stumpf and L. D. Grant, eds.), pp. 120–133, Karger, Basel.

Shillito, E. E., 1970, The effect of parachlorophenylalanine on social interaction of male rats, *Br. J. Pharmacol.* **38**:305.

Sicuteri, F., 1974, Serotonin and sex in man, *Pharmacol. Res. Commun.* **6**:403.

Simpkins, J. W., Kalra, P. S., and Kalra, S. P., 1980, Effects of testosterone on catecholamine turnover and LHRH contents in the basal hypothalamus and preoptic area, *Neuroendocrinology* **30**:94.

Södersten, P., and Ahlenius, S., 1972, Female lordosis behavior in estrogen-primed male rats treated with *p*-chlorophenylalanine or alpha-methyl-p-tyrosine, *Horm, Behav.* **3**:181.

Södersten, P., Berge, O. G., and Hole, L., 1978, Effects of *p*-chloroamphetamine and 5,7-dihydroxytryptamine on the sexual behavior of gonadectomized male and female rats, *Pharmacol. Biochem. Behav.* **9**:499.

Soulairac, A., and Soulairac, M.-L., 1961, Action de la réserpine sur le comportement sexuel du rat mâle, *C. R. Soc. Biol. (Paris)* **155**:1010.

Soulairac, A., and Soulairac, M.-L., 1962, Effets de l'administration chronique de réserpine sur le comportement sexuel du rat mâle, *Ann. Endocrinol.* **23**:281.

Soulairac, A., and Soulairac, M.-L., 1971, Action de la serotonin sur le comportement sexuel du rat mâle, *C. R. Soc. Biol. (Paris)* **165**:253.

Soulairac, M.-L., 1963, Étude expérimentale des régulations hormono-nerveuses de comportement sexuel du rat mâle, *Ann. Endocrinol.* 24 (Suppl. 1):1.

Soulairac, M.-L., and Soulairac, Á., 1975, Monoaminergic and cholinergic control of sexual behavior in the male rat, in: *Sexual Behavior—Pharmacology and Biochemistry* (M. Sandler and G. L. Gessa, eds.), pp. 99–116, Raven Press, New York.

Stein, L., Wise, C. D., and Berger, B. D., 1973, Antianxiety action of benzodiazepines: Decrease in activity of serotonin neurons in the punishment system, in, *The Benzodiazepines* (S. Garratini, ed.), pp. 299–325, Raven Press, New York.

Stumpf, W. E., Sar, M., and Keefer, D. A., 1975, Atlas of estrogen target cells in rat brain, in: *Anatomical Neuroendocrinology* (W. E. Stumpf, and L. D. Grant, eds.), pp. 104–119, Karger, Basel.

Tagliamonte, A., Tagliamonte, P., Gessa, G. L., and Brodie, B. B., 1969, Compulsive sexual activity induced by *p*-chlorophenylalanine in normal and pinealectomized male rats, *Science* **166**:1433.

Tagliamonte, A., Fratta, W., del Fiacco, M., and Gessa, G. L., 1974, Possible stimulatory role of brain dopamine in the copulatory behavior of male rats, *Pharmacol. Biochem. Behav.* **2**:257.

Uphouse, L. L., Wilson, J. R., and Schlesinger, K., 1970, Induction of estrus in mice: The possible role of adrenal progesterone, *Horm. Behav.* **1**:255.

Van de Poll, N. E., Van Dis. H., and Bermond, B., 1977, The induction of mounting behavior in female rats by *p*-chlorophenylalanine, *Eur. J. Pharmacol.* **41**:225.

Van Loon, G. R., 1973, Brain catecholamines and ACTH secretion, in: *Frontiers in Neuroendocrinology* (W. F. Ganong and L. Martini, Eds.), pp. 209–247, Oxford University Press, New York.

Ward, I. L., 1972, Female sexual behavior in male rats treated prenatally with an anti-androgen, *Physiol. Behav.* **8**:53.

Ward, I. L., Crowley, W. R., Zemlan, F. P., and Margules, D. L., 1975, Monoaminergic mediation of female sexual behavior, *J. Comp. Physiol. Psychol.* **88**:53.

Weiner, R. I., and Ganong, W. F., 1978, Role of brain monoamines and histamine on regulation of anterior pituitary secretion, *Physiol. Rev.* **58**:905.

Whalen, R. E., Gorzalka, B., and DeBold, J. F., 1975, Methodologic considerations in the study of animal sexual behavior, in: *Sexual Behavior: Pharmacology and Biochemistry* (M. Sandler and G. L. Gessa, eds.), pp. 33–50, Raven Press, New York.

Wirz-Justice, A., Hackmann, E., and Lichsteiner, M., 1974, The effect of oestradiol dipropionate and progesterone on monoamine uptake in rat brain, *J. Neurochem.* **22**:187.

Wise, C. D., Berger, B. D., and Stein, L., 1973, Evidence of alpha-noradrenergic reward receptors and serotonergic punishment receptors in the rat brain, *Biol. Psychiatry* **6**:3.

Young, W. C., 1961, The hormones and mating behavior, in: *Sex and Internal Secretions*, Vol. II (W. C. Young, ed.), pp. 1173–1239, Williams & Wilkins, Baltimore.

Young, W. C., 1969, Psychobiology of sexual behavior in the guinea pig, in: *Advances in the Study of Behavior* (D. S. Lehrman, R. A. Hinde, and E. Shaw, eds.), pp. 1–110, Academic Press, New York.

Zemlan, F. P., 1978, The influence of *p*-chloroamphetamine and *p*-chlorophenylalanine on female mating behavior, *Am. N. Y. Acad. Sci* **305**:621.

Zemlan, F. P., and Adler, N. T., 1977, Hormonal control of female reproductive behavior in the rat, *Horm. Behav.* **9**:345.

Zemlan, F. P., Ward, I. L., Crowley, W. R., and Margules, D. L., 1973, Activation of lordotic responding in female rats by suppression of serotonergic activity, *Science* **179**:1010.

Zemlan, F. P., Trulson, M. E., Howell, R., and Hoebel, B. G., 1977, Influence of *p*-chloroamphetamine on female sexual reflexes and brain monoamine levels, *Brain Res.* **123**:347.

Zigmond, M. J., and Stricker, E. M., 1974, Ingestive behavior following damage to central dopamine neurons: Implications for homeostasis and recovery of function, in: *Neuropsychopharmacology of Monoamines and their Regulatory Enzymes* (E. Usdin, ed.), pp. 385–402, Raven Press, New York.

Zitrin, A., Beach, F. A., Barchas, J. D., and Dement, W. C., 1970, Sexual behavior of male cats after administration of parachlorophenylalanine, *Science* **170**:868.

Zucker, J., 1966, Facilitatory and inhibitory effects of progesterone on sexual responses of spayed guinea pigs, *J. Comp. Physiol. Psychol.* **62**:376.

15

Cellular Biochemistry of Hormone Action in Brain and Pituitary

BRUCE S. McEWEN

I. INTRODUCTION

With the introduction of tritium-labeling techniques for steroid hormones in the late 1950s, the investigation of the cellular biochemistry of hormone action made enormous advances. More recent development of iodination procedures for thyroid hormone and protein hormones has made possible the investigation of the action of these hormones at the molecular level. We are now in a position to see the broad outlines of two major modes of hormone action on target cells, and a discussion of this topic forms the central theme around which this chapter revolves.

Application of these procedures to a study of hormone interactions with pituitary and brain cells has had two principal effects on our understanding of how these tissues function. First, the realization that hormones may enter the brain from the blood and act on neurons by mechanisms that appear to be similar, if not identical, to those operating in the rest of the organism helps to destroy long-standing myths about the "separation" of mind and body. In other words, the brain is a tissue like any other body tissue and is amenable to molecular and cellular biochemical investigations by the same techniques. Second, the influence of hormones on events in the genome of the cell makes possible the understanding of long-term influences of hormones on brain development and adult brain function. Thus, hormones function at least in part as mediators of long-term functional adaptations of brain and pituitary

BRUCE S. McEWEN • Laboratory of Neuroendocrinology, The Rockefeller University, New York, New York 10021.

cells. We shall, however, note the distinction between the reversible, "activational" adjustments of mature brain and pituitary to hormonal signals (see Chapters 11 and 13) and the apparently irreversible "organizational" actions of hormones on developing tissues (see Chapters 7 and 8). It is of fundamental importance to understand how these differential effects of the same hormone may be produced at the genomic level.

II. CELLULAR MECHANISMS OF HORMONE ACTION

Hormones may be divided into two major classes based on their cellular mechanism of action: steroid hormones and thyroid hormone, which interact with receptors located in the cytoplasm; and amino acid derivatives and polypeptide and protein hormones, which interact with cell surface receptors (Fig. 1).

In many cases, the latter interactions (between proteinaceous hormones and cell surface receptors) lead to increases of cyclic 3',5'-AMP (cyclic AMP), which appears to be an intracellular "second messenger" for carrying out at least some of the hormone effects within the cell (Robinson *et al.,* 1971). In the heart ventricle, epinephrine promotes increased cyclic AMP levels and cardiac acceleration. Acetylcholine, on the other hand, decreases heart contractility and increases ventricular levels of another cyclic nucleotide, cyclic 3',5'-GMP. The occurrence, in other tissues, of an "antagonism" between hormone-sensitive levels of cyclic AMP and cyclic GMP has led to the speculation that cyclic AMP and cyclic GMP are antagonistic intracellular "second messengers"

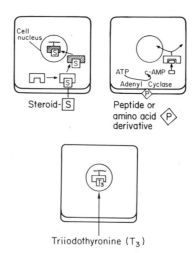

Figure 1. Schematic summary of three principal cellular mechanisms of hormone–target cell interactions.

(Goldberg *et al.*, 1973). Although the antagonistic relationship is not altogether so clear for tissues other than the heart, the hypothesis provides a valuable conceptual framework for experimental work.

The best examples for understanding cyclic AMP mediation of cellular metabolism are the stimulation of glycogen breakdown and inhibition of glycogen formation in skeletal muscle by epinephrine. These are accomplished by the following steps: (a) epinephrine stimulation of cyclic AMP generation via adrenergic receptors on the cell surface; (b) interaction of cyclic AMP with a class of enzymes, protein phosphokinases, capable of attaching phosphate to a variety of protein substrates (Activation of the protein phosphokinase occurs when cyclic AMP binds to a regulatory subunit and causes it to dissociate from the enzyme.); and (c) the protein phosphokinase catalyzing the phorphorylation of phosphorylase kinase. This enzyme in turn catalyzes phosphorylation of glycogen phosphorylase, which is thereby activated to cleave glycogen. The protein phosphokinase also catalyzes the phosphorylation of glycogen synthetase, thereby rendering it inactive, and thereby inhibits the storage of glycogen. It is interesting that acetylcholine may reverse these events and may do so by stimulating cyclic GMP formation. The mechanism by which cyclic GMP accomplishes this reversal remains to be elucidated.

The activation of protein phosphokinases by cyclic AMP (and possibly in specific instances by cyclic GMP) appears to be the means by which this cyclic nucleotide initiates a variety of intracellular events by causing phorphorylation of diverse protein substrates, including enzymes (see above), histones of the cell nucleus, and membrane proteins (Langan, 1973).

Steroid hormone interactions with chromosomes have been shown to lead to increased production of mRNAs for specific proteins (O'Malley and Means, 1974). In the oviduct, estradiol increases production of mRNA for ovalbumin, and progesterone increases production of mRNA for avidin. In the liver, glucocorticoids have been shown to increase mRNA production for tryptophan oxygenase (Schultz *et al.*, 1973). In other cases, genomic interactions of steroid hormones have been demonstrated morphologically in the case of ecdysone, an invertebrate hormone (Berendes, 1967), and also by the blockade of their effects with inhibitors of RNA and protein synthesis. The mechanism of steroid hormone interaction with intracellular receptor sites (Fig. 1) consists of five steps (see McEwen and Luine, 1979): (a) passive diffusion of steroid across the cell membrane; (b) binding to a cytoplasmic "receptor" protein; (c) changes induced by the steroid in the size and shape of this receptor; (d) penetration of hormone–receptor complex into the nucleus; and (e) interaction of this complex with the chromosomes. Only the last step is enigmatic: one group of results suggests that the interaction is with acidic (nonhistone) proteins of the cell nuclei; another body of information points to DNA as the primary site of interaction. Whatever the case, the interaction is believed to increase the number of initiation sites for mRNA formation, as exemplified by estrogen stimulation of the production of mRNA for ovalbumin in the oviduct of the chick.

Triiodothyronine (T_3) penetrates into the brain and other tissues (Hagen and Solberg, 1974) and binds with high affinity to limited capacity sites in cell nuclei of a large number of rat tissues (Oppenheimer *et al.*, 1974). There is no known cytosol protein required for binding of T_3 by cell nuclei. These observations suggest a mode of action of thyroid hormone that is similar in respect to a genomic effect to that of steroid hormones (Fig. 1).

III. METHODS FOR MEASURING RECEPTORS

Histological techniques, including immunocytochemistry and autoradiography, permit a high degree of spatial resolution which is useful in determining the cell types that bind or contain a particular hormone. Autoradiography is particularly useful for steroid hormones (see Chapter 16) where a cell nuclear receptor localization provides a clear-cut image. Immunocytochemistry is of use for localizing peptide hormones such as LRF, TRF, and somatostatin (see Sternberger, 1974, for methods).

Biochemical techniques for peptide and steroid receptor localization permit characterization of the receptors as well as the bound hormone, and it is the purpose of this section to review methodological aspects of typical biochemical receptor measurements.

A. Cell Surface Receptors for Releasing Hormones in Pituitary as Revealed by Biochemical Analysis

The first and foremost problem is the synthesis of biologically active, labeled peptide of high specific radioactivity. Once this is done, the measurement of binding is relatively simple. In one recent study, Grant *et al.*, (1973a) synthesized TRF labeled with [^{3}H]proline, one of three constituent amino acids, at a specific activity of 40 Ci/mmol and verified its biological activity. Labeled TRF was then incubated with intact mouse pituitary tumor cells that secrete TSH or with osmotically lysed cells (membrane fragments). At the end of the incubation, suspensions of cells or membranes were rapidly filtered onto Whatman GF/c filters. The cells or membranes, which are retained on the filters, were washed with physiological saline and then counted for radioactivity. Bound radioactivity was graphed as a function of the [^{3}H]-TRF concentration in the incubation medium and also in the form of a Scatchard plot (y axis = bound hormone; x axis = bound hormone/unbound hormone) in which analysis of the y and x intercepts yields the dissociation constant:

$K_d =$ [Free Hormone] [Free Receptor]

[Hormone–Receptor Complex]

(K_d = concentration at which half of the receptors are occupied by hormone). Analysis of the intercepts also gives the saturation capacity, the amount of hormone that would be bound at infinite hormone concentration. In this particular study, two K_ds were observed (2×10^{-8} M and 5×10^{-7} M), indicating the likely existence of dual binding sites.

Competition studies were run with unlabeled analogs of TRF, each added in a range of concentrations, thus permitting one to evaluate their K_d of binding from the concentration at which 50% of [³H]-TRH binding was observed. One of the analogues, which is also more potent than natural TRH in eliciting TSH secretion, has an eight- to tenfold lower K_d (i.e., a higher binding affinity).

Studies of the binding of [³H]-LRH and its analogues to pituitary membranes have revealed another class of interactions with receptors, namely, binding of analogues that are not themselves potent agonists but that antagonize LRH action (Grant *et al.*, 1973b). Like [³H]-TRH binding, the binding of [³H]-LRH to pituitary receptors shows two saturation points: one, of low capacity and high affinity ($K_d = 2 \times 10^{-9}$M), that corresponds to the half-maximal biological potency of LRH; the second, of lower affinity ($K_d = 2 \times 10^{-8}$ M) and higher capacity, that binds inactive as well as active LRH analogs. Only the high-affinity binding site shows specificity toward LRH agaonists or antagonists and is therefore more likely to be the true receptor site.

B. Steroid Hormone Receptors in Brain and Pituitary

As noted above, a primary subcellular site of action for steroid hormones is the cell nucleus, and thus a considerable part of the identification of a steroid hormone receptor revolves around the isolation of highly purified cell nuclei. This is easily accomplished even for small amounts of brain and pituitary tissue (as little as 10–15 mg wet weight), since these tissues lack components like the heavy connective tissue of myofibrils that make specimens of skeletal muscle, skin, and uterus so difficult to disjoin. Our procedure for cell fractionation is diagrammatically summarized in Fig. 2 (McEwen and Zigmond, 1972). Nuclear isolation is used in experiments where [³H]steroids are either administered *in vivo* of incubated with intact cells or tissue slices *in vitro*. As far as is presently known, steroid hormones do not associate with specific receptor sites in isolated nuclei except by exchange with steroids on receptor complexes already in the nucleus (Clark *et al.*, 1972). The reason for this is that steroid receptors do not appear to exist in cell nuclei (at least not in tightly bound form) in the absence of hormone.

Once hormone–receptor complexes enter the nucleus, they may be extracted from isolated nuclei by 0.3–0.4 M NaCl or KCl solutions; these extracted complexes are generally obtained in smaller molecular sizes than the complexes that may be extracted from the soluble portion (i.e., cytosol receptors) of the tissue (see below). In fact, the conversion of a large complex to a smaller one may be one precondition for the tight association of the complex with the chromatin (O'Malley and Means, 1974).

CELL FRACTIONATION

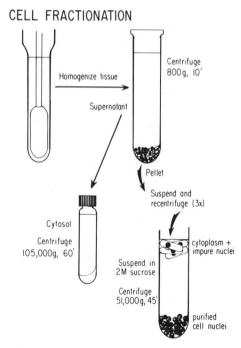

Figure 2. Flow diagram of a procedure for cell fractionation used in obtaining "cytosol" and purified cell nuclear fractions of tissues.

The soluble receptors of the so-called cytosol fraction (see Fig. 2) as well as those extracted from cell nuclei may be assayed by a variety of methods (see King and Mainwaring, 1974). There are four principal methods: (a) molecular sieving, (b) ultracentrifugation, (c) isoelectric focusing, and (d) adsorption either of hormone–receptor complex or of unbound hormone. In all cases, the result is the separation of bound from unbound hormone.

1. Gel filtration or molecular sieving uses the grossly different molecular weights of hormone (*ca.* 300) and receptor (*ca.* 50,000) to achieve a separation. Sephadex G25, G50, or G100 (Pharmacia) are often used as are Biogel P10, P30, or P60 (Biorad Laboratories). Separations by this method are more time-consuming than adsorption assays, but molecular sieves (e.g., Sephadex G200 or Biogel A5M) that have large pores and, therefore, higher thresholds for excluding molecules on the basis of size may be used together with density gradient centrifugation to obtain information about molecular size and shape (Siegel and Monty, 1966).

2. In sucrose density gradient centrifugation, stable gradients of 5–20% sucrose in appropriate buffers provide an excellent medium for the separation of high molecular weight hormone–receptor complexes from free steroid by the faster sedimentation velocity of the former in a centrifugal field. Molecular weights are estimated from the positions in the gradient of "marker" proteins of known molecular weight (Martin and Ames, 1961). The accuracy of these

estimates requires that both markers and receptors have spherical shapes and that they have similar buoyant densities (i.e., are not complexed with lipids or nucleic acids that would, respectively, decrease or increase the density of the complex). Typical "S" values (the S or Svedberg coefficient is a measure of molecular size) for estrogen–receptor complexes from pituitary and brain cytosol are around 8 (corresponding to a molecular weight in excess of 200,000); those for cell nuclear complexes are 5–7 S. Uterine receptors binding [³H]estradiol are 8–9 S (cytosol, low salt; mol.wt. 240,000), 4.5 and 5.3 S (cytosol, high salt; mol.wt. 60,000 and 120,000, respectively) and 5 S (cell nuclear, high salt; mol.wt. 60,000 subunit complexed with an unknown factor, mol.wt. 60,000, which does not itself bind estradiol). For details see Luine and McEwen (1978). Glucocorticoid–receptor complexes in brain cytosol have a maximal S value around 7 (Chytil and Toft, 1972).

3. In isoelectric focusing, a stable pH gradient is created with amphoteric organic molecules in an electric field in a supporting medium such as poly-acrylamide (Haglund, 1971). Proteins in this gradient migrate to positions where they are at their isoelectric points (pI, i.e., the pH where they have no net charge). For example, glucocorticoid–receptor complexes in liver cytosol have a pI of 7.1 before activation at 25°C for 30 min, and a pI of 6.1 after activation (Kalimi *et al.*, 1975). This increase of net positive charge with activation results from a conformational change of the receptor and may be responsible for the increased binding of the activated receptor to DNA (see below).

4. In adsorbtion techniques, popular adsorbing agents for unbound [³H]steroid include activated charcoal and Sephadex LH-20. The [³H]-steroid–receptor complexes remain intact, probably because the hormone is "wrapped" inside the receptor molecule, and the rate-limiting step is the un-folding of the receptor molecule rather than the "off rate" of the hormone from its binding site. In contrast to receptors, the fetoneonatal estrogen-binding protein, a serum protein that binds [³H]estradiol without "wrapping" it up (Raynaud *et al.*, 1971), loses its bound hormone when brought into contact with Sephadex LH-20 (Barley *et al.*, 1974). LH-20, which has been more useful than activated charcoal in our laboratory, consists of beads of hydroxypropy-lated dextran gel (Joustra *et al.*, 1967). In an aqueous medium with LH-20 in a small column consisting of a pasteur pipet packed with glass wool, the free [³H]steroid is retained by the beads, and the hormone–receptor complex passes through the column. The use of small columns and a two-step procedure of loading and then eluting permits the processing of 40–50 samples in a single run. Thus, the evaluation of the K_d and binding capacity for several samples is possible from the hormone concentration dependence of the binding, evaluated in the form of a Scatchard plot (see Section III.A). Data for [³H]es-tradiol binding by uterine, brain, and pituitary cytosol is summarized in Table 1.

Adsorbtion of the hormone–receptor complex that leaves the free steroid to be washed away may be accomplished with adsorbants that capitalize on special properties of the receptors. For example, estrogen receptors from the

Table 1. Characteristics of Estradiol Binding to
Soluble Receptors in Rat Tissues[a]

Tissue	Binding capacity (sites/mg tissues $\times$ 10^{-8})	K_d (M $\times$ 10^{10})
Cerebral cortex	0.18 $\pm$ 0.03	1.66 $\pm$ 0.65
Amygdala	0.83 $\pm$ 0.04	1.08 $\pm$ 0.16
Hypothalamus	1.98 $\pm$ 0.12	1.48 $\pm$ 0.27
Pituitary	65 $\pm$ 6	0.69 $\pm$ 0.05
Uterus	61 $\pm$ 9	1.76 $\pm$ 0.21

[a] K_d, equilibrium dissociation constant, and binding capacity are evaluated from Scatchard plots of the concentration dependence of *in vitro* binding of [^{3}H]estradiol-17β to cytosol receptors. Data from Ginsburg *et al.* (1974).

uterus, pituitary, and brain and glucocorticoid–receptor complexes from the brain have been quantitatively precipitated by protamine sulfate, a polycation, thus indicating that the receptor molecules have many negative charges (see McEwen *et al.*, 1972b; King and Mainwaring, 1974). The negative charges undoubtedly also account for the binding of the hormone–receptor complex to DE-52, an anion exchange resin used in chromatography (see Kalimi *et al.*, 1975). The "activation" step, which is caused by warming of the cytosol in the presence of the hormone and involves conformational changes in the receptor, does not always involve an increased negativity of net charge. As noted above, liver glucocorticoid–receptor complexes shift in a positive direction with activation. The significance of these shifts in pI with respect to binding to DNA (a polyanion) remains to be determined.

The binding of steroid–receptor complexes to DNA linked to cellulose and to isolated cell nuclei increases as a result of activation. DNA binding has been proposed as a means of purifying hormone–receptor complexes (Irving and Mainwaring, 1974). Since increases in DNA binding with activation *in vitro* resemble the "activation" and cell nuclear binding that occurs in the intact cell, it is tempting to regard DNA binding as a model of the natural process. Yet, there are reasons to be cautious about making such conclusions. For example, bacterial as well as mammalian DNA is bound by the receptor, thus demonstrating a lack of species specificity. Cell nuclear binding *in vitro* does not appear to be prevented by saturation of cell nuclear sites *in vivo*, indicating that the *in vitro* and *in vivo* "acceptor" sites may not be the same (see Williams, 1975).

C. Thyroid Hormone Receptors in Pituitary and Brain

As noted earlier, thyroid hormone receptors are detected in cell nuclei (Samuels *et al.*, 1974; DeGroot and Torresani, 1975). There is no clear-cut evidence at present that soluble (cytosol) receptors are involved in cell nuclear binding. Purified cell nuclei, isolated by methods similar to that described in Fig. 2, are incubated in 0.25 or 0.32 M sucrose containing 1–2 mM Mg and/or

CaCl$_2$, 0.01–0.02 M Tris–HCl buffer, pH 7.4 or pH 7.85 with 2 × 10^{-11} M [^{125}I]-triiodothyronine (T$_3$) at 20°C or 37°C for 30–60 min and then reisolated by centrifugation and washing of the pellet with the buffer. Nonsaturable binding is estimated as cell-nuclear-associated radioactivity in incubations containing [^{125}I]-T$_3$ plus a 100-fold or greater excess of unlabeled T$_3$. This nonsaturable component may be subtracted from the binding measured in the absence of unlabeled hormone to give the true saturable binding.

In addition to these *in vitro* methods for demonstrating T$_3$ binding, there are *in vivo* experiments that have revealed cell nuclear receptor sites in brain tissue as well as pituitary, liver, and kidney after infusing [^{125}I]-T$_3$ via the tail vein. As shown in Table 2, pituitary binding is exceptionally high, and brain cell nuclear binding is moderate (Oppenheimer *et al.*, 1974).

The affinities of receptors in various tissues for T$_3$ are similar to each other, suggesting (but by no means proving) that the same kind of receptor may be present throughout the body. The relationship between T$_3$ binding and a biological effect is perhaps best documented for cultured rat pituitary cells, where T$_3$ concentrations between 10^{-11} and 10^{-10} M stimulate glucose utilization. Thyroxine, i.e., tetraiiodothyronine (T$_4$), is approximately tenfold less potent than T$_3$ (Samuels *et al.*, 1973). In agreement with these data, the nuclear receptors of these cells show a marked preference for T$_3$ over T$_4$ and have an equilibrium binding constant for T$_3$ of 10^{-11} to 10^{-10} M.

If cell nuclei are isolated from tissues unstimulated by exogenous T$_3$ and then extracted by 0.4 M KCl solutions, and if these extracts are incubated with [^{125}I]-T$_3$ under *K* values buffer, time, and temperature similar to those used for demonstrating T$_3$ receptors in intact cell nuclei, T$_3$ binding sites can be demonstrated (Samuels *et al.*, 1974). These solubilized T$_3$ binding sites show a marked affinity for purified eukaryotic DNA (MacLeod and Baxter, 1975). As is the case for steroid receptor binding to DNA, the functional significance of this T$_3$–receptor interaction with DNA is not clear. However, such interaction may occur in the intact cell and may underlie the genomic effects of the hormone.

Table 2. Triiodothyronine (T$_3$) Binding to Cell Nuclei in Rat Tissues[a]

Tissue	Binding capacity	
	(ng/mg DNA)	(Relative to liver)
Liver	0.61	1.00
Brain	0.27	0.44
Heart	0.40	0.65
Spleen	0.018	0.03
Testis	0.0023	0.004
Kidney	0.53	0.87
Anterior pituitary	0.79	1.30

[a] Data from Oppenheimer *et al.* (1974).

IV. FUNCTIONAL ASPECTS OF HORMONE–RECEPTOR INTERACTIONS IN MATURE NEUROENDOCRINE TISSUES

Having described briefly the characteristics of the hormone receptors and the biochemical methods for measuring them, let us now consider how their action in pituitary and brain fits in with the cellular mechanisms of action described earlier. Where such information is not yet available, as in the case of releasing hormone action on behavior, we shall consider the more fundamental question of the possible neural or nonneural site of these effects.

A. Releasing Hormones

1. Pituitary

As one might expect from the likely existence of cell surface receptors for releasing hormones in pituitary, interest in releasing factor action on this tissue centers around the possible mediation of their effects by cyclic AMP (see Chapter 13). Synthetic LRH at concentrations from 10 ng to 1 μg/ml increased cyclic AMP concentrations in rat anterior pituitary incubated *in vitro* within 1 min and increased LH and FSH release into the medium within 15 min (Kaneko *et al.*, 1973). Theophylline, an inhibitor of cyclic AMP degradation, enhanced the LH release stimulated by a hypothalamic extract that presumably contained natural LRH (Wakabayashi *et al.*, 1973). Furthermore, in this study dibutyryl cyclic AMP (a longer-acting derivative) added together with theophylline stimulated release of LH.

In contrast to the effects of LRH, somatostatin (growth hormone release inhibiting factor) leads to a 50% reduction of cyclic AMP accumulation in anterior pituitary tissue during the first 2 min of incubation *in vitro* (Borgeat *et al.*, 1974). It remains to be shown whether stimulation (or inhibition) of cyclic AMP formation is a universal feature of releasing hormone action and a necessary condition for the secretion of trophic hormones by the pituitary.

2. Brain

The releasing hormones are secretory products of neurons and are stored and released by nerve endings in the median eminence. In addition, two releasing hormones, TRH (Winokur and Utiger, 1974; Jackson and Reichlin, 1974; Oliver *et al.*, 1974) and somatostatin (Patel *et al.*, 1975) are reported to exist in regions of the brain other than the hypothalamus. It is therefore of considerable interest whether, in addition to their effects on the pituitary, certain releasing hormones may have some neurotransmitter function in the brain. It should be noted that releasing hormone actions and distribution may be more widespread in the body than heretofore believed, since somatostatin has recently been shown to inhibit gastrin release *in vitro* (Hayes *et al.*, 1975), to reduce basal insulin secretion in a number of species (Koerker *et al.*, 1974), and to be present in pancreatic islet cells (Patel *et al.*, 1975).

More important for the present discussion is the fact that exogenous, systemically administered LRH, TRH, somatostatin, and MIF have been reported to alter neurochemical parameters and/or behavior. For example, MIF has been shown to potentiate L-DOPA-induced reactivity and irritability and to antagonize decreased activity induced by oxotremorine in hypophysectomized mice (Plotnikoff *et al.*, 1971, 1972). Angiotensin and TRH, in higher doses than MIF, also potentiates effects of L-DOPA and 5-hydroxytryptophan (Huidobro-Toro *et al.*, 1974). Thyrotropin-releasing hormone also increases cerebral norepinephrine turnover in normal rats, an effect that is not prevented by thyroidectomy, although T_3 in normal rats also enhances hypothalamic norepinephrine turnover (Keller *et al.*, 1974). Thyrotropin-releasing hormone also has been reported to induce hypothermia in intact cats, an effect also produced by norepinephrine and serotonin, whereas LRH and MIF are without effect (Metcalf, 1974). Finally, several interesting effects of TRH and somatostatin, opposite to each other with respect to LD_{50}s of several drugs, have recently been reported (Brown and Vale, 1975).

Luteotropin-releasing hormone is known to potentiate lordosis behavior in ovariectomized and also in hypophysectomized–ovariectomized rats primed with subthreshold doses of estrogen (Moss and McCann, 1973; Pfaff, 1973). Still another effect of a peptide hormone, vasopressin, on behavior is related to the establishment of long-term passive avoidance memory in rats (van Wimersma Greidanus *et al.*, 1975). Finally, angiotension, a hormone, is known to facilitate drinking (Epstein and Hsiao, 1975).

The data presented above suggest that peptidic hormones can affect behavior, presumably by altering the central nervous system. There is also direct evidence for these humoral substances acting on nervous tissue. Thyrotropin-releasing hormone, LRH, and somatostatin, applied iontophoretically to neurons in various brain regions including hypothalamus, inhibit the activity of some of these neurons (Dyer and Dyball, 1974; Renaud and Martin, 1975; Renaud *et al.*, 1975). Such effects are consistent with, but by no means a proof of, neurotransmitter function for these peptides. As noted above, the distribution in the brain of TRH and possibly also of somatostatin suggests a role for these peptides other than as a releasing or release-inhibiting hormone. What does remain obscure in the actions of these studies of hypothalamic peptides is the site of action of exogenously applied peptides in altering neural processes and behavior. There is uncertainty as to how readily these hormones can enter the brain from the blood (see Dupont *et al.*, 1975; Epstein and Hsiao, 1975) and concern over the rapidity with which these peptides can be inactivated by lytic enzymes in the blood. In some cases, e.g., angiotensin-induced drinking, some effects of these peptides may be mediated by the circumventricular organs (e.g., the subfornical organ) (Epstein and Hsiao, 1975). Studies of the cellular mechanism of action of releasing hormones on cells other than pituicytes must wait until their sites of action are more clearly established.

B. Thyroid Hormone

1. Pituitary

Thyrotrophs in the pituitary apparently respond to the thyroid hormone, since the pituitary is the site of the negative feedback effects of thyroid hormone in regulating TSH secretion (Reichlin *et al.*, 1972). In addition, the number of growth-hormone-secreting cells in the pituitary decreases markedly during the 2–3 weeks after thyroidectomy (Schooley *et al.*, 1966). Pituitary tumor cells that secrete growth hormone respond to T_3 and to higher doses of T_4 by showing increased glucose utilization (Samuels *et al.*, 1973). Dose–response studies with thyroid hormone analogues reveal parallels between their action and receptor-binding properties.

2. Brain

Unlike the peptide hormones, there is no question that T_3 and T_4 are able to enter the brain from the blood (Hagen and Solberg, 1974). Moreover, brain cells contain nuclear receptor sites of the type found in pituitary, liver, and kidney (see Section III.C). In spite of this, the mature brain does not respond to alterations in thyroid state with dramatic (or even significant) changes in oxygen consumption or glucose utilization (Ford, 1968). Yet, the mature rat brain does show alterations in cholinesterase activity as a function of thyroid state (Ling, 1970). T_4 treatment of euthyroid mice results in increased turnover of brain catecholamines as well as an apparently increased sensitivity of brain catecholamine receptors (Engström *et al.*, 1974). These effects may be related to the reported acceleration and potentiation of the clinical antidepressant effects of imipramine (Schildkraut *et al.*, 1971).

C. Steroid Hormones: Topography of Receptors

An important consideration in relating steroid hormone receptors to hormonal influences on the brain is the regional distribution of various receptor systems within the brain. The estradiol receptor system is the best studied from a functional point of view. For example, implantation of crystalline estradiol into brain regions having high receptor levels is effective in modifying gonadotropin secretion and facilitating lordosis behavior (Lisk, 1967). Let us now consider topographical and functional aspects of receptor systems for five classes of steroids.

1. Glucocorticoids

The glucocorticoid corticosterone concentrates in cell nuclei of hippocampus, septum, and amygdala of adrenalectomized rats (see McEwen *et al.,* 1972a). This pattern has also been observed in the Pekin duck, the guinea pig, and the rhesus monkey (see Luine and McEwen, 1978). By autoradiography, it appears that neurons are the predominant cellular sites of [³H] corticosterone accumulation (see McEwen *et al.,* 1972a; Warembourg, 1975), but glial cells are also known to respond to glucocorticoids and appear to have some glucocorticoid receptors (deVellis *et al.,* 1974).

Soluble glucocorticoid "receptors" in rat brain, high-affinity binding proteins of high molecular weight, have a regional topography resembling the topography of cell nuclear "receptor" sites for [³H] corticosterone (McEwen *et al.,* 1972b; Grosser *et al.,* 1973). These brain receptors are distinguishable from the serum binding protein transcortin which functions as a carrier for glucocorticoids in the blood. It has recently become apparent that the tritiated form of the well-known, clinically useful glucocorticoid, dexamethasone, distributes itself differently from [³H]corticosterone when infused into the tail vein of adrenalectomized rats. It accumulates predominantly in pituitary tissue, is retained by pituitary cell nuclei at least five times better than [³H] corticosterone, and labels hippocampal "receptors" about one-sixth as well as [³H]corticosterone (deKloet *et al.,* 1975). This unexpected result may have some bearing on the potency of dexamethasone with respect to suppressing pituitary ACTH secretion (for discussion, see deKloet *et al.,* 1975). Glucocorticoid receptors in the brain may mediate a number of effects that have been observed following systemic glucocorticoid administration. These effects include suppression of hippocampal single unit electrical activity, suppression of REM sleep, restoration of normal thresholds of detection and recognition of sensory stimuli, affective disorders, and alterations of extinction rates of appetitively and aversively motivated behaviors (see McEwen *et al.,* 1975c).

2. Mineralocorticoids

Proteins capable of binding [³H]deoxycorticosterone and [³H]aldosterone have been described in rat brain (Swaneck *et al.,* 1969; Lassman and Mulrow, 1974; Anderson and Fanestil, 1976). Indeed, the brain appears to be capable of responding to mineralocorticoids in its regulation of specific salt hunger (see Fregly and Waters, 1966). A confounding factor in the study of mineralocorticoid receptors is the fact that glucocorticoid-binding proteins in the brain have a moderate ability to bind mineralocorticoids. It will be necessary in future work to devise means of distinguishing, both by hormonal specificity and by physical separation of binding proteins, between glucocorticoid receptors and *bona fide* mineralocorticoid binding sites.

3. Progestins

Progesterone, like testosterone (see Section III.C.4) is likely to undergo one of a number of metabolic transformations in the body (see Luine and McEwen, 1978). The conversion to 5α-dihydroprogesterone occurs in brain and pituitary tissue and appears to be carried out by the same enzyme responsible for the 5α reduction of testosterone. Another progesterone metabolite, 20α-hydroxyprogesterone, is produced by ovarian tissue and may also be produced in brain and pituitary. The progesterone story is thus, like that of testosterone, complicated by the question of metabolites that may mediate the hormonal effects.

Studies of the fate of systematically injected [³H]progesterone and [³H]20α-OH-progesterone have shown highest uptake to occur in the midbrain region, somewhat lower uptake in hypothalamus, and still lower uptake in cerebral cortex and hippocampus of rat and guinea pig brains (Wade and Feder, 1972; Wade *et al.*, 1973). Midbrain and hypothalamus in guinea pig are both sites where progesterone implants exert effects on mating that resemble the physiological effects of the hormone given systemically. This pattern of uptake is, however, similar to that observed for [³H]corticosterone and [³H]estradiol in guinea pig brains when binding sites are saturated either by endogenous or exogenous hormones. These facts have suggested that an interaction of the steroid with lipids in the brain, and not with specific receptors, determines the pattern of uptake. Attempts to saturate and thereby reveal limited-capacity binding sites for [³H]progesterone using unlabeled progesterone have proven uniformly unsuccessful and have tended to suggest that specific progesterone binding sites may be so few in number as to escape detection.

Several pieces of evidence support the existence of progesterone receptors in the brain and pituitary. First, Sar and Stumpf (1973) have reported autoradiographic localization of binding of radioactivity injected as [³H]progesterone in neurons of the basomedial hypothalamus of the spayed, estrogen-primed guinea pig. Second, Leavitt *et al.*, (1977) reported the existence of macromolecular [³H]progesterone-binding components with S values in the

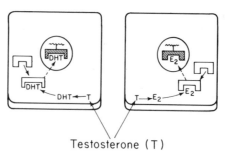

Testosterone (T)

Figure 3. Schematic diagram of the target cell transformations of testosterone (T) now known to occur in brain tissue. DHT, 5α-dihydrotestosterone; E₂, estradiol-17β.

range of 6–7 S in pituitary and hypothalamus from estrogen-primed rats. Third, Kato and Onouchi (1977), Moguilewsky and Raynaud (1978), and MacLusky *et al.* (1980) have described macromolecular binding sites for [³H]-R5020, a synthetic progestin, in rat pituitary and brain tissue. One important feature of these binding sites for R5020 (MacLusky and McEwen, 1980), which is also suggested by the work of Leavitt *et al.*, (1977), is that estrogen induces their appearance in pituitary, hypothalamus, and preoptic area of the rat. Some evidence for cell nuclear binding of [³H]-R5020 has also been published (Blaustein and Wade, 1978), suggesting that these receptors function in the manner of other steroid receptor systems.

4. Androgens

Binding of labeled testosterone by pituitary and brain tissue of the rat is less intense than that of labeled estradiol, but in general, the same brain regions are most heavily labeled by the two hormones (see Luine and McEwen, 1978). Autoradiographic studies reveal that approximately 15% of rat pituitary cells, mostly basophils, are labeled after a [³H]testosterone injection, whereas, as noted above, 60–80% of the cells are labeled after [³H]estradiol. In the medial preoptic area of the rat, a majority of the cells are labeled by both [³H]testosterone and [³H]estradiol. This clearly indicates overlap of cells binding the two labels, but the overlap may in turn be explained by the conversion of [³H]testosterone to [³H]estradiol (aromatization).

The conversion of testosterone to either 5α-dihydrotestosterone (5α-DHT) or estradiol appears increasingly to be of major significance in androgenic influences on neuroendocrine function and behavior (see Luine and McEwen, 1978). 5α-DHT formation occurs predominantly in mes- and diencephalon and in pituitary of the rat, and formation in the latter structure is under feedback control by gonadal secretion (Denef *et al.*, 1973). Estrogen formation occurs predominantly in limbic structures (but not in pituitary) of fetal as well as neonatal and adult members of a variety of species (Naftolin *et al.*, 1975). This aromatization also appears to be influenced by gonadal secretion.

The conversion of testosterone to either estradiol or 5α-reduced metabolites makes difficult the interpretation of any labeling experiment with [³H]testosterone unless the radioactive metabolites are recovered (Fig. 3). With respect to estradiol as a metabolite, male rat brains are known to contain estrogen "receptors" with a topography closely resembling that in female rat brains (Mauer and Woolley, 1974), and [³H]estradiol has been recovered from brain cell nuclei after *in vivo* [³H]testosterone administration to adult males (Lieberburg and McEwen, 1975b, 1977). With respect to 5α-DHT as a metabolite, several laboratories have presented evidence for soluble androgen-binding macromolecules in brain and pituitary (see Luine and McEwen, 1978, for references).

5. Estrogens

Putative receptor sites for estradiol are found in pineal, in anterior pituitary, and in a number of brain regions: predominently in basomedial hypothalamus, medial preoptic area, and corticomedial amygdala; to a lesser extent in midbrain central gray, ventral hippocampus and spinal cord (see Luine and McEwen, 1978). Autoradiography not only reveals neurons to be labeled in these CNS regions (see Chapter 16) but also reveals the detailed topography of these "estrophilic neurons" within these CNS regions. Within the anterior pituitary of the rat, 60–80% of the cells are labeled after a [³H]estradiol injection (Stumpf, 1968). The topography of estrophilic neurons in the rat CNS is similar to that observed in brains of other vertebrates, e.g., fish, amphibia, birds, and mammals including primates (see Chapter 16).

Soluble estrogen receptors in brain and pituitary are similar to those found in uterus, having a sedimentation coefficient in sucrose density gradients of $ca.$ 8 S at low ionic strength, a high affinity ($K_d = 10^{-10}$ M) for estradiol-17β (see Table 1), and a preference for active estrogens such as estradiol-17β and diethylstilbestrol (see Luine and McEwen, 1978). Cell nuclear accumulation of labeled [³H]estradiol in $vivo$ is observed in pituitary and in brain regions, paralleling the autoradiographically determined distribution of estrophilic neurons (Pfaff and Keiner, 1973; McEwen et $al.$, 1975a).

D. Steroid Hormones: Functioning of Receptors

The implied action of cell nuclear steroid hormone–receptor complexes is the regulation of genomic activity, especially the production of RNA molecules along a DNA template (transcription). According to this scheme, secondary changes in cellular protein synthesis, directed by the altered population of messenger RNA molecules, would be responsible for hormone effects on cellular structure and function. We shall now consider evidence in support of this mechanism of action using the best-understood example of steroid hormones action on brain and pituitary function, the effects of estradiol. (For details and references, the reader should consult Luine and McEwen, 1978.)

1. Temporal Aspects

A fundamental clue to the mechanism of estrogen action is the temporal relationship between estrogen levels in blood and on receptors and the appearance of estrogen effects. Estradiol levels rise during early proestrus; this rise in circulating steroids precedes by several hours both the surge of pituitary LH and the onset of behavioral estrus. There is also a lag of 20–30 hr between the injection of estrogen and the facilitation of lordosis responding and an LH surge, respectively. The duration of [³H]estradiol retention on brain and pituitary cell nuclear "receptors" following a single injection of 10 μg appears to be less than 12 hr, and the intervening time, up to the appearance of the physiological effect, would seem to correspond to a sequence of metabolic events initiated by the hormone. Thus estrogen's effect should not be conceptualized so much as that of a "stimulus" (required at the time the response occurs) but rather as a "permissive agent" (increasing the probability that appropriate stimuli occurring after an induction period will elicit the response). It is important to emphasize the essential role of the appropriate exteroceptive stimuli (e.g., the male's palpating the female's flanks to elicit lordosis and the day–night light cycle's inducing ovulation); the hormone does not by itself induce the physiological response.

2. Pharmacological Intervention

Another important piece of evidence for genomic involvement in estrogen action is the effectiveness of an RNA synthesis inhibitor, actinomycin D, in preventing both estrogen induction of lordosis and the occurrence of the LH surge. Actinomycin D must be given before estradiol to block the LH surge and is effective 6–12 hr after estradiol (but not later) in blocking estrogen's facilitation of behavioral estrus. In these latter experiments, actinomycin D was administered intracranially and led to reversible morphological alterations of the nucleolar structure, the disappearance of which could be correlated with the reappearance some days later of estrogen sensitivity. Evidence for the participation of translation (protein synthesis) in mediating the effects of estrogen is provided by studies of intracranially applied cycloheximide. This drug inhibits protein formation and produces reversible blockade of lordosis facilitation. Cycloheximide was, like actinomycin D, effective only when applied from 6 hr before to 12 hr after estradiol treatment.

Another tool for analyzing the nature of estrogen–receptor interaction is the use of antiestrogenic compounds (such as clomiphene, MER-25, and CI628) to prevent both the LH surge and behavioral estrus. These antiestrogens are known to bind to the steroid receptors, thus making them unavailable to the natural estrogen. As in the case of actinomycin D, these antiestrogens must be given before or shortly after estrogen treatment to be effective on behavior; they therefore must be given on diestrus day 2 of the normal cycling female to block the LH surge.

3. Neurochemical Evidence

Correlative studies of estrogen effects on pituitary and brain RNA and protein metabolism using radioactive tracers provide some evidence for altered metabolic states resulting from enhanced estrogen secretion or from estrogen administration (see Luine and McEwen, 1978). Measurements of brain and pituitary enzyme activities as a function of estrogen treatment also point to a variety of "inductive" chemical effects on cellular metabolism. Where these effects have been examined in some detail, they appear to be the direct result of estrogen action at the receptor level, although the definitive proof of this relationship is lacking. Thus, an "inductive" neurochemical effect of estrogen may underlie a "permissive" action at the physiological level. That is, quantitative changes on the neurochemical level may underlie qualitative changes on the physiological level. Resolution of any paradox implicit in the juxtaposition of the terms "inductive" and "permissive" may rest on the fact that none of the neurochemical changes are increases from undetectable levels of a gene product. Rather, they appear to be increases (or decreases) in level or activity of a constituent that is already present in substantial amount in the absence of the hormonal stimulus. Modulation in the amount of these constituents might be thought of as a means of "tuning" neuronal systems, i.e., of increasing (or decreasing) the functional efficiency of specific neural circuits. For a discussion of neural circuits that are involved in the mediation of the estrogen-dependent lordosis response, the reader is referred to the work of Pfaff (Pfaff *et al.*, 1973; McEwen and Pfaff, 1973).

With respect to biochemical changes in the pituitary that correlate with estradiol levels, hypophyseal RNA levels were reported to be lowest during diestrus and to be highest in proestrus or estrus (Convey and Reece, 1969; Robinson and Leavitt, 1971). The changes in RNA concentrations were ascribed to the action of estrogen, since ovariectomy reduced concentrations of RNA in pituitary, and replacement therapy with estradiol restored normal RNA levels (Robinson and Leavitt, 1971). An excellent protein marker of estrogen action in the pituitary is the enzyme glucose-6-phosphate dehydrogenase (G6PDH), which is the first enzyme of the pentose phosphate pathway of glucose metabolism. This pathway is a source of reducing equivalents for reductive biosynthesis and of pentose sugars for nucleoside triphosphate and RNA synthesis (Luine *et al.*, 1974, 1975a). The enzyme, which is also elevated in the uterus and in the hypothalamus, is elevated in the pituitary by estradiol-17β and diethylstilbestrol but not by estradiol-17α or testosterone (Luine *et al.*, 1974). The "action spectrum" of these four steroids thus parallels the specificity of intracellular estrogen receptors. Estradiol elevation of G6PDH activity in pituitary is blocked by the antiestrogen MER-25, and this action is in keeping with—and in fact is predicted by—a cell nuclear receptor action of estradiol (Luine *et al.*, 1975a).

An important physiological effect of estrogen on the pituitary is the facilitation of its sensitivity to LH-RH. Increased sensitivity is seen in the course of the estrous cycle on the afternoon of proestrus, following elevation of circulating estrogen levels (Gordon and Richlin, 1974; Cooper *et al.*, 1974), and is observed 14 or more hours after estradiol administration to ovariectomized or intact rats (Vilchez-Martinez *et al.*, 1974, Libertun *et al.*, 1974). These effects of estradiol may be mediated by alterations in the amount or availability of the LH-RH receptor (Spona, 1974).

Although there have been a number of reports of altered levels of labeling of RNA following estrogen, these data are somewhat conflicting, thus precluding a coherent picture (see Luine and McEwen, 1978). One reason for this confusion may be the high rate of RNA synthesis independent of hormonal stimulation. Another factor is the relatively low density of estrogen-responsive cells in neural tissue. Autoradiographic studies of amino acid incorporation into protein in brain cells as a function of estrogen stimulation have presented a more coherent picture (see Luine and McEwen, 1978). In studies that monitor fluctuations of endogenous estrogen levels, it appears that estrogen-dependent increases in amino acid incorporation into proteins are restricted, for the most part, to those brain regions that contain putative estradiol receptor sites. If estradiol is given exogenously, particularly in large amounts, other brain regions respond with an increased or decreased incorporation rate. It is presently not known whether these more widespread changes in incorporation represent alterations in the amino acid pool size rather than altered rates of protein formation. Studies of brain enzyme activities as a function of estrogen treatment of ovariectomized rats have pointed to effects that are, so far as is presently known, specific to receptor-containing brain regions (Luine et al., 1974, 1975a,b).

Among the enzymes that change are oxidative enzymes such as glucose-6-phosphate dehydrogenase (in basomedial hypothalamus) and isocitrate and maleate dehydrogenases (in basomedial hypothalamus and corticomedial amygdala). The activity of monoamine oxidase, using serotonin as a substrate, is decreased by estrogen replacement therapy in basomedial hypothalamus and corticomedial amygdala, whereas the activity of choline acetyltransferase is increased in medial preoptic area and corticomedial amygdala by estrogen treatment (Luine et al., 1975b). The activities of hypothalamic peptidases have been shown to change during the estrous cycle and are increased by estrogen replacement therapy in ovariectomized rats (Heil et al., 1971; Kuhl et al., 1974; Griffiths and Hooper, 1973, 1974). It remains to be seen whether these effects relate to the modulation of releasing hormone activities, since in one case the enzyme undergoing estrogen-dependent alteration inactivates LH-RH (Griffiths and Hooper, 1973, 1974).

Of primary interest in the ultimate understanding of estrogen action on sexual behavior and neuroendocrine function are the estrogenic effects on neurotransmitter metabolism and action. For references concerning neurotransmitter systems and their physiological implications in reproductive function, the reader should consult Chapters 4 and 14. The actual evidence for hormonal effects at the neurochemical level is relatively scanty.

a. Catecholamines

Estrogen suppression of dopamine-stimulated gonadotropin release *in vitro* in a combined median eminance–pituitary system was prevented by protein synthesis inhibitors. On the other hand, stimulation by dopamine of gonadotropin release *in vivo* was shown to depend on prior estrogen priming (see McCann and Moss, 1975). In this regard, low doses of estradiol have been reported to increase the turnover of tuberoinfundibular dopamine (Fuxe et al.,

1969), but dopamine turnover is also reported to be reduced during proestrus (see McCann and Moss, 1975), when estrogen titers have reached their peak. Resolution of this apparent discrepancy may well depend on elucidation of the time dependence of effects of a single estradiol injection and clarification of dose–response characteristics since, as noted earlier in this section, there is a lag period between the presence of estradiol on its receptors and its physiological effects.

Norepinephrine turnover is reported to be highest during states of high gonadotropin release, for example, during proestrus or as a result of gonadectomy (see Chapter 13). A single estradiol injection 56 hr before sacrifice followed by a single progesterone injection 6 hr before sacrifice is reported to decrease norepinephrine turnover especially in the preoptic–anterior hypothalamic region of the rat brain, and these effects parallel the decreased gonadotropin secretion that results (Bapna *et al.*, 1971). Again as in the case of dopamine turnover, the relationships of hormone amount and time are undoubtedly complex and beyond the scope of the present discussion. Nevertheless, it is worth while to note that current opinion favors a positive role for norepinephrine in the triggering of the LH surge and an inhibitory role for dopamine in prolactin secretion (see McCann and Moss, 1975).

It is worthwhile to note that two studies have reported increases after gonadectomy of hypothalamic activity of tyrosine hydroxlase (TH), the rate-limiting enzyme of catecholamine biosynthesis (Beattie *et al.*, 1972; Kizer *et al.*, 1974). However, neither report was able to establish which gonadal steroids are involved in maintaining normal TH levels or whether the increase in enzyme activity occurs by a direct steroid action or by an indirect effect, perhaps analogous to the reserpine or stress induction of this enzyme (Thoenen *et al.*, 1969).

b. Serotonin

Studies in the rat have been unable to show changes in the turnover of this putative neurotransmitter in the hypothalamus following combined estradiol plus progesterone treatment in ovariectomized rats (Bapna *et al.*, 1971). However, Gradwell *et al.* (1975) reported decreased serotinin turnover in ovariectomized–adrenalectomized rhesus monkeys as a result of either estradiol or testosterone replacement therapy. These authors did not localize the precise brain region involved. Again, it must be pointed out that the time dependence of gonadal steroid effects has not been systematically investigated in either species, nor have the regional changes in serotonin metabolism been thoroughly investigated. However, it is quite apparent that there are important gonadal steroid influences on serotonin metabolism that await to be elucidated.

c. Acetylcholine

Acetylcholine metabolism may be influenced by estradiol, as suggested by the observations cited earlier that choline acetyltransferase activity is increased in the medial preoptic area and corticomedial amygdala of female rats by estrogen replacement therapy (Luine *et al.,* 1975b). These observations, however, must be extended to include other parameters of acetylcholine metabolism and to include a study of physiological levels of estradiol before a role for this transmitter system in the normal action of this hormone can be accepted.

d. General

The variety of possible neurochemical effects of estradiol serve to generate a working hypothesis or model of steroid hormone action on neurons. First, there are alterations in oxidative metabolism of neural tissue, and of the pituitary as well, that may provide increased amounts of energy for neuronal function. The alteration in metabolism may also provide reducing equivalents for reductive biosynthesis of lipids and pentose sugars for RNA synthesis. Second, there may be hormone-induced alterations in biosynthetic and degradative enzymes for neurotransmitters and releasing hormones. In such cases, it might be expected that part of the "inductive lag" in the manifestation of hormonal effects would be occupied by the time required for the axonal or dendritic transport of the newly synthesized enzymes. Third, there may also be hormonally induced alterations in the number of postsynaptic receptors for neurotransmitters. At the present time the only evidence supporting this third effect relates to the sensitivity of the pituitary to LH-RH (see Section IV.D), but future work will undoubtedly yield interesting results as techniques for quantitatively measuring these receptors become available.

V. DEVELOPMENT ACTIONS OF HORMONES

A. Thyroid Hormone

The most clear-cut evidence for thyroid hormone action on the brain comes from studies of brain development, for it appears that both hyper- and hypothyroid states result in abnormalities of brain structure, chemistry, and behavior. In the rat, thyroid hormone deficiency from birth retards myelinization and development of the neuropil and decreases respiratory activity of brain tissue (Hamburgh, 1968). Thyroidectomy before day 10 impairs body temperature regulation permanently (Hamburgh, 1968). This is especially significant since body temperature is one of the most important regulators of thyroid function throughout adult as well as neonatal life.

Although both RNA and protein content in cerebrum and cerebellum are lower in rats made hypothyroid at birth, total DNA in each structure is normal at day 35 after cell proliferation has ceased, suggesting that the absence of thyroid hormones does not reduce total cell number but does reduce cell size. In contrast, administration of T_3 to euthyroid rats at birth decreases total cell number in cerebrum and cerebellum (Balasz, 1971).

Both norepinephrine levels and tyrosine hydroxylase fail to show normal development increases in neonatally radiothyroidectomized rats (Rastogi and Singhal, 1974). With respect to synapse formation, the cerebellum has been studied under both hyperthyroid and hypothyroid conditions (Nicholson and Altman, 1972). Total numbers of synaptic profiles are decreased in hypothyroid rats after 10 days of age following chemical thyroidectomy at birth. Hyperthyroidism is associated with an initial increase in synaptic density and number followed by a reduction in number of synaptic profiles after 21 days of age. Interesting parallels with synapse formation are reported for learning in rats as a result of neonatal hypothyroidism; hyperthyroid rats show an initial acceleration in learning ability but are poorer than euthyroid controls later in life (Eayrs, 1964).

These changes in cellular morphology following thyroid hormone manipulation must reflect underlying physiological changes in the CNS. It is most attractive to postulate that receptors of the type discussed earlier in connection with thyroid hormone action on mature tissues mediate the developmental effects as well. Evidence on this point is not available, although a recent report indicates that the newborn dog brain contains some triiodothyronine receptors; these receptors, however, appear to be fewer in number than in the adult brain (Hagen *et al.*, 1975).

B. Gonadal Steroids

In addition to their reversible activational effects in adult animals, gonadal steroids are capable of permanently altering reproductive tract and neural development when applied to these tissues during a critical period of fetal or early neonatal life (Chapters 5–8). In considering the cellular biochemistry of these effects the two most important questions are the chemical nature of the agonists and the type of "receptors" mediating their effects. Although it is clear that testosterone is the active secretory product of the testes during the critical period for sexual differentiation (see Chapter 5), it may not be the actual agent for inducing developmental changes. In the urogenital tract of the rabbit, 5α-dihydrotestosterone, a product of testosterone metabolism in a number of androgen target tissues, promotes male differentiation of the urogenital sinus (the anlage of the prostate) and the urogenital tubercle (the anlage of the external genitalia). Furthermore, 5α-reductase, which produces 5α-DHT, is present prior to the onset of testosterone synthesis by the gonads (see Wilson, 1973; Schultz and Wilson, 1974). In the Wolffian duct (the anlage of the epididimus, the vas deferens, and the seminal vesicle), the appearance of 5α-DHT formation follows the differentiation of this tissue to its irreversible stage of development, and thus testosterone itself (which is required for this differentiation) or some other metabolite than 5α-DHT is responsible for initiating irreversible differentiation of this embryonic tissue (Wilson, 1973).

In the brain of the rat and hamster, 5α-DHT is ineffective in inducing sexual differentiation, whereas estradiol and a number of synthetic estrogens are able to promote developmental changes similar to those seen as a result of testicular secretion or testosterone administration (see Plapinger and McEwen, 1978). The fetal or neonatal brain is capable of converting [³H]testosterone to [³H]estradiol (see Lieberburg and McEwen, 1975a; Plapinger and McEwen, 1978 for references). The fact that [³H]estradiol, as a metabolite of [³H]testosterone in 5-day-old male and female rats, is retained and concentrated by cell nuclei of the hypothalamus and limbic brain regions and not the cerebral cortex indicates that the neonatal brain contains estrogen receptors (Lieberburg and McEwen, 1975a). This influence has been supported by direct measurements of receptor-like proteins in cytosols of neonatal rat brains (Barley *et al.*, 1974) and by *in vivo* cell nuclear labeling experiments utilizing high doses of [³H]estradiol or lower doses of two synthetic ³H-labeled estrogens (McEwen *et al.*, 1975b).

The reason for using the high doses of [³H]estradiol to demonstrate neonatal estrogen receptors in the studies just described is that another estrogen-binding system, present in fetal and neonatal plasma and cerebrospinal fluid, prevents low doses of [³H]estradiol from reaching the intracellular receptor sites (see McEwen *et al.*, 1975b). This fetoneonatal estrogen-binding protein is presumed to serve a protective function for the sensitive fetal and neonatal tissues; presumably the fetoneonatal protein prevents the potential masculinizing effect of maternal estrogen (see Plapinger and McEwen, 1978). Synthetic estrogens such as 11β-methoxy-17α-ethynyl-17β-estradiol (RU2858) and diethylstilbestrol (DES) are bound less well than estradiol-17β by the fetoneonatal protein. These analogues are observed to be more effective at lower doses than estradiol-17β in labeling neonatal brain cell nuclear receptors (McEwen *et al.*, 1975b) and in promoting sexual differentiation (Ladosky, 1967; Doughty *et al.*, 1975; see also Plapinger and McEwen, 1978).

Autoradiographic evidence lends support to these observations by showing the accumulation in neonatal rat brains of radioactivity injected es [³H]testosterone in neurons of preoptic area, hypothalamus, and amygdala and by showing competition for this uptake by unlabeled estradiol as well as testosterone, but not by unlabeled DHT (Sheridan *et al.*, 1974b). A virtually identical pattern of neural uptake has been reported for [³H]estradiol in neonatal brains and has been shown to be reduced by unlabeled testosterone and estradiol (Sheridan *et al.*, 1974a). The significance of cerebral aromatization of testosterone for brain sexual differentiation is suggested by experiments showing that an inhibitor of aromatization and an estrogen antagonist both interfere with this process when given during the first few days of postnatal life (McEwen *et al.*, 1977).

The permanent development effects of neonatally administered testosterone and estrogens on brain function clearly implicate the genome as an important agent, if not a direct site of action, in these effects. Experiments demonstrating the existence of cell nuclear "receptor" sites for estrogens begin to fill in the molecular basis of hormone-dependent differentiation. In the remainder of this section we will describe biochemical and morphological observations dealing with the mechanism of these organizing effects.

One approach to the study of genomic involvement is to use inhibitors of DNA, RNA, and protein synthesis in an attempt to block neonatal hormone effects. Using anovulatory sterility as the end point of androgen action, Kobayashi and Gorski (1970) found that subcutaneous administration of actinomycin D or puromycin 2–4 hr after 30 μg testosterone propionate (TP) in 5-day-old female rats significantly reduced the number of anovulatory animals on day 45. All TP-treated animals were anovulatory at day 90, however, indicating that the antibiotics were only partially effective. In a subsequent study, Gorski and Shryne (1972) reported that intrahypothalamic cycloheximide (in cocoa butter) on day 5 attenuated effects of 30 μg TP in producing anovulatory sterility measured on day 45; again the drug given on day 5 had no effect on sterility measured on day 90. In that study, other antibiotics given intracranially were ineffective. However, Barnea and Lindner (1972) found that intrahypothalamic treatment with protein synthesis inhibitors (puromycin and cycloheximide) as well as nucleic acid synthesis inhibitors (hydroxyurea and 5-bromo-deoxyuridine) all were ineffective in blocking TP-induced anovulatory sterility. Unlike the Gorski and Shryne study, Barnea and Lindner used a higher dose of TP (100 μg) and infused the inhibitors in a large volume of saline (10 μl).

A recent report by Salaman and Birkett (1974) indicates successful attenuation of TP-induced anovulatory sterility measured at day 80–90 by RNA, protein, and DNA synthesis inhibitors given subcutaneously on postnatal day 4 when they were injected together with TP and again 6 hr later. Hydroxyurea, a DNA synthesis inhibitor with effects on overall RNA synthesis, and α-amanitin, an inhibitor of messenger RNA synthesis attenuated effects of 30, 80, and 200 μg of TP. Puromycin and actinomycin D were generally less effective in the doses used. It should also be noted that α-amanitin and hydroxyurea were by themselves ineffective in inducing anovulatory sterility.

Promising as these experiments are, they raise many questions. (a) Are the primary effects ascribed to these inhibitors actually the reasons for their effects, or are other metabolic side effects responsible? (b) Is the brain necessarily the site of action of these drugs in view of the lesser success of intracranial application of the drugs? (c) What is the critical exposure time to TP during which such drugs must be effective?

With respect to the first question, it is at least possible to point to alterations in RNA and protein metabolism in the brain associated with gonadal secretion or gonadal steroid administration during the first days of postnatal life. In one study, testosterone administration to 2-day-old female rats significantly decreased the incorporation of [^{3}H]uridine into RNA in all brain regions within 4 hr except the anterior hypothalamus and medial amygdala (Clayton *et al.*, 1970). The authors attributed special significance to the sparing action in anterior hypothalamus and amygdala in view of the presumed importance of these areas in the regulation of gonadotropin secretion. Westley and Salaman

(1975) also observed decreases in [^{3}H]uridine incorporation of 25–50% into hypothalamic RNA lasting from 2–10 hr after the administration of 1 mg of testosterone propionate to 4-day-old female rats.

Yet another study reported increases in [^{3}H]leucine incorporation into neurons of the arcuate nucleus 24 hr after castration of full-term fetal male rats (Nakai *et al.*, 1971). These authors preferred to interpret their results as indicating that "the hypothalamic–pituitary–testicular axis begins to function before birth." Another brief report indicated increased incorporation of [^{35}S]methionine in thalamus and amygdala at 12 and 24 hr after TP treatment of 3-day-old female rats (Darrah *et al.*, 1961). In no case is there any compelling evidence that these changes reflect early events in sexual differentiation, but the evidence does indicate that the neonatal brain does respond, directly or indirectly, to androgen treatment.

Direct evidence for androgen effects on brain differentiation comes from implantation of testosterone into the brains of neonatal female rats. Nadler (1968, 1972, 1973) found that TP implants in the regional ventromedial and arcuate nuclei of 5-day-old female rats were most effective in inducing anovulatory sterility and reducing female sexual receptivity. Subcutaneous implants of TP were ineffective as were implants in a great many other brain regions. Hayashi and Gorski (1974) reported anovulatory sterility from implantation of TP bilaterally into both ventromedial–arcuate and anterior hypothalamic sites of 3-day-old female rats. Using a removable implant, they found that 48–72 hr of exposure to TP were most effective, and this result implies that drugs that are used to attenuate TP effects must be allowed to act for a considerable length of time. Thus, unsuccessful inhibitor experiments performed thus far may have failed to produce a sufficiently long period of macromolecular synthesis inhibition.

The brain TP implantation experiments present a strong argument in favor of a neural target located in the hypophysiotropic area. Support for this comes from morphological studies indicating enlargement of cell nuclear volumes in neurons of the preoptic area and ventromedial nucleus in female (compared to male) rats during the last 2 days of fetal life (Dörner and Staudt, 1969). More detailed information as to the morphological consequences of sexual differentiation comes from the work of Raisman and Field (1973) showing a sexual dimorphism in the relative number of synapses from non-amygdaloid projections to shafts and spines of preoptic area dendrites. In these studies, castration of male rats 12 hr (but not 7 days) after birth successfully prevented the male patterns from appearing; and treatment of females with TP on day 4 (but not on day 16) induced a male pattern of preoptic morphology (Raisman and Field, 1973).

The hypophysiotropic area may not be the only neural target of neonatal androgen or estrogen action, since two studies have shown selective inhibitory effects of [^{3}H]lysine incorporation into cerebellar Purkinje neurons of adult rats resulting from neonatal treatment with estradiol and with testosterone (Litteria and Thorner, 1974a,b). In these studies, however, the sex difference in [³H]lysine incorporation into these cells is, if anything, in the opposite direction, males having higher incorporation than females (Litteria and Throner, 1974b). Consequently, the physiological significance of these results remains in question. Litteria (1973) and Litteria and Throner (1975) have also reported that neonatal androgen treatment of females and estrogen treatment of males significantly reduces [³H]lysine incorporation into neurons of arcuate, paraventricular, periventricular, and supraoptic nuclei but is without effect in other preoptic and hypothalamic nuclei. Suggestive as these results may be, there is again no necessary connection between these effects and sexual differentiation of the brain. In view of the observations of Johnson (1972) that true sex reversal of plasma and pituitary levels of gonadotropin has never been demonstrated by neonatal TP treatment of females or by neonatal castration of males (see also Plapinger and McEwen, 1978), it is perhaps wise to require a steroid-induced effect on the neonatal brain to recapitulate a natural sex difference. The Raisman and Field study cited above is perhaps the only solid example at the morphological level that so far meets this criterion.

A neurochemical sex difference that partially meets this criterion is a transient evaluation of brain serotonin (5-HT) levels around the 10th to 14th postnatal day of life in female compared to male rats (Ladosky and Garziri, 1970; Giulian *et al.*, 1973). Castration of males on day 1 resulted in significant (Ladosky and Gaziri, 1970) or nonsignificant (Giulian *et al.*, 1973) elevations of brain 5-HT on day 12 compared to intact males. Injection of TP in sesame oil into females on day 1 resulted in reduced brain 5-HT measured on day 12 compared to intact males. Injection of TP in sesame oil into females on day 1 resulted in reduced brain 5-HT measured on day 12 and 14 compared to oil-injected females (Ladosky and Gaziri, 1970; Giulian *et al.*, 1973).

Several exceptions were found, however, to the apparent parallel of 5-HT changes to sexual differentiation (Giulian *et al.*, 1973). First, estrogen, which also masculinizes the brain, has opposite effects to androgens on 5-HT levels: ovariectomy of females on day 1 resulted in a significant reduction of brain 5-HT on day 12 compared to intact females; and injection of estradiol or diethylstilbestrol on day 1 elevated brain 5-HT measured on days 3, 12, and 14 in females and days 8 and 12 in males. Second, DHT, which is not capable of masculinizing the brain, reduced 5-HT levels to a similar degree as did TP.

It would thus appear that sex differences in brain 5-HT levels are related to some other maturational processes than sexual differentiation per se. In this connection, it is important to note that other factors besides gonadal hormones influence maturation of the brain 5-HT system. Giulian *et al.*, (1974) showed that 15 min chilling on an ice bath (a common anaesthetic treatment for surgery) on postnatal day 1 resulted in elevated 5-HT levels around day 16. The elevation is independent of the sex of the animal and occurs later than the abovementioned sex difference. Adrenal secretion is apparently not the mediator of the effect. It is also worthwhile to note that neonatally cold-stressed animals show the typical effects of "neonatal handling" as adults, i.e., increased activity scores in an open field and decreased reaction to handling (Giulian *et al.*, 1974).

VI. CONCLUSION

It is only too evident that we have just begun to understand the cellular biochemistry of hormone action on the developing and mature brain. The broad outlines of two fundamental cellular mechanisms of hormone action have become apparent. One mechanism, for protein hormones and certain amino acid derivatives such as epinephrine, appears to involve cell surface receptors that mediate the production of intracellular "second messengers" such as cyclic AMP and cyclic GMP. The other mechanism for steroid and thyroid hormones involves intracellular receptors that appear to operate at the genomic level. Genomic effects of steroid hormones such as estradiol appear to account for the delayed "activation" of behavioral estrus and of ovulation and may well result in altered neuronal and synaptic efficiency within developmentally fixed neural pathways.

Genomic interactions also appear to be involved in the "organizational" actions of gonadal steroids during brain development; and the developing brain contains receptor sites for at least one steroid, estradiol, that are similar, if not identical, to those found in adult brain tissue. If, indeed, these receptors do mediate the developmental effects of gonadal steroids, then the difference between "activational" and "organizational" effects must involve the state of differentiation of the target neurons themselves. According to this notion, the immature cell genome is less permanently fixed in terms of genes that may be turned on or off, and the hormone–receptor interaction during the critical period can provide a signal that permanently alters the pattern of gene expression of those cells and directs the pattern of neural connections formed by those cells.

ACKNOWLEDGMENTS. The work performed in this laboratory was supported by research grant NS-07080 from The National Institutes of Health, and by Rockefeller Foundation grant RF70095 for research in reproductive biology. I would like to thank Ms. Freddi Berg for editorial assistance in the preparation of this chapter.

REFERENCES

Anderson, N. S. III, and Fanestil, D. D., 1976, Corticoid receptors in rat brain: Evidence for an aldosterone receptor, *Endocrinology* **98**:676.
Balasz, R., 1971, Effects of hormones on the biochemical maturation of the brain, in: *Influence*

of Hormones on the Nervous System, Proceedings of the International Society of Psychoneuroendocrinology, Brooklyn, 1970 (D.H. Ford, ed.), pp. 150–164, Karger, Basel.

Bapna, J., Neff, N. H., and Costa, E., 1971, A method for studying norepinephrine and serotonin metabolism in small regions of rat brain: Effect of ovariectomy on amine metabolism in anterior and posterior hypothalamus, *Endocrinology* **89**:1345.

Barley, J., Ginsburg, M., Greenstein, B. D., Maclusky, N. J., Thomas, P. J., 1974, A receptor mediating sexual differentiation? *Nature* **252**:259.

Barnea, A., and Lindner, H. R., 1972, Short-term inhibition of macromolecular synthesis and androgen-induced sexual differentiation of the rat brain, *Brain Res.* **45**:479.

Beattie, C. W., Rodgers, C. H., and Soyka, L. F., 1972, Influence of ovariectomy and ovarian steroids on hypothalamic tyrosine hydroxylase activity in the rat, *Endocrinology* **91**:276.

Berendes, H. D., 1967, The hormone ecdysone as effector of specific changes in the pattern of gene activities of drosophilia hydei, *Chromosoma* **22**:274.

Blaustein, J. D., and Wade, G. N., 1978, Progestin binding by brain and pituitary cell nuclei and female rat sexual behavior, *Brain Res.* **140**:360.

Borgeat, P., Labrie, F., Drouin, J., and Bélanger, A., 1974, Inhibition of adenosine 3′,5′-monophosphate accumulation in anterior pituitary gland *in vitro* by growth hormone-release inhibiting hormone, *Biochem. Biophys. Res. Commun.* **56**:1052.

Brown, M., and Vale, W., 1975, Central nervous system effects of hypothalamic peptides, *Endocrinology* **96**:1333.

Chytil, F., and Toft, D., 1972, Corticoid binding component in brain, *J. Neurochem.* **19**:2877.

Clark, J. H., Anderson, J., and Peck, E. J., Jr., 1972, Receptor–estrogen complex in the nuclear fraction of rat uterine cells during the estrous cycle, *Science* **176**:528.

Clayton, R. B., Kogura, J., and Kraemer, H. C., 1970, Sexual differentiation of the brain: Effects of testosterone on brain RNA metabolism in newborn female rats, *Nature* **226**:810.

Convey, E. M., and Reece, R. P., 1969, Influence of the estrous cycle on the nucleic acid content of the rat anterior pituitary, *Proc. Soc. Exp. Biol. Med.* **132**:878.

Cooper, K. J., Fawcett, C. P., and McCann, S. M., 1974, Variations in pituitary responsiveness to a luteinizing hormone/follicle stimulating hormone releasing factor (LH-RF/FSH-RF) preparation during the rat estrous cycle, *Endocrinology* **95**:1293.

Darrah, H. K., MacKinnon, P. C. B., and Rogers, A. W., 1961, Sexual differentiation in the brain of the neonatal rat, *J. Physiol. (Lond.)* **218**:22P.

DeGroot, L. J., and Torresani, J., 1975, Triiodothyronine binding to isolated liver cell nuclei, *Endocrinology* **96**:357.

deKloet, R., Wallach, G., and McEwen, B. S., 1975, Differences in corticosterone and dexamethasone binding to rat brain and pituitary, *Endocrinology* **96**:598.

Denef, C., Magnus, C., and McEwen, B. S., 1973, Sex differences and hormonal control of testosterone metabolism in rat pituitary and brain, *J. Endocrinol.* **59**:605.

deVellis, J., McEwen, B. S., Cole, R., and Inglish, D., 1974, Relations between glucocorticoid binding and glycerolphosphate dehydrogenase induction in a rat glial cell line, *Trans. Am. Soc. Neurochem.* **5**:125.

Dörner, G., and Staudt, J., 1969, Perinatal structural sex differentiation of the hypothalamus in rats, *Neuroendocrinology* **5**:103.

Doughty, C.. Booth, J. E., McDonald, P. G., and Parrott, R. F., 1975, Effects of oestradiol-17β, oestradiol benzoate and the synthetic oestrogen, RU2858 on sexual differentiation in the neonatal female rat, *J. Endocrinol.* **67**:419–424.

Dupont, A., Labrie, F., Pelletier, G., Puviani, R., Coy, D. H., Schally, A. V., and Kastin, A. J., 1975, Distribution of radioactivity in the organs of the rat and mouse after injection of L-^{3}H-prolyl-L-leucyl-L-glycinamide, *J. Endocrinol.* **63**:243.

Dyer, R. G., and Dyball, R. E. J., 1974, Evidence for a direct effect of LRF and TRF on a single unit activity in the rostral hypothalamus, *Nature* **252**:486.

Eayrs, J. T., 1964, Endocrine influence on cerebral development, *Arch. Biol. (Liege)* **75**:529.

Engström, G., Svensson, T. H., and Waldeck, B., 1974, Thyroxine and brain catecholamines: Increased transmitter synthesis and increased receptor sensitivity, *Brain Res.* **77**:471.

Epstein, A. N., and Hsiao, S., 1975, Angiotensin as dipsogen, in: *Control Mechanisms of Drinking* (G.

Peters, J. T. Fitzsimmons, and L. Peters-Haefeli, eds.), Springer-Verlag, pp. 108–116, New York.

Ford, D. H., 1968, Central nervous system–thyroid interrelationships, *Brain Res.* **7**:329.

Fregly, M. J., and Waters, I. W., 1966, Effect of mineralocorticoids on spontaneous sodium chloride appetite of adrenalectomized rats, *Physiol. Behav.* **1**:65.

Fuxe, K., Hökfelt, T., and Nilsson, O., 1969, Castration, sex hormones and tuberinfundibular dopamine neurons, *Neurodendocrinology* **5**:107–120.

Ginsburg, M., Greenstein, B. D., MacLusky, N. J., Morris, I. D., and Thomas, P. J., 1974, An improved method for the study of high-affinity steroid binding: Oestradiol binding in brain and pituitary, *Steroids* **23**:773.

Giulian, D., Pohorecky, L. A., and McEwen, B. S., 1973, Effects of gonadal steroids upon brain 5-hydroxy-tryptamine levels in the neonatal rat, *Endocrinology* **93**:1329.

Giulian, D., McEwen, B. S., and Pohorecky, L. A., 1974, Altered development of the rat brain serotonergic system after disruptive neonatal experience, *Proc. Natl. Acad. Sci. USA* **74**:4106.

Goldberg, N. D., O'Dea, R. F., and Haddox, M. K., 1973, Cyclic GMP, in: *Advances in Cyclic Nucleotide Research,* Vol. 3 (P. Greengard and G. A. Robison, eds.), pp. 155–223, Raven Press, New York.

Gordon, J. H., and Reichlin, S., 1974, Changes in pituitary responsiveness to luteinizing hormone-releasing factor during the rat estrous cycle, *Endocrinology* **94**:974.

Gorski, R. A., and Shryne, J., 1972, Intracerebral antibiotics and androgenization of the neonatal female rat, *Neuroendocrinology* **10**:109.

Gradwell, P. B., Everitt, B. J., and Herbert, J., 1975, 5-Hydroxytryptamine in the central nervous system and sexual receptivity of female rhesus monkeys, *Brain Res.* **88**:281.

Grant, G., Vale, W., and Guillemin, R., 1973a Characteristics of the pituitary binding sites for thyrotropin-releasing factor, *Endocrinology* **92**:1629.

Grant, G., Vale, W., and Rivier, J., 1973b, Pituitary binding sites for ³H-labeled luteinizing hormone releasing factor (LRF), *Biochem. Biophys. Res. Commun.* **50**:771.

Griffiths, E. C., and Hooper, K. C., 1973, Changes in hypothalamic peptidase activity during the oestrous cycle in the adult female rat, *Acta Endocrinol. (Kbh.)* **74**:41.

Griffiths, E. C., and Hooper, K. C., 1974, Peptidase activity in different areas of the rat hypothalamus, *Acta Endocrinol. (Kbh.)* **77**:10.

Grosser, B. I., Stevens, W., and Reed, D. J., 1973, Properties of corticosterone-binding macromolecules from rat brain cytosol, *Brain Res.* **57**:387.

Hagen, G. A., and Solberg, L. A., Jr., 1974, Brain and cerebrospinal fluid permeability to intravenous thyroid hormones, *Endocrinology* **95**:1398.

Hagen, G. A., Fleshman, J. W., and Diuguid, L. I., 1975, Newborn brain triiodothyronine (T₃) receptors and cooperative binding effect, *Program, The Endocrine Society 5th Annual Meeting, New York June 18–20, 1975,* abstract #387.

Haglund, H., 1971, Isoelectric focusing in pH gradients—a technique for fractionation and characterization of ampholytes, *Methods Biochem. Anal.* **19**:1.

Hamburgh, M., 1968, An analysis of the action of thyroid hormone on development based on *in vivo* and *in vitro* studies, *Gen. Comp. Endocrinol.* **10**:198.

Hayashi, S., and Gorski, R. A., 1974, Critical exposure time for androgenization by intracranial crystals of testosterone propionate in neonatal female rats, *Endocrinology* **94**:1161.

Hayes, J. R., Johnson, D. G., Koerker, D., and Williams, R. H., 1975, Inhibition of gastrin release by somatostatin *in vitro, Endocrinology* **96**:1374.

Heil, H., Meltzer, V., Kuhl, H., Abraham, R., and Taubert, H. D., 1971, Stimulation of L-cystine-aminopeptidase activity by hormonal steroids and steroid analogs in the hypothalamus and other tissues of the female rat, *Fertil. Steril.* **22**:181.

Huidobro-Toro, J. P., Scotti de Carolis, A., and Longo, V. G., 1974, Action of two hypothalamic factors (TRH, MIF) and of angiotensin II on the behavioral effects of L-DOPA and 5-hydroxytryptophan in mice, *Pharmacol. Biochem. Behav.* **2**:105.

Irving, R., and Mainwaring, W. I. P., 1974, Partial purification of steroid–receptor complexes by DNA–cellulose chromatography and isoelectric focusing, *J. Steroid Biochem.* **5**:711.

Jackson, I. M. D., and Reichlin, S., 1974, Thyrotropin-releasing hormone (TRH): Distribution in hypothalamic and extrahypothalamic brain tissues of mammalian and submammalian chordates, *Endocrinology* **95**:854.

Johnson, D. C., 1972, Sexual differentiation on gonadotropin patterns, *Am. Zool.* **12**:193.

Joustra, M., Söderquist, B., and Fischer, L., 1967, Gel filtration in organic solvents, *J. Chromatogr.* **28**:21.

Kalimi, M., Colman, P., and Feigelson, P., 1975, The "activated" hepatic glucocorticoid–receptor complex, *J. Biol. Chem.* **250**:1080.

Kaneko, T., Saito, S., Oka, H., Oda, T., and Yanaihara, N., 1973, Effects of synthetic LH-RH and its analogs on rat anterior pituitary cyclic AMP and LH and FSH release, *Metabolism* **22**:77.

Kato, J., and Onouchi, T., 1977, Specific progesterone receptors in the hypothalamus and anterior hypophysis of the rat, *Endocrinology* **101**:920.

Keller, H. H., Bartholini, G., and Pletscher, A., 1974, Enhancement of cerebral noradrenaline turnover by thyrotropin-releasing hormone, *Nature* **248**:528.

King, R. J. B., and Mainwaring, W. I. P., 1974, *Steroid–Cell Interactions*, University Park Press, Baltimore.

Kizer, J. S., Palkovits, M., Zivih, J., Brownstein, M., Saavedra, J. M., and Kopin, I. M., 1974, The effect of endocrinology manipulations on tyrosine hydroxylase and dopamine-β-hydroxylase activities in individual hypothalamic nuclei of the adult male rat, *Endocrinology* **95**:799.

Kobayashi, F., and Gorski, R. A., 1970, Effects of antibiotics on androgenization of the neonatal female rat, *Endocrinology* **86**:285.

Koerker, D. J., Ruch, W., Chideckel, E., Palmer, J., Goodner, C. J., Ensinck, J., and Gale, C. C., 1974, Somatostatin: Hypothalamic inhibitor of the endocrine pancreas, *Science* **184**:482.

Kuhl, H., Rosniatowski, C., Oen, S., and Taubert, H., 1974, Sex steroids stimulate the activity of hypothalamic arylamidases in the rat, *Acta Endocrinol. (Kbh.)* **76**:1.

Ladosky, W., 1967, Anovulatory sterility in rats neonatally injected with stilbestrol, *Endokrinologie* **52**:259.

Ladosky, W., and Gaziri, L. C. J., 1970, Brain serotonin and sexual differentiation of the nervous system, *Neuroendocrinology* **6**:168.

Langan, T. A., 1973, Protein kinases and protein kinase substrates, in: *Advances in Cyclic Nucleotide Research*, Vol. 3 (P. Greengard and G. A. Robison, eds.), pp. 99–153, Raven Press, New York.

Lassman, M. N., and Mulrow, P. J., 1974, Deficiency of deoxycorticosterone-binding protein in the hypothalamus of rats resistant to deoxycorticosterone-induced hypertension. *Endocrinology* **94**:1541.

Leavitt, W. W., Chen, T. J., and Allen, T. C., 1977, Regulation of progesterone receptor formation by estrogen action, *Ann. N. Y. Acad. Sci.* **286**:210.

Libertun, C., Cooper, K. J., Fawcett, C. P., and McCann, S. M., 1974, Effects of ovariectomy and steroid treatment on hypophyseal sensitivity to purified LH-releasing factor (LRF), *Endocrinology* **94**:518.

Lieberburg, I., and McEwen, B. S., 1975a, Estradiol-17β: A metabolite of testosterone recovered in cell nuclei from limbic areas of neonatal rat brains, *Brain Res.* **85**:165.

Lieberburg, I., and McEwen, B. S., 1975b, Estradiol-17β: A metabolite of testosterone recovered in cell nuclei from limbic areas of adult male rat brains, *Brain Res.* **91**:171.

Lieberburg, I., and McEwen, B. S., 1977, Brain cell nuclear retention of testosterone metabolites, 5α-dihydrotestosterone and estradiol-17β in adult rats, *Endocrinology* **100**:588.

Ling, A. S. C., 1970, The influence of the thyroid gland on brain cholinesterase activity of mature rats, *Brain Res.* **22**:73.

Lisk, R. D., 1967, Sexual behavior: Hormonal control, in: *Neuroendocrinology*, Vol. 2 (L. Martini and W. F. Ganong, eds), pp. 197–239, Academic Press, New York.

Litteria, M., 1973, Inhibitory action of neonatal androgenization on the incorporation of ^{3}H-lysine in specific hypothalamic nuclei of the adult female rat. *Exp. Neurol.* **41**:395.

Litteria, M., and Thorner, M. W., 1974a, Inhibition in the incorporation of ^{3}H-lysine in the Purkinje cells of the adult female rat after neonatal androgenization, *Brain Res.* **69**:170.

Litteria, M., and Thorner, M. W., 1974b, Inhibitory effect of neonatal estrogenization on the incorporation of ^{3}H-lysine in the Purkinje cells of the adult male and female rat. *Brain Res.* **80**:152.

Litteria, M., and Thorner, M. W., 1975, Inhibitory action of neonatal estrogenization on the incorporation of ^{3}H-lysine into proteins of specific hypothalamic nuclei in the adult male rat, *Brain Res.* **90**:179.

Luine, V. N., Khylchevskaya, R. I., and McEwen, B. S., 1974, Oestrogen effects on brain and pituitary enzyme activities, *J. Neurochem.* **23**:925.

Luine, V. N., Khylchevskaya, R. I., and McEwen, B. S., 1975a, Effect of gonadal hormones on enzyme activities in brain and pituitary of male and female rats, *Brain Res.* **86**:283.

Luine, V. N., Khylchevskaya, R. I., and McEwen, B. S., 1975b, Effect of gonadal steroids on activities of monoamine oxidase and choline acetylase in rat brain, *Brain Res.* **86**:293.

MacLeod, K. M., and Baxter, J. D., 1975, DNA binding of thyroid hormone receptors, *Biochem. Biophys. Res. Commun.* **62**:577.

MacLusky, N. J., and McEwen, B. S., 1980, Progestin receptors in rat brain: Distribution and properties of cytoplasmic progestin binding sites, *Endocrinology* **106**:192–202.

Martin, R. G., and Ames, B. N., 1961, A method for determining the sedimentation behavior of enzymes: Application to protein mixtures, *J. Biol. Chem.* **236**:1372.

Maurer, R. A., and Woolley, D. E., 1974, Demonstration of nuclear ^{3}H-estradiol binding in hypothalamus and amygdala of female, androgenized-female, and male rats, *Neuroendocrinology* **16**:137.

McCann, S. M., and Moss, R. L., 1975, Putative neurotransmitters involved in discharging gonadotropin-releasing neurohormones and the action of LH-releasing hormone on the CNS, *Life Sci.* **16**:833.

McEwen, B. S., and Luine, V. N., 1979, Specificity, mechanisms, and functional significance of steroid-receptor interactions in the brain and pituitary, in: *Biologie Cellulaire des Processus Neurosécrétoires Hypothalamiques, CNRS Colloque Internationaux du CNRS No. 280,* pp. 239–265, CNRS, Paris.

McEwen, B. S., and Pfaff, D. W., 1973, Chemical and physiological approaches to neuroendocrine mechanisms: Attempts at integration, in: *Frontiers in Neuroendocrinology* (W. F. Ganong and L. Martini, eds.), pp. 267–335, Oxford University Press, New York.

McEwen, B. S., and Zigmond, R. E., 1972, Isolation of brain cell nuclei, in: *Research Methods in Neurochemistry,* Vol. 1 (N. Marks and R. Rodnight, eds.), pp. 140–161, Plenum Press, New York.

McEwen, B. S., Zigmond, R. E., and Gerlach, J. L., 1972a, Sites of steroid binding and action in the brain, in: *Structure and Function of Nervous Tissue,* Vol. 5 (G. H. Bourne, ed.), pp. 205–291, Academic Press, New York.

McEwen, B. S., Magnus, C., and Wallach, G., 1972b, Soluble corticosterone-binding macromolecules extracted from rat brain, *Endocrinology* **90**:217.

McEwen, B. S., Pfaff, D. W., Chaptal, C., and Luine, V., 1975a, Brain cell nuclear retention of ^{3}H-estradiol doses able to promote lordosis: Temporal and regional aspects, *Brain Res.* **86**:155.

McEwen, B. S., Plapinger, L., Chaptal, C., Gerlach, J., and Wallach, G., 1975b, Role of fetoneonatal estrogen binding proteins in the association of estrogen with neonatal brain cell nuclear receptors, *Brain Res.* **96**:400–406.

McEwen, B. S., Gerlach, J. L., and Micco, D. J., Jr., 1975c, Putative glucocorticoid receptors in hippocampus and other regions of the rat brain, in: *The Hippocampus: A Comprehensive Treatise* (R. Isaacson and K. Pribram, eds.), pp. 285–322, Plenum Press, New York.

McEwen, B. S., Lieberburg, I., Chaptal, C., and Krey, L. C., 1977, Aromatization: Important for sexual differentiation of the neonatal rat brain, *Horm. Behav.* **9**:249–263.

Metcalf, G., 1974, TRH: A possible mediator of thermoregulation, *Nature* **252**:310.

Moguilewsky, M., and Raynaud, J. P., 1978, Progestin binding sites in the rat hypothalamus, pituitary, and uterus, *Steroids* **30**:99–109.

Moss, R. L., and McCann, S. M., 1973, Induction of mating behavior in rats by luteinizing hormone-releasing factor, *Science* **181**:177.

Nadler, R. D., 1968, Maculinization of female rats by intracranial implantation of androgen in infancy, *J. Comp. Physiol. Psychol.* **66**:157.

Nadler, R. D., 1972, Intrahypothalamic exploration of androgen-dependent brain loci in neonatal female rats, *Trans. N. Y. Acad. Sci. Ser. II* **34**:572.

Nadler, R. D., 1973, Further evidence on the intrahypothalamic locus for androgenization of female rats, *Neuroendocrinology* **12**:110.

Naftolin, F., Ryan, K. J., Davies, I. J., Reddy, V. V., Flores, F., Kuhn, M., White, R. J., Takaoka, Y., and Wolin, L., 1975, The formation of estrogens by central neuroendocrine tissues, *Recent Prog, Horm. Res.* **31**:295.

Nakai, T., Kigawa, T., and Sakamoto, S., 1971, ^{3}H-Leucine uptake of hypothalamic nuclei in fetal male rats and its fluctuation after castration, *Endocrinol. Jpn.* **18**:353.

Nicholson, J. L., and Altman, J., 1972, Synaptogenesis in the rat cerebellum: Effects of early hypo-and hyperthyroidism, *Science* **176**:530.

Oliver, C., Eskay, R. L., Ben-Jonathan, N., and Porter, J. C., 1974, Distribution and concentration of TRH in the rat brain, *Endocrinology* **95**:540.

O'Malley, B. W., and Means, A. R., 1974, Female steroid hormones and target cell nuclei, *Science* **183**:610.

Oppenheimer, J. H., Schwartz, H. L., and Surks, M. I., 1974, Tissue differences in the concentration of triiodothyronine nuclear binding sites in the rat: Liver, kidney, pituitary, heart, brain, spleen and testis, *Endocrinology* **95**:897.

Patel, Y. C., Weir, G. C., and Reichlin, S., 1975, Anatomic distribution of somatostatin (SRIF) in brain and pancreatic islets as studied by radioimmunoassay (RIA), in: *Program, The Endocrine Society 57th Annual Meeting, New York, June 18–20, 1975,* abstract #154, J. B. Lippincott, Philadelphia.

Pfaff, D. W., 1973, Luteinizing hormone-releasing factor potentiates lordosis behavior in hypophysectomized ovariectomized female rats, *Science* **182**:1148.

Pfaff, D. W., and Keiner, M., 1973, Atlas of estradiol-concentrating cells in the central nervous system of the female rat, *J. Comp. Neurol.* **151**:121.

Pfaff, D., Lewis, C., Diakow, C., and Keiner, M., 1973, Neurophysiological analysis of mating behavior responses as hormone-sensitive reflexes, in: *Progesss in Physiological Psychology,* Vol. 5 (E. Stellar and J. M. Sprague, eds.), pp. 253—297, Academic Press, New York.

Plapinger, L., and McEwen, B. S., 1978, Gonadal steroid–brain interactions in sexual differentiation, in: *Biological Determinants of Sexual Behavior* (J. Hutchison, ed.), pp. 153–218, John Wiley and Sons, New York and London.

Plotnikoff, N. P., Kastin, A. J., Anderson, M., and Schally, A. V., 1971, DOPA potentiation by a hypothalamic factor, MSH release inhibiting hormone (MIF), *Life Sci.* **10**:1279.

Plotnikoff, N. P., Kastin, A. J., Anderson, M., and Schally, A. V., 1972, Oxotremorine antagonism by a hypothalamic hormone, melanocyte-stimulating hormone release inhibiting factor (MIF), *Proc. Soc. Exp. Biol. Med.* **140**:811.

Raisman, G., and Field, P. M., 1973, Sexual dimorphism in the neuropil of the preoptic area of the rat and its dependence on neonatal androgen, *Brain Res.* **54**:1.

Rastogi, R. B., and Singhal, R. L., 1974, Alterations in brain norepinephrine and tyrosine hydroxylase activity during experimental hypothyroidism, *Brain Res.* **81**:253.

Raynaud, J. P., Mercier-Bodard, C., and Baulieu, E. E., 1971, Rat estradiol binding plasma protein (EBP), *Steroids* **18**:767.

Reichlin, S., Martin, J. B., Mitnick, M. A., Boshaus, R. L., Grimm, Y., Bollinger, J., Gordon, J., and Malacara, J., 1972, The hypothalamus in pituitary–thyroid regulation, *Recent Prog. Horm. Res.* **28**:229.

Renaud, L. P., and Martin, J. B., 1975, Thyrotropin releasing hormone (TRH): Depressant action on central neuronal activity, *Brain Res.* **86**:150.

Renaud, L. P., Martin, J. B., and Brezeau, P., 1975, Depressant action of TRH, LH-RH and somatostatin on activity of central neurons, *Nature* **255**:233.

Robinson, J. A., and Leavitt, W. W., 1971, Estrogen related changes in anterior pituitary RNA levels, *Proc. Soc. Exp. Biol. Med.* **139**:471.

Robison, G. A., Butcher, R. W., and Sutherland, E. W., 1971, *Cyclic AMP,* Academic Press, New York.

Salaman, D. F., and Birkett, S., 1974, Androgen-induced sexual differentiation of the brain is blocked by inhibitors of DNA and RNA synthesis, *Nature* **247**:109.

Samuels, H. H., Tsai, J. S., and Cintron, R., 1973, Thyroid hormone action: A cell culture system responsive to physiological concentrations of thyroid hormones, *Science* **181**:1253.

Samuels, H. H., Tsai, J. S., and Casanova, J., 1974, Thyroid hormone action: *In vitro* demonstration of putative receptors in isolated nuclei and soluble nuclear extracts, *Science* **184**:1188.

Sar, M., and Stumpf, W. E., 1973, Neurons of the hypothalamus concentrate ^{3}H-progesterone or its metabolites, *Science* **182**:1266.

Schildkraut, J. J., Winokur, A., Draskoczy, P. R., and Hensle, J. H., 1971. Changes in norepinephrine turnover in rat brain during chronic administration of imipramine and protriptyline: A possible explanation for the delay in onset of clinical antidepressant effects, *Am. J. Psychiatry* **127**:1032.

Schooley, R. A., Friedkin, S., and Evans, E. S., 1966, Re-examination of the discrepancy between acidophil numbers and growth hormone concentration in the anterior pituitary gland following thyroidectomy, *Endocrinology* **79**:1053.

Schultz, F. M., and Wilson, J. D., 1974, Virilization of the Wolffian duct in the rat fetus by various androgens, *Endocrinology* **94**:979.

Schutz, G., Beato, M., and Feigelson, P., 1973, Messenger RNA for hepatic tryptophan oxygenase: Its partial purification, its translation in a heterologous cell-free system, and its control by glucocorticoid hormones, *Proc. Natl. Acad. Sci. USA* **70**:1218.

Sheridan, P. J., Sar, M., and Stumpf, W. E., 1974a, Autoradiographic localization of ^{3}H-estradiol or its metabolites in the central nervous system of the developing rat, *Endocrinology* **94**:1386.

Sheridan, P. J., Sar, M., and Stumpf, W. E., 1974b, Interaction of exogenous steroids in the developing rat brain, *Endocrinology* **95**:1749.

Siegel, L. M., and Monty, K. J., 1966, Determination of molecular weights and fractional ratios of proteins in impure systems by use of gel filtration and density gradient centrifugation. Application to crude preparations of sulfite and hydroxylamine reductases, *Biochim. Biophys. Acta* **112**:346.

Spona, J., 1974, LH-RH interaction with the pituitary plasma membrane is affected by sex steroids, *FEBS Lett.* **39**:221.

Sternberger, L. A., 1974, *Immunocytochemistry,* Prentice Hall, Englewood Cliffs.

Stumpf, W. E., 1968, Cellular and subcellular ^{3}H-estradiol localization in the pituitary by autoradiographs, *Z. Zellforsch.* **92**:23.

Swaneck, G. E., Highland, E., and Edelman, I. S., 1969, Stereospecific nuclear and cytosol aldosterone-binding proteins of various tissues, *Nephron* **6**:297.

Thoenen, H., Mueller, R. A., and Axelrod, J., 1969, Trans-synaptic induction of adrenal tyrosine hydroxylase, *J. Pharmacol. Exp. Ther.* **169**:249.

Van Wimersma Greidanus, T. B., Dogterom, J., and de Wied, D., 1975, Intraventricular administration of anti-vasopressin serum inhibits memory consolidation in rats, *Life Sci.* **16**:637.

Vilchez, Martinez, J. A., Arimura, A., Debeljuk, L., Schally, A. V., 1974, Biphasic effect of estradiol benzoate on the pituitary responsiveness to LH-RH, *Endocrinology* **94**:1300.

Wade, G. N., and Feder, H. H., 1972, [1,2-^{3}H]Progesterone uptake by guinea-pig brain and uterus: Differential localization, time-course of uptake and metabolism and effects of age, sex, estrogen-priming and competing steroids, *Brain Res.* **45**:525.

Wade, G. N., Harding, C. F., and Feder, H. H., 1973, Neural uptake of [1,2-^{3}H]progesterone in ovariectomized rats, guinea pigs and hamsters: Correlation with species differences in behavioral responsiveness, *Brain Res.* **61**:357.

Wakabayashi, K., Date, Y., and Tamaoki, B.-I., 1973, On the mechanism of action of luteinizing hormone-releasing factor and prolactin release inhibiting factor, *Endocrinology* **92**:698.

Warembourg, M., 1975, Radioautographic study of the rat brain after injection of [1,2-^{3}H]corticosterone, *Brain Res.* **89**:61.

Westley, B. R. and Salaman, D. F., 1975, Incorporation of ^{3}H-uridine into RNA in the hypothalamus of the neonatal rat. *J. Endocrinol.* **64**:58P.

Williams, D. L., 1975, The estrogen receptor: A minireview, *Life Sci.* **15**:583.

Wilson, J. D., 1973, Testosterone uptake by the urogenital tract of the rabbit embryo, *Endocrinology* **92**:1192.

Winokur, A., and Utiger, R. D., 1974, Thyrotropin-releasing hormone: Regional distribution in rat brain, *Science* **185**:265.

16

Autoradiographic Technique for Steroid Hormone Localization

Application to the Vertebrate Brain

JOAN I. MORRELL AND DONALD W. PFAFF

I. INTRODUCTION

Autoradiographic procedures can be used to locate cells that concentrate steroid hormones. The autoradiographic demonstration of steroid concentration has been used for studies on the uterus and other tissues, but it is an especially useful technique when applied to the brain. The brain is made up of cells heterogenous in structure and function, and thus the anatomical detail obtainable with autoradiography is an especially important advantage in this organ.

With this technique, it is readily possible to study the whole brain for the topography of steroid-concentrating cells. By serial sectioning, one can examine regions of the brain in detail without the hindrance of excessively small tissue samples. The brain–endocrine interaction demonstrated is very specific, and the autoradiographic technique can be considered a "staining" method for this functional interaction.

In autoradiographic studies with steroid hormones, it is presumed that the accumulated radioactivity visualized in the light microscope results from the binding of a tritiated steroid hormone to a receptor protein in the cell. There is

JOAN I. MORRELL and DONALD W. PFAFF • Department of Psychology, The Rockefeller University, New York, New York 10021.

a considerable body of biochemical data that supports this and furnishes chemical detail about the steroid receptor protein and the sequence of steroid–receptor interaction (see Chapter 15). The cells that concentrate sex steroid hormones (Pfaff, 1968) as well as adrenal steroid hormones (Gerlach and McEwen, 1972) have been examined with the technique to be described. This chapter is concerned primarily with the use of autoradiography for sex steroid hormone localization.

The sex steroids are slightly water soluble and hence are diffusible in most histological procedures. Therefore, autoradiographic procedures for steroid-concentrating cells avoid steps where diffusion might take place. Basically, this involves using unfixed, unembedded, frozen sections applied to dry emulsion-coated slides.

Brain sites containing cells that concentrate sex steroids are frequently studied with other techniques, and such studies have shown involvement of these sites in behavioral or neuroendocrine function. In the rat brain, for example, the areas of highest [^{3}H]estradiol concentration are areas that have been demonstrated to regulate behavioral or neuroendocrine events (Pfaff and Keiner, 1973; McEwen and Pfaff, 1973). Similar examples can be found with the areas of highest [^{3}H]estradiol or testosterone concentration in the brain of anuran amphibian, *Xenopus laevis* (Kelly *et al.*, 1975; Morell *et al.*, 1975b). These and other species will be discussed in Section IV of this chapter. That section will show that the presence of sex-steroid-concentrating cells in the brain is a general phenomenon among vertebrates and that there are striking similarities in the topography of hormone-concentrating neurons from species to species.

II. PROCEDURES FOR PRODUCTION OF STEROID HORMONE AUTORADIOGRAMS

The production of autoradiograms has been divided into five major steps in this section. Steroid hormone autoradiograms require long exposure times, and mistakes are discovered only at the end of the procedure. Each step in the procedure requires special care, for one error could ruin months of work. Autoradiography includes steps analogous to the processes used to produce a black-and-white photograph, but it is technically more demanding. For example, light, dirt, inappropriate temperatures, and humidity are all greater problems during the production of a good quality autoradiogram. The darkroom used for autoradiography must be well regulated for constant temperature and humidity. A safelight equipped with Kodak No. 2 red filter and a 15-watt bulb can be no closer than 3 feet from the autoradiograms. The Thomas Duplex safelight with sodium vapor light source and FBD and FOB filters (7 feet above autoradiograms) increases the overall background slightly but is acceptable if greater visibility is essential and if precautions are taken to minimize exposure of the emulsion to the safelight.

The steps for steroid autoradiogram production outlined below (Fig. 1) have been used successfully in this laboratory to localize estradiol- and testosterone-concentrating neurons in a wide variety of vertebrate species (see Section IV).

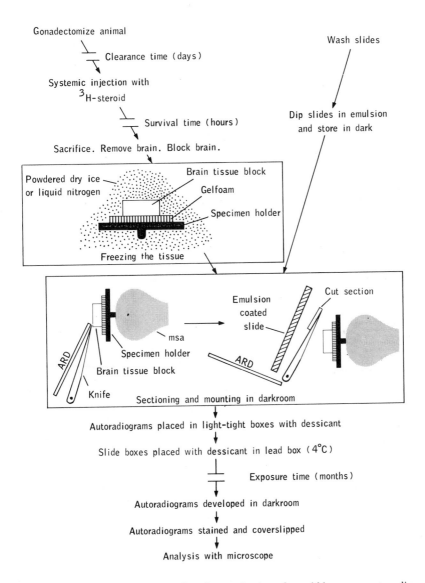

Figure 1. Diagram of steps in the procedure for production of steroid hormone autoradiograms. Sequence of procedures follows direction of arrows from top to bottom of figure. A R D, antiroll device (part of microtome); msa, microtome sliding attachment.

A. Preparation of Emulsion-Coated Slides

Microscope slides are washed for 1 hr in hot water and detergent, rinsed for 2 hr or longer in hot running water, rinsed in distilled water, and dried in an oven overnight. All further steps in this section are completed in the darkroom with one safelight, minimizing exposure of the emulsion to the safelight.

Nuclear track emulsion (Kodak NTB-2 or 3) is stored in the cold until ready for use. When the emulsion is to be used to coat slides, it is melted in a water bath at 43°C. The melted emulsion is then poured into a weighted cylinder which is kept at 43°C in the water bath. The cleaned slides are dipped into the emulsion. The dipped emulsion-coated slides are dried in a place not exposed to the safelight.

The dry emulsion-coated slides are then loaded into black plastic slide boxes that are light-tight and contain a desiccant. The slides are stored in the dark and kept dry until used.

B. Isotope Administration, Brain Removal, and Freezing

Animals are gonadectomized 2 days to 1 week before isotope administration. This reduces levels of endogenous hormone that would compete with the tritiated hormone for cellular binding sites. Quadruply tritiated sex steroid of high specific activity (80–110 Ci/mmol) is administered to the animal by an intraperitoneal, intramuscular, intravenous, or subcutaneous route. The dose, calculated per unit of body weight, must yield blood levels within the physiological range for the hormone. Testosterone or estradiol doses in the range of 25 to 200 μCi per 100 g body weight have resulted in readily detectable labeled cells in the brains of several species: rat (Pfaff and Keiner, 1973), hamster (Floody and Pfaff, 1974), Rhesus monkey (Pfaff *et al.*, 1974; Gerlach *et al.*, 1975), mink (Morrell and Pfaff, 1975); the amphibians *Xenopus laevis* (Kelley *et al.*, 1975; Morrell *et al.*, 1975b) and *Rana pipiens* (Kelley and Pfaff, 1975a); the chaffinch (Zigmond *et al.*, 1973), the zebra finch (Arnold *et al.*, 1975), the chicken (Barfield *et al.*, 1975); and, in the teleost, the green sunfish.

The length of time between radioactive steroid administration and sacrifice is selected so that at sacrifice, the level of isotope circulating in the blood has decreased from its peak value and is low. The best way to determine this interval is by scintillation counting of blood samples from animals sacrificed at regular intervals after injection of isotope.

When the animal is sacrificed, brain removal is done as quickly as possible. When the brain is freed from the skull, it is placed on a glass surface that is cooled by ice. The brain is blocked in such a way as to give convenient block sizes and planes of section. Each tissue block is placed on a specimen holder that has been prepared by freezing wet gelfoam onto the surface. The specimen holder is frozen with dry ice or liquid nitrogen. The brain block is placed in the desired orientation on this gelfoam surface and is then frozen quickly with finely powdered dry ice or liquid nitrogen (Fig. 1). The frozen tissue block and holder are then placed in the cryostat (previously cooled to −19°C) and allowed to equilibrate to cryostat temperature. If the tissue is frozen too slowly, the morphology of the tissue will be disrupted. Freezing too rapidly can cause the block of tissue to crack.

C. Sectioning and Mounting Autoradiograms in the Darkroom

For sectioning between −17° and −20°C, a Harris International Equipment Co. enclosed cryostat (Model CTD) or a similar piece of equipment can be used. Sections are usually cut at 4 or 6 μm. The antiroll device, the part of the cryostat that helps to keep the sections flat during cutting, is moved away from the knife when sections are mounted (Fig. 1). A section is cut and then mounted on an emulsion-coated slide by lowering the slide carefully toward the knife until the section adheres to it. Pressure on the emulsion-coated slide must be avoided, since this will result in poor morphology of the section and greatly increased autoradiographic background (pressure artifact).

D. Exposure, Developing, and Staining Procedures

During exposure, autoradiograms are stored in light-tight black slide boxes that have tightly fitting tops and contain desiccant. During the exposure period, the slide boxes are stored at 4°C in a lead box containing desiccant. Freezing the sections is also acceptable. The time necessary for adequate exposure of the emulsion to the β emission particles usually ranges between 4 and 12 months, depending on the amount of isotope used and bound. The number of grains under labeled cells is proportional to the length of exposure. A few "test" slides can be removed and developed to allow a judgment to be made about the intensity of labeling and to determine the optimum time of exposure.

After an appropriate exposure time, the slides are removed from the cold and developed in the darkroom in Kodak D-19 ® Developer (16 °C), rinsed in Kodak Liquid Hardener® (18°–21°C), and fixed in Kodak fixer (18°–21°C). The sections can then be stained with, for example, cresyl violet or hematoxylin and eosin methods. It is possible to lose grains from a developed emulsion, and each new staining method should be tested for this.

E. Controls for Autoradiographic Artifact

In addition to being sensitive to light and nuclear emissions, nuclear track emulsion is sensitive to mechanical and chemical interaction with the sections applied to it (Rogers, 1973). Mechanical forces produced by the tissue drying on the emulsion or by pressure applied during mounting can cause high background. Chemical interactions that cause artifact are referred to as positive or negative "chemography." Positive chemography is an artifactual grain reduction, resulting in an increased number of grains under the tissue. Negative chemography is a fading of the latent image, often associated with high humidity (Leblond et al., 1963) and resulting in an artifactual decrease in the number of grains under a section. Some types of tissue are more likely to produce chemography than others. The possibility of artifact must be ruled out in each study by preparation of appropriate control sections.

It is best to prepare a control, nonradioactive brain with each group of experimental, radioactive brains. As a control for artifactual grain reduction, sections from a nonradioactive brain are taken and treated in all respects the same as the radioactive sections. After the sections are developed, no grain accumulations under the cells should be visible.

As a control for negative chemography, sections mounted on emulsion-coated slides are intentionally exposed to light. After developing, the emulsion appears entirely black. If there were any fading of the latent image because of tissue–emulsion interactions, light spots where reduced grains are "missing" would be visible with the microscope. Some control sections for positive and negative chemography should be developed with each batch of auto-radiograms.

III. ANALYSIS OF AUTORADIOGRAMS

Autoradiograms are analyzed in this laboratory by systematic scanning with a light microscope for accumulation of black grains in the emulsion layer under stained cells, primarily cell nuclei (Figs. 2 and 3). The emulsion consists of a suspension of silver halide—mostly silver bromide—crystals in gelatin. Beta particles emitted from the tritiated hormone ionize the silver crystals; these are subsequently reduced during developing and thereby become visible (Fig. 2) (Pelc et al., 1965).

A cell body is defined as labeled when the number of grains accumulated under it exceed a fixed quantitative criterion. This criterion is a ratio of grains under the cell body to grains under an adjacent cell-sized area. When the value of the ratio for a given cell is five or greater, that cell is defined as labeled. Because this criterion requires that the number of reduced grains associated with a labeled cell far exceed the distribution of grains in the "background" (i.e., usually >> 6 standard deviations above mean background), false positive designations of cells as labeled are highly improbable (Fig. 3).

Grains defined as "background" (i.e., grains under the neuropil) have two origins: background caused by the [^{3}H]steroid hormone itself or its metabolites and degradation products, and background from other sources. Background in the first category is caused by tritiated hormone or metabolites that lies outside the cell nucleus and cell body and which may or may not be bound in a physiologically significant way. Background in the second category results from light or other incident radiation, from chemography or from pressure exerted when the tissue was applied to the slide. The procedures outlined above minimize the background in this category.

Usually, the microscopic analysis is concerned with the location and number of labeled cells with respect to defined nuclear groups as seen with standard stains. After the sections have been scanned systematically with a microscope, the exact positions of labeled cells are plotted on an anatomically detailed drawing of the section. This method allows serial sections throughout entire brains to be examined systematically with high, cell-by-cell resolution.

Production of good quality photographs is valuable for illustration of autoradiographic results. The major problem is that the grains are in the emulsion, below the plane of focus of the stained cell. Kodak Color Photomicrography film (#PCF 135-36) and Kodak Panatomic X black-and-white film (FX-135-36) are generally satisfactory for photomicrography of autoradiograms.

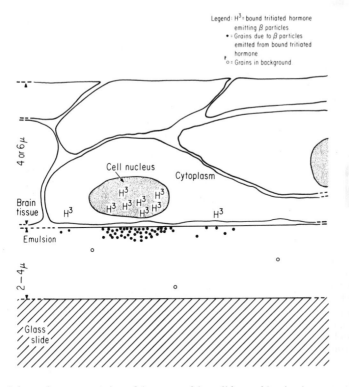

Figure 2. Schematic representation of tissue–emulsion–slide combination in an autoradiogram as viewed from the side. Drawing depicts the cellular localization of the tritiated hormone and the localized effect of the β emission on the emulsion below.

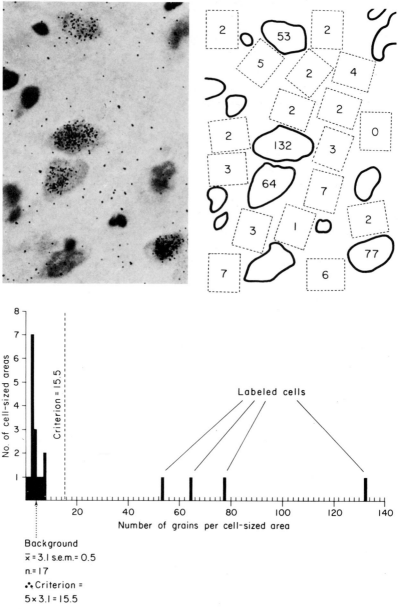

Figure 3. An example of the method used to evaluate steroid hormone autoradiograms. A photomicrograph of estrogen-concentrating cells in monkey brain, a tracing of that photomicrograph, and a histogram of quantitative results from the photomicrograph are shown. Top left: photomicrograph of labeled cells in the ventromedial nucleus of the hypothalamus of a female Rhesus monkey, 2.5 hr following intravenous infusion of [³H]estradiol. Silver grains are concentrated over four lightly stained cell bodies. Top right: tracing of the adjacent micrograph, showing the outlines of all cells (heavy solid black lines) as well as the outlines of 17 cell-sized areas of neuropil counted to determine "background" (light dashed lines). Numbers are the grain counts over labeled cells and cell-sized areas of neuropil. Bottom: histogram showing the distribution of grain counts in the photomicrograph (top left), as recorded in the tracing (top right). Compare the bars showing background grain counts to the dashed line showing criterion for labeled cells (five times mean background) and to the bars showing grain counts for the labeled cells.

IV. EXPERIMENTAL FINDINGS AFTER STEROID AUTORADIOGRAPHY BY THE TECHNIQUE DESCRIBED

A. Concentration of Estradiol and Testosterone by Neurons Is a Common Phenomenon among Vertebrates

With the autoradiographic technique described, the brains of the rat (Pfaff and Keiner, 1973), Rhesus monkey (Gerlach *et al.*, 1975; Pfaff *et al.*, 1974), hamster (Floody and Pfaff, 1974), mink (Morrell and Pfaff, 1975), the frogs, *Xenopus laevis* (Kelley *et al.*, 1975; Morrell *et al.*, 1975b) and *Rana pipines* (Kelley and Pfaff, 1975), the sunfish (Pfaff *et al.*, 1980), and three species of birds, the chaffinch (Zigmond *et al.*, 1973), the zebra finch (Arnold *et al.*, 1975), and the chicken (Barfield *et al.*, 1975) have been explored for sex steroid concentration sites. Such sites have been demonstrated in each of the species studied.

B. Striking Similarities across Species in the Neuroanatomical Distribution of Sex-Hormone-Concentrating Cells

The topographical pattern of major sex steroid concentration sites is very similar from species to species. The neuroanatomical areas that show sex steroid concentration in all species examined are (a) the preoptic area, (b) the tuberal region of the hypothalamus, (c) limbic forebrain structures (e.g., amygdala, lateral septum), and (d) specific portions of the mesencephalon deep to the tectum.

The species that have been examined for sex-steroid-concentrating sites in the brain are members of widely diverse classes within the vertebrate phylum. In the face of this diversity, the basically similar neuroanatomical pattern of sex steroid concentration is especially notable.

A small number of additional sex steroid concentration sites can be termed species specializations. For example, in the anuran amphibian, *Xenopus laevis*, large cells of the posterior lateral medulla, proposed to be the nucleus of cranial nerves IX–X, concentrate testosterone (Kelley *et al.*, 1975; Morrell *et al.*, 1975b). This is also true in the related anuran amphibian *Rana pipiens* (Kelley and Pfaff, 1975a).

C. Estradiol- and Testosterone-Concentrating Neurons Are Found in Brain Regions That Have Been Implicated in the Control of Hormone-Dependent Functions

Information has been gathered in most of the species examined by a variety of experimental techniques that demonstrates a behavioral (see Kelley and Pfaff, 1978) or neuroendocrine function for many of the estradiol and testosterone concentration sites. Sex-steroid-binding sites in the vertebrates examined and some of their functional correlates have been reviewed (see Morrell *et al.*, 1975a). As examples, concentration sites in four of the species that have been examined are discussed below.

Major sites of [³H]estradiol or [³H]testosterone (Pfaff, 1968; Pfaff and Keiner, 1973) concentration in the brain of the rat are in the medial preoptic area, anterior hypothalamic area, arcuate nucleus, ventromedial nucleus of the hypothalamus, and the ventral premammillary nucleus. Further concentrations of labeled cells are found in the lateral septum, bed nucleus of the stria terminalis, in the medial and cortical amygdaloid nuclei, and in the central gray of the mesencephalon. Although the overall topography of estradiol-concentrating cells is very similar to that of the cells labeled by [³H]testosterone injection, the number of labeled cells and the intensity of labeling are less with testosterone. The known behavioral and neuroendocrine functions for the uptake sites have been discussed at length (Pfaff and Keiner, 1973; McEwen and Pfaff, 1973).

The locations of [³H]estradiol-concentrating cells in the brain of the Rhesus monkey have also been examined (Pfaff *et al.*, 1974; Gerlach *et al.*, 1975) (Fig. 3). Labeled cells have been found in the lateral septum, bed nucleus of the stria terminalis, medial preoptic area, and in the anterior nucleus, the ventromedial nucleus (Fig. 3), and the arcuate nucleus of the hypothalamus. The medial amygdala and the subfornical organ also contained labeled cells. Extensive analysis of the anterior pituitary showed 30–50% of the basophils to be labeled, and 5–20% of the acidophils were labeled.

In another study, [³H]estradiol or [³H]testosterone was administered to male and female *Xenopus laevis* (Kelley *et al.*, 1975; Morrell *et al.*, 1975b). Estradiol was concentrated by cells within the telencephalon, specifically ventral lateral septum and amygdala, the ventral striatum, nucleus accumbens, in the anterior preoptic area (APOA), the ventral infundibular nucleus (VIN), the ventral thalamus, and the anterior torus semicircularis. Testosterone was primarily concentrated by cells in the APOA, the VIN, a dorsal tegmental area of the medulla (DTAM), and in large cells of the posterior medulla proposed to be the nucleus of cranial nerves IX–X. The topographical pattern of hormone concentration depended on which hormone was administered and not on the genetic sex of the frog. These autoradiographic findings are the first demonstration of the topography of sex steroid concentration in an amphibian. Several of the areas of sex steroid concentration have been established to be involved in control of mating behavior or the neuroendocrine events of reproduction (see review by Kelley and Pfaff, 1975b).

The green sunfish *(Lepomis cyanellus)* is currently being examined for [³H]testosterone-concentrating sites in the brain (Pfaff *et al.*, 1980). So far the analysis shows androgen-concentrating cells in the preoptic area, the tuberal nucleus of the median lobe (hypothalamic), (Fig. 4), and specific segments of the anterior pituitary. The hormone-concentrating cells in the POA are found

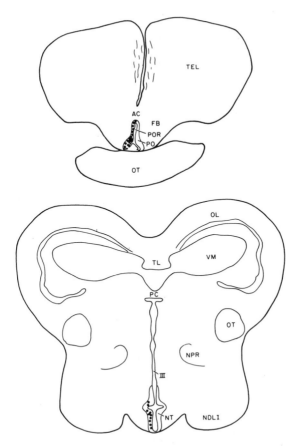

Figure 4. Top: transverse section through the brain (telencephalon) of the green sunfish, *Lepomis cyanellus,* showing labeled cells in the preoptic area following injection of [³H]testosterone. The left side of the figure shows the precise positions of labeled cells in this section, each black dot (●) indicating one labeled cell. The right side of the figure shows anatomical structures indicated with abbreviations. Nomenclature is from Demski *et al.* (1975). Bottom: transverse section through the diencephalon of the sunfish at the level of the anterior portion of nucleus tuberalis, showing testosterone-concentrating cells in nucleus tuberalis. Conventions as for top section of this figure. Abbreviations: AC, anterior commissure; FB forebrain bundles; NDLI, nucleus diffuses lobi inferioris; NPR, nucleus prerotundus; NT, nucleus tuberal; OL; optic lobe; OT, optic tract; PC, posterior commissure; PO, preoptic area; POR, preoptic recess of third ventricle; TEL, telencephalon; TH, thalamus, TL, torus longitudinalis; VM, ventricle of the midbrain; III, third ventricle.

where sperm release has been electrically stimulated in this same species (Demski *et al.,* 1975).

In conclusion, autoradiographic studies have shown the generality across vertebrates of sex-steroid-concentrating neurons: their existence, their precise locations in limbic and hypothalamic structures (Fig. 5), and their likely connection with the control of behavioral and endocrine events in reproduction.

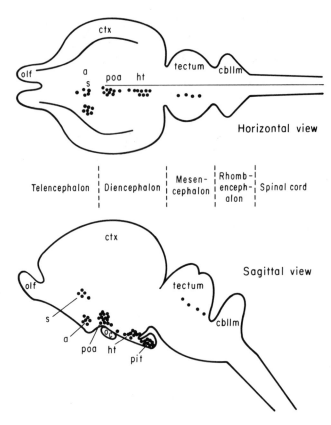

Figure 5. Abstract representation of a "generalized vertebrate brain" showing locations of estradiol- and testosterone-concentrating neurons common to all vertebrates so far studied. The schematic drawings show a horizontal view and a sagittal view. Black dots represent groups of steroid-concentrating cells. Features of the distribution of [³H]estradiol and [³H]testosterone that are common across vertebrates include labeled cells in the limbic telencephalon (e.g., septum, amygdala, or archistriatum), preoptic area, tuberal hypothalamic nuclei, and specific subtectal loci in the mesencephalon. [Nauta and Karten (1970) was used as a reference for generalized view of vertebrate brain.] Abbreviations: a, amygdala or archistriatum; cbllm, cerebellum; ctx, cortex (nonmammalian—general cortex; mammals—neocortex); ht, nuclei in tuberal region of hypothalamus; oc, optic chiasm; olf, olfactory bulb; pit, pituitary; POA, preoptic area; S, septum; tectum, (nonmammalian—optic tectum and inferior colliculus; mammalian—superior colliculus and inferior colliculus). .

REFERENCES

Arnold, A. P., Nottebohm, F, and Pfaff, D. W., 1975, Hormone concentrating cells in vocal control and other areas of the brain of the zebra finch, *(Poephila guttata), J. Comp. Neurol.* **165**:487–512.
Barfield, R., Ronay, G., and Pfaff, D. W., 1975, Autoradiographic localization of androgen-concentrating cells in the brain of the chicken, *Neuroendocrinology* **26**:297–311.

Demski, L. S., Bauer, D. H., and Gerald, J. W., 1975, Sperm release evoked by electrical stimulation of the fish brain: A functional–anatomical study, *J. Exp. Zool.* **191**:215.

Floody, O. R., and Pfaff, D. W., 1974, Steroid hormones and aggressive behavior: Approaches to the study of hormone-sensitive brain mechanisms for behavior, in: *Aggressive Behavior*, Vol. 52. *Research Publications, Association for Research in Nervous and Mental Disease* (S. Frazier, ed.), pp. 149–185, Waverly Press, Boston.

Gerlach, J. L., and McEwen, B. S., 1972, Rat brain binds adrenal steroid hormones: Radioautography of hippocampus with corticosterone, *Science* **175**:1133.

Gerlach, J. L., McEwen, B. S., Pfaff, D. W., Moskovitz, S., Ferin, M., Carmel, P. W., and Zimmerman, E. A., 1975, Cells in regions of Rhesus monkey and pituitary retain radioactive estradiol, corticosterone and cortisol differentially, *Brain Res.* **103**:603–612.

Kelley, D. B., and Pfaff, D. W., 1975, Locations of steroid hormone-concentrating cells in the central nervous system of *Rana pipiens*, in: *Society for Neuroscience Fifth Annual Meeting*, p. 438, New York.

Kelley, D. B., and Pfaff, D. W., 1978, Generalizations from comparative studies on neuroanatomical and endocrine mechanisms for sex behavior, in: *Biological Determinants of Sexual Behavior* (J. B. Hutchison, ed.), pp. 225–254, John Wiley and Sons, Chichester.

Kelley, D. B., Morrell, J. I., and Pfaff, D. W., 1975, Autoradiographic localization of hormone-concentrating cells in the brain of an amphibian, *Xenopus laevis*. I. Testosterone, *J. Comp. Neurol.* **164**:47–62.

Leblond, C. P., Kopriwa, B., and Messier, B., 1963, Radioautography as a histochemical tool, in: *Histochemistry and Cytochemistry, Proceedings of the First International Congress* (R. Wegmann, ed.), pp. 1–31, MacMillan, New York.

McEwen, B. S., and Pfaff, D. W., 1973, Chemical and physiological approaches to neuroendocrine mechanisms: Attempts at integration, in: *Frontiers in Neuroendocrinology* (W. F. Ganong and L. Martini, eds.), pp. 267–335, Oxford University Press, London.

Morrell, J. I., and Pfaff, D. W., 1975, Autoradiographic localization of ^{3}H-estradiol uptake in the brain of the female mink *Mustela vison*, *Anat. Rec.* **181**:430.

Morrell, J. I., Kelley, D. B., and Pfaff, D. W., 1975a, Sex steroid binding in the brains of vertebrates: Studies with light microscopic autoradiography, in: *Brain-Endocrine Interaction II. The Ventricular System, Proceedings of the Second International Symposium, Shizuaka* (K. M. Knigge, D. E. Scott, H. Kobayashi, and S. Ishii, eds.), pp. 230–256, Basel, Karger.

Morrell, J. I., Kelley, D. B., and Pfaff, D. W., 1975b, Autoradiographic localization of hormone-concentrating cells in the brain of an amphibian, *Xenopus laevis*. II. Estradiol. *J. Comp. Neurol.* **164**:63–78.

Nauta, W. J. H., and Karten, H. J., 1970, A general profile of the vertebrate brain, with sidelights on the ancestry of cerebral cortex, in: *The Neurosciences, Second Study Program* (F. O. Schmitt, ed.), pp. 7–26, The Rockefeller University Press, New York.

Pelc, S. R., Appleton, T. C., and Welton, M. E., 1965, State of light autoradiography, in: *The Use of Radioautography in Investigating Protein Synthesis, Symposia of the International Society for Cell Biology*, Vol. 4 (C. P. Leblond, ed.), pp. 9–22, Academic Press, New York and London.

Pfaff, D. W., 1968, Autoradiographic localization of radioactivity in rat brain after injection of tritiated sex hormones, *Science* **161**:1355.

Pfaff, D. W., and Keiner, M., 1973, Atlas of estradiol-concentrating cells in the central nervous system of the female rat, *J. Comp. Neurol.* **151**:121.

Pfaff, D. W., Moskovitz, S., Gerlach, J., McEwen, B., Carmel, P., Ferin, M., and Zimmerman, E., 1974, Autoradiographic localization of cells which bind estradiol or corticosterone in the brain and pituitary of the female rhesus monkey, in: *Proceedings of the 26th International Congress of Physiological Sciences, New Delhi*, abstract #843:281, Thompson Press, New Delhi.

Rogers, A. W., 1973, *Techniques of Autoradiography*, Elsevier, Amsterdam.

Zigmond, R. E., Nottebohm, F., and Pfaff, D. W., 1973, Androgen-concentrating cells in the midbrain of a songbird, *Science* **179**:1005.

17

Electrophysiological Effects of Steroid Hormones in Brain Tissue

DONALD W. PFAFF

I. INTRODUCTION

The two previous chapters in this book have given autoradiographic and biochemical evidence of hormone concentration by cells in specific portions of the brain. The notion of a "hormone receptor," in its usual sense, includes not only the idea of a specific, saturable, energy-dependent accumulation process, but also the idea that this hormone accumulation mediates effects of the hormone on the tissue in question. To demonstrate and characterize steroid hormone receptors in brain, therefore, it is necessary to describe physiological effects of the hormones in brain tissue. Neurophysiological data are summarized in this chapter. Where possible, they are compared with each other and with relevant behavioral phenomena.

Experiments on single-unit activity (as opposed to multiunit activity or wave recordings) are emphasized here because much work has shown that neurons near each other may have different physiological properties. If the separate responses of such heterogeneous cells were mixed together with unselective recording methods, their individual properties would be obscured. For some purposes, this would be unfortunate. Therefore, in this and many other laboratories, the electrical activity of an individual neuron is carefully isolated with extracellular recording procedures, using microelectrodes (micropipettes or finely etched metal electrodes) and high quality micromanipulators to allow small, well-controlled electrode movements. Most

DONALD W. PFAFF • Department of Psychology, The Rockefeller University, New York, New York 10021.

experiments have been done using animals anesthetized with urethane. Some work suggests that this anesthetic interferes only minimally with hypothalamic electrophysiology. It is possible to record hormone effects in unanesthetized, freely moving animals (for instance, Pfaff *et al.,* 1971), but in such animals prepared for chronic recording, the collection of data is very slow, and many discriminating (and technically difficult) electrophysiological experiments can not be done. It appears that chronic recording will be the ideal technique when a system is fairly well understood physiologically from experiments with anesthetized animals, and the hypotheses of relations to behavioral responses remain to be tested.

Two fairly new electrophysiological approaches have not yet been used much in studies of steroid hormone effects but will surely play a large role in the near future. One is the microelectrophoresis of substances onto nerve cells: driving dissolved ionized material from the micropipette into the cell's environment by application of an electrical potential. The second is the identification of a site of axonal projection of the cell recorded by electrically stimulating the axon and causing an antidromic action potential to be recorded ("backfiring" the neuron). Increasing technical sophistication in electrophysiological studies of the hypothalamus have given, and hopefully will continue to give, more detailed information about hormone-sensitive nerve cells.

II. ESTRADIOL

In recent years, a considerable amount of work has shown that the firing rates of nerve cells in the preoptic area and hypothalamus, as well as in limbic forebrain structures, vary during the estrous cycle of the rat. Thus, Kawakami *et al.* (1970) have reported an elevation in firing rates on the afternoon on the day of proestrus, during the "critical period" for the determination of ovulation. Similarly, Terasawa and Sawyer (1969) recorded elevations in the rate of multiunit activity in the arcuate nucleus of the hypothalamus that were correlated with the occurrence of ovulation. Dyer *et al.* (1972) recorded single unit activity in the brains of female rats on different days of their estrous cycle. Firing rates were higher on the day of proestrus for neurons in the ventral portion of a hypothalamic region, which, according to the convention in this chapter, is designated the medial anterior hypothalamus. The conclusions of that experiment were similar to those reported by Moss and Law (1971). The fact that circulating hormones were acting in these experiments directly on hypothalamic tissue was indicated by similar experiments in which an island of hypothalamic tissue was prepared surgically (Cross and Dyer, 1971). Because similar variations of anterior hypothalamic neuronal activity were seen throughout the estrous cycle in the "hypothalamic islands" as in the intact preparation (higher firing rates during proestrus), it was concluded that indirect influences from other brain regions did not play an important role.

Further, following attempts to antidromically identify hypothalamic neurons by stimulation in the ventromedial–arcuate region, it was suggested that those neurons in the ventral medial anterior hypothalamus that increase firing rates during proestrus are not the neurons that project to the arcuate nucleus region (Dyer, 1973).

Fluctuations in neuronal activity during the estrous cycle presumably are correlated with one or more of the hormones whose blood levels also vary during the cycle. However, a simpler situation for analyzing effects of estradiol is to use ovariectomized animals with or without systemic estrogen injections. Studies reviewed below used this strategy, and the review focuses almost exclusively on studies with rats to avoid possible complications resulting from species differences. Wherever possible, single-unit recording studies using microelectrodes are treated, because it is known that adjacent hypothalamic neurons can have different functional properties (Pfaff and Gregory, 1971b).

Several single-unit recording studies have shown that firing rates of neurons in the medial anterior hypothalamus, ventromedial nucleus, or arcuate nucleus are, on the average, increased by estrogen. Recording in ovariectomized female rats, Kawakami et al. (1971) showed increases caused by estrogen in the firing rates of arcuate neurons. In the medial anterior hypothalamus, Cross and Dyer (1972) showed increases in resting discharge rates following estradiol injection in ovariectomized rats. In spayed female cats, multiunit activity in the ventromedial nucleus and the medial anterior hypothalamus tends to be more responsive to peripheral stimuli following estrogen treatment, and there is a definite shift in response direction toward excitation (Alcaraz et al., 1969). For neurons in the ventromedial nucleus and the medial anterior hypothalamus of ovariectomized female rats, Bueno and Pfaff (1975) have compared single-unit activity in long-term estrogen-treated rats with that in untreated control preparations. In estrogen-treated females, there was a significantly greater number of ventromedial hypothalamic units with recordable spontaneous activity (Fig. 1). Among units recorded in anterior and ventromedial hypothalamus, those in estrogen-treated preparations tended to be more responsive (with excitatory responses) to peripheral somatosensory stimuli (Fig. 2). Yagi (1973) found neurons in the medial anterior hypothalamus whose activity was briefly raised after systemic estradiol injection, whereas he found no units whose activity was simply inhibited by estradiol.

These results appear to show that the predominant electrophysiological effect of estradiol in the arcuate and ventromedial hypothalamic nuclei and in the medial anterior hypothalamus is one of excitation. This would agree nicely with the increased activities of glycolytic enzymes found in the basomedial and anterior hypothalamus following estradiol treatment of ovariectomized female rats (Luine et al., 1974, 1975b).

Interestingly, recent results have shown that the predominant effect of estradiol in preoptic tissue of ovariectomized female rats might be different from that in the basomedial and anterior hypothalamus. Lincoln (1967)

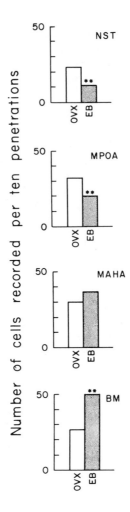

Figure 1. Comparison of single unit recordings from estradiol-treated (EB) and untreated (OVX) ovariectomized female rats. Numbers of neurons with recordable spontaneous activity are plotted, normalized according to the number of electrode penetrations through each anatomical structure. Estradiol depressed resting discharge rates in the medial preoptic area and nucleus of the stria terminalis, while it elevated resting discharge in the basomedial hypothalamus. Abbreviations: NST, bed nucleus of stria terminalis; MPOA, medial preoptic area; MAHA, medial anterior hypothalamus; BM, basomedial hypothalamus (combination of arcuate, ventromedial, and dorsomedial nucleus recording sites). Definitions according to the Lönig and Klippel atlas. Differences between estrogen-treated and untreated ovariectomized female rats: $**p < 0.01$. (Reprinted with permission from Bueno and Pfaff, 1975.)

showed that estradiol treatment of ovariectomized rats is followed by lower spontaneous activity of units in the preoptic region, in the most anterior portion of the medial anterior hypothalamus, and in the lateral septum. Probing of the vaginal cervix produced inhibition of preoptic neurons in estrogen-treated animals (Lincoln and Cross, 1967). In similar experiments recording

Stimuli:

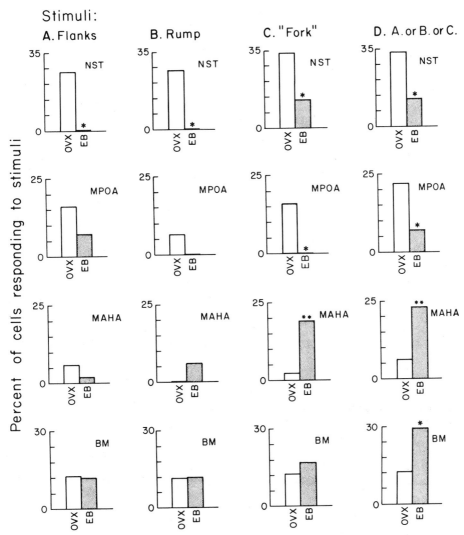

Figure 2. Percent of neurons responding to somatosensory stimuli plotted for each neuroanatomical structure (definitions and abbreviations as in Fig. 1). "Fork" stimuli (C) were brief applications of pressure on the skin of the perineum, tail base, and posterior rump; in the unanesthetized, hormone-primed female rat, these stimuli would elicit lordosis. Part D shows percentages of neurons that would respond to at least one of the somatosensory stimuli A, B, or C. Differences between responsiveness of neurons in estradiol-treated (EB) and untreated (OVX) female rat recording samples: *p <0.05; **p <0.01. (Reprinted with permission from Bueno and Pfaff, 1975.)

estrogen-dependent increases in arcuate activity in ovariectomized rats, Kawakami *et al.*, (1971; Table 8.1) saw no changes or mixed changes in preoptic neuron discharge following estrogen treatment. Following long-term estrogen treatment of ovariectomized rats, Bueno and Pfaff (1975) were able to find fewer preoptic units with recordable spontaneous activity (Fig. 1), and those found were less responsive to peripheral somatosensory stimuli than units in control, untreated preparations (Fig. 2). Yagi (1970, 1973) looked for changes in single-unit activity in the preoptic area at short latencies after systemic estradiol injections. Some of the units showed complicated, biphasic responses to estrogen. However, it was notable that many preoptic units decreased their activity to very low levels shortly after estradiol injection, and in some cases activity remained low throughout the duration of recording. Even some of the preoptic units that showed an increase following estrogen subsequently dropped to very low levels of firing for a long time.

From this pattern of estradiol-dependent neurophysiological changes found by Yagi, it appears that the overall effect of estrogen in the preoptic area would be a net decrease in spontaneous firing rates. In a similar study on ovariectomized female rats, Whitehead and Ruf (1974) also found units in the periods following intravenous administration of estrogens. In biochemical studies (Luine *et al.*, 1974), also, it was noted that estradiol-induced increases in glycolytic enzyme activity in the basomedial hypothalamus were not seen in tissue samples including the medial preoptic area and nucleus of the stria terminalis.

From the studies just reviewed and others using electrophysiological (Kawakami and Kubo, 1971) and neurochemical (Luine *et al.*, 1975a) methods, it is evident that the overall effect of systemically injected estradiol on preoptic neurons is different from that on neurons in the anterior hypothalamus, ventromedial nucleus, and arcuate nucleus. Single-unit activity seems to be lowered in the preoptic region following systemic estrogen treatment but raised in the anterior hypothalamus and ventromedial and arcuate nuclei (Table 1). Some corresponding enzymatic changes are also seen.

It should be noted that the preponderant effects of systemic estrogen treatment in the preparations studied may actually be a combination of direct effects on the very neurons recorded and indirect effects initiated elsewhere in the nervous system and transmitted synaptically to the neurons recorded. The only way to dissociate these two types of effects would be to restrict estrogen application to the neuron recorded. Attempts to do this have not been successful because the lack of ionization of estradiol makes it difficult to drive iontophoretically, and in any case it might be difficult to record from the cell long enough for the hormone effect to be registered when applied that way.

Another difficulty encountered in these recording experiments has to do with the heterogeneity of nerve cells that are near each other. Even within a small histological region, spontaneous firing rates of different neurons near each other may vary widely (Kawakami and Kubo, 1971; Yagi and Sawaki, 1973; Bueno and Pfaff, 1975). It seems likely that adjacent neurons within the hypothalamus or preoptic area might have different physiological properties and play different roles in hypothalamic circuits. In future studies, such neurons will have to be identified as belonging to different groups.

The difference between estrogen effects on preoptic neurons and anterior–ventromedial–arcuate hypothalamic neurons appears to correspond nicely to differences in the roles these two tissue regions play in the control of

Table 1. Comparison of Estradiol Effects in Brain[a] and Tissue Effects on Lordosis in Ovariectomized Female Rats[b]

	Estradiol effect on single unit firing	Estradiol effect on glycolytic enzymes	Effect of lesion on lordosis behavior	Effect of electrical stimulation on lordosis behavior
Preoptic region	↓	0	↑	↓
Anterior and basomedial hypothalamus	↑	↑	↓	

[a] Estradiol administered systemically. Effects may be combinations of direct action on preoptic or hypothalamic neurons and indirect actions.
[b] ↑, Increase; ↓, decrease; 0, no change.

female reproductive behavior in rats. Lesions in the medial preoptic region in hormone-treated ovariectomized female rats actually can enhance lordosis behavior (Law and Meagher, 1958; Powers and Valenstein, 1972). Electrical stimulation in the medial preoptic region disrupts the performance of lordosis in hormone-treated ovariectomized female rats (Moss *et al.*, 1974) and hamsters (Malsbury and Pfaff, 1973, 1975). In contrast, lesions in the medial anterior hypothalamus (Brookhart *et al.*, 1941; Singer, 1968; Law and Meagher, 1958) or ventromedial nucleus of the hypothalamus (Dorner *et al.*, 1969; Kennedy and Mitra, 1963; Kow *et al.*, 1974a) have the opposite effect from preoptic lesions—they reduce the performance of lordosis in female rats and other rodents. It seems, therefore, that estrogen acting on anterior hypothalamic or ventromedial hypothalamic neurons would promote lordosis by increasing neural activity of cells that have a facilitatory effect on lordosis (Table 1). Estrogen acting on preoptic neurons would be promoting lordosis by inhibiting activity in tissue that has an inhibitory effect on lordosis.

III. TESTOSTERONE

Less information has been gathered on the effects of androgenic hormones in brain tissue, compared to the great amount of work on ovarian hormones. Following systemic injection of [³H]testosterone, there does appear to be accumulation of radioactive hormone by cells in preoptic tissue and some other brain regions as measured by autoradiographic (Pfaff, 1968; Sar and Stumpf, 1973) and biochemical (McEwen *et al.*, 1970a,b) techniques (see Chapter 15). Testosterone can have striking effects on single unit activity in the preoptic region of castrated male rats, whether administered locally in the preoptic area or systemically (Pfaff and Pfaffmann, 1969). It is especially interesting, therefore, that at least for choline acetyltransferase, testosterone administration can cause a significant increase in enzymatic activity in the medial preoptic area even under conditions where there is no effect in the basomedial hypothalamus (Luine *et al.*, 1975a).

Neurophysiological effects of testosterone in the preoptic area fit well with much existing data on the control of male reproductive behavior in rats. Lesions of preoptic tissue cause striking deficits in male copulatory behavior (Heimer and Larsson, 1966; Lisk, 1968). Electrical stimulation of the medial preoptic area facilitates copulation in male rats (Malsbury, 1971). Implantation of testosterone in the medial preoptic area can facilitate male sex behavior in castrated male rats (Davidson, 1966; Lisk, 1967). In fact, integrity of medial preoptic tissue seems to be a requirement for the normal performance of male courtship or copulatory behavior in a wide variety of vertebrate species (see Kelley and Pfaff, 1975, for review). From the pattern of single-unit electrophysiological effects of testosterone (Pfaff and Gregory, 1971a,b), it has been argued that testosterone does not affect sensory coding of input to the preoptic area but rather alters some aspect of the animal's "motivated response" to that input (Pfaff et al., 1972).

Thus, the data that exist seem to relate neurons in the preoptic region to testosterone effects and the activation of male sex behavior. This may be contrasted with the previous section, in which it was suggested that hypothalamic tissue posterior to the preoptic area is required for the normal performance of female mating behavior and is activated by estrogens.

IV. CORTICOSTERONE

Work with cell-fractionation (McEwen et al., 1970c) and autoradiographic (Gerlach and McEwen, 1972) techniques has given ample demonstration of selective corticosterone accumulation by nerve cells in the hippocampus (see Chapter 15). With single unit recording methods, it is possible to see effects of systemically injected corticosterone on firing rates of hippocampal pyramidal neurons (Pfaff et al., 1971). The long time course of this electrophysiological effect is consistent with the notion that it is mediated by intracellular biosynthetic events. The various behavioral mechanisms in which the hippocampus might participate have not been spelled out very clearly. At present, therefore, it is more difficult to guess the possible behavioral correlates of corticosterone effects in hippocampus than it has been for estradiol and testosterone in the hypothalamus and preoptic area.

V. PROGESTERONE

To date, there is no convincing evidence that progesterone receptors exist in the brain—that is, binding similar in strength and specificity to that of estradiol has not been demonstrated. Nevertheless, behavioral effects of progesterone implantation in brain have been reported. Indeed, several authors have reported effects of systemic progesterone injections on the electrical activity of single units in the hypothalamus (Barraclough and Cross, 1963; Ramirez *et al.*, 1967; Komisaruk *et al.*, 1967; Beyer *et al.*, 1967; Lincoln, 1969). Matters not completely resolved include the question of the extent to which progesterone affects cells outside the hypothalamus and the question of how specific the effects of progesterone are on individual hypothalamic neurons (i.e., are all responses of the neuron affected or just responses related to reproductive processes?). Since the effect of progesterone on lordosis behavior of female rats can be mimicked by drugs that interfere with serotonergic function, it has been suggested (Kow *et al.*, 1974b) that progesterone inhibits the activity of neurons in serotonergic pathways, which themselves inhibit the performance of lordosis.

VI. OUTLOOK

It is hoped that neurophysiological studies of steroid hormone effects will show precisely how hormones affect neuroendocrine function and behavioral responses. However, there are many steps between the demonstration of a hormone-sensitive hypothalamic cell and the attainment of that goal. For instance, we must know where the axons of hormone-sensitive cells project in order to see where the outputs that are governed by hormones could impinge on behavior control circuits. With reference to the control of lordosis behavior in female rats, the axonal projections of anterior hypothalamic neurons have just recently been determined (Conrad and Pfaff, 1975). Many other questions remain about the anatomical pattern of outputs of specific portions of the hypothalamus. Finally, the location and physiology of brainstem and spinal cord circuits that govern well-defined behavioral responses must be studied in detail to understand how fluctuating hypothalamic outputs could affect their operation in a physiologically significant and adaptive way (for instance, for studies on the lordosis reflex, see Pfaff *et al.*, 1972, 1973). With this information in hand, it may be possible to see (and, importantly, to rule out hypotheses about) how individual neurons mediate the influences of steroid hormones on specific behavioral responses.

REFERENCES

Alcaraz, M., Guzman-Flores, C., Salas, M., and Beyer, C., 1969, Effect of estrogen on the responsivity of hypothalamic and mesencephalic neurons in the female cat, *Brain Res.* **15**:439.

Barraclough, C., and Cross, B., 1963, Unit activity in the hypothalamus of the cyclic female rat: Effect of genital stimuli and progesterone, *J. Endocrinol.* **26**:339.

Beyer, C., Ramirez, V. D., Whitmoyer, D. E., and Sawyer, C. H., 1967, Effects of hormones on the electrical activity of the brain in the rat and rabbit, *Exp. Neurol.* **18**:313.

Brookhart, J. M., Dey, F. L., and Ranson, S. W., 1941, The abolition of mating behavior by hypothalamic lesions in guinea pigs, *Endocrinology* **28**:561.

Bueno, J., and Pfaff, D. W., 1976, Single unit recording in hypothalamus and preoptic area of estrogen-treated and untreated ovariectomized female rats, *Brain Res.* **101**:67.

Conrad, L. C. A., and Pfaff, D. W., 1975, Axonal projections of anterior hypothalamic neurons, *J. Comp. Neurol.*

Cross, B. A., and Dyer, R. G., 1971, Cyclic changes in neurons of the anterior hypothalamus during the rat estrous cycle and the effect of anesthesia, in: *Steroid Hormones and Brain Function, UCLA Forum in Medical Sciences,* Number 15 (C. H. Sawyer and R. A. Gorski, eds.), pp. 95–102, University of California Press, Los Angeles.

Cross, B. A., and Dyer, R. G., 1972, Ovarian modulation of unit activity in the anterior hypothalamus of the cyclic rat, *J. Physiol. (Lond.)* **222**:25P.

Davidson, J. M., 1966, Activation of the male rat's sexual behavior by intracerebral implantation of androgen, *Endocrinology* **79**:783.

Dorner, G., Docke, F., and Hinz, G., 1969, Homo- and hypersexuality in rats with hypothalamic lesions, *Neuroendocrinology* **4**:20.

Dyer, R. G., 1973, An electrophysiological dissection of the hypothalamic regions which regulate the pre-ovulatory secretion of luteinizing hormone in the rat, *J. Physiol. (Lond.)* **234**:421.

Dyer, R. G., Pritchett, C. J., and Cross, B. A., 1972, Unit activity in the diencephalon of female rats during the oestrous cycle, *J. Endocrinol.* **53**:151.

Gerlach, J. L., and McEwen, B. S., 1972, Rat brain binds adrenal steroid hormone: Radioautography of hippocampus with corticosterone, *Science* **175**:1133.

Heimer, L., and Larsson, K., 1966, Impairment of mating behavior in male rats following lesions in the preoptic–anterior hypothalamic continuum, *Brain Res.* **3**:248.

Kawakami, M., and Kubo, K., 1971, Neuro-correlate of limbic–hypothalamo–pituitary–gonadal axis in the rat: Change in limbic–hypothalamic unit activity induced by vaginal and electrical stimulation, *Neuroendocrinology* **7**:65.

Kawakami, M., Terasawa, E., and Ibuki, T., 1970, Changes in multiple unit activity of the brain during the estrous cycle, *Neuroendocrinology* **6**:30.

Kawakami, M., Terasawa, E., Ibuki, T., and Manaka, M., 1971, Effects of sex hormones and ovulation-blocking steroids and drugs on electrical activity of the rat brain, in: *Steroid Hormones and Brain Function, UCLA Forum in Medical Sciences,* Number 15 (C.H. Sawyer and R. A. Gorski, eds.), pp. 79–93, University of California Press, Los Angeles.

Kelley, D. B., and Pfaff, D. W., 1978, Generalizations from comparative studies on neuro anatomical and endocrine mechanisms of reproductive behavior, in: *Biological Determinants of Sexual Behavior* (J. Hutchison, ed.), pp. 225–254, Wiley, New York.

Kennedy, G. C., and Mitra, J., 1963, Hypothalamic control of energy balance and the reproductive cycle in the rat, *J. Physiol. (Lond.)* **166**:395.

Komisaruk, B. R., McDonald, P. G., Whitmoyer, D. I., and Sawyer, C. H., 1967, Effects of progesterone and sensory stimulation on EEG and neuronal activity in the rat, *Exp. Neurol.* **19**:494.

Kow, L.-M., Malsbury, C. W., and Pfaff, D. W., 1974a, Effects of medial hypothalamic lesions on the lordosis response in female hamsters, *Proc. Soc. Neurosci.* 291 (abstract #365).

Kow, L.-M., Malsbury, C., and Pfaff, D. W., 1974b, Effects of progesterone on female reproductive behavior in rats: Possible modes of action and role in behavioral sex differences, in: *Reproductive Behavior* (W. Montagna and W. Sadler, eds.), pp. 179–210, Plenum Press, New York.

Law, T., and Meagher, W., 1958, Hypothalamic lesions and sexual behavior in the female rat, *Science* **128**:1626.

Lincoln, D. W., 1967, Unit activity in the hypothalamus, septum and preoptic area of the rat: Characteristics of spontaneous activity and the effect of oestrogen, *J. Endocrinol.* **37**:177.

Lincoln, D. W., 1969, Effects of progesterone on the electrical activity of the forebrain, *J. Endocrinol.* **45**:585.

Lincoln, D. W., and Cross, B. A., 1967, Effect of oestrogen on the responsiveness of neurones in the hypothalamus, septum and preoptic area of rats with light-induced persistent oestrus, *J. Endocrinol.* **37**:191.

Lisk, R. D., 1967, Neural localization for androgen activation of copulatory behavior in the male rat, *Endocrinology* **80**:754.

Lisk, R. D., 1968, Copulatory activity of the male rat following placement of preoptic–anterior hypothalamic lesions, *Exp. Brain Res.* **5**:306.

Luine, V. N., Khylchevskaya, R. I., and McEwen, B. S., 1974, Oestrogen effects on brain and pituitary enzyme activities, *J. Neurochem.* **23**:925.

Luine, V. N., Khylchevskaya, R. I., and McEwen, B. S., 1975a, Effect of gonadal steroids on activities of monoamine oxidase and choline acetylase in rat brain, *Brain Res.* **86**:293.

Luine, V. N., Khylchevskaya, R. I., and McEwen, B. S., 1975b, Effect of gonadal hormones on enzyme activities in brain and pituitary of male and female rats, *Brain Res.* **86**:283.

Malsbury, C. W., 1971, Facilitation of male rat copulatory behavior by electrical stimulation of the medial preoptic area, *Physiol. Behav.* **7**:797.

Malsbury, C., and Pfaff, D. W., 1973, Suppression of sexual receptivity in the hormone-primed female hamster by electrical stimulation of the medial preoptic area, *Proc. Soc. Neurosci.* 122 (abstract).

Malsbury, C. W., Pfaff, D. W., and Malsbury, A. M., 1980, Suppression of sexual receptivity in the female hamster: Neuroanatomical projections from preoptic and anterior hypothalamic electrode sites, *Brain Res.* **181**:267.

McEwen, B., Pfaff, D. W., and Zigmond, R. E., 1970a, Factors influencing sex hormone uptake by rat brain regions: II. Effects of neonatal treatment and hypophysectomy on testosterone uptake, *Brain Res.* **21**:17.

McEwen, B. S., Pfaff, D. W., and Zigmond, R. E., 1970b, Factors influencing sex hormone uptake by rat brain regions: III. Effects of competing steroids on testosterone uptake, *Brain Res.* **21**:29.

McEwen, B. S., Weiss, J. M., and Schwartz, L. S., 1970c, Retention of corticosterone by cell nuclei from brain regions of adrenalectomized rats, *Brain Res.* **17**:471.

Moss, R. L., and Law, O. T., 1971, The estrous cycle: Its influence on single unit activity in the forebrain, *Brain Res.* **30**:435.

Moss, R. L., Paloutzian, R. F., and Law, O. T., 1974, Electro-chemical stimulation of forebrain structures and its effect on copulatory as well as stimulus-bound behavior in ovariectomized hormone-primed rats, *Physiol. Behav.* **12**:997.

Pfaff, D. W., 1968, Autoradiographic localization of radioactivity in rat brain after injection of tritiated sex hormones, *Science* **161**:1355.

Pfaff, D. W., and Gregory, E., 1971a, Olfactory coding in olfactory bulb and medial forebrain bundle of normal and castrated male rats, *J. Neurophysiol.* **34**:208.

Pfaff, D. W., and Gregory, E., 1971b, Correlation between preoptic area unit activity and the cortical EEG: Difference between normal and castrated male rats, *Electroencephalogr. Clin. Neurophysiol.* **31**:223.

Pfaff, D. W., and Pfaffmann, C., 1969, Olfactory and hormonal influences on the basal forebrain of the male rat, *Brain Res.* **15**:137.

Pfaff, D. W., Silva, M. T. A., and Weiss, J. M., 1971, Telemetered recording of hormone effects on hippocampal neurons, *Science* **172**:394.

Pfaff, D. W., Lewis, C., Diakow, C., and Keiner, M., 1972, Neurophysiological analysis of mating behavior responses as hormone-sensitive reflexes, in: *Progress in Physiological Psychology*, Vol. 5 (E. Stellar and J. M. Sprague, eds.), pp. 253–297, Academic Press, New York.

Pfaff, D. W., Diakow, C., Zigmond, R. E., and Kow, L.-M., 1973, Neural and hormonal determinants of female mating behavior in rats, in: *The Neurosciences*, Vol. III (F. O. Schmitt and F. G. Worden, eds.), pp. 621–646, M. I. T. Press, Cambridge, Massachusetts.

Powers, B., and Valenstein, E. S., 1972, Sexual receptivity: Facilitation by medial preoptic lesions in female rats, *Science* **175**:1003.

Ramirez, V. D., Komisaruk, B. R., Whitmoyer, D. I., and Sawyer, C. H., 1967, Effects of hormones and vaginal stimulation on the EEG and hypothalamic units in rats, *Am. J. Physiol.* **212**:1376.

Sar, M., and Stumpf, W. E., 1973, Autoradiographic localization of radioactivity in the rat brain after the injection of 1,2-³H-testosterone, *Endocrinology* **92**:251.

Singer, J. J., 1968, Hypothalamic control of male and female sexual behavior in female rats, *J. Comp. Physiol. Psychol.* **66**:738.

Terasawa, E., and Sawyer, C. H., 1969, Changes in electrical activity in the rat hypothalamus related to electrochemical stimulation of adenohypophyseal function, *Endocrinology* **85**:143.

Whitehead, S. A., and Ruf, K. B., 1974, Responses of antidromically identified preoptic neurons in the rat to neurotransmitters and to estrogen, *Brain Res.* **79**:185.

Yagi, K., 1970, Effects of estrogen on the unit activity of the rat hypothalamus, *J. Physiol. Soc. Jpn.* **32**:692.

Yagi, K., 1973, Changes in firing rates of single preoptic and hypothalamic units following an intravenous administration of estrogen in the castrated female rat, *Brain Res.* **53**:343.

Yagi, K., and Sawaki, Y., 1973, Feedback of estrogen in the hypothalamic control of gonadotrophin secretion, in: *Neuroendocrine Control* (K. Yagi and S. Yoshida, eds.), pp. 297–325, University of Toyko Press, Tokyo.

Appendix

A Gross Anatomical Study of the Peripheral Nerves Associated with Reproductive Function in the Female Albino Rat

PETER REINER, JOHN WOOLSEY, NORMAN ADLER, and ADRIAN MORRISON

I. INTRODUCTION

Although there are a number of excellent anatomical studies of central neuro-endocrine mechanisms, there is no single comprehensive dissection guide to the peripheral neural apparatus. The purpose of this appendix is to provide a clear description of the peripheral neuroanatomy associated with reproductive function in the female rat.

This guide deals with six major peripheral nerves: femoral, genitofemoral, pelvic, hypogastric, pudendal, and caudal cutaneous femoral. The anatomy of these nerves has been described in various species, including the albino rat, following Langley and Anderson's classic paper of 1896 (see Bradley and Teague, 1972; Carlson and DeFeo, 1965; Greene, 1968; Hebel and Stromberg, 1976; Kollar, 1952; Langworthy, 1965; Purinton *et al.*, 1973). However, gaps in these anatomical descriptions still exist. For example, some studies are primarily devoted to electrophysiology, and the accompanying anatomical descriptions were limited to the service of specific physiological experiments. Furthermore, the anatomical studies cited often are large and do not provide great detail on the peripheral genital apparatus per se. Finally, there is no single

PETER REINER and ADRIAN MORRISON • School of Veterinary Medicine, University of Pennsylvania, Philadelphia, Pennsylvania 19104. JOHN WOOLSEY • Leidy Laboratories, University of Pennsylvania, Philadelphia, Pennsylvania 19104   NORMAN ADLER • Department of Psychology, University of Pennsylvania, Philadelphia, Pennsylvania 19104.

source that pulls all of the information together in one place with accompanying diagrams for use by investigators in reproductive anatomy and physiology.

In order to facilitate understanding of the various nerves, muscles, organs, etc. discussed below, we have used the nomenclature with which most readers are familiar, that used by Greene (1968). In order to insure accuracy, we have followed Greene's terminology with the nomenclature used in *Nomina Anatomica Veterinaria* (World Association of Veterinary Anatomists, 1973), placed in parentheses, as well as using the *NAV* nomenclature in all figures. Figure 1 gives the major anatomical landmarks used for orientation and provides a useful reference throughout. Although anterior and posterior are used to facilitate comparison with the standard work by Greene, the accepted terminology for quadrupeds is cranial and caudal (World Association of Veterinary Anatomists, 1973). Anterior and posterior are now reserved for upright, bipedal animals.

II. METHODS

One hundred female rats were dissected in order to ascertain the anatomical relationships of the nerves innervating urogenital structures as well as other areas associated with reproductive function. The animals were sacrificed by overdose of anesthetic. All dissections were performed on fresh specimens in order to enhance the contrast between nervous and connective tissue. Nerves were followed from their origin at the spinal cord to the organs and muscles that they innervated with the aid of a Zeiss stereoscopic dissecting microscope. All animals were approached from the ventral aspect, and the descriptions are based upon that approach.

III. RESULTS

A. Femoral Nerve

The femoral nerve (N. femoralis) is formed by contributions from the third and fourth lumbar nerves (Greene, 1968). It travels caudolaterally, dorsal to the psoas muscle group and ventral to the body of M. iliacus. The nerve has been divided into two divisions: anterior (Ramus musculares) and posterior (N. saphenus).

The anterior division consists of those nerve branches given off to M. psoas major and M. iliacus, as the femoral nerve passes between the fascial planes separating the two (Fig. 2). It then continues on to innervate M. pectineus, passing dorsal to the external iliac vein (Vena iliaca externus), and enters the muscle on its dorsal side prior to the final branching as shown in Fig. 2.

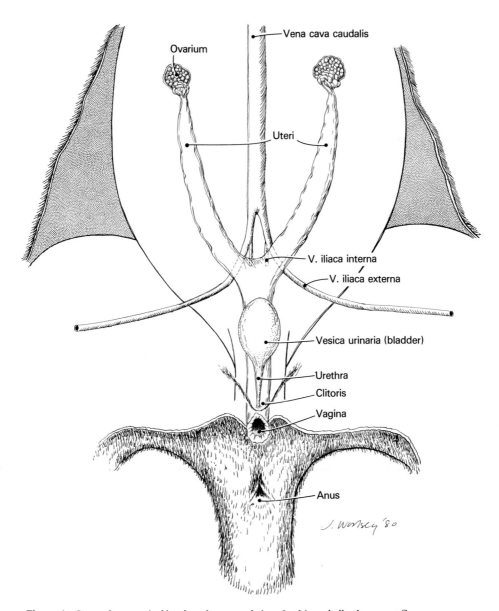

Figure 1. General anatomical landmarks, ventral view. In this and all subsequent figures, nomenclature used will be that found in *Nomina Anatomica Veterinaria* (World Association of Veterinary Anatomists, 1973). Abbreviations: A, Arteria; L, Ligamentum; M, Musculus; MM, Musculi; N, Nervus; V, Vena.

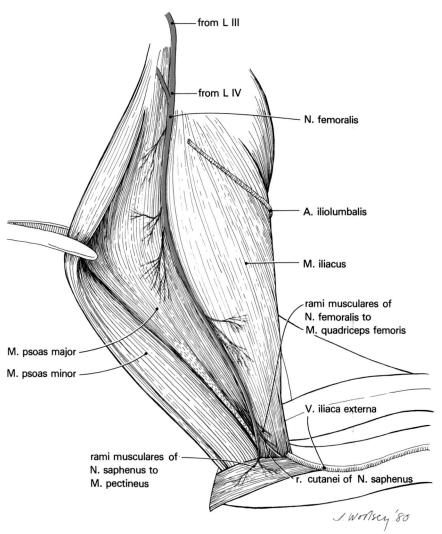

Figure 2. Nervus femoralis, ventral view, with MM. psoas reflected medially.

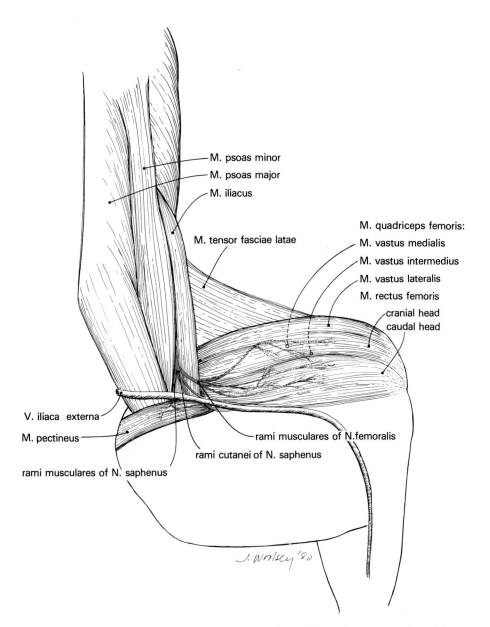

M. psoas minor
M. psoas major
M. iliacus

M. tensor fasciae latae

M. quadriceps femoris:
M. vastus medialis
M. vastus intermedius
M. vastus lateralis
M. rectus femoris
cranial head
caudal head

V. iliaca externa
M. pectineus

rami musculares of N. femoralis

rami cutanei of N. saphenus

rami musculares of N. saphenus

J. Woolsey '80

Figure 3. Nervus femoralis, ventral view, with innervation of M. pectineus and MM. quadriceps detailed.

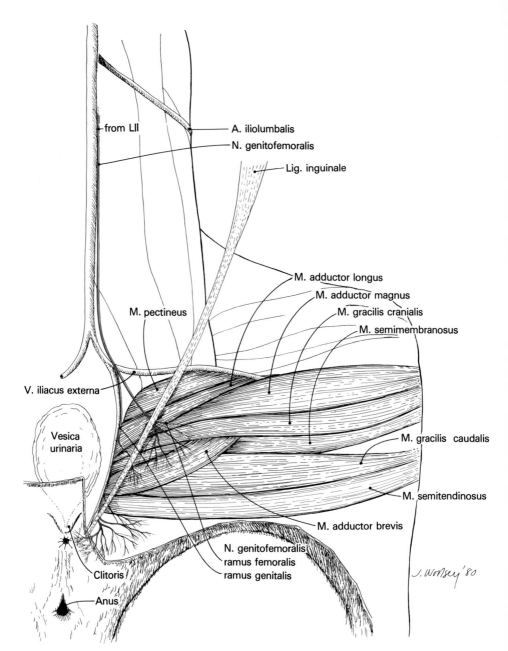

Figure 4. Nervus genitofemoralis, ventral view.

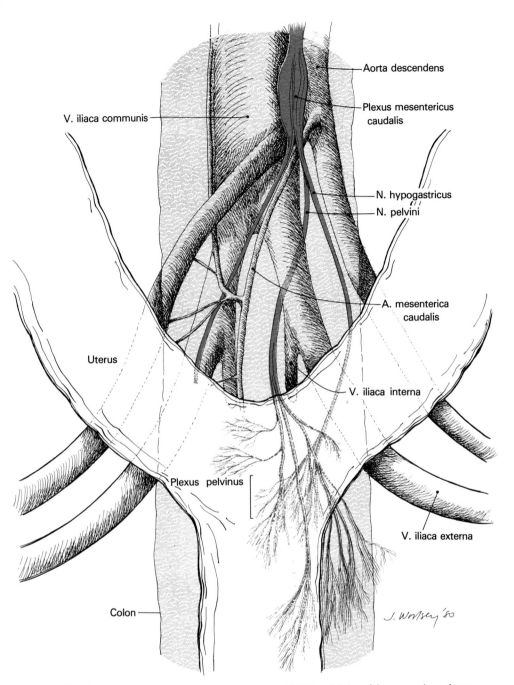

Figure 5. Plexus pelvinus, ventral view, with course of NN. pelvini and hypogastricus shown.

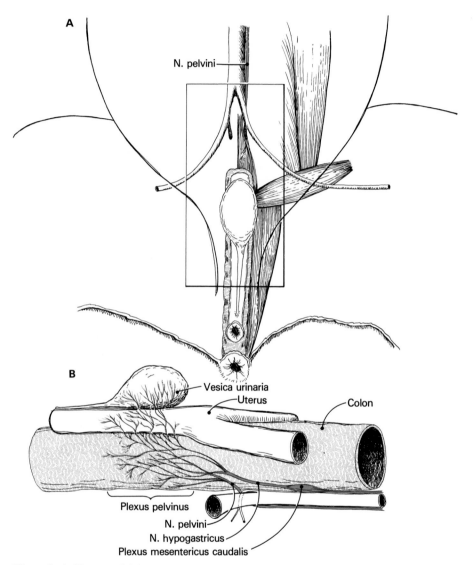

Figure 6. A, Nervus pelvini, ventral view, detail of course alongside Vena cava caudalis. B, Plexus pelvini, lateral view.

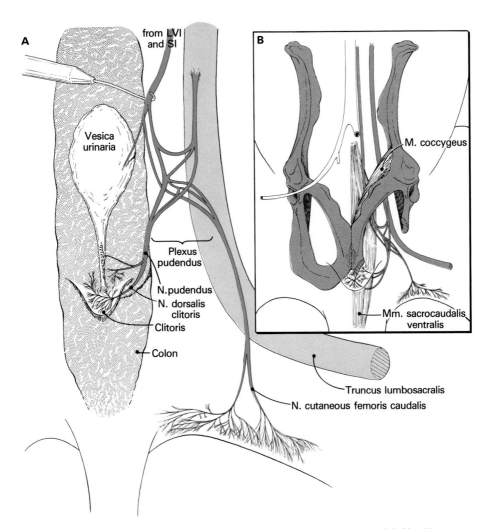

Figure 7. A, Nervus pudendus, ventral view, with detail of innervation of caudal skin (N. cutaneous femorus caudalis) and the urethra and clitoris (N. dorsalis clitoris). B, Nervus pudendus with relationship to M. coccygeus; MM. sacrocaudalis ventralis are detailed.

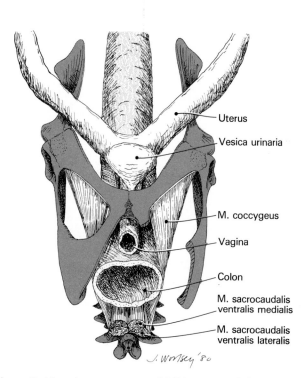

Figure 8. Musculus coccygeus and MM. sacrocaudalis ventralis, oblique caudocranial view.

The posterior division also splits into two divisions: a muscular branch (Ramus musculares and the saphenous nerve (Ram cutanei). The saphenous nerve is well-known and needs no further description here (we refer the reader to Greene, 1968). The muscular branch innervates M. quadriceps femoris (Fig. 3). M. quadriceps femoris is the well-known muscle group situated in the upper thigh and is composed of four muscles: M. vastus lateralis, M. vastus intermedius, M. vastus medialis, and M. rectus femoris. The distribution of the innervation to these muscles is detailed in Fig. 3.

B. Genitofemoral Nerve

The genitofemoral nerve (N. genitofemoralis) emerges at the level of L2 and travels caudally along the border between the psoas muscle group and the aorta. Just caudal to the aortal bifurcation (Fig. 4), it divides into two branches that pass ventral to the common iliac vein (Vena ilaca communis): the external spermatic (Ramus genitalis) and the lumboinguinal branch (Ramus femoralis). The latter branch innervates the skin of the cranial femoral triangle, the area overlying the muscles innervated by the posterior division of the femoral nerve (see Fig. 3). The external spermatic branch travels farther caudally, giving off branches to the skin of the caudal femoral triangle, through the inguinal canal, and finally innervates the skin immediately adjacent to the genitalia as well as the Labium majus (Labium pudendi) Greene, 1968).

C. Pelvic and Hypogastric Nerves

These two nerves must be described together in order to understand their anatomical relationship. The two nerves intermingle in the pelvic plexus (Plexus pelvinus) (Figs. 5, 6B) located on the lateral wall of the rectum, dorsal to the uterine junction. The hypogastric nerve (N. hypogastricus) emerges as a bilaterally paired nerve from the inferior mesenteric plexus (Plexus mesentericus caudalis) (Fig. 5), a ganglion located on the ventral surface of the inferior mesenteric artery (A. mesenterica caudalis) at the bifurcation of the aorta (Marshall, 1970).

The inferior mesenteric plexus is one of a network of sympathetic plexus and ganglia that more or less cover the ventral surface of the aorta and Vena cava (Kuntz, 1965). They receive input from the sympathetic chain ganglia via the lumbar splanchnic nerves (Nn. splanchnici lumbales). From the inferior mesenteric plexus, the nerve travels laterally and caudally, usually within a mass of fatty tissue, more or less defining the side of an ellipse formed by the iliacal vessels and the uteri. It descends dorsally from the level of the dorsal extent of the uterus to the lateral surface of the colon as it explodes into the pelvic plexus.

The pelvic nerve (N. pelvini) provides the parasympathetic component of the plexus (Bradley *et al.*, 1974; Carlson and DeFeo, 1965; Langworthy, 1965). The nerve emerges from S1 and S2 and travels caudally and slightly laterally. It runs immediately ventral to the pudenal nerve (N. pudendus) and traverses medial to the internal iliac vein (Vena iliaca interna) as the latter descends dorsally. From there, it arches medially, coming to rest on the lateral surface of the colon. (Fig. 6A).

The pelvic plexus is a delicate structure in the female rat. From the plexus, fine strands innervate the rectum, vagina, clitoris, urethra, urinary bladder, and cervix (Langworthy, 1965). Much work has been devoted to the details of visceral innervation via the pelvic plexus both extrinsically and intrinsically (Bradley and Teague, 1972; Langley and Anderson, 1896; Marshall, 1970; Purinton *et al.*, 1973). For details, we refer the reader to these papers.

D. Pudendal and Caudal Cutaneous Femoral Nerves

Fibers arising from L6 and S1 that ultimately contribute to the pudendal plexus form a trunk that travels caudally just deep to the pelvic nerve. In fact, between the vertebrae and the internal iliacal vessels, they run duplicate courses, the only difference being that the trunk lies dorsal (i.e., "deep" in our figures) to the pelvic nerve along the way. As the pelvic nerve rises caudal to the internal iliac (Fig. 6A), the trunk dives dorsally under the ascending ramus of the pubis (Ramus cranialis os pubis), traveling between the coccygeus muscle (M. coccygeus) and the caudal flexors (Mm. sacrocaudalis ventralis) (Fig. 7B). As the trunk continues caudally, deep to the obturator foramen (Foramen obturatorum), it meets collaterals from the lumbosacral trunk (Truncus lumbosacralis) in the so-called pudendal plexus (Plexus pudendus) (Fig. 7A). The Ramus musculi coccygei, a series of delicate fibers innervating the coccygeus muscle, is given off just prior to the plexus.

The plexus itself is a fine structure that can easily be separated into its component parts. A narrow branch of the lumbosacral trunk interacts with the pudendal trunk to produce the plexus which lies deep to the caudolateral aspect of the obturator foramen. From there, two nerve groups emerge. Laterally, the caudal cutaneous femoral nerve (N. cutaneous femoris caudalis) travels to the caudal extent of the animal, innervating the skin that lies in the trough formed between the tail and thigh itself (Greene, 1968; Langley and Anderson, 1896). The medial nerve group is that of the pudendal nerve itself (N. pudendus), innervating the urethra and colon with fine branches while sending a prominent branch, the dorsal nerve of the clitoris (N. dorsalis clitoris), beneath the symphysis pubis to innervate the clitoris.

A brief mention of the relationship of the muscles of the pelvic diaphragm and the caudal flexors to the appropriate nerves will aid the reader in orienting himself and understanding the overall topography. The caudal flexors, brevis (M. sacrocaudalis ventralis lateralis) and longus (M. sacrocaudalis ventralis medialis), are shown in Fig. 8. They take their origins from the lumbar vertebrae as far cranially as L5 and insert upon and throughout the tail (Greene, 1968). The coccygeus muscle is also illustrated in Fig. 8. It arises from the ventrocaudal ilium and inserts upon the tail with the caudal flexors (Green, 1968). The muscle known as Levator ani in many texts is absent in the female rat after day 18 of neonatal life (Hebel and Stromberg, 1976). The pudendal nerve travels medial to the coccygeus, within the pelvic diaphragm, to reach its ultimate destination. It is therefore necessary to remove much of the ventral aspect of the pelvis in order to properly visualize its intrapelvic course.

REFERENCES

Bradley, W. E., and Teague, C. T., 1972, Electrophysiology of pelvic and pudendal nerves in the cat, *Exp. Neurol.* **35**:378.

Bradley, W. E., Timm, G. W., and Scott, F. B., 1974, Innervation of the detrusor muscle and urethra, *Urol. Clin. North Am.* **1**(1):3.

Carlson, R. R., and DeFeo, V. J., 1965, Role of the pelvic nerve vs. the abdominal sympathetic nerves in the reproductive function of the female rat, *Endocrinology* **77**:1014.

Greene, E. C., 1968, Anatomy of the rat, *Trans. Am. Philosoph. Soc.* **XXVII**:1.

Hebel, R., and Stromberg, M. W., 1976, *Anatomy of the Laboratory Rat,* Williams & Wilkins, Baltimore.

Kollar, E. J., 1952, Reproduction in the female rat after pelvic nerve neuroectomy, *Anat. Rec.* **115**:641.

Kuntz, A., 1965, *Autonomic Nervous System,* Third Edition, Lea & Febiger, Philadelphia.

Langley, J. N., and Anderson, H. K., 1896, The innervation of the pelvic and adjoining viscera. Part VII: Anatomical observations, *J. Physiol. (Lond.)* **20**:372.

Langworthy, O. R., 1965, Innervation of the pelvic organs of the rat, *Invest. Urol.* **2**:491.

Marshall, J. M., 1970, Adrenergic innervation of the female reproductive tract: Anatomy, physiology and pharmacology, *Ergeb. Physiol.* **62**:6.

Purinton, P. T., Fletcher, T. F., and Bradley, W. E., 1973, Gross and light microscopic features of the pelvic plexus in the rat, *Anat. Rec.* **175**:697.

World Association of Veterinary Anatomists, 1973, *Nomina Anatomica Veterinaria,* Second Edition, International Committee on Veterinary Nomenclature, Vienna.

Index